Exam Preparatory Manual for Undergraduates
FORENSIC MEDICINE AND TOXICOLOGY
(Theory, Practical and MCQs)

Exam Preparatory Manual for Undergraduates
FORENSIC MEDICINE AND TOXICOLOGY
(Theory, Practical and MCQs)

As per the Competency-based Medical Education Curriculum

Third Edition

Dekal V
Professor and Head
Department of Forensic Medicine and Toxicology
Meenakshi Medical College Hospital and Research Institute
Enathur, Kanchipuram, Tamil Nadu, India

Foreword
TKK Naidu

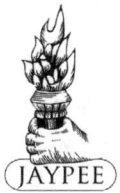

JAYPEE BROTHERS MEDICAL PUBLISHERS

The Health Sciences Publisher
New Delhi | London

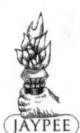 **Jaypee Brothers Medical Publishers (P) Ltd**

Headquarters
Jaypee Brothers Medical Publishers (P) Ltd
EMCA House, 23/23-B
Ansari Road, Daryaganj
New Delhi 110 002, India
Landline: +91-11-23272143, +91-11-23272703
+91-11-23282021, +91-11-23245672
Email: jaypee@jaypeebrothers.com

Corporate Office
Jaypee Brothers Medical Publishers (P) Ltd
4838/24, Ansari Road, Daryaganj
New Delhi 110 002, India
Phone: +91-11-43574357
Fax: +91-11-43574314
Email: jaypee@jaypeebrothers.com

Overseas Office
J.P. Medical Ltd
83, Victoria Street, London
SW1H 0HW (UK)
Phone: +44 20 3170 8910
Fax: +44 (0)20 3008 6180
Email: info@jpmedpub.com

Website: www.jaypeebrothers.com
Website: www.jaypeedigital.com

© 2024, Jaypee Brothers Medical Publishers

The views and opinions expressed in this book are solely those of the original contributor(s)/author(s) and do not necessarily represent those of editor(s) and publishers of the book.

All rights reserved. No part of this publication may be reproduced, stored or transmitted in any form or by any means, electronic, mechanical, photocopying, recording or otherwise, without the prior permission in writing of the publishers.

All brand names and product names used in this book are trade names, service marks, trademarks or registered trademarks of their respective owners. The publisher is not associated with any product or vendor mentioned in this book.

Medical knowledge and practice change constantly. This book is designed to provide accurate, authoritative information about the subject matter in question. However, readers are advised to check the most current information available on procedures included and check information from the manufacturer of each product to be administered, to verify the recommended dose, formula, method and duration of administration, adverse effects and contraindications. It is the responsibility of the practitioner to take all appropriate safety precautions. Neither the publisher nor the author(s)/editor(s) assume any liability for any injury and/or damage to persons or property arising from or related to use of material in this book.

This book is sold on the understanding that the publisher is not engaged in providing professional medical services. If such advice or services are required, the services of a competent medical professional should be sought.

Every effort has been made where necessary to contact holders of copyright to obtain permission to reproduce copyright material. If any have been inadvertently overlooked, the publisher will be pleased to make the necessary arrangements at the first opportunity.

Inquiries for bulk sales may be solicited at: jaypee@jaypeebrothers.com

Exam Preparatory Manual for Undergraduates: Forensic Medicine and Toxicology (Theory, Practical and MCQs)

First Edition: 2015
Second Edition: 2018
Third Edition: **2024**

ISBN: 978-93-5696-731-1

Printed at: Sterling Graphics Pvt. Ltd.

About CBME Curriculum

Competency-Based Medical Education (CBME) was introduced by the National medical Commission (NMC) to create a medical graduate who is a **clinician, leader, and member of the healthcare team**, a communicator, a lifelong learner and with attributes of professionalism and ethics.

As per the CBME curriculum, the syllabus has not changed; the change is only in the teaching learning methods and assessment of the student's competency. Competency is **the capability to apply or use a set of related knowledge, skills, and abilities required to successfully perform the task.**

CBME is an outcomes-based approach to the **design, implementation, and evaluation** of medical education programs and the assessment of learners, using competencies or observable abilities. The goal of CBME is to ensure that all learners achieve the desired out-comes during their training.

The CBME curriculum is **designed to identify the desired outcomes, define the level of performance for each competency, and develop a framework for assessing competencies.** The CBME curriculum **emphasizes on the complex outcomes of a learning process** (i.e., **knowledge, skills,** and **attitudes**) to be applied by learners) rather than mainly focusing on what learners are expected to learn about in terms of traditionally defined subject content.

This third edition of the book maintains the **originality of serving as** *Exam Preparatory Manual* along with that **appropriate competency** to be gained by every learner, which are incorporated at the beginning of every chapter.

The seven basic competencies to be gained by every medical graduate are:

1. Ability to inspire and motivate others
2. Convey high-integrity and honesty
3. The ability to analyze issues and problem solve
4. Drives for results
5. Strong communication skills
6. Teamwork and collaboration
7. Technical and professional expertise

Objectives of the Indian Graduate Medical Training Program

The undergraduate medical education program is designed with a goal to create an "Indian Medical Graduate" (IMG) possessing requisite knowledge, skills, attitudes, values, and responsiveness so that she or he may function appropriately and effectively as a physician of first contact of the community while being globally relevant.

Foreword

The third edition of the textbook *Exam Preparatory Manual for Undergraduates: Forensic Medicine and Toxicology (Theory, Practicals and MCQs)* by Dr Dekal V is a lucid elucidation of the essence of medico-legal aspects of medical practice, which is essential knowledge, any, compulsory knowledge, for all medical students and practicing doctors irrespective of their specialty.

Law and medicine are the world's oldest noble professions that are claimed to have been wedded long ago, transforming into a science of facts assisting to resolve the social evils. Professor Dr Dekal V is head of the department of Forensic Medicine and Toxicology at Meenakshi Medical College and Research Institute Kanchipuram, Tamil Nadu, India. He has profound experience and knowledge to compile and revise this book. His research publications available in the world forensic literature have earned many honors conferred on to him by the various authorities in India.

I have gone through this revamped third edition of the textbook *Exam Preparatory Manual for Undergraduates: Forensic Medicine and Toxicology (Theory, Practicals and MCQs)* by Dr Dekal V. The book has very useful information for the medical and law students and for the practicing physicians and legal professionals. The publisher's efforts to come out with the third edition clearly spell out the popularity of the book. Innumerable references cited in each chapter construe the scientific base for the book. The book also includes worthy appendices at the end, comprising of completely revised theory topics as per the CBME curriculum, covered all the practical exercises and viva-voce questions and MCQs.

The format and the printing of the book have been of very high order. The language is simple and easy to understand. The book should be kept in the clinic of every practicing doctor. This would be a blessing as a ready reference in the courtroom as well. I see a bright future for this book. I feel it may help the exam-going student as well. I wish the book all the success.

I am sure that the third edition of the book too will get very good reception. My best wishes to Professor Dr Dekal V.

TKK Naidu
MD (Forensic Medicine) LLB DFM PGDMLS
Professor and Head
Department of Forensic Medicine
Vice Principal
Prathima Institute of Medical Sciences
Karimnagar, Telangana, India

Preface to the Third Edition

I am very happy to come out with the third edition of this textbook *Exam Preparatory Manual for Undergraduates: Forensic Medicine and Toxicology (Theory, Practical and MCQs)* after a reasonable long period of time of 5 years since the second edition. I would first like to thank all my colleagues who recommended my book and to the students who with hope studied my book and scored excellent marks. I mainly wish to thank "M/s Jaypee Brothers Medical Publishers (P) Ltd, New Delhi, India" who made it possible to make the book enter every part of India and the rest of the world.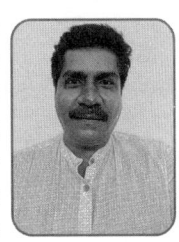

There have been many new amendments to law in the recent years; a lot of recent advances have taken place in the subject of Forensic Medicine. The Medical Council has been replaced by the National Medical Commission (NMC), and the system of teaching has totally changed from the traditional teaching methods to Competency-Based Medical Education (CBME) which was introduced by the NMC in 2019. Because of all this, the need for the new edition of the book has become mandatory to enable the student to learn the subject in accordance with the CBME curriculum.

The readers and faculty who were reading this book know well that this is the only book on the subject of Forensic Medicine which satisfies all the needs of the subject, mainly Theory, Practical, Viva-Voce, and MCQs. The book is also very useful for various competitive examinations like NEET-PG/NEXT. The syllabus has not changed, but the teaching learning methods have totally changed. This book enables the reader to gain the necessary competencies as prescribed by the NMC.

The major change is in the examination pattern. The total marks have been set up as 200, out of which 100 marks are given for MCQs and Theory and 100 marks for practical and viva-voce examinations. This has been made universally the same in all the universities of India. Efforts are made to include the maximum number of MCQs in each chapter. Hence, there is a need for a reasonably exhaustive book which covers all the topics as per the CBME curriculum.

Thus, now the book will serve all the aspects of learning such as to know, know how, reproduce, demonstrate how to do under supervision and does the task independently. All the chapters are written in accordance with the syllabus prescribed by the NMC along with all the competencies as specified by the NMC which will help one to apply the skills in real-time life scenarios.

The competencies that the students are expected to gain during the course of learning every topic have been tabulated at the beginning of each chapter and the competency number is quoted against each question. I wish the readers the best experience of studying the book, gain reasonable knowledge, score excellent marks in exams, and also apply the skills throughout their lifetime.

With best wishes
Dekal V

Preface to the First Edition

Writing a book on Forensic Medicine is my lifetime ambition. The basic aim of me taking up this subject is to bring a reasonable standard of uniform Medico-Legal Services throughout the country, a good ethical practice of medicine, and also to bring life to the outdated term "Medical Etiquette".

Working on this project of writing a book was a slow and studious process, and I started doing it very soon after I completed my postgraduate. I also wanted to be sure that my book should not be just an addition to the series of books in Forensic Medicine. I wanted to come out with a book which is student friendly, short, and precise; covers all the aspects of the subject, theory and practicals; and help the students to face the exams with confidence as well as learn the basic skills, thus helping them to apply these throughout their lifetime. All my dreams came true when M/s Jaypee Brothers Medical Publishers (P) Ltd, New Delhi, India joined hands with me and gave me the opportunity to write this excellent student-friendly textbook.

Only doctors who possess the basic degree of MBBS are called medical experts in the court of law, so allopathic physicians apart from the basic duty of curing patients of their ailments have yet another important responsibility, which is to fight for social justice by enlightening the court by the truth based on strong scientific proof. To be frank only by the knowledge of this subject of Forensic Medicine and of course pathology, emergency medicine and surgery, we the allopathic physicians stand distinct in the huge crowd of doctors, but only a very few of us recognize this fact.

Even though plenty of forensic medicine experts are available in the country, yet nearly 90% of the Medico-Legal workload of the country is still being carried out by the doctors who do not possess a postgraduate degree in Forensic Medicine. Ultimately, they have to depend upon the knowledge gained by them in the second year of their MBBS course.

This book is entitled as *Exam Preparatory Manual for Undergraduates: Forensic Medicine and Toxicology* and is prepared in accordance with the syllabus prescribed by the Medical Council of India (MCI). All the chapters in this book are carefully written for easy understanding and are presented in a question-and-answer format, to help the students understand how the questions would be asked in exams and what they are expected to write as answer for each question.

Even though the book is in a question-and-answer format, it carries all the points which a standard textbook is expected to contain—questions in the form of topics/headings and answers in the form of explanations; thus, students can study only this book which would be more than enough for the undergraduate medical examination and they would be rewarded back with excellent marks.

For the welfare of the students, an important set of practical exercises is also discussed; thus, the students can also prepare well for their practical exams. This book will serve all the needs of the students for theory, practical, and viva-voce examinations.

Apart from the medical students, this book will also be useful for the investigation team, judiciary, and other branches of students who need to have knowledge of forensic medicine, such as students of criminology, criminal justice, and forensic science.

Dekal V

Acknowledgments

My heartful special thanks to:
Dr RC Siddesh, MD, PGDMLE, Associate Professor of FMT, SS Institute of Medical Sciences, Davanagere, Karnataka, for his endless contributions to the 3rd edition of this book.

Next, I wish to acknowledge my senior professors, colleagues, students, and well wishers.

- Dr V Rajasekar, Dean and Professor of Radiology, Meenakshi Medical College and Research Institute, Kanchipuram, Chennai.
- Dr TKK Naidu MD, LLB, DFM, PGDMLS, Professor and Head of FMT and Vice Principal, Prathima Institute of Medical Sciences, Karimnagar (TS).
- Dr Ananda K, *Formerly* Professor and Head of FMT, Kempegowda Institute of Medical Sciences, Bangalore.
- Dr K Thangaraj, *Formerly* Professor and Head of FMT, SRM Medical College, Chennai.
- Dr P Sampath Kumar, Professor and Head of FMT, Saveetha Medical College, Chennai.
- Dr B Santha Kumar, *Formerly* Director of Forensic Medicine, Tamil Nadu.
- Dr Manohar, Professor and Head of FMT, SRM Medical College, Chennai.
- Dr P Parasakthi, Director of Forensic Medicine, Government Madras Medical College, Chennai.
- Dr R Selvakumar, Professor and Head of FMT, Sree Balaji Medical College, Chennai.
- DR Jai Singh, Professor and Head of FMT, Government Coimbatore Medical College.
- Dr BC Shivakumar, Professor and Head of FMT, Sapthagiri Medical College Bangalore.
- Dr Vijaynath, Professor and Head of FMT, ESI Medical College, Bangalore.
- Dr Jagannatha SR, Professor and Head of FMT, Kempegowda Institute of Medical Sciences, Bangalore.
- Dr Balaji Singh, Professor and Head of FMT, ACS Medical College, Chennai.
- Dr Priyadarshee Pradhan, Professor and Head of FMT, Sri Ramachandra Medical College, Chennai.
- Dr Anand Kumar, Professor of FMT, ACS Medical College, Chennai.
- Dr P Vedanayagam, Professor and Head of FMT, Bhaarath Medical College, Chennai.
- Dr P Shruthi, Professor in FMT, Saveetha Medical College, Chennai.
- Dr Geethanjali, Professor and Head of FMT, Government Villupuram Medical College.
- Dr Sudarshan, Professor and Head of FMT, Lalithambigai Medical College, Chennai.
- Dr Sanjeev, Professor of FMT, SRM Medical College, Chennai.
- Dr Rajamani Bheema Rao, Vel Tech Medical College, Chennai.
- Dr Priyadharshini, Associate Professor, Government Stanley Medical College, Chennai.
- Dr Vinoth Kumar, Associate Professor of FMT, Sree Balaji Medical College, Chennai.
- Dr Manigandaraj, Associate Professor and i/c Head of FMT, Government Chengalpattu Medical College.
- Dr Naveen, Senior Assistant Professor and i/c Head of FMT, Government Thiruvarur Medical College.
- Dr Karthikeyan, Senior Assistant Professor of FMT, Government Chengalpattu Medical College.

- Dr Nanda Kumar, Senior Assistant Professor of FMT, Government Erode Medical College.
- Dr Karpagam Dekal, Zonal Medical officer, Corporation of Chennai.
- Dr R Dhuvaraga, Post-Graduate of FMT, SRM Medical College, Chennai
- Dr D Priyadarshini, Post-Graduate in FMT, ACS Medical College, Chennai.
- Mr Loganathan, Scientific Officer in FMT, Government Madras Medical College, Chennai.
- Mr V Baskaran and Family, BS Enterprises and DR Properties, Chennai.

Special Acknowledgments to Our Publishers

I am very grateful to the whole team of M/s Jaypee Brothers Medical Publishers (P) Ltd, New Delhi, India, who helped and guided me, Shri Jitendar P Vij (Group Chairman), Mr Ankit Vij (Managing Director), Mr MS Mani (Group President), Dr Madhu Choudhary (Director-Educational Publishing), Ms Pooja Bhandari [Director-Production (Books and Journals)], Ms Sunita Katla (Executive Assistant to Group Chairman and Publishing Manager), Mr Ajay Kumar Sharma [Deputy General Manager (Books and Journals)], Ms Samina Khan (Executive Assistant to Director-Educational Publishing), Dr Upma Tomar (Development Editor), Mr Rajesh Sharma (Production Coordinator), Mr Sumit Kumar (Cover Visualizer) and their team members, for all their support to work in this project and make it a success. Without their cooperation, I could not have completed this project.

Contents

Section 1: Medical Jurisprudence

1. Introduction and Scope of Forensic Medicine 3
2. The Indian Legal System 6
3. Medical Ethics and the Law 23
4. Consent and Medical Negligence 47

Section 2: Personal Identity

5. Identification of the Living and Dead 61
6. Trace Evidences and Forensic Science Laboratory 81

Section 3: Forensic Pathology

7. Medico-Legal Autopsy 93
8. Thanatology: Death and its Causes 109
9. Postmortem Changes 119
10. Violent Asphyxial Deaths 135
11. Death due to Starvation 160

Section 4: Forensic Traumatology

12. Mechanical Injuries 165
13. Regional Injuries 185
14. Medico-Legal Aspects of Injuries 198
15. Thermal Injuries 210
16. Forensic Ballistics 223
17. Electrical and Lightening Injuries 235

Section 5: Sexual Jurisprudence

18. Virginity 243
19. Impotence, Sterility and Artificial Insemination 247
20. Pregnancy and Delivery 253
21. Abortion and MTP Act 1971 261
22. Infant Deaths 268
23. Sexual Offences and Paraphilias 277

Section 6: Forensic Psychiatry

24. Symptoms of Psychiatry and Mental Health Act 1987 293

Section 7: Medical Toxicology

25. General Considerations of Poisoning 311
26. Agricultural Poisons 327
27. Corrosive Poisons 335
28. Metallic and Inorganic Irritants Poisons 343
29. Organic Irritant Poisons 360
30. Neurotoxic Poisons 376
31. Cardiac Poisons 400
32. Asphyxiants 404
33. Miscellaneous Poisons 410

Section 8: Practical Examination

Exercise 1. Age Estimation by Dentition 419
Exercise 2. Age Estimation by Radiology 422
Exercise 3. Examination of Skeletal Remains 432
Exercise 4. Wound Certificate 439
Exercise 5. Drunkenness 442
Exercise 6. Sexual Offence Certificates 445
Exercise 7. Examination of the Accused of Rape 449
Exercise 8. Fetal Examination 451
Exercise 9. Leave Certificate and Certificate of Fitness 453
Exercise 10. Death Certificate 455
Exercise 11. Postmortem Certificate 457
Exercise 12. Spotters 460

Index *467*

Competency Table

Competency No.	Competency: The student should be able to	Domain K/S/A/C	Level K/KH/ SH/P	Core Y/N	Suggested teaching learning method	Suggested assessment method	Vertical integration	Chapter No.
FM1.1	Demonstrate knowledge of basics of forensic medicine like definitions of forensic medicine, clinical forensic medicine, forensic pathology, state medicine, legal medicine and medical jurisprudence	K	KH	N	Lecture/ small group discussion	Written/viva voce		1
FM1.2	Describe history of forensic medicine	K	KH	N	Lecture/ small group discussion	Written/viva voce		1
FM1.3	Describe legal procedures including criminal procedure code, Indian Penal Code, Indian Evidence Act, civil and criminal cases, inquest (police inquest and magistrate's inquest), cognizable and noncognizable offences	K	KH	N	Lecture/ small group discussion	Written/viva voce		2
FM1.4	Describe courts in India and their powers: Supreme Court, High Court, sessions court, Magistrate's court, labour court, family court, executive magistrate court and juvenile justice board	K	KH	N	Lecture/ small group discussion	Written/viva voce		2

Competency Table

Competency No.	Competency: The student should be able to	Domain K/S/A/C	Level K/KH/ SH/P	Core Y/N	Suggested teaching learning method	Suggested assessment method	Vertical integration	Chapter No.
FM1.5	Describe Court procedures including issue of summons, conduct money, types of witnesses, recording of evidence oath, affirmation, examination in chief, cross examination, re-examination and court questions, recording of evidence and conduct of doctor in witness box	K	KH	N	Lecture/ small group discussion moot court	Written/viva voce		2
FM1.6	Describe offenses in court including perjury; court strictures vis-avis medical officer	K	KH	N	Lecture/ small group discussion	Written/viva voce		2
FM1.7	Describe dying declaration and dying deposition	K	KH	N	Lecture/ Small Group Discussion	Written/viva voce		2
FM1.8	Describe the latest decisions/ notifications/ resolutions/ circulars/standing orders related to medico-legal practice issued by Courts/ Government authorities, etc.	K	KH	N	Lecture/ small group discussion	Written/viva voce	Radio-diagnosis, general surgery, general medicine, pediatrics	2
FM2.1	Define, describe and discuss death and its types including somatic/clinical/ cellular, molecular and brain-death, cortical death and brainstem death	K	KH	Y	Lecture/ Small Group Discussion	Written/viva voce	Pathology	8
FM2.2	Describe and discuss natural and unnatural deaths	K	KH	Y	Lecture/ small group discussion	Written/viva voce	Pathology	8

Competency Table

Competency No.	Competency: The student should be able to	Domain K/S/A/C	Level K/KH/ SH/P	Core Y/N	Suggested teaching learning method	Suggested assessment method	Vertical integration	Chapter No.
FM2.3	Describe and discuss issues related to sudden natural deaths	K	KH	Y	Lecture/ small group discussion	Written/viva voce	Pathology	8
FM2.4	Describe salient features of the organ transplantation and the human organ transplant (amendment act 2011) and discuss ethical issues regarding organ donation	K	KH	Y	Lecture/ small group discussion	Written/viva voce AETCOM		8
FM2.5	Discuss moment of death, modes of death—coma, asphyxia and syncope	K	KH	N	Lecture/ small group discussion	Written/viva voce	Pathology	8, 17
FM2.6	Discuss presumption of death and survivorship	K	KH	N	Lecture/ small group discussion	Written/viva voce		8
FM2.7	Describe and discuss suspended animation	K	KH	N	Lecture/ small group discussion	Written/viva voce		8
FM2.8	Describe and discuss postmortem changes including signs of death, cooling of body, postmortem lividity, rigor mortis cadaveric spasm, cold stiffening and heat stiffening	K	KH	Y	Lecture/ small group discussion autopsy, doap session	Written/viva voce OSPE		9
FM2.9	Describe putrefaction, mummification, adipocere and maceration	K	KH	Y	Lecture/ small group discussion autopsy, DOAP session	Written/viva voce OSPE		9

Competency Table

Competency No.	Competency: The student should be able to	Domain K/S/A/C	Level K/KH/SH/P	Core Y/N	Suggested teaching learning method	Suggested assessment method	Vertical integration	Chapter No.
FM2.10	Discuss estimation of time since death	K	KH	Y	Lecture/small group discussion autopsy, DOAP session	Written/viva voce OSPE		9
FM2.11	Define and discuss autopsy procedures including postmortem examination, different types of autopsies, aims and objectives of postmortem examination	K	KH	Y	Lecture/small group discussion autopsy, DOAP session	Written/viva voce OSPE	Pathology	7
FM2.12	Describe the legal requirements to conduct post-mortem examination and procedures to conduct medico-legal postmortem examination	K	KH	Y	Lecture/small group discussion autopsy, DOAP session	Written/viva voce OSPE	Pathology	7
FM2.13	Describe and discuss obscure autopsy	K	KH	Y	Lecture/small group discussion	Written/viva voce	Pathology	7
FM2.14	Describe and discuss examination of clothing, preservation of viscera on postmortem examination for chemical analysis and other medico-legal purposes, post-mortem artefacts	K	KH	Y	Lecture/small group discussion autopsy DOAP session	Written/viva voce OSPE		7

Competency Table

Competency No.	Competency: The student should be able to	Domain K/S/A/C	Level K/KH/SH/P	Core Y/N	Suggested teaching learning method	Suggested assessment method	Vertical integration	Chapter No.
FM2.15	Describe special protocols for conduction of medico-legal autopsies in cases of death in custody or following violation of human rights as per National Human Rights Commission Guidelines	K	KH	N	Lecture/ small group discussion autopsy, DOAP session	Written/viva voce OSPE		7
FM2.16	Describe and discuss examination of mutilated bodies or fragments, charred bones and bundle of bone	K	KH	N	Lecture/ small group discussion DOAP session	Written/viva voce OSPE		7
FM2.17	Describe and discuss exhumation	K	KH	N	Lecture/ small group discussion autopsy, DOAP session	Written/viva voce OSPE		7
FM2.18	Crime scene investigation:- describe and discuss the objectives of crime scene visit, the duties and responsibilities of doctors on crime scene and the reconstruction of sequence of events after crime scene investigation	K	KH	Y	Lecture/ small group discussion	Written/viva voce		6
FM2.20	Define, classify and describe asphyxia and medico-legal interpretation of postmortem findings in asphyxial deaths	K	KH	N	Lecture/ small group discussion autopsy, DOAP session	Written/viva voce OSPE		10

Competency Table

Compe-tency No.	Competency: The student should be able to	Domain K/S/A/C	Level K/KH/SH/P	Core Y/N	Suggested teaching learning method	Suggested assessment method	Vertical integration	Chapter No.
FM2.21	Describe and discuss different types of hanging and strangulation including clinical findings, causes of death, post-mortem findings and medico-legal aspects of death due to hanging and strangulation including examination, preservation and dispatch of ligature material	K	KH	N	Lecture/small group discussion autopsy, DOAP session	Written/viva voce OSPE		10
FM2.22	Describe and discuss patho-physiology, clinical features, postmortem findings and medico-legal aspects of traumatic asphyxia, obstruction of nose and mouth, suffocation and sexual asphyxia	K	KH	Y	Lecture/small group discussion autopsy, DOAP session	Written/viva voce OSPE		10
FM2.23	Describe and discuss types, pathophysiology, clinical features, postmortem findings and medico-legal aspects of drowning, diatom test and gettler's test	K	KH	Y	Lecture/small group discussion autopsy, DOAP session	Written/viva voce OSPE		10
FM2.24	Thermal deaths: Describe the clinical features, postmortem finding and medico-legal aspects of injuries due to physical	K	KH	N	Lecture/small group discussion/autopsy, DOAP session	Written/viva voce		15

Competency Table xxiii

Competency No.	Competency: The student should be able to	Domain K/S/A/C	Level K/KH/ SH/P	Core Y/N	Suggested teaching learning method	Suggested assessment method	Vertical integration	Chapter No.
	agents like heat (heat-hyperpyrexia, heat stroke, sun stroke, heat exhaustion/ prostration, heat cramps [miner's cramp] or cold (systemic and localized hypothermia, frostbite, trench foot, immersion foot)							
FM2.25	Describe types of injuries, clinical features, pathophysiology, postmortem findings and medico-legal aspects in cases of burns, scalds, lightening, electrocution and radiations	K	KH	N	Lecture / small group discussion autopsy, DOAP session	Written/viva voce	General Surgery	15
FM2.26	Describe and discuss clinical features, postmortem findings and medico-legal aspects of death due to starvation and neglect	K	KH	N	Lecture/ small group discussion	Written/viva voce		11
FM2.27	Define and discuss infanticide, foeticide and stillbirth	K	KH	Y	Lecture/ small group discussion	Written/viva voce	Pediatrics	22
FM2.28	Describe and discuss signs of intrauterine death, signs of live birth, viability of fetus, age determination of fetus, DOAP session of ossification centres, hydrostatic test, sudden infants death syndrome and munchausen's syndrome by proxy	K	KH	Y	Lecture/ small group discussion autopsy, DOAP session	Written/viva voce OSCE	Pediatrics, human anatomy	22

Competency Table

Competency No.	Competency: The student should be able to	Domain K/S/A/C	Level K/KH/ SH/P	Core Y/N	Suggested teaching learning method	Suggested assessment method	Vertical integration	Chapter No.
FM3.1	Define and describe corpus delicti, establishment of identity of living persons including race, sex, religion, complexion, stature, age determination using morphology, teeth-eruption, decay, bite marks, bones-ossification centres, medico-legal aspects of age	K	KH	N	Lecture/ small group discussion/ bedside clinic/DOAP session	Written/viva voce skill assessment	Human anatomy	5
FM3.2	Describe and discuss identification of criminals, unknown persons, dead bodies from the remains-hairs, fibers, teeth, anthropometry, dactylography, foot prints, scars, tattoos, poroscopy and superimposition	K	KH	N	Lecture/ small group discussion	Written/viva voce		5, 6, 14
FM3.3	Mechanical injuries and wounds: Define, describe and classify different types of mechanical injuries, abrasion, bruise, laceration, stab wound, incised wound, chop wound, defense wound, self-inflicted / fabricated wounds and their medico-legal aspects	K	KH	Y	Lecture/ small goup discussion bedside clinic, DOAP session	Written/viva voce OSPE	General surgery	12

Competency Table

Competency No.	Competency: The student should be able to	Domain K/S/A/C	Level K/KH/ SH/P	Core Y/N	Suggested teaching learning method	Suggested assessment method	Vertical integration	Chapter No.
FM3.4	Define injury, assault and hurt. Describe IPC pertaining to injuries	K	KH	N	Lecture/ small group discussion	Written/viva voce		14
FM3.5	Describe accidental, suicidal and homicidal injuries. Describe simple, grievous and dangerous injuries. Describe antemortem and postmortem injuries	K	KH	N	Lecture/ small group discussion	Written/viva voce		14
FM3.9	Describe different types of firearms including structure and components, along with description of ammunition propellant charge and mechanism of fire-arms, different types of cartridges and bullets and various terminology in—caliber, range, choking	K	KH	N	Lecture/ small group discussion	Written/viva voce	General surgery ortho-paedics	16
FM3.10	Describe and discuss wound ballistics-different types of firearm injuries, blast injuries and their interpretation, preservation and dispatch of trace evidences in cases of fire-arm and blast injuries, various tests related to confirmation of use of fire-arms	K	KH	N	Lecture/ small group discussion bed side clinic, DOAP session	Written/viva voce OSCE	General Surgery Ortho-paedics	16

Competency Table

Compe-tency No.	Competency: The student should be able to	Domain K/S/A/C	Level K/KH/SH/P	Core Y/N	Suggested teaching learning method	Suggested assessment method	Vertical integration	Chapter No.
FM3.11	Describe and discuss regional injuries to head (Scalp wounds, fracture skull, intracranial hemorrhages, coup and contrecoup injuries), neck, chest, abdomen, limbs, genital organs, spinal cord and skeleton	K	KH	N	Lecture/small group discussion/bedside clinic/autopsy DOAP session	Written/viva voce/OSCE/OSPE	General surgery ortho-pedics	13
FM 3.12	Describe and discuss injuries related to fall from height and vehicular injuries—primary and secondary impact, secondary injuries, crush syndrome, railway spine	K	KH	N	Lecture/small group discussion/bedside clinic/autopsy DOAP session	Written/viva voce OSCE/OSPE	General surgery ortho-paedics	13
FM3.13	Describe different types of sexual offences. Describe various sections of IPC regarding rape including definition of rape (Section 375 IPC), punishment for rape (Section 376 IPC) and recent amendments notified till date	K	KH	Y	Lecture/small group discussion	Written/viva voce/OSCE/OSPE	Obstetrics and gynecology	23
FM3.14	Describe and discuss the examination of the victim of an alleged case of rape, and the preparation of report, framing the opinion and preservation and dispatch of trace evidences in such cases	K	KH	Y	Lecture/small group discussion bedside clinic, DOAP session	Written/viva voce/OSCE	Obstetrics and gynecology	23

Competency Table **xxvii**

Competency No.	Competency: The student should be able to	Domain K/S/A/C	Level K/KH/SH/P	Core Y/N	Suggested teaching learning method	Suggested assessment method	Vertical integration	Chapter No.
FM3.15	Describe and discuss examination of accused and victim of sodomy, preparation of report, framing of opinion, preservation and despatch of trace evidences in such cases	K	KH	Y	Lecture/small group discussion bedside clinic, DOAP session	Written/viva voce/OSCE	Obstetrics and gynecology psychiatry	6, 23
FM3.16	Describe and discuss adultery and unnatural sexual offences sodomy, incest, lesbianism, buccal coitus, bestiality, indecent assault and preparation of report, framing the pinion and preservation and despatch of trace evidences in such cases	K	KH	Y	Lecture/small group discussion	Written/viva voce	Obstetrics and gynecology psychiatry	23
FM3.17	Describe and discuss the sexual perversions fetishism, transvestism, voyeurism, sadism, necrophagia, masochism, exhibitionism, frotteurism, necrophilia	K	KH	N	Lecture/small group discussion	Written/viva voce	Obstetrics and gynecology psychiatry	23
FM3.18	Describe anatomy of male and female genitalia, hymen and its types. Discuss the medico-legal importance of hymen. Define virginity, defloration, legitimacy and its medico-legal importance	K	KH	Y	Lecture/small group discussion	Written/viva voce	Gynecology	18

Competency Table

Competency No.	Competency: The student should be able to	Domain K/S/A/C	Level K/KH/ SH/P	Core Y/N	Suggested teaching learning method	Suggested assessment method	Vertical integration	Chapter No.
FM3.19	Discuss the medico-legal aspects of pregnancy and delivery, signs of pregnancy, precipitate labour, superfoetation, superfecundation and signs of recent and remote delivery in living and dead	K	KH	Y	Lecture/small group discussion	Written/viva voce	Obstetrics and gynecology	20
FM3.20	Discuss disputed paternity and maternity	K	KH	Y	Lecture/small group discussion	Written/viva voce	Obstetrics and gynecology	20
FM3.22	Define and discuss impotence, sterility, frigidity, sexual dysfunction, premature ejaculation. Discuss the causes of impotence and sterility in male and female	K	KH	Y	Lecture/small group discussion	Written/viva voce	Obstetrics and gynecology, general medicine	19
FM3.23	Discuss sterilization of male and female, artificial insemination, test tube baby, surrogate mother, hormonal replacement therapy with respect to appropriate national and state laws	K	KH	Y	Lecture / small group discussion	Written/viva voce	Obstetrics and Gynaecology	19
FM3.27	Define, classify and discuss abortion, methods of procuring MTP and criminal abortion and complication of abortion. MTP Act 1971	K	KH	N	Lecture/small group discussion	Written/viva voce	Obstetrics and gynecology AETCOM	21

Competency Table

Compe-tency No.	Competency: The student should be able to	Domain K/S/A/C	Level K/KH/SH/P	Core Y/N	Suggested teaching learning method	Suggested assessment method	Vertical integration	Chapter No.
FM3.28	Describe evidences of abortion - living and dead, duties of doctor in cases of abortion, investigations of death due to criminal abortion	K	KH	N	Lecture/small group discussion	Written/viva voce	Obstetrics and gynecology, pathology	21
FM3.29	Describe and discuss child abuse and battered baby syndrome	K	KH	Y	Lecture/small group discussion	Written/viva voce	Pediatrics	22
FM4.1	Describe medical ethics and explain its historical emergence	K	KH	Y	Lecture/small group discussion	Written/viva voce	AETCOM	3
FM4.2	Describe the Code of Medical Ethics 2002 conduct, etiquette and ethics in medical practice and unethical practices and the dichotomy	K	KH	Y	Lecture/small group discussion	Written/viva voce	AETCOM	3
FM4.3	Describe the functions and role of National Medical Commission and State Medical Councils	K	KH	Y	Lecture/small group discussion Moot Court	Written/viva voce	AETCOM	3
FM4.4	Describe the National Medical Commission Register	K	KH	Y	Lecture/small group discussion	Written/viva voce	AETCOM	3
FM4.5	Rights/privileges of a medical practitioner, penal erasure, infamous conduct, disciplinary Committee, disciplinary procedures, warning notice and penal erasure	K	KH	Y	Lecture/small group discussion	Written/viva voce	AETCOM	3

Competency Table

Competency No.	Competency: The student should be able to	Domain K/S/A/C	Level K/KH/SH/P	Core Y/N	Suggested teaching learning method	Suggested assessment method	Vertical integration	Chapter No.
FM4.6	Describe the Laws in Relation to medical practice and the duties of a medical practitioner towards patients and society	K	KH	Y	Lecture/small group discussion	Written/viva voce	AETCOM	3
FM4.7	Describe and discuss the ethics related to HIV patients	K	KH	Y	Lecture/small group discussion	Written/viva voce	AETCOM	3
FM4.8	Describe the Consumer Protection Act-1986 (Medical Indemnity Insurance, Civil Litigations and Compensations), Workman's Compensation Act and ESI Act	K	KH	Y	Lecture/small group discussion	Written/viva voce	AETCOM	3, 4
FM4.9	Describe the medicolegal issues in relation to family violence, violation of human rights, NHRC and doctors	K	KH	N	Lecture/small group discussion	Written/viva voce	AETCOM	3
FM4.10	Describe communication between doctors, public and media	K	KH	Y	Lecture/small group discussion	Written/viva voce	AETCOM	3
FM4.11	Describe and discuss euthanasia	K	KH	Y	Lecture/small group discussion	Written/viva voce	AETCOM	3
FM4.12	Describe legal and ethical issues in relation to stem cell research				Lecture/small group discussion	Written/viva voce	Pharmacology AETCOM	3
FM4.13	Describe social aspects of medico-legal cases with respect to victims of assault, rape, attempted suicide, homicide, domestic violence, dowry-related cases	K	KH	Y	Lecture/small group discussion	Written/viva voce	AETCOM	3

Competency Table

Compe-tency No.	Competency: The student should be able to	Domain K/S/A/C	Level K/KH/SH/P	Core Y/N	Suggested teaching learning method	Suggested assessment method	Vertical integration	Chapter No.
FM4.14	Describe and discuss the challenges in managing medico-legal cases including development of skills in relationship management—human behaviour, communication skills, conflict resolution techniques	K	KH	Y	Lecture/small group discussion	Written/viva voce	AETCOM	3
FM4.15	Describe the principles of handling pressure—definition, types, causes, sources and skills for managing the pressure while dealing with medico-legal cases by the doctor	K	KH	Y	Lecture/small group discussion	Written/viva voce	AETCOM	3
FM4.16	Describe and discuss bioethics	K	KH	Y	Lecture/small group discussion	Written/viva voce		3
FM4.17	Describe and discuss ethical principles: Respect for autonomy, nonmalfeasance beneficence and justice	K	KH	Y	Lecture/small group discussion	Written/viva voce	Pharma-cology AETCOM	3
FM4.18	Describe and discuss medical negligence including civil and criminal negligence, contributory negligence, corporate negligence, vicarious liability, res ipsa loquitor, prevention of medical negligence and defenses in medical negligence litigations	K	KH	N	Lecture/small group discussion	Written/viva voce		4

Competency Table

Competency No.	Competency: The student should be able to	Domain K/S/A/C	Level K/KH/ SH/P	Core Y/N	Suggested teaching learning method	Suggested assessment method	Vertical integration	Chapter No.
FM4.19	Define Consent. Describe different types of consent and ingredients of informed consent. Describe the rules of consent and importance of consent in relation to age, emergency situation, mental illness and alcohol intoxication	K	KH	N	Lecture/ small group discussion	Written/viva voce		4
FM4.20	Describe therapeutic Privilege, malingering, therapeutic misadventure, professional secrecy, human experimentation	K	KH	N	Lecture/ small group discussion Moot Court	Written/viva voce		4
FM4.21	Describe products liability and medical indemnity insurance	K	KH	N	Lecture/ small group discussion	Written/viva voce		4
FM4.23	Describe the modified declaration of Geneva and its relevance	K	KH	Y	Lecture/ small group discussion	Written/viva voce	Pharma-cology AETCOM	3
FM4.24	Enumerate rights, privileges and duties of a registered medical practitioner. Discuss doctor-patient relationship: professional secrecy and privileged communication	K	KH	Y	Lecture/ small group discussion	Written/viva voce		3

Competency Table

Competency No.	Competency: The student should be able to	Domain K/S/A/C	Level K/KH/ SH/P	Core Y/N	Suggested teaching learning method	Suggested assessment method	Vertical integration	Chapter No.
FM4.25	Clinical research and ethics. Discuss human experimentation including clinical trials	K	KH	N	Lecture/ small group discussion	Written/viva voce	Pharma-cology AETCOM	3
FM4.26	Discuss the constitution and functions of ethical committees	K	KH	Y	Lecture/ small group discussion	Written/viva voce	Pharmacology AETCOM	3
FM4.27	Describe and discuss ethical guidelines for biomedical research on human subjects and animals	K	KH	N	Lecture/ small group discussion	Written/viva voce	Pharmacology AETCOM	3
FM4.28	Demonstrate respect to laws relating to medical practice and ethical code of conduct prescribed by medical council of India and rules and regulations prescribed by it from time to time	A and C	SH	Y	Lecture/ small group discussion	Written/viva voce	–	3
FM4.29	Demonstrate ability to communicate appropriately with media, public and doctors	A and C	KH SH	Y	Lecture/ small group discussion	Written/viva voce	–	3
FM4.30	Demonstrate ability to conduct research in pursuance to guidelines or research ethics	A and C	KH SH	Y	Lecture/ small group discussion	Written/viva voce	–	3
FM5.1	Classify common mental illnesses including post-traumatic stress disorder (PTSD)	K	KH	N	Lecture/ small group discussion	Written/viva voce	Psychiatry	24

Competency Table

Compe-tency No.	Competency: The student should be able to	Domain K/S/A/C	Level K/KH/ SH/P	Core Y/N	Suggested teaching learning method	Suggested assessment method	Vertical integration	Chapter No.
FM5.2	Define, classify and describe delusions, hallucinations, illusion, lucid interval and obsessions with exemplification	K	KH	N	Lecture/small group discussion	Written/viva voce	Psychiatry	24
FM5.3	Describe civil and criminal responsibilities of a mentally ill person	K	KH	N	Lecture/small group discussion	Written/viva voce	Psychiatry	24
FM5.4	Differentiate between true insanity from feigned insanity	K	KH	N	Lecture/small group discussion	Written/viva voce	Psychiatry	24
FM5.5	Describe and discuss delirium tremens	K	KH	N	Lecture/small group discussion	Written/viva voce	Psychiatry General Medicine	24
FM5.6	Describe the Indian Mental Health Act, 1987 with special reference to admission, care and discharge of a mentally ill person	K	KH	N	Lecture/small group discussion	Written/viva voce	Psychiatry	24
FM8.1	Describe the history of toxicology	K	KH	Y	Lecture/small group discussion	Written/viva voce	Pharmacology	25
FM8.2	Define the terms toxicology, forensic toxicology, clinical toxicology and poison	K	KH	Y	Lecture/small group discussion	Written/viva voce	Pharmacology	25
FM8.3	Describe the various types of poisons, toxicokinetics, and toxicodynamics and diagnosis of poisoning in living and dead	K	KH	Y	Lecture/small group discussion	Written/viva voce	Pharmacology	25
FM8.4	Describe the laws in relations to poisons including NDPS Act, medico-legal aspects of poisons	K	KH	Y	Lecture/small group discussion	Written/viva voce	Pharmacology	25

Competency No.	Competency: The student should be able to	Domain K/S/A/C	Level K/KH/SH/P	Core Y/N	Suggested teaching learning method	Suggested assessment method	Vertical integration	Chapter No.
FM8.5	Describe medico-legal autopsy in cases of poisoning including preservation and dispatch of viscera for chemical analysis	K	KH	Y	Lecture/small group discussion, autopsy, DOAP session	Written/viva voce	Pharmacology	25
FM8.6	Describe the general symptoms, principles of diagnosis and management of common poisons encountered in India	K	KH	Y	Lecture/small group discussion bedside clinic, DOAP session	Written/viva voce	Pharmacology	25, 33
FM8.7	Describe simple bedside clinic tests to detect poison/drug in a patient's body fluids	K	KH	Y	Lecture, small group discussion, bedside clinic, DOAP session	Written/viva voce/OSCE	Pharmacology, general medicine	25
FM8.8	Describe basic methodologies in treatment of poisoning: Decontamination, supportive therapy, antidote therapy, procedures of enhanced elimination	K	KH	Y	Lecture, small group discussion, bedside clinic, DOAP session	Written/viva voce OSCE	Pharmacology, general medicine	25
FM8.9	Describe the various types of poisons, toxicokinetics, and toxicodynamics and diagnosis of poisoning in living and dead	K	KH	Y	Lecture/small group discussion	Written/viva voce	Pharmacology	25
FM8.10	Describe the general principles of analytical toxicology and give a brief description of analytical methods available for toxicological analysis.	K	KH	Y	Lecture, small group discussion	Written/viva voce	25	25

Competency Table

Compe-tency No.	Competency: The student should be able to	Domain K/S/A/C	Level K/KH/SH/P	Core Y/N	Suggested teaching learning method	Suggested assessment method	Vertical integration	Chapter No.
	Chromatography – thin layer chromato-graphy, gas chromato-graphy, liquid chromatography and atomic absorption spectroscopy							
FM9.1	Describe general principles and basic methodologies in treatment of poisoning: Decontamination, supportive therapy, antidote therapy, procedures of enhanced elimination with regard to: caustics: Inorganic-sulfuric, nitric, and hydrochloric acids; organic-carbolic acid (phenol), oxalic and acetylsalicylic acids	K	KH	Y	Lecture, small group discussion, bed side clinic, autopsy, DOAP session	Written/viva voce OSCE	Pharma-cology, general medicine	27
FM9.2	Describe general principles and basic methodologies in treatment of poisoning: Decontamination, supportive therapy, antidote therapy, procedures of enhanced elimination with regard to phosphorus, Iodine, barium	K	KH	Y	Lecture, small group discussion, bedside clinic, autopsy, DOAP session	Written/viva voce OSCE	Pharma-cology, general medicine	28

Competency Table xxxvii

Competency No.	Competency: The student should be able to	Domain K/S/A/C	Level K/KH/SH/P	Core Y/N	Suggested teaching learning method	Suggested assessment method	Vertical integration	Chapter No.
FM9.3	Describe general principles and basic methodologies in treatment of poisoning: Decontamination, supportive therapy, antidote therapy, procedures of enhanced elimination with regard to arsenic, lead, mercury, copper, iron, cadmium and thallium	K	KH	Y	Lecture, small group discussion, bedside clinic, autopsy, DOAP session	Written/viva voce OSCE	Pharmacology, general medicine	28
FM9.4	Describe general principles and basic methodologies in treatment of poisoning: Decontamination, supportive therapy, antidote therapy, procedures of enhanced elimination with regard to ethanol, methanol, ethylene glycol	K	KH	Y	Lecture, Small group discussion, bedside clinic, autopsy, DOAP session	Written/viva voce/ OSCE	Pharmacology, general medicine	30
FM9.5	Describe general principles and basic methodologies in treatment of poisoning: Decontamination, supportive therapy, antidote therapy, procedures of enhanced elimination with regard to organophosphates, Carbamates, organochlorines, pyrethroids, paraquat, aluminum and zinc phosphide	K	KH	Y	Lecture, small group discussion, bedside clinic, autopsy, DOAP session	Written/viva voce OSCE	Pharmacology, general medicine	26

Competency Table

Competency No.	Competency: The student should be able to	Domain K/S/A/C	Level K/KH/SH/P	Core Y/N	Suggested teaching learning method	Suggested assessment method	Vertical integration	Chapter No.
FM9.6	Describe general principles and basic methodologies in treatment of poisoning: Decontamination, supportive therapy, antidote therapy, procedures of enhanced elimination with regard to ammonia, carbon monoxide, hydrogen cyanide and methyl-isocyanate, tear (riot control) gases	K	KH	Y	Lecture, small group discussion, bedside clinic, autopsy, DOAP session	Written/viva voce OSCE	Pharmacology, general medicine	32
FM10.1	Describe general principles and basic methodologies in treatment of poisoning: decontamination, supportive therapy, antidote therapy, procedures of enhanced elimination with regard to: Neuro-psychotoxicology barbiturates, benzodiazepins phenytoin, lithium, aloperidol, neuroleptics, tricyclics. Narcotic Analgesics,	K	KH	Y	Lecture, small group discussion, bed side clinic, autopsy, DOAP session	Written/viva voce/ OSCE	Pharmacology, general medicine	30, 31
FM11.1	Describe features and management of Snake bite, scorpion sting, bee and wasp sting and spider bite	K	KH	Y	Lecture, small group discussion, autopsy	Written/viva voce	General medicine	29

Compe-tency No.	Competency: The student should be able to	Domain K/S/A/C	Level K/KH/ SH/P	Core Y/N	Suggested teaching learning method	Suggested assessment method	Vertical integration	Chapter No.
FM12.1	Describe features and management of abuse/ poisoning with following camicals: Tobacco, cannabis, amphetamines, cocaine, hallucinogens, designer drugs and solvent	K	KH	Y	Lecture, small group discussion, autopsy	Written/viva voce/ OSCE	Pharma-cology, general medicine	30
FM14.7	To identify and draw medico-legal inference from common poisons e.g. datura, castor, cannabis, opium, aconite copper sulphate, pesticides compounds, marking nut, oleander, Nux vomica, abrus seeds, snakes, capsicum, calotropis, lead compounds and tobacco.	K	KH	Y	Small group discussion, DOAP session	Log book/ viva voce	General medicine	29
Practical Excercise								
FM14.1	Examine and prepare medico-legal report of an injured person with different etiologies in a simulated/ supervised environment	K	KH	Y	Bedside clinic (ward/ casualty), small group discussion	Log book/ skill station/ viva voce/ OSCE	General surgery ortho-pedics	Exer-cise-4
FM14.4	Conduct and prepare report of estimation of age of a person for medico-legal and other purposes and prepare medico-legal report in a simulated/ supervised environment	K	KH	Y	Small roup discussion, demons-tration,	Log book/ skill station /viva voce/ OSCE	Radiology	Exer-cise-1

Competency Table

Competency No.	Competency: The student should be able to	Domain K/S/A/C	Level K/KH/ SH/P	Core Y/N	Suggested teaching learning method	Suggested assessment method	Vertical integration	Chapter No.
FM14.5	Conduct and prepare postmortem examination report of varied etiologies (at least 15) in a simulated/ supervised environment	K	KH	Y	Small group discussion, autopsy, DOAP session	Log book/ skill station/ viva voce/ OSCE		Exercise-11
FM14.9	Demonstrate examination of and present an opinion after examination of skeletal remains in a simulated/ supervised environment	K	KH	Y	Small group discussion, DOAP session	Log book/ skill station/ viva voce		Exercise-3
FM14.10	Demonstrate ability to identify and prepare medico-legal inference from specimens obtained from various types of injuries e.g. contusion, abrasion, laceration, fire-arm wounds, burns, head injury and fracture of bone	K	KH	Y	Small group discussion, DOAP session	Log book/ skill station/ viva voce/ OSCE		Exercise-12
FM14.11	To identify and describe weapons of medicolegal importance which are commonly used e.g. lathi, knife, kirpan, axe, gandasa, gupti, farsa, dagger, bhalla, razor and stick. Able to prepare report of the weapons brought by police and to give opinion regarding injuries present on the person as described in injury report/	K	KH	Y	Small group discussion, DOAP session	Log book/ skill station/ vViva voce/ OSCE		Exercise-12

Competency Table

Competency No.	Competency: The student should be able to	Domain K/S/A/C	Level K/KH/ SH/P	Core Y/N	Suggested teaching learning method	Suggested assessment method	Vertical integration	Chapter No.
	PM report so as to connect weapon with the injuries. (prepare injury report/PM report must be provided to connect the weapon with the injuries)							
FM14.12	Describe the contents and structure of bullet and cartridges used and to provide medico-legal interpretation from these	K	KH	Y	Small group discussion, DOAP session	Log book/ skill station/ viva voce/OSCE		Exercise-12
FM14.13	To estimate the age of fetus by postmortem examination	K	KH	Y	Small group discussion, DOAP session	Theory/clinical assessment/ viva voce		Exercise-8
FM14.14	To examine and prepare report of an alleged accused in rape/unnatural sexual offence in a simulated/ supervised environment	K	KH	Y	Small group discussion, DOAP session	Log book/ Skill station/viva voce/ OSCE	OBG	Exercise-6,7
FM14.16	To examine and prepare medico-legal report of drunk person in a Simulated/ supervised environment	K	KH	Y	Small group discussion, bed side clinic, DOAP session	Log book/ skill station/ viva voce/ OSCE		Exercise-5
FM14.17	To identify and draw medico-legal inference from common poisons e.g. datura, castor, cannabis, opium, aconite copper sulphate, pesticides compounds, marking nut, oleander, nux vomica, abrus seeds, snakes, capsicum, calotropis, lead compound and tobacco	K	KH	Y	Small group discussion, DOAP session	Log book/ viva voce		Exercise-12

Plate 1

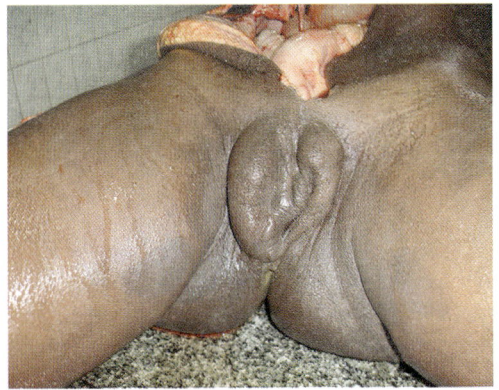

Fig. 5.1: Female pseudohermaphroditism.

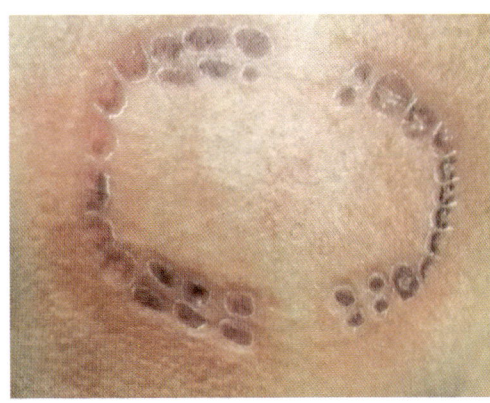

Fig. 5.2: Human bite mark showing the impression of all the 32 teeth.

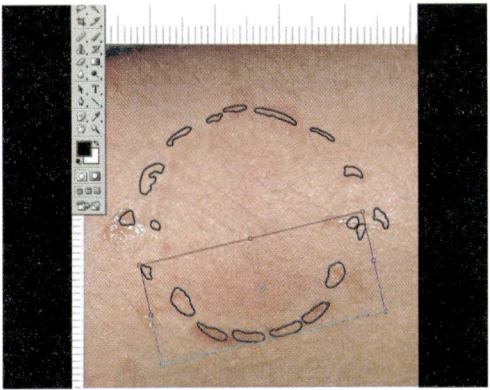

Fig. 5.3: Marking the bite marks and measuring the various dimensions for positive identification of the assailant.

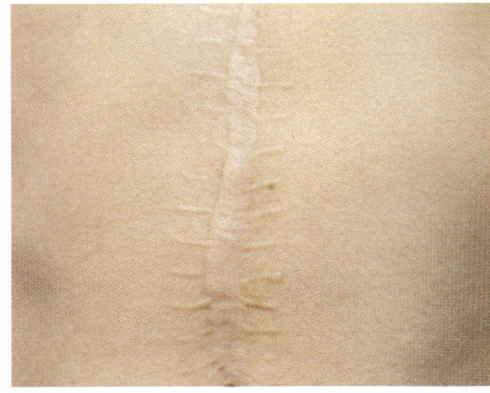

Fig. 5.4: Surgical incised wound scar of laparotomy, an unique feature of identification.

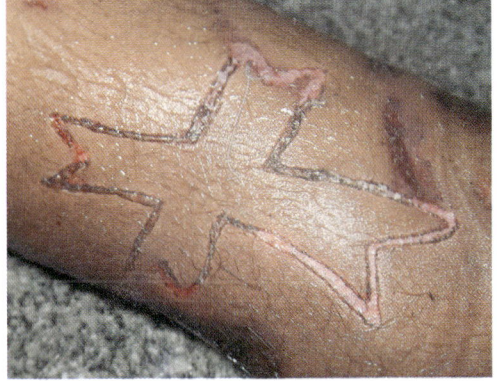

Fig. 5.5: Unique scar bearing the symbol of a cross, mode of infliction is suicidal.

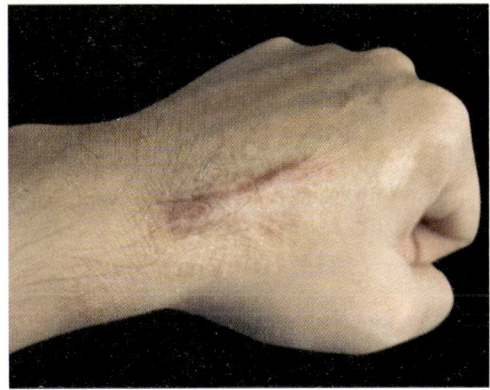

Fig. 5.6: Keloid formation on a pre-existing scar.

Plate 2

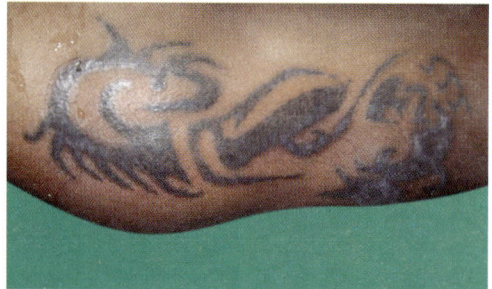

Fig. 5.7: Tattoo mark a unique tool of identification.

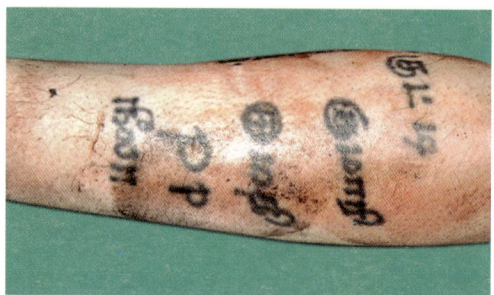

Fig. 5.8: Tattoo mark, especially useful for identification of decomposed bodies; well visible after skin slippage.

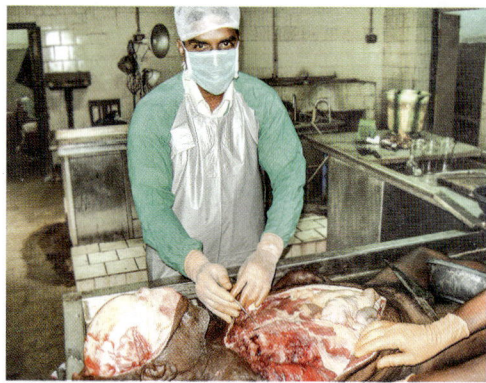

Fig. 7.1: Dissection of internal organs during autopsy.

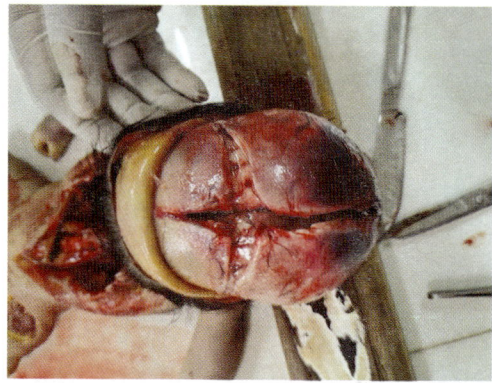

Fig. 7.2: Fetal skull dissection.

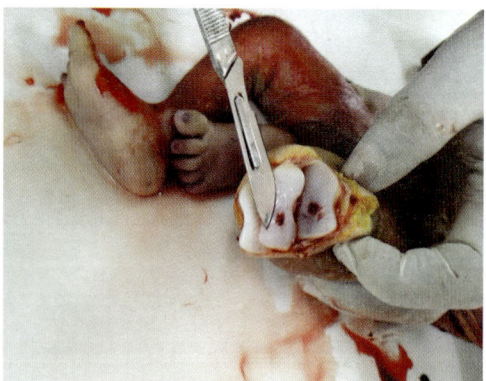

Fig. 7.3: Demonstration of ossification center in femur during autopsy–full term fetus.

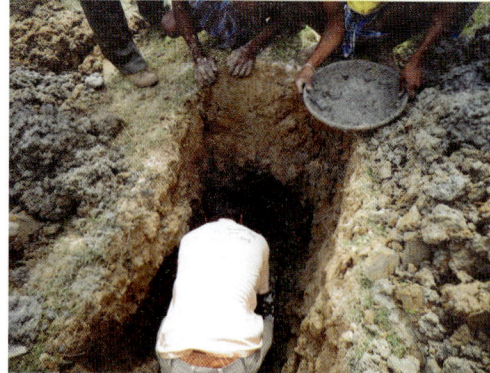

Fig. 7.4: Exhumation.

Plate 3

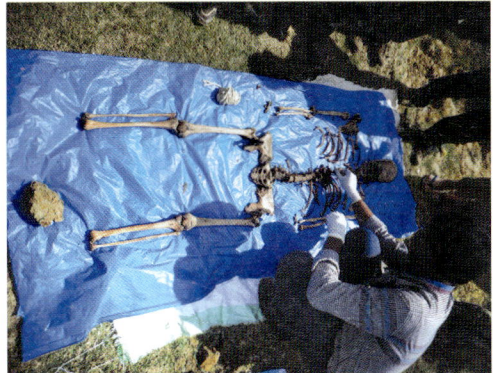

Fig. 7.5: Reconstruction of the body after exhumation with the recovered skeletal remains.

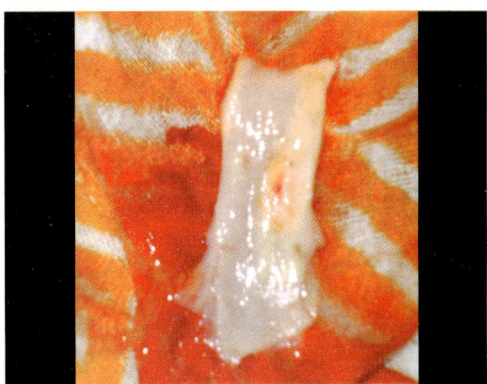

Fig. 8.1: Dissection of lumen of left coronary artery, showing thrombosis.

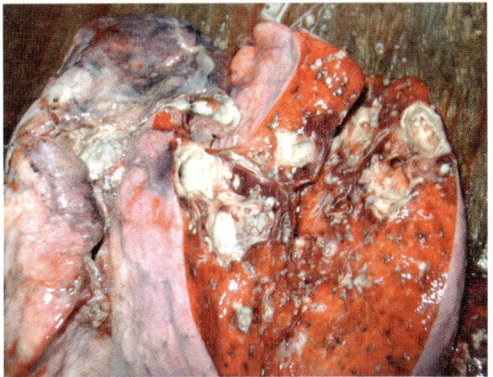

Fig. 8.2: Cross section of the lung, showing multiple cavities filled with pus interspersed with firm yellowish septum—a case of chronic pulmonary tuberculosis.

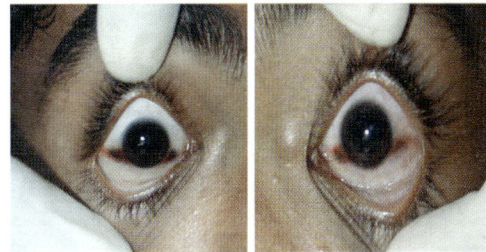

Fig. 9.1: Tache Noire sclerotica.

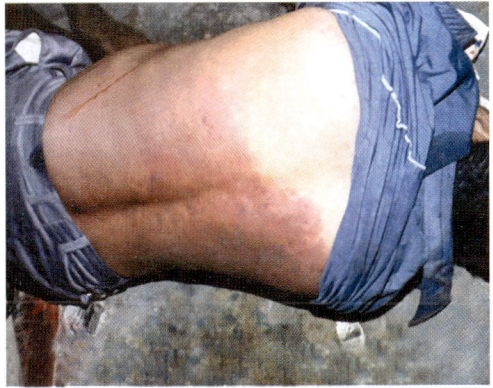

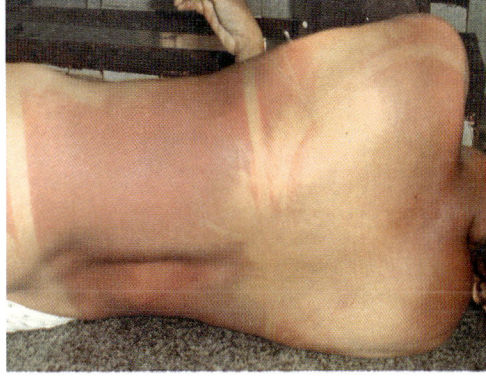

Figs. 9.2 and 9.3: Fixed postmortem staining with areas of contact flattening time since death is more than 6 hours.

Plate 4

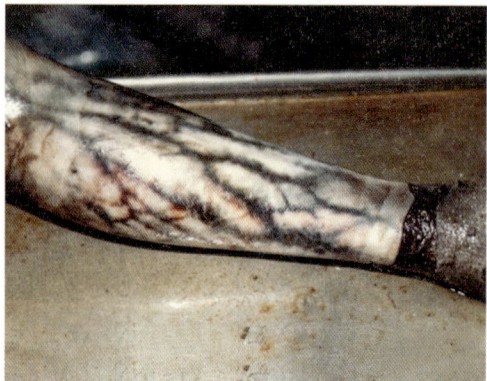

Fig. 9.4: Marbling of veins.

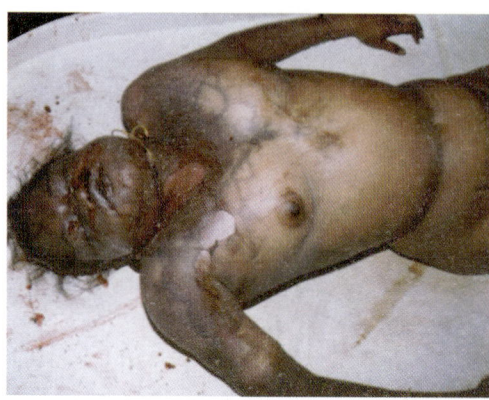

Fig. 9.5: Postmortem purge with gas stiffening.

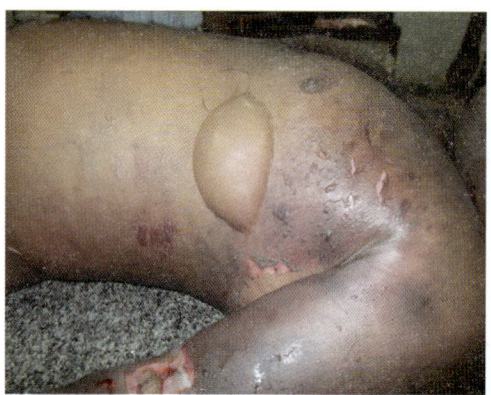

Fig. 9.6: Postmortem blister formation.

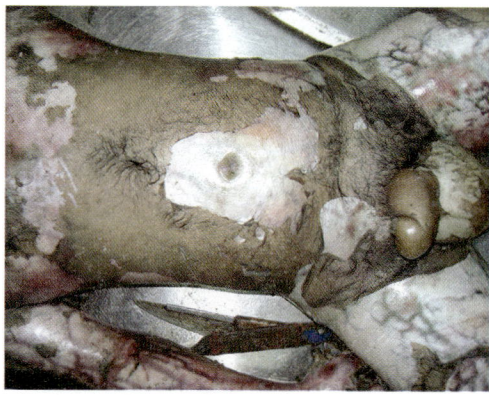

Fig. 9.7: Postmortem peeling of cuticle of skin with gas stiffening.

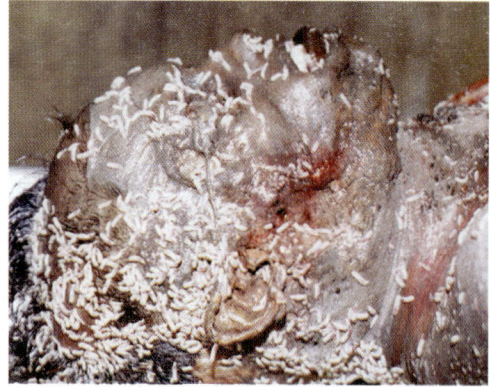

Fig. 9.8: Fully grown maggots crawling over the face.

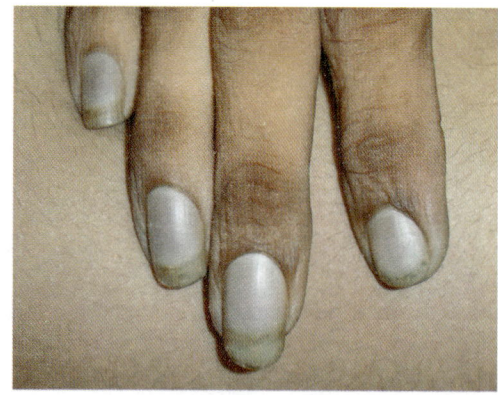

Fig. 10.1: Cyanosis of finger nails.

Plate 5

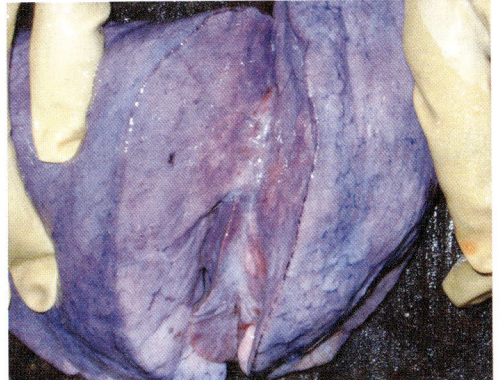

Fig. 10.2: Congestion of lungs.

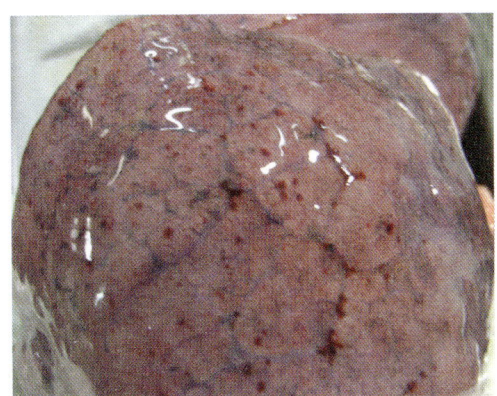

Fig. 10.3: Petechial hemorrhage.

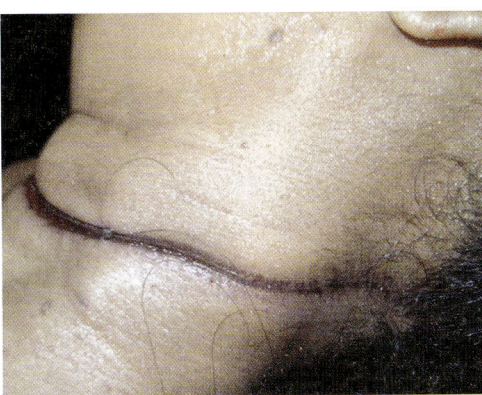

Fig. 10.4: Oblique ligature abrasion of hanging caused by a string.

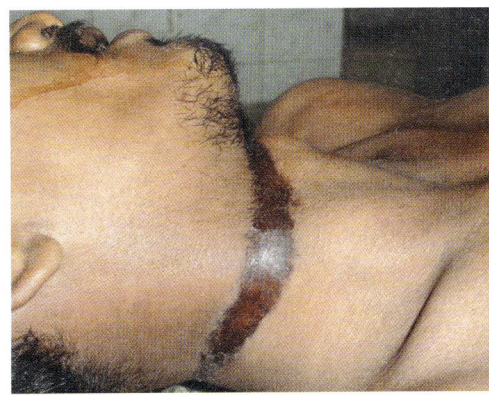

Fig. 10.5: Ligature abrasion of hanging.

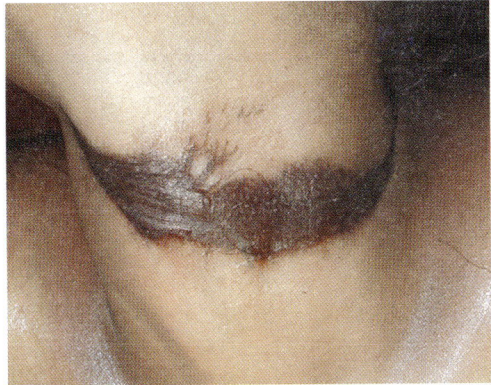

Fig. 10.6: Broad ligature abrasion of hanging caused by twisted clothing. Note the color of the abrasion—antemortem ligature abrasion of hanging.

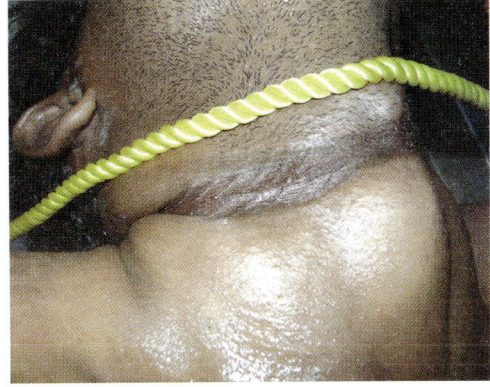

Fig. 10.7: Ligature abrasion of hanging caused by nylon rope. The material can be compared with abrasion—imprint ligature abrasion.

Plate 6

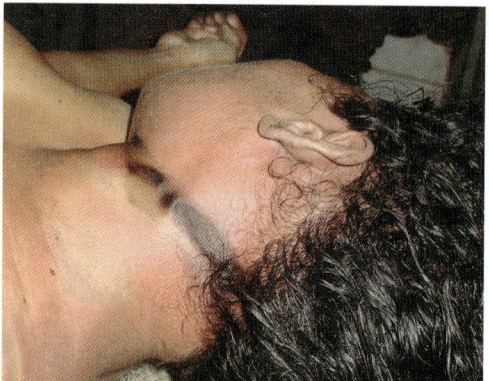

Fig. 10.8: Oblique ligature abrasion–note the postmortem staining above the ligature mark.

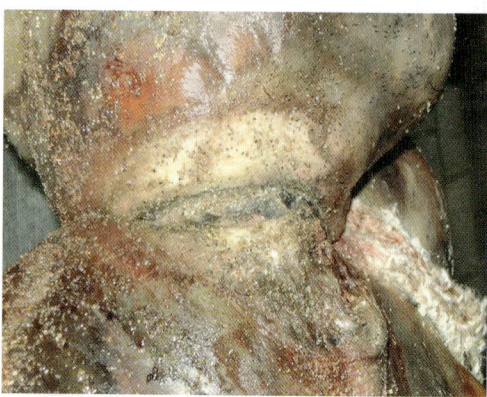

Fig. 10.9: Horizontal ligature abrasion of strangulation. Note: Even when the body has under gone reasonable degree of decomposition still the ligature mark is visible.

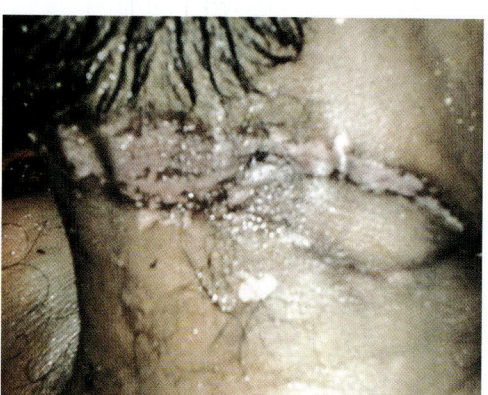

Fig. 10.10: Ligature strangulation–completely encircling ligature mark around the neck.

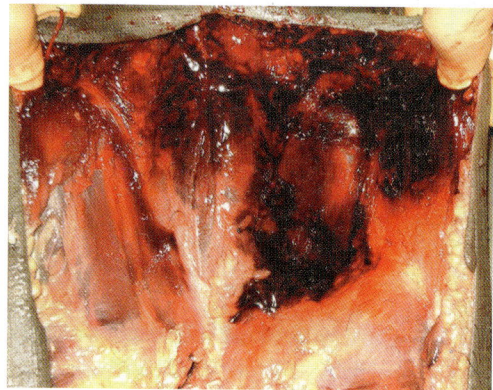

Fig. 10.11: Neck dissection in ligature strangulation. Note, the extensive extravasation of blood in the neck muscles trachea.

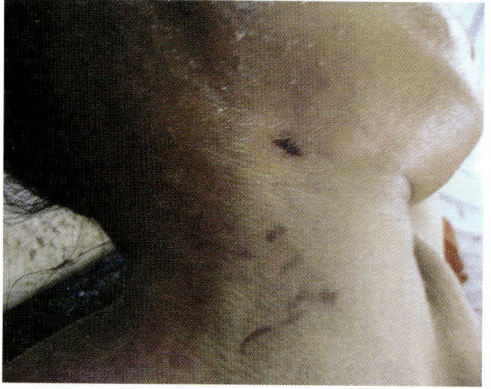

Fig. 10.12: Throttling–pressure abrasion and nail marks around the neck in case of throttling.

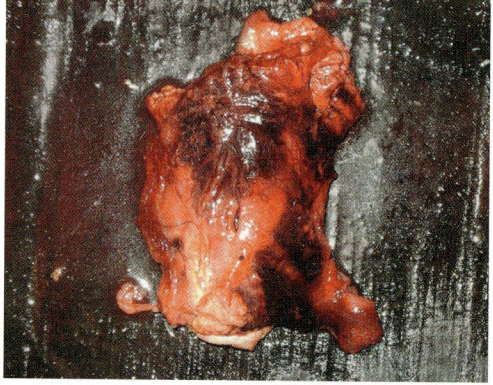

Fig 10.13: Extravasation on the posterior pharyngeal wall—a cased of throttling.

Plate 7

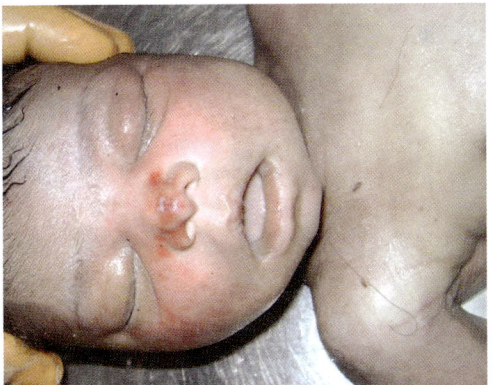

Fig. 10.14: Pressure abrasion and contusion around the mouth and nostrils–a case of smothering.

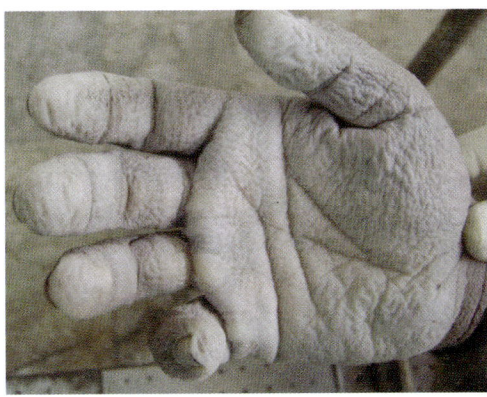

Fig. 10.15: Washerwoman's hand: A nonspecific external sign of death due to drowning.

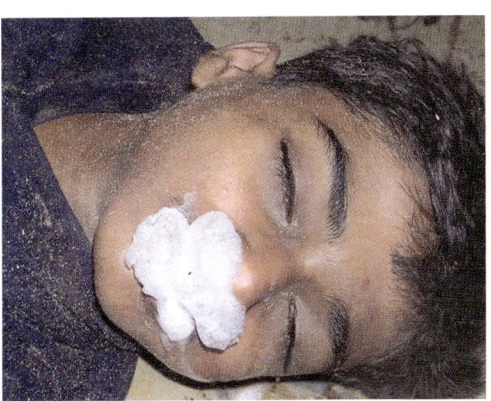

Fig. 10.16: Froth in the mouth and nostrils (the sign of drowning)—a case of sea water drowning.

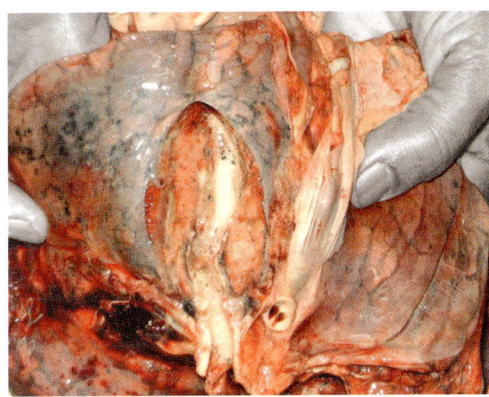

Fig. 10.17: Dissection of lung in case of death due to drowning—dissection along the bronchial tree, showing fine white, tenacious froth in the secondary bronchioles.

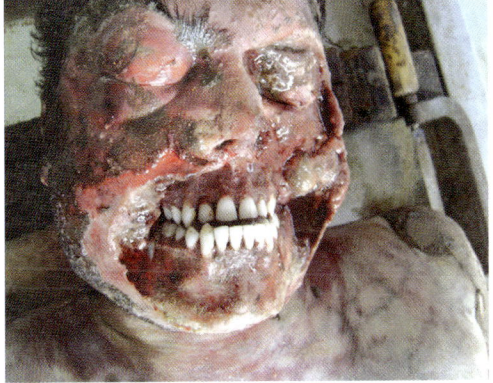

Fig. 10.18: A Case of drowning: Body recovered after 2 to 3 days—mutilation of the body by aquatic animals.

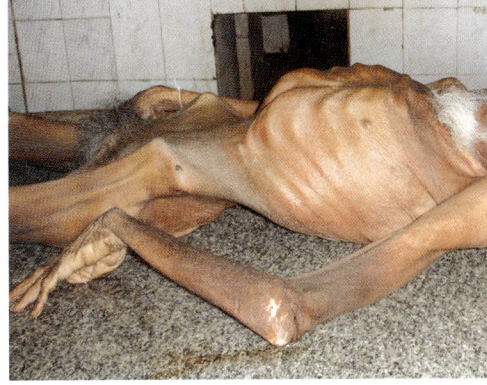

Fig. 11.1: Death due to starvation.

Plate 8

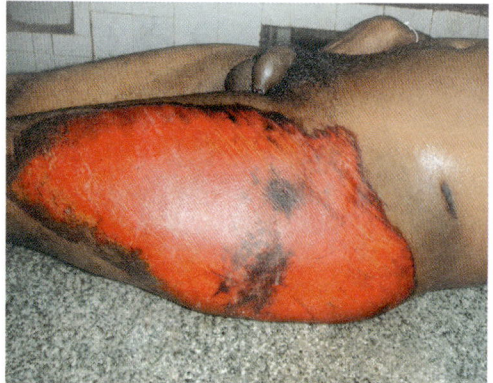

Fig. 12.1: Grazed abrasion caused in a road traffic accident.

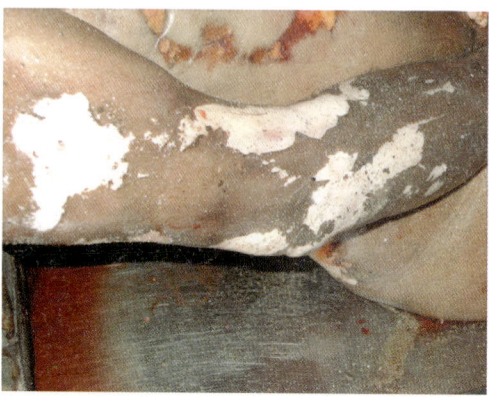

Fig. 12.2: Postmortem abrasion.

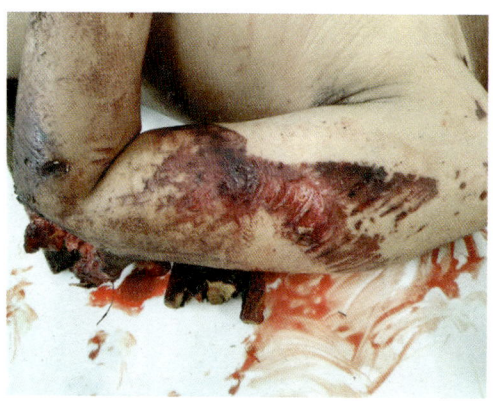

Fig. 12.3: Grazed abrasion (gravel rash).

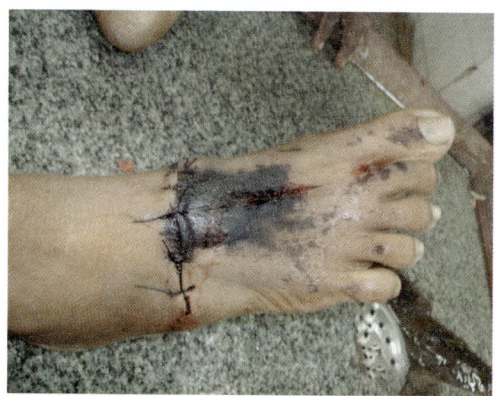

Fig. 12.4: Superficial contusion.

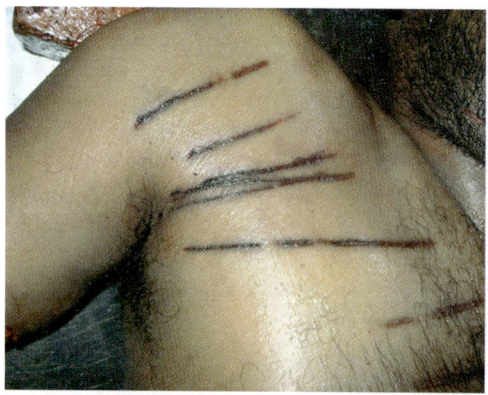

Fig. 12.5: Patterned contusion.

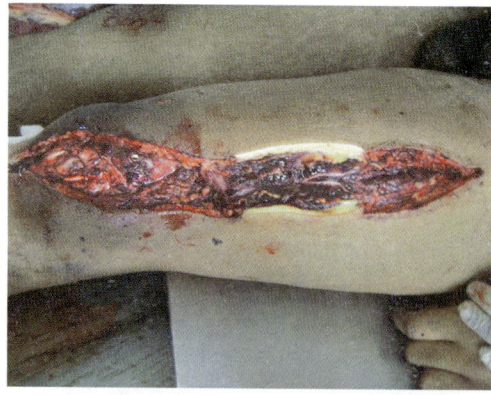

Fig. 12.6: Deep contusion.

Plate 9

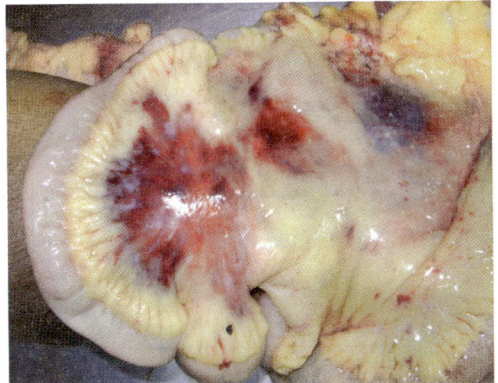

Fig. 12.7: Internal contusion.

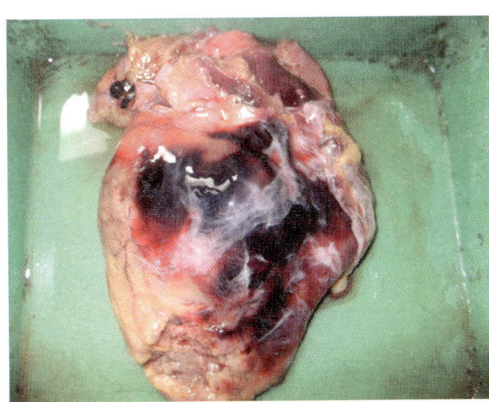

Fig. 12.8: Contusion of heart.

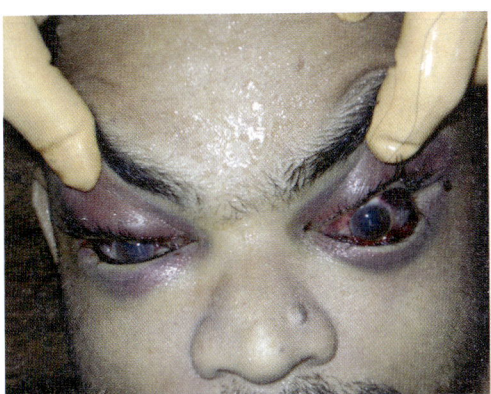

Fig. 12.9: Ectopic contusion.

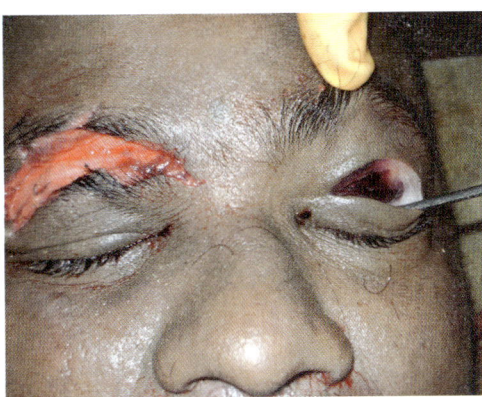

Fig. 12.10: Ectopic contusion–dissection of the eyelids to demonstrate the contusion; also there is laceration on the eyebrow of the opposite eye.

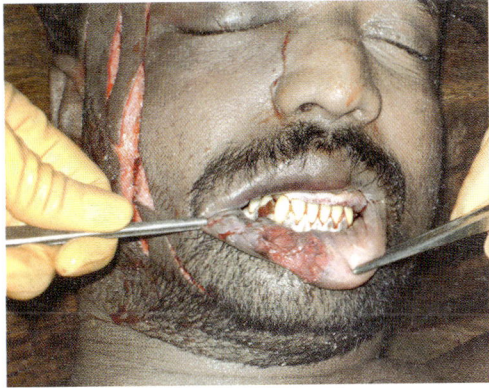

Fig. 12.11: Laceration of inner surface of lips caused by teeth.

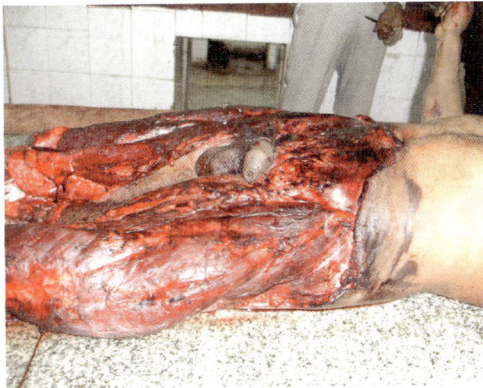

Fig. 12.12: Crush laceration of thigh caused in road traffic accident.

Plate 10

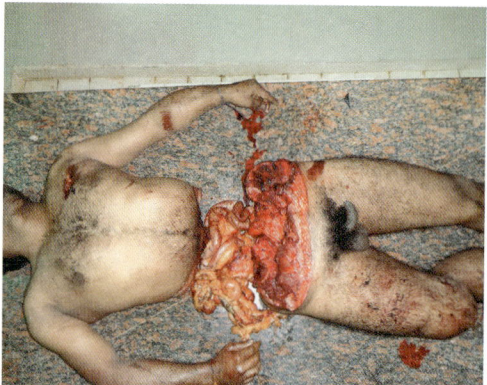

Fig. 12.13: Transaction of the body in a run-over train accident.

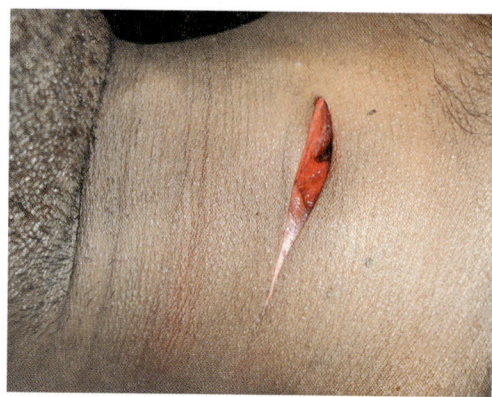

Fig. 12.14: Incised wound with tailing of wound.

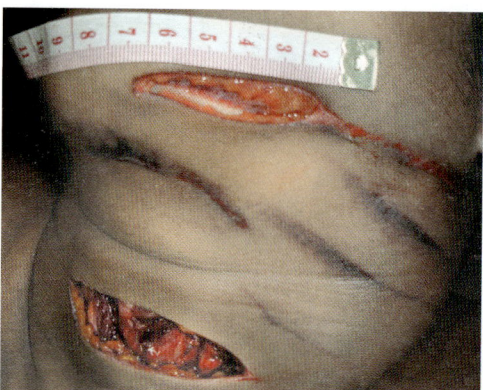

Fig. 12.15: Multiple incised wounds on the neck.

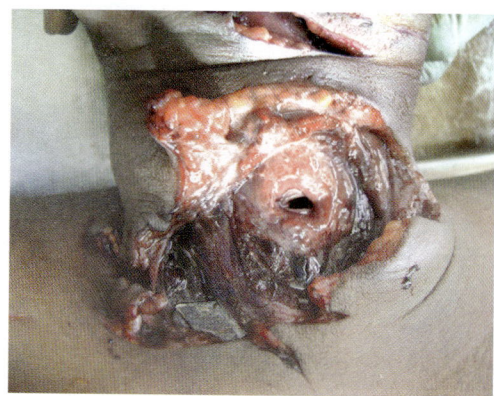

Fig. 12.16: Multiple overlapping incised wounds on the neck.

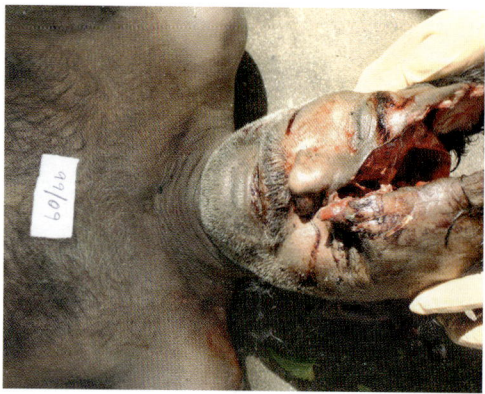

Fig. 12.17: Cut wound.

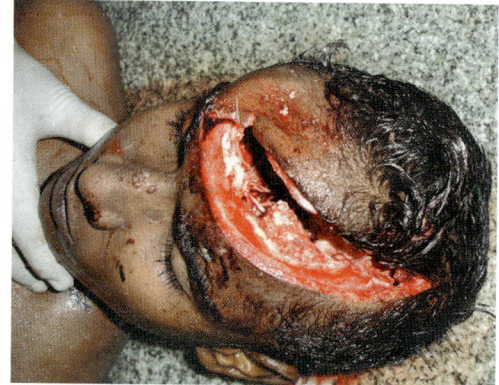

Fig. 12.18: Chop wound.

Plate 11

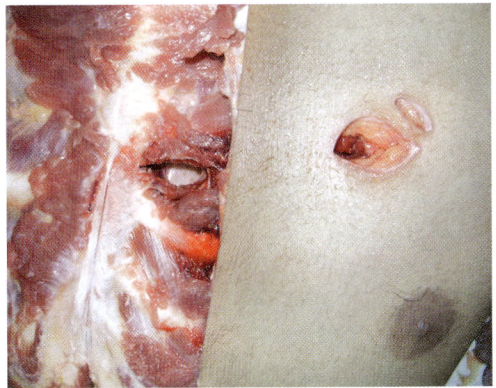

Fig. 12.19: Stab wound on the chest, the wound enters into the thoracic cavity through the intercostal space.

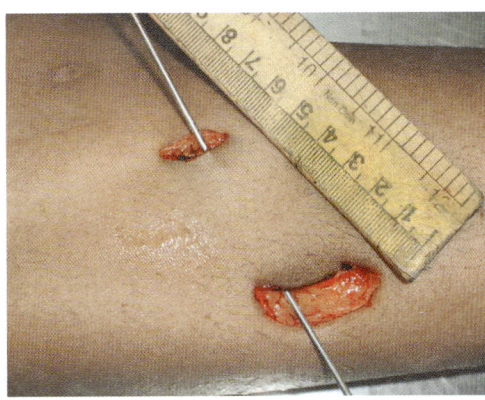

Fig. 12.20: Probing of stab wound on the thigh, to demonstrate the tract of the wound.

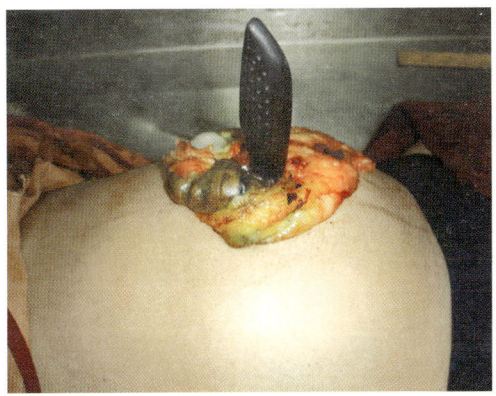

Fig. 12.21: Stab wound on the abdomen.

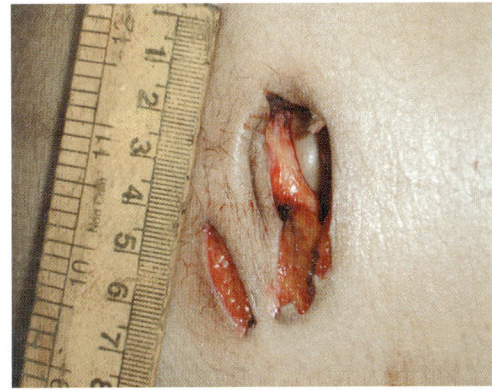

Fig. 12.22: Multiple stab wounds on the abdomen.

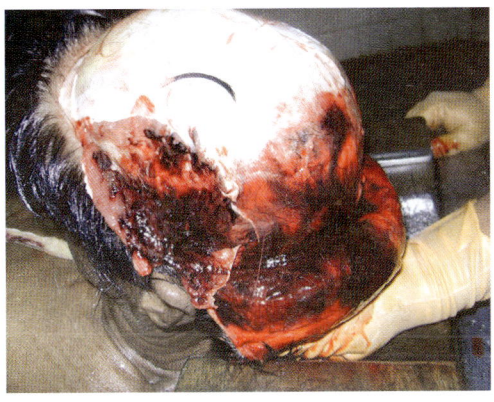

Fig. 13.1: Scalp contusion.

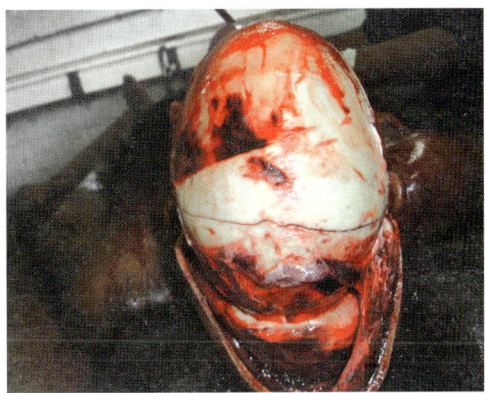

Fig. 13.2: Fissured fracture.

Plate 12

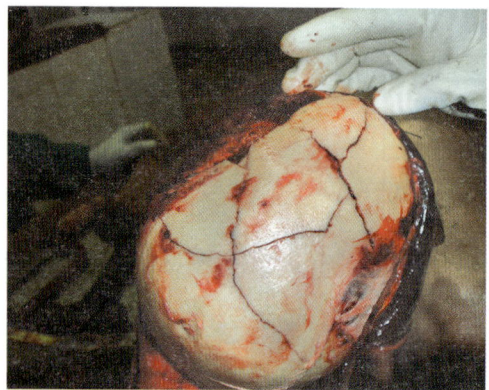

Fig. 13.3: Comminuted fracture.

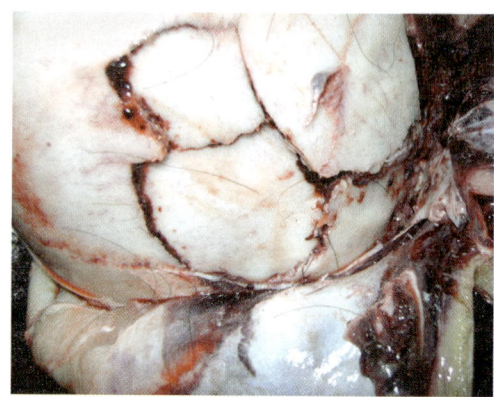

Fig. 13.4: Depressed fracture.

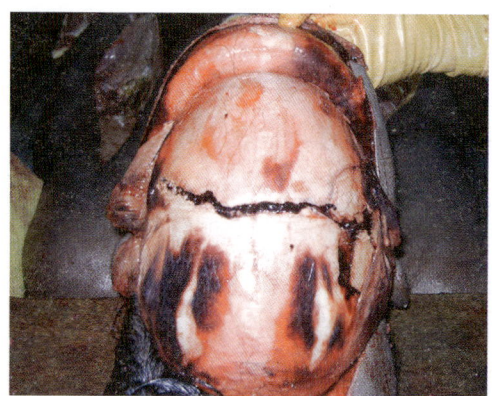

Fig. 13.5: Sutural fracture.

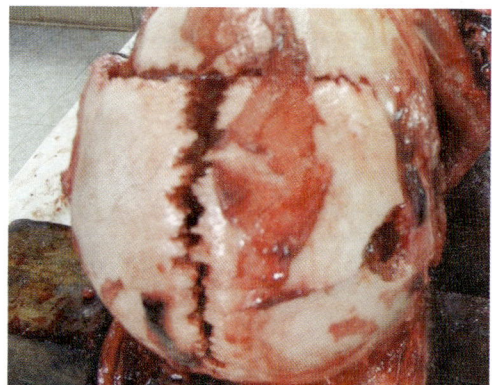

Fig. 13.6: Diastatic fracture.

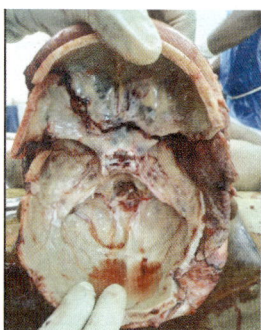

Fig. 13.7: Fracture base of skull on the anterior cranial fossa.

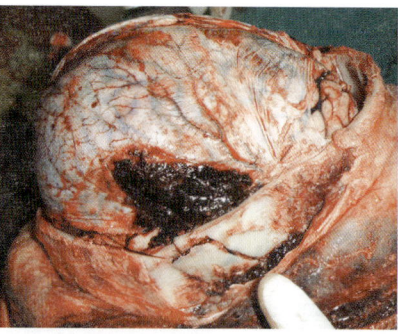

Fig. 13.8: Extra-dual hemorrhage.

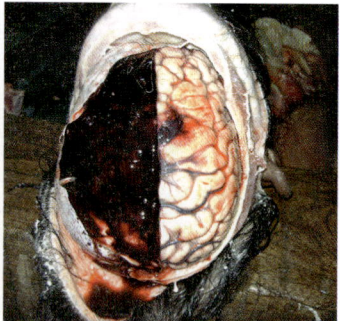

Fig. 13.9: Subdural hemorrhage.

Plate 13

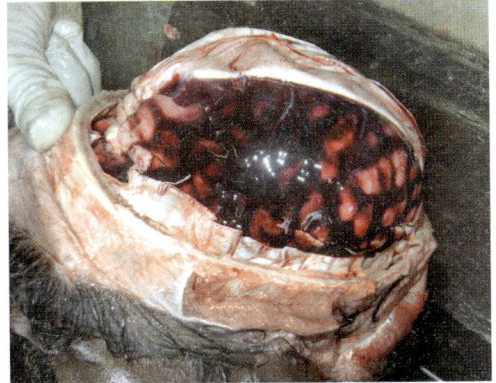

Fig. 13.10: Subarachnoid hemorrhage.

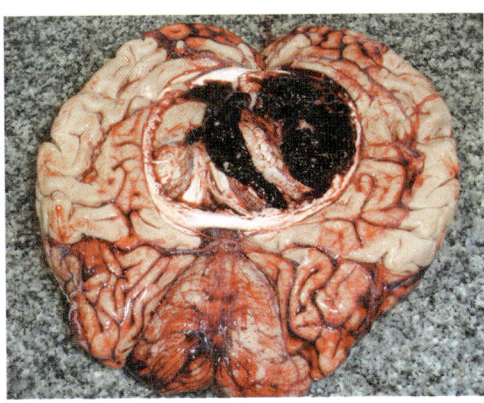

Fig. 13.11: Intracerebral hemorrhage.

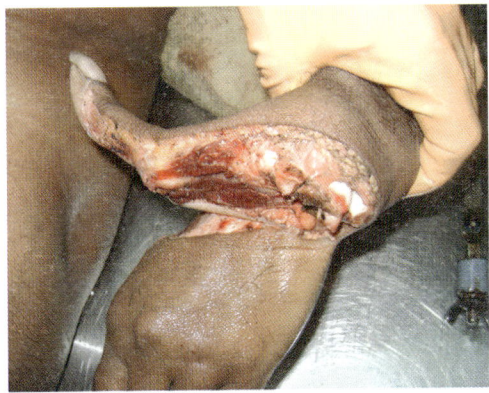

Fig. 14.1: Defense wound.

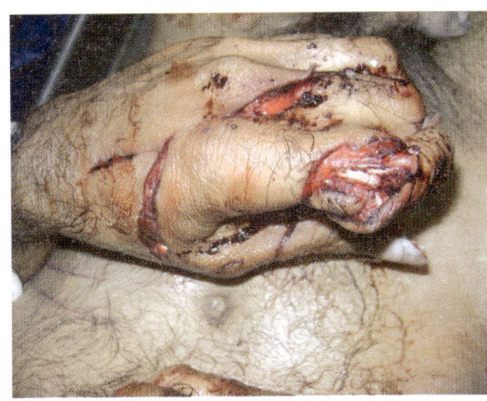

Fig. 14.2: Multiple cut wounds—defense wounds.

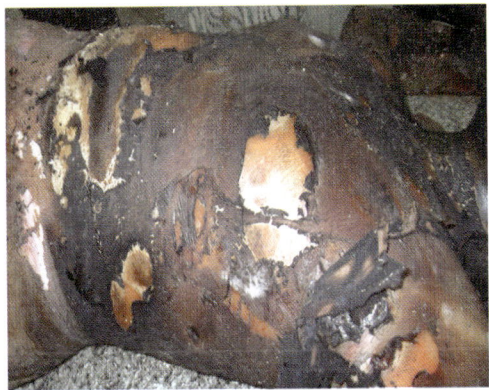

Fig. 15.1: Extensive superficial burns with charring.

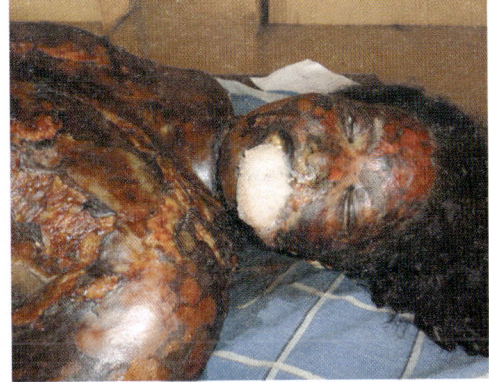

Fig. 15.2: Dermo-epidermal burns exposing underlying pink dermis—antemortem burns.

Plate 14

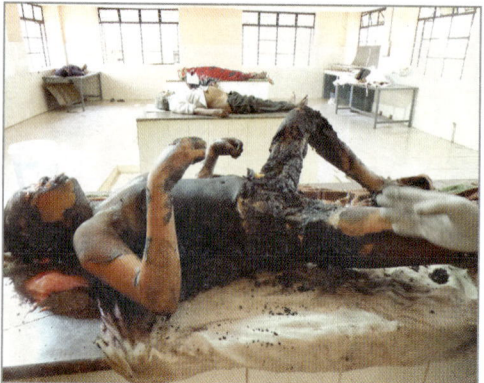

Fig. 15.3: Burns with heat stiffening—pugilistic attitude.

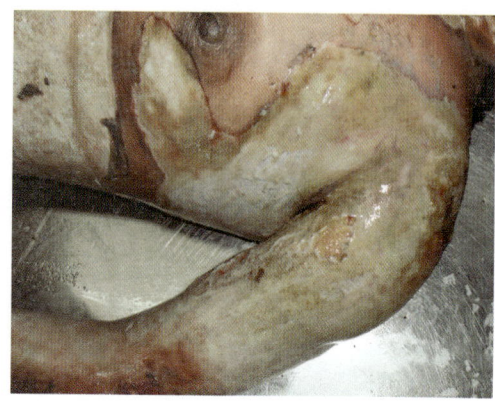

Fig. 15.4: Infected burns—death due to septicemia.

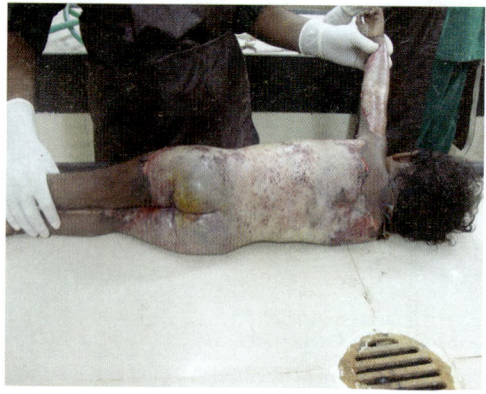

Fig. 15.5: Infected scalds.

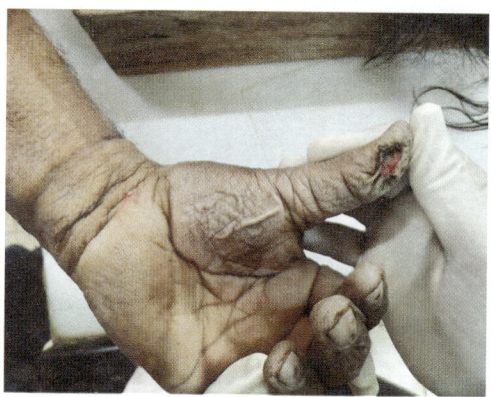

Fig. 17.1: Electrical entry wound on the hands.

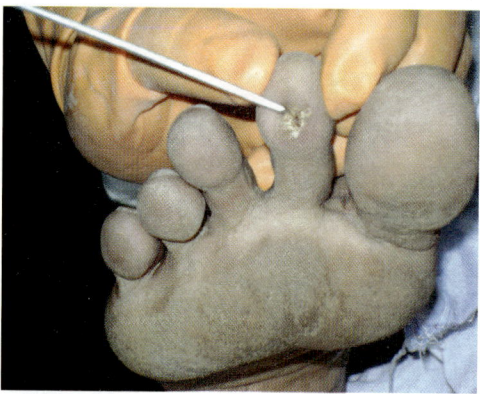

Fig. 17.2: Electrical exit wound on the sole of foot.

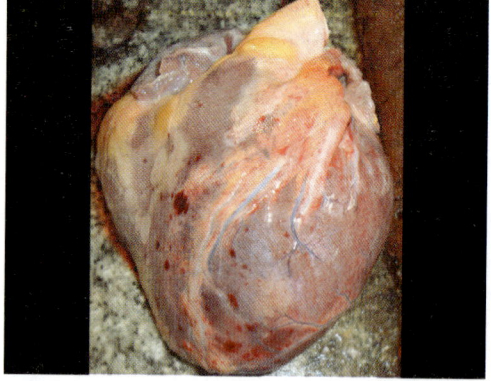

Fig. 17.3: Peticho-ecchymotic hemorrhage on the surface of left ventricle of heart—a case of death due to electrocution.

Plate 15

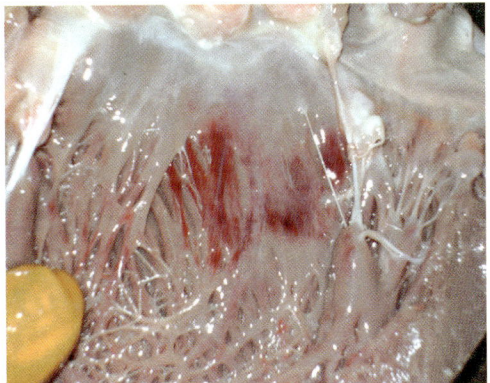

Fig. 17.4: Intraventricular hemorrhage in electrocution.

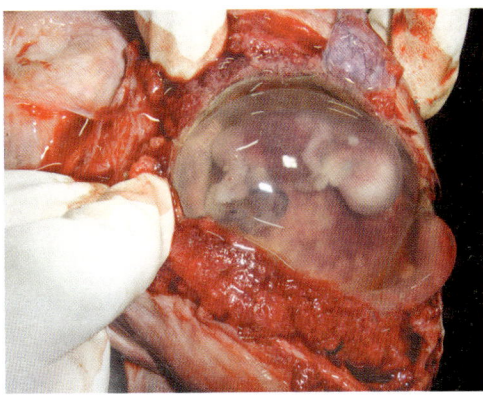

Fig. 20.1: Fetus of 3 months gestation present inside the uterus in the amniotic fluid sac.

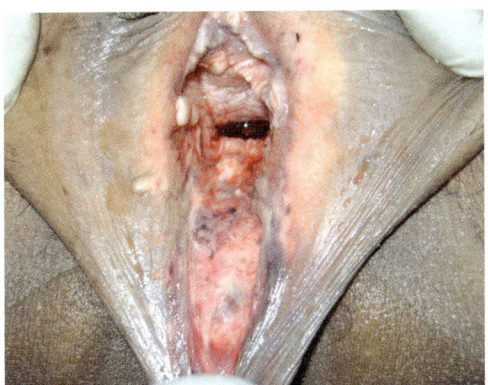

Fig. 20.2: Bruising and tear in the perineum.

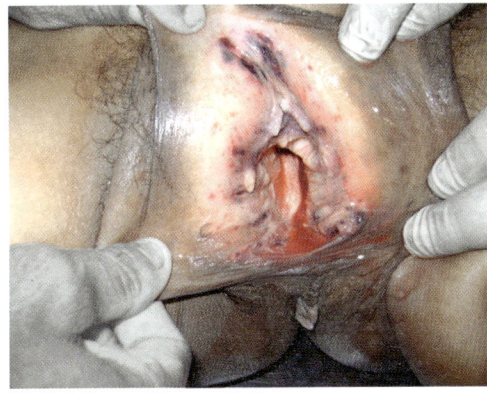

Fig. 20.3: Bruising of the vaginal wall with tear in the perineum.

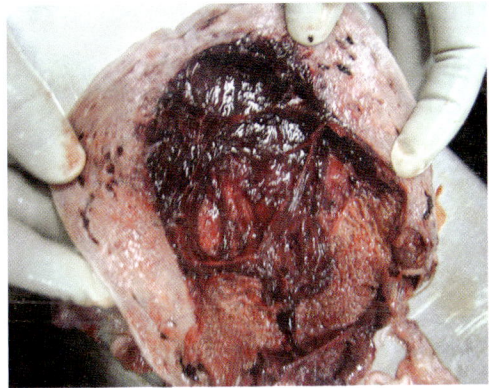

Fig. 20.4: Inner surface of uterus showing retained placenta.

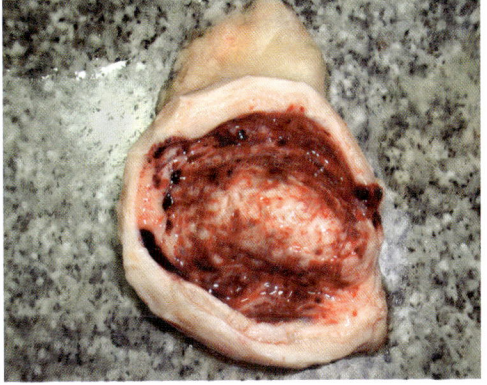

Fig. 20.5: Inner surface of uterus showing irregular nodular areas of placental attachment.

Plate 16

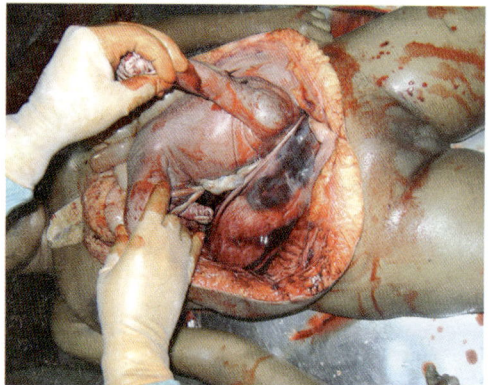

Fig. 20.6: Prolonged obstructed labor resulted in rupture of the uterus and the dead fetus is present in the abdominal cavity with bruising of the peritoneum.

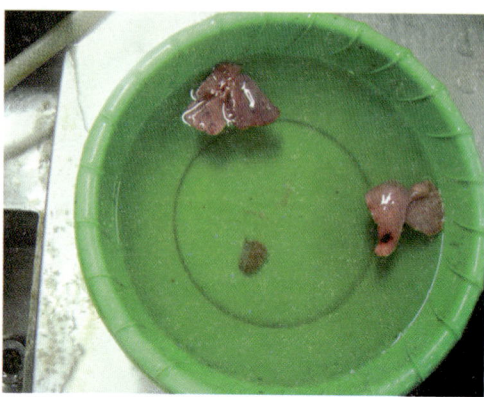

Fig. 22.1: Whole lung is put in water with liver as control.

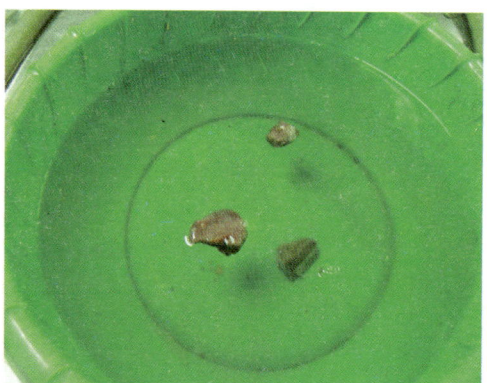

Fig. 22.2: Pieces of lung after squeezing are put into water with liver as control. Pieces of lung floats and liver sinks–positive hydrostatic test, indicating live birth.

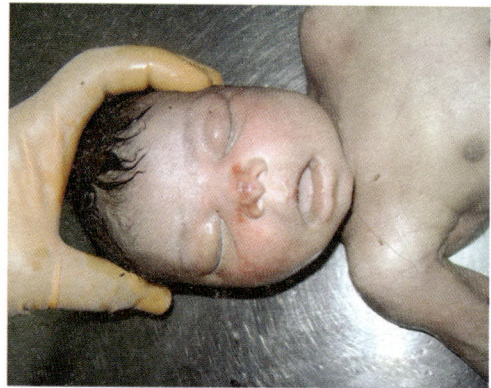

Fig. 22.3: A case of smothering showing bruising of nostrils.

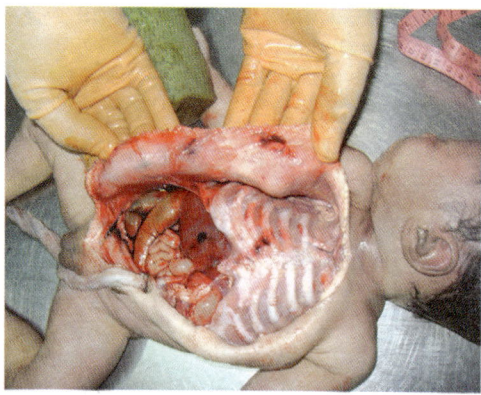

Fig. 22.4: Punctured wound on the right side of abdomen entering into the liver.

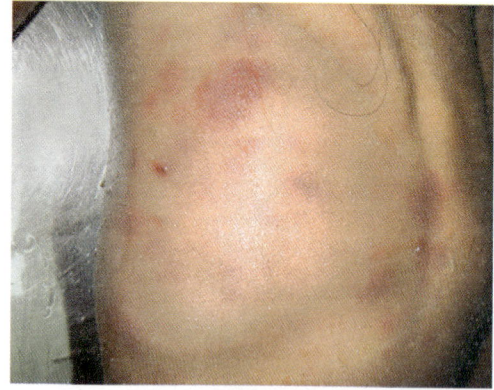

Fig. 22.5: The multiple bruises on chest and abdomen caused by poking with the fingers (six penny bruises).

Plate 17

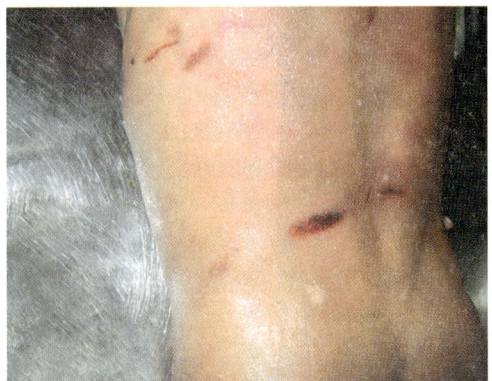

Fig. 22.6: Linear bruise caused by whipping with blunt weapon like a stick.

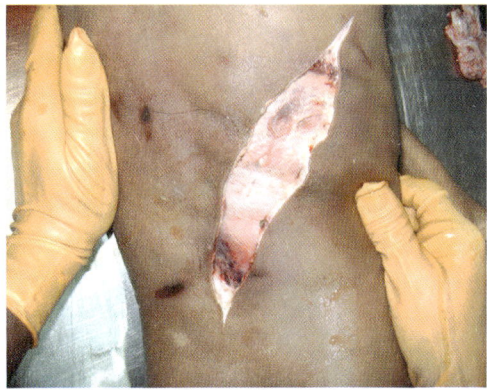

Fig. 22.7: Demonstration of the bruises of the underlying subcutaneous tissues and muscles by dissection.

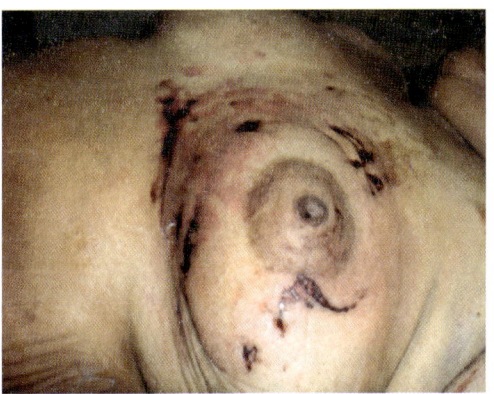

Fig. 23.1: Multiple contusions on the breast produced by biting and scratches by finger nails of the assailant.

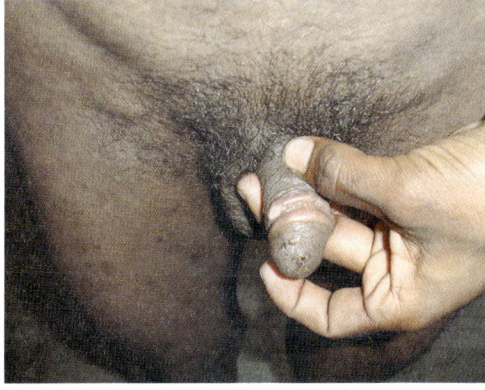

Fig. 23.2: Presence of injuries on the glans penis and ulcer on the skin coving the glans penis.

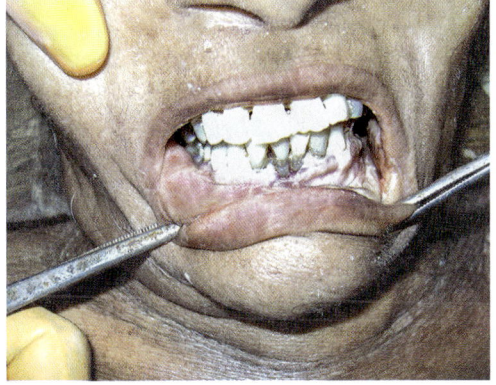

Fig. 27.1: Chalky white teeth in sulfuric acid poisoning.

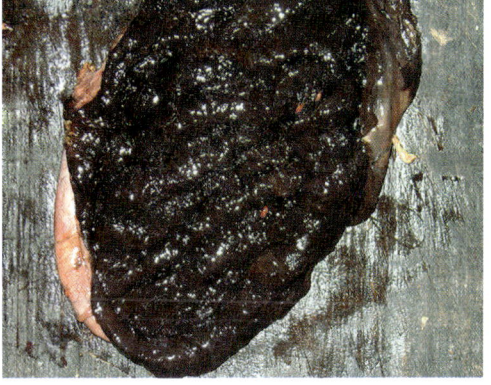

Fig. 27.2: Erosion and necrosis of stomach mucosa in case of sulfuric acid poisoning.

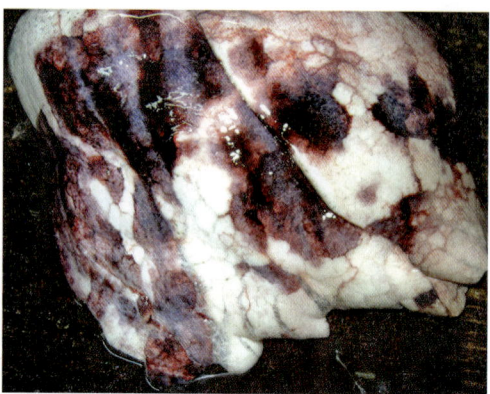

Fig. 27.3: Lung—inhalation of mixture of acids (cleaning acid): Alternative areas of bleeding (corrosion and rupture of arteries) and pale lung parenchyma caused by inhalation while the victim consumed the cleaning acid to commit suicide—a treated case died after 20 days of poisoning near the recovery period; CT could not pick up the lung finding and the patient suddenly collapsed and died after a heavy bout of hemoptysis.

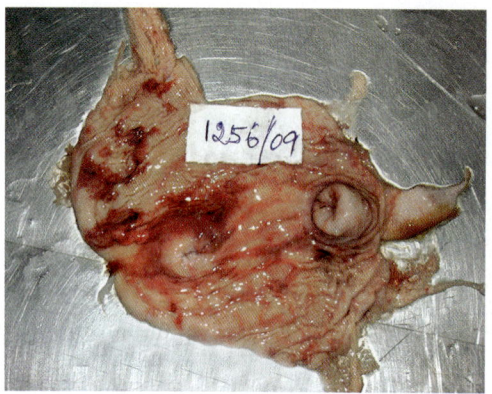

Fig. 27.4: Kerosene poisoning—diffuse submucosal hemorrhages in stomach.

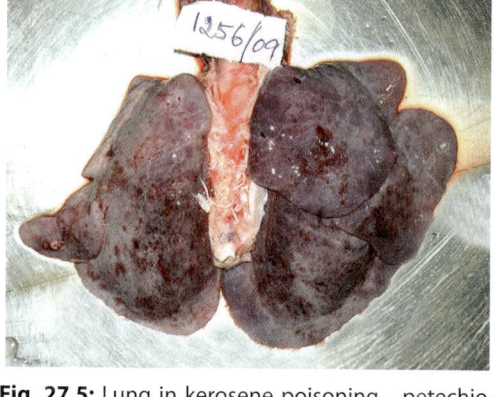

Fig. 27.5: Lung in kerosene poisoning—petechio-ecchymotic hemorrhages more concentrated on the upper lobe; the child died of aspiration pneumonitis.

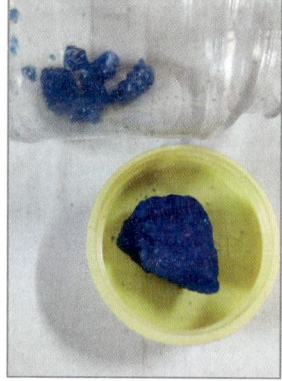

Fig. 28.1: Metallic irritant poison (copper sulphate).

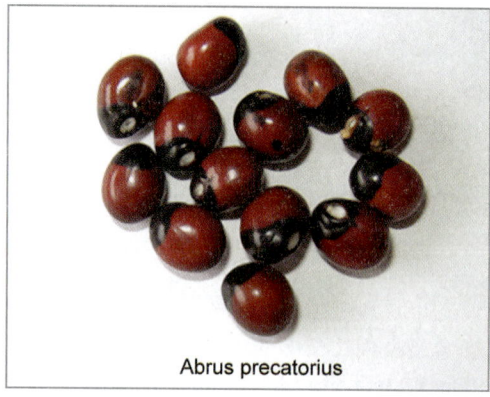

Fig. 29.1: Abrus precatorius.

Plate 19

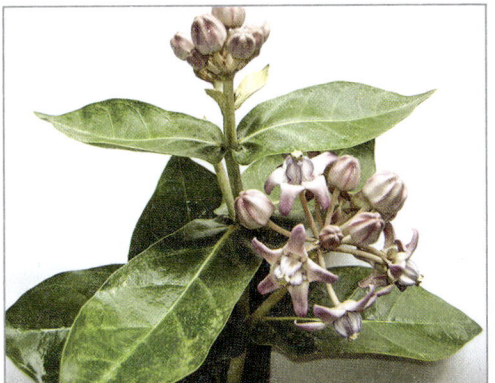

Fig. 29.2: Calotropis.

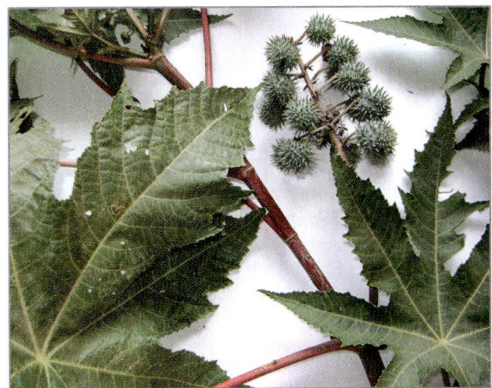

Fig. 29.3: Castor plant (ricinus communis).

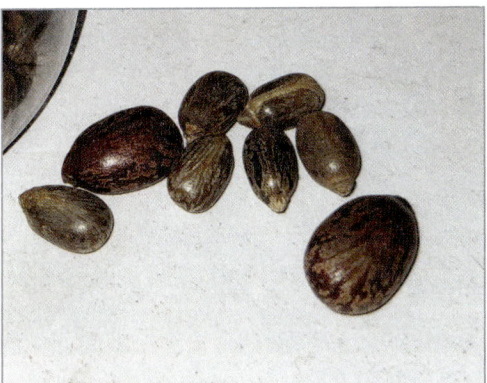

Fig. 29.4: Ricinus communis/castor seeds.

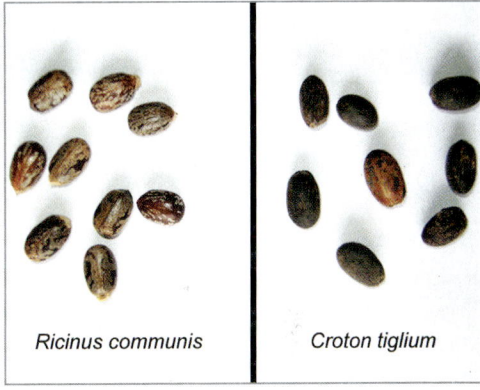

Fig. 29.5: Castor and croton seeds.

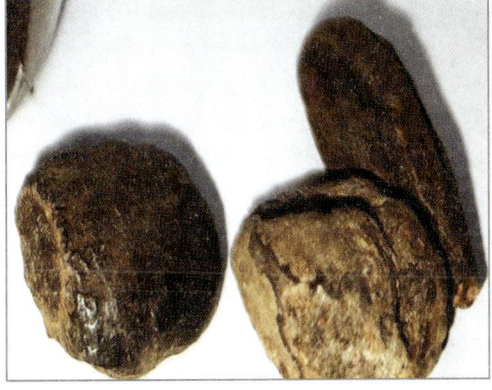

Fig. 29.6: Semecarpus anacardium (marking nut).

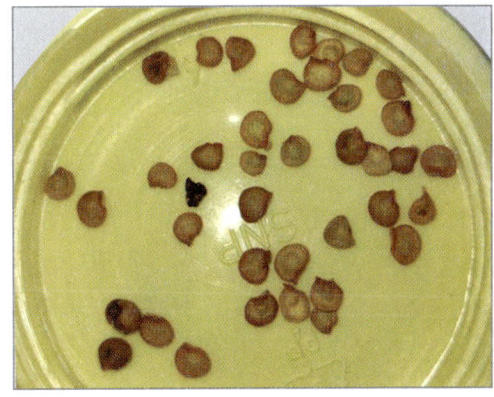

Fig. 29.7: Capsicum seeds.

Plate 20

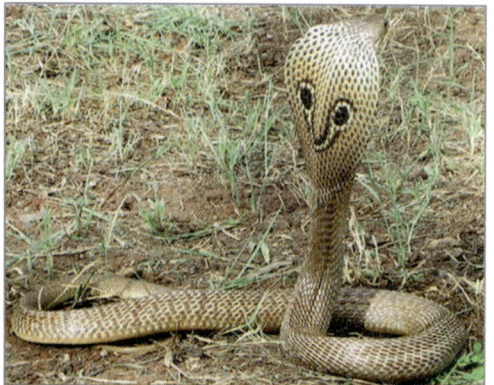

Fig. 29.8: Cobra (Elapidae).

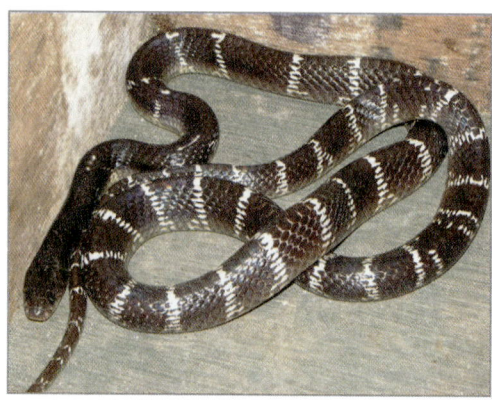

Fig. 29.9: Viperidae.

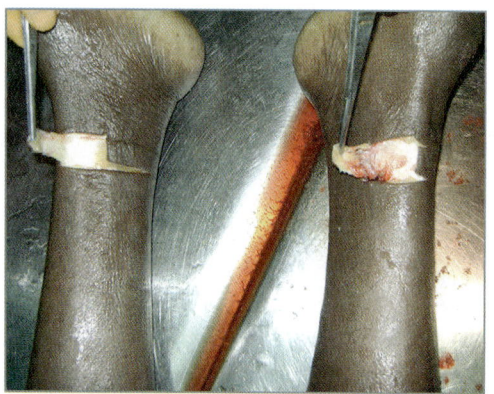

Fig. 29.11: Dissection of the bitten area demonstrating bruising of the underlying subcutaneous tissues. The opposite limb is also dissected as a control, which shows no bruising.

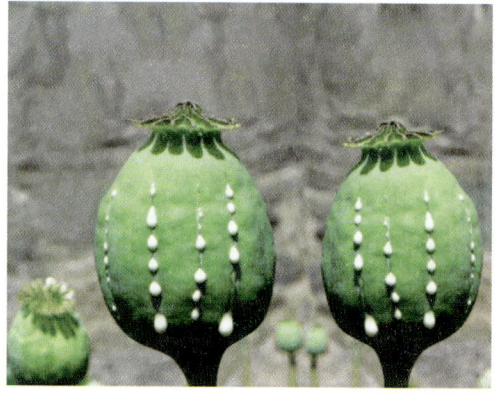

Fig 30.1: Papaver somniferum/poppy.

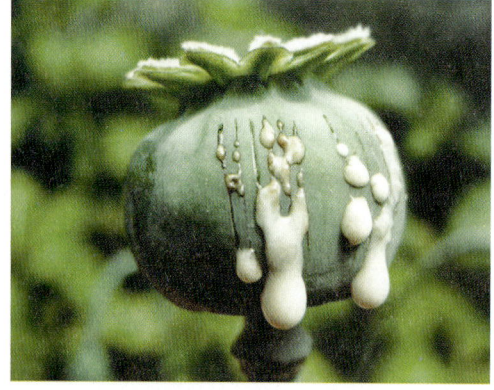

Fig 30.2: Poppy capsule.

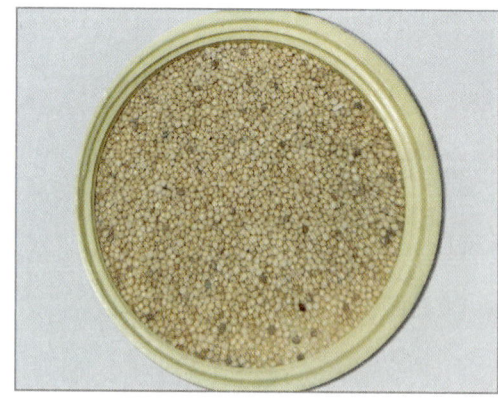

Fig 30.3: Poppy seeds.

Plate 21

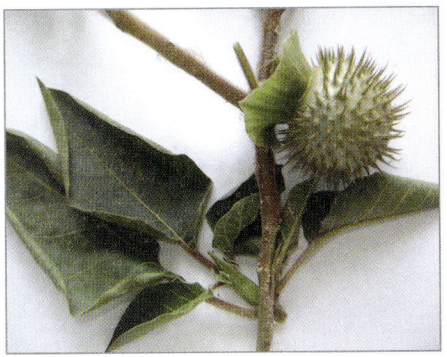

Fig 30.4: Datura plant with fruit (thorn apple).

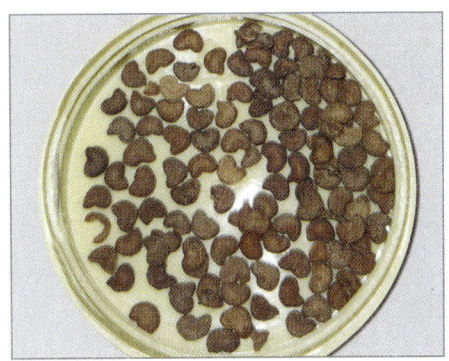

Fig. 30.5: Datura seeds.

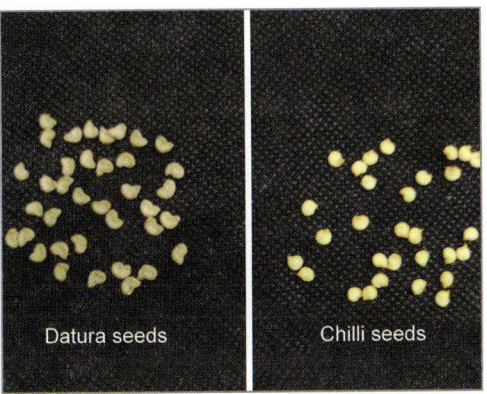

Fig. 30.6: Datura seeds and chilli seeds.

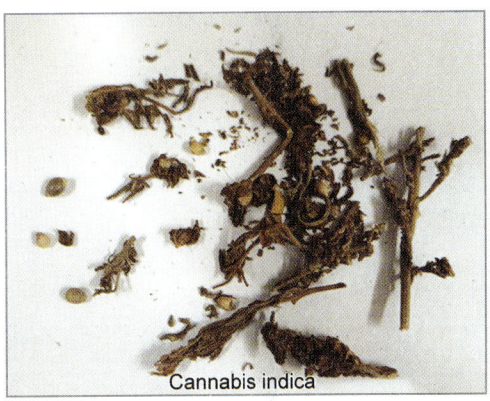

Fig. 30.7: Cannabis indica.

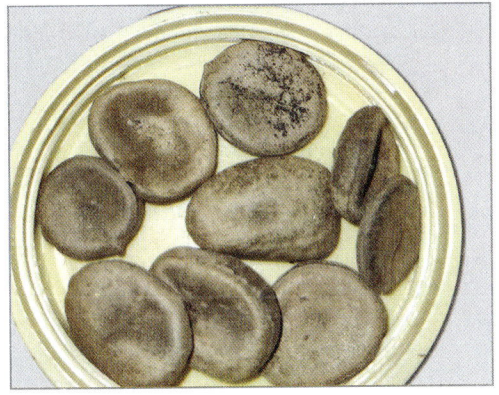

Fig 30.8: Nux vomica seeds.

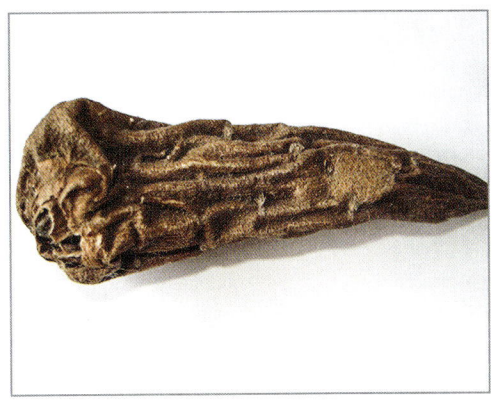

Fig. 31.1: Aconite root (Monk's Hood).

Plate 22

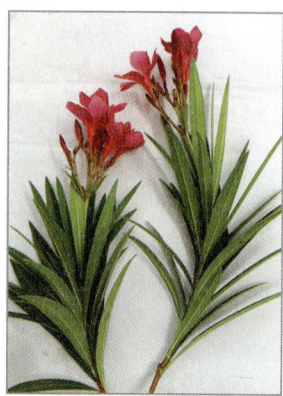

Fig. 31.2: Nerium odorum.

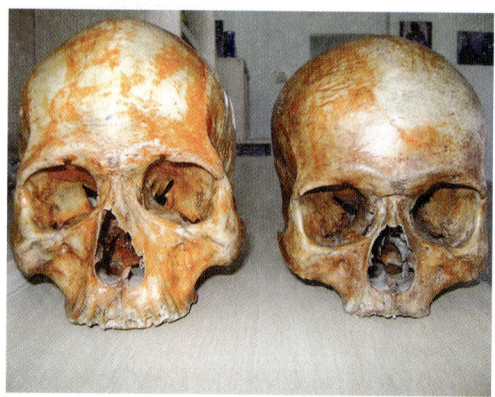

Fig. E3.1: *Skull:* Male and female skull: Sloping forehead, square and low placed orbits, large cheek bones and prominent supraorbital ridges features of male skull; steep forehead, highly placed orbits, less prominent supraorbital ridges and less prominent muscular markings—features of female skull.

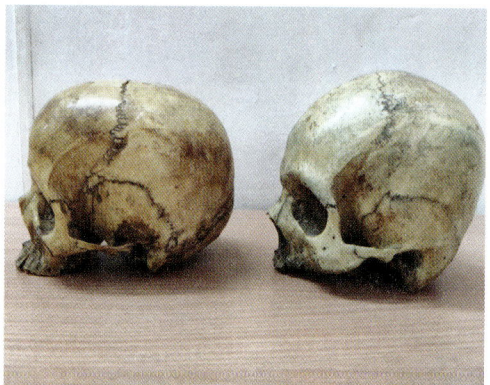

Fig. E3.2: *Skull lateral view:* Female and male skull: Vertical forehead, more prominent parietal eminence and less prominent zygomatic arch—features of female skull; sloping forehead, less prominent parietal eminence and more prominent zygomatic arch—features of male skull.

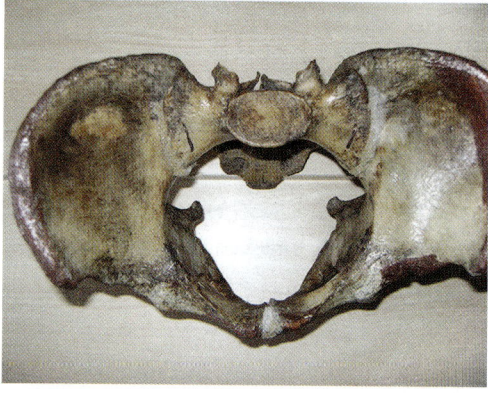

Fig. E3.3: *Male pelvis:* Deep funnel shaped and small pelvic inlet.

present days. Almost all the offences against the human body requires medical opinion in order to deliver an impeccable justice in the court of law. The primary interest is to provide the source of information about medical science to confine the needs of the law.
- Forensic medicine is mostly an exercise of common sense combined with the application of knowledge and experience acquired in other branches of medicine.
- Forensic medicine involves:
  i. Observation of facts,
  ii. Collection of evidence,
  iii. Interpretation of the scene of crime and
  iv. Reconstruction of the events based on medicolegal examination.
- In all cases of crime involving human body, e.g., homicide, suicide, assault, sexual offences, criminal abortion, traffic accidents, poisoning, etc., the help of the medical officer is sought by the investigative agency. In all such cases, the doctor will be required to appear in the court as an expert witness and depose evidence.
- In some cases, as in cases of sudden death, the authorities will have to depend completely on the medical witness in establishing the cause of death.
- A properly prepared physician often finds his court room experience educative. The physician must bear testimony within the limits of science. The attitude of the scientific witness should be the same whether he is called by the prosecution or by the defense.
- The sole obligation of the medical witness is to present the truth as he sees it, adding nothing, withholding nothing and distorting nothing. The doctor must be honest, unbiased and truthful, for the confidence is inspired by honesty and success depends on *confidence.*

WHAT ARE THE CIRCUMSTANCES A DOCTOR MAY BE CALLED TO THE COURT?

- A doctor may be called to the court to testify:
  i. As an ordinary witness who saw something happen.
  ii. As a medical practitioner who treated the patient.
  iii. As an expert witness to give opinion on matters of science.

MULTIPLE CHOICE QUESTIONS

1. **Medical jurisprudence means:**
   a. Knowledge of medicine required for lawyers
   b. Knowledge of law required for doctors for medical practice
   c. Knowledge of medicine required for doctors
   d. Knowledge of law required for legal practice
2. **"Medical etiquette" deals with:**
   a. The conventional laws of the courtesy observed between members of the medical profession
   b. Legal responsibilities of the physician
   c. The study and application of the effects of violence or unnatural disease in its various forms
   d. The moral principles which should guide members of the medical profession in their dealings

ANSWERS

1. b   2. a

2
CHAPTER

The Indian Legal System

KEY WORDS

Inquest, Police inquest, Magistrate inquest, Coroner's court, Criminal courts in India, cognizable offences, Supreme court, High court, Sessions court, Magistrate court, Labor court, Family court, summons, conduct money, court procedures, witness, exert witness, evidence, documentary evidence, medical evidence, dying declaration, compos mentis, dying deposition, perjury, hostile witness, leading question, Government standing orders for medicolegal cases.

FM1.3	Describe legal procedures including criminal procedure code, Indian Penal Code, Indian Evidence Act, civil and criminal cases, inquest (police inquest and Magistrate's inquest), Cognizable and noncognizable offences.
FM1.4	Describe courts in India and their powers: Supreme court, High court, Sessions court, Magistrate's court, Labor court, Family court, Executive magistrate court and Juvenile justice board.
FM1.5	Describe court procedures including issue of summons, conduct money, types of witnesses, recording of evidence oath, affirmation, examination in chief, cross-examination, re-examination and court questions, recording of evidence and conduct of doctor in witness box.
FM1.6	Describe offenses in court including perjury; court strictures vis-a-vis medical officer.
FM1.7	Describe dying declaration and dying deposition.
FM1.8	Describe the latest decisions/notifications/resolutions/circulars/standing orders related to medicolegal practice issued by Courts/Government authorities, etc.

INTRODUCTION

The legal system in India is governed by **(FM1.3)**.

Indian Penal Code (IPC) Formed in the Year 1860 (FM1.3)

- It deals with substantial criminal laws of India. It defines various offences and prescribes punishment for all offences.
- Hence, when a case is booked under IPC the doctor who conducts any examination and issues certificate should remember that the case will come to court for trial and he has to go to court and depose evidence at later stage.

Criminal Procedure Code (CrPC) Formed in the Year 1973 (FM1.3)

- It stipulates the duties of the police/enquiry officer, in their dealings with the offender during interrogation and in the investigation of death. CrPC lays down guidelines on how to investigate a case, the procedure of arrest, interrogation and detention of an accused person.
- When a case is booked under CrPC, it indicates the investigation is on progress and may get changed to sections of IPC if any crime is involved.

Indian Evidence Act (IEA) Formed in 1872 (FM1.3)

- It deals with laws of evidence and applies to any court whether civil or criminal. Evidence means and includes anything which the court permits or required to be produced before the court by the witnesses.
- Every case has to be proved by means of evidences. The outcome of any case depends upon the quality of the evidences to prove or disprove any issue beyond any reasonable doubt in the courts of law.

Case Laws

Legal principles derived from judicial decisions. It is different from statutory laws enacted by the legislature; but accepted as precedence in similar types of cases in future.

Civil Case (FM1.3)

- Civil case is dispute between two parties. The person who brings the proceedings in the court is called the "Complainant" and against whom the complaint is made is the "Defendant".
- Both the complainant and the defendant have to arrange lawyers on their behalf and argue the case. Based on the evidences produced the judicial magistrate gives the judgment.

Criminal Case (FM1.3)

- Criminal case is a case filed by the Government against a person (accused) who is said to have committed any crime. A crime is disobedience of law. When the Government releases in the Gazette from that time it becomes law. If anyone bypasses any of the provisions of the law he is said to have committed a crime. When a crime is committed by someone the Government (Police–People empowered to enforce the law in the society) files the case under appropriate sections of IPC and proceeds with further action as per the provisions of the law.
- In criminal case, the prosecution (Government lawyer) has to prove the case with appropriate evidences beyond any reasonable doubt so that the judge will award the punishment as the provisions of IPC. The accused person has to arrange a lawyer (Defense Lawyer) on his behalf to disprove the crime or prove that he has not committed any crime.

DEFINE INQUEST. WHAT ARE THE VARIOUS TYPES OF INQUEST? DESCRIBE THE PROCEDURE OF POLICE INQUEST? (FM1.3)

Inquest (in-in; quasitus—to seek) (to seek into): Inquest is defined as the preliminary legal inquiry into the cause, manner and circumstances of any unnatural, sudden and suspicious death.

Types of Inquest

There are basically four types of inquest prevalent throughout the world and they are:
  i. Police inquest
  ii. Magistrate inquest
  iii. Coroner's inquest
  iv. Medical examiner system of inquest

- In India, there are only two types of inquest (police inquest and magistrate inquest).
- Section 174 CrPC deals with police inquest and section 176 CrPC deals with magistrate inquest.

Police Inquest

- This is the commonest type of inquest conducted in India.
- The officer in charge of a police station, not below the rank of sub-inspector (called the investigation officer of that particular case), on receipt of information of a death, informs the executive magistrate and proceeds to the place where the dead body is found.
- Conducts the inquest in the presence of two reliable witnesses, who should be respectable persons of the society (**Panchas**). He comes to a conclusion regarding the apparent cause of death, as judged by him and prepares a report called the inquest report (**Panchanama**).
- If death is purely due to disease (natural death) he may hand over the body to the relatives for disposal of the body according to their religious customs. If death is unnatural or if the investigation officer suspects any foul play or the cause of death is not known, then he sends the body to the nearest authorized autopsy center for postmortem examination, along with a copy of the inquest report.

WHAT IS MAGISTRATE INQUEST AND WHEN IT IS CONDUCTED? (FM1.3)

Magistrate Inquest

It is the inquest conducted by the executive magistrate appointed by the state government. The executive magistrates are people of the revenue department not below the rank of Tehsildar, District Revenue Officer (DRO), Revenue Divisional Officer (RDO), PA to Collector or the District Collector can all act as executive magistrates. The executive magistrate conducts inquest in the following circumstances:

- **Dowry deaths:** Unnatural death of a female within 7 years of marriage.
- Death in police custody
- Death during police interrogation
- Death due to police firing
- Death in a psychiatric hospital/mental asylum
- Exhumation
- As per Section 176 CrPC, in any case of death the magistrate may/can conduct an inquest instead of or in addition to the police inquest.

DESCRIBE CORONER'S INQUEST AND MEDICAL EXAMINER SYSTEM OF INQUEST (TABLE 2.1)

Coroner's Inquest

- Coroner is a person qualified either in medicine or law or both, appointed by the government.
- He conducts the inquest in all unnatural and suspicious deaths.
- He is empowered to summon any person for enquiry.
- Coroner's court is a court of enquiry, but he is not empowered to conduct a trial.
- After the enquiry the coroner forwards all documents to the magistrate court and

TABLE 2.1: Differences between coroner's court and magistrate court.

Coroner's court	Magistrate court
Court of inquiry	Court of trail
Can summon a witness, issue warrant and impose fine	Do
Court of inquiry and hence cannot award any punishment	Court of trail and hence punishment is awarded after trail

Plate 23

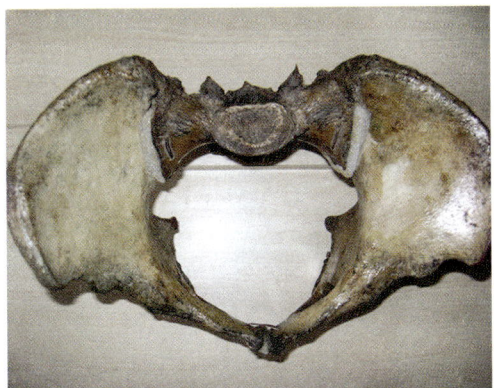

Fig. E3.4: *Female pelvis:* Flat bowl shaped and large pelvic inlet.

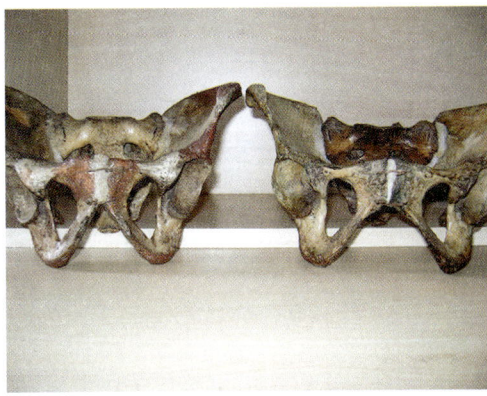

Fig. E3.5: *Male and female pelvis:* Less vertical ileum and "V" shaped subpubic angle in male. More vertical ileum and "U" shaped large subpubic angle in female.

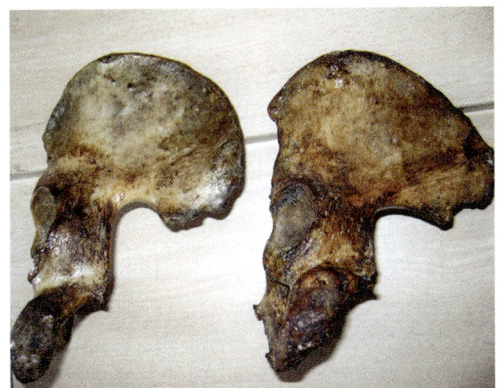

Fig. E3.6: *Male and female pelvic bone:* Note the sciatic notch; narrow, deep and "V" shaped in male; wide, shallow and "U" shaped in female. The only sex diagnostic feature in bones even before puberty, as the pelvic bone by nature is designed for delivery in females.

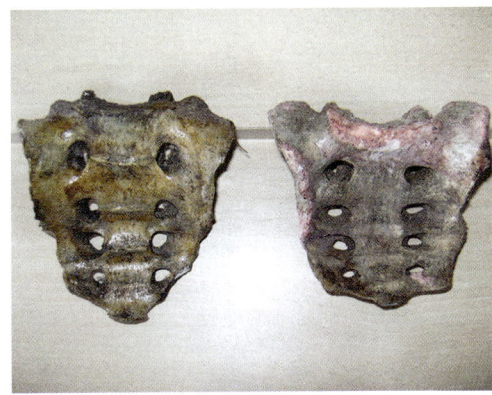

Fig. E3.7: *Sacrum:* Male and female; tall, narrow and uniformly curved in male and short, broad and curved only in the lower portion in female.

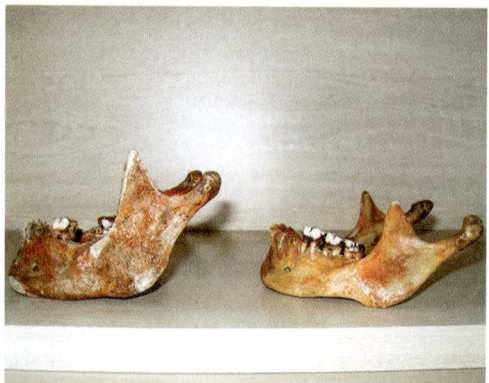

Fig. E3.8: *Mandible:* Male and female; large condyles and less obtuse angle of ramus in male and small condyles and more obtuse angled in female.

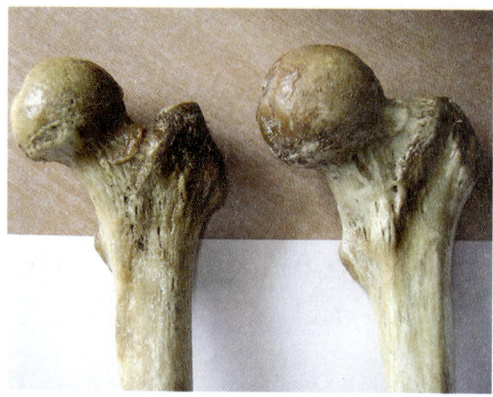

Fig. E3.9: *Femur:* Female and male; head is small, less obtuse angle with the shaft and the head forms less than two third of the sphere in female. Head is large, more obtuse angle with the shaft and the head forms more than two third of the sphere in male.

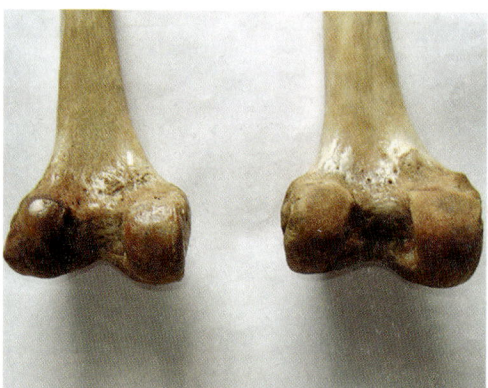

Fig. E3.10: *Condyles of femur:* Female and male; condyles are small and the bicondylar width is 67 to 76 mm in female. Condyles are large and the bicondylar width is 74 to 89 mm in male.

SECTION 1

Medical Jurisprudence

SECTION OUTLINE

Chapter 1: Introduction and Scope of Forensic Medicine
Chapter 2: The Indian Legal System
Chapter 3: Medical Ethics and the Law
Chapter 4: Consent and Medical Negligence

- In India, there are only two types of inquest (police inquest and magistrate inquest).
- Section 174 CrPC deals with police inquest and section 176 CrPC deals with magistrate inquest.

Police Inquest

- This is the commonest type of inquest conducted in India.
- The officer in charge of a police station, not below the rank of sub-inspector (called the investigation officer of that particular case), on receipt of information of a death, informs the executive magistrate and proceeds to the place where the dead body is found.
- Conducts the inquest in the presence of two reliable witnesses, who should be respectable persons of the society (**Panchas**). He comes to a conclusion regarding the apparent cause of death, as judged by him and prepares a report called the inquest report (**Panchanama**).
- If death is purely due to disease (natural death) he may hand over the body to the relatives for disposal of the body according to their religious customs. If death is unnatural or if the investigation officer suspects any foul play or the cause of death is not known, then he sends the body to the nearest authorized autopsy center for postmortem examination, along with a copy of the inquest report.

WHAT IS MAGISTRATE INQUEST AND WHEN IT IS CONDUCTED? (FM1.3)

Magistrate Inquest

It is the inquest conducted by the executive magistrate appointed by the state government. The executive magistrates are people of the revenue department not below the rank of Tehsildar, District Revenue Officer (DRO), Revenue Divisional Officer (RDO), PA to Collector or the District Collector can all act as executive magistrates. The executive magistrate conducts inquest in the following circumstances:

- **Dowry deaths:** Unnatural death of a female within 7 years of marriage.
- Death in police custody
- Death during police interrogation
- Death due to police firing
- Death in a psychiatric hospital/mental asylum
- Exhumation
- As per Section 176 CrPC, in any case of death the magistrate may/can conduct an inquest instead of or in addition to the police inquest.

DESCRIBE CORONER'S INQUEST AND MEDICAL EXAMINER SYSTEM OF INQUEST (TABLE 2.1)

Coroner's Inquest

- Coroner is a person qualified either in medicine or law or both, appointed by the government.
- He conducts the inquest in all unnatural and suspicious deaths.
- He is empowered to summon any person for enquiry.
- Coroner's court is a court of enquiry, but he is not empowered to conduct a trial.
- After the enquiry the coroner forwards all documents to the magistrate court and

TABLE 2.1: Differences between coroner's court and magistrate court.

Coroner's court	Magistrate court
Court of inquiry	Court of trail
Can summon a witness, issue warrant and impose fine	Do
Court of inquiry and hence cannot award any punishment	Court of trail and hence punishment is awarded after trail

Criminal Procedure Code (CrPC) Formed in the Year 1973 (FM1.3)

- It stipulates the duties of the police/enquiry officer, in their dealings with the offender during interrogation and in the investigation of death. CrPC lays down guidelines on how to investigate a case, the procedure of arrest, interrogation and detention of an accused person.
- When a case is booked under CrPC, it indicates the investigation is on progress and may get changed to sections of IPC if any crime is involved.

Indian Evidence Act (IEA) Formed in 1872 (FM1.3)

- It deals with laws of evidence and applies to any court whether civil or criminal. Evidence means and includes anything which the court permits or required to be produced before the court by the witnesses.
- Every case has to be proved by means of evidences. The outcome of any case depends upon the quality of the evidences to prove or disprove any issue beyond any reasonable doubt in the courts of law.

Case Laws

Legal principles derived from judicial decisions. It is different from statutory laws enacted by the legislature; but accepted as precedence in similar types of cases in future.

Civil Case (FM1.3)

- Civil case is dispute between two parties. The person who brings the proceedings in the court is called the "Complainant" and against whom the complaint is made is the "Defendant".
- Both the complainant and the defendant have to arrange lawyers on their behalf and argue the case. Based on the evidences produced the judicial magistrate gives the judgment.

Criminal Case (FM1.3)

- Criminal case is a case filed by the Government against a person (accused) who is said to have committed any crime. A crime is disobedience of law. When the Government releases in the Gazette from that time it becomes law. If anyone bypasses any of the provisions of the law he is said to have committed a crime. When a crime is committed by someone the Government (Police–People empowered to enforce the law in the society) files the case under appropriate sections of IPC and proceeds with further action as per the provisions of the law.
- In criminal case, the prosecution (Government lawyer) has to prove the case with appropriate evidences beyond any reasonable doubt so that the judge will award the punishment as the provisions of IPC. The accused person has to arrange a lawyer (Defense Lawyer) on his behalf to disprove the crime or prove that he has not committed any crime.

DEFINE INQUEST. WHAT ARE THE VARIOUS TYPES OF INQUEST? DESCRIBE THE PROCEDURE OF POLICE INQUEST? (FM1.3)

Inquest (in-in; quasitus—to seek) (to seek into): Inquest is defined as the preliminary legal inquiry into the cause, manner and circumstances of any unnatural, sudden and suspicious death.

Types of Inquest

There are basically four types of inquest prevalent throughout the world and they are:
  i. Police inquest
  ii. Magistrate inquest
  iii. Coroner's inquest
  iv. Medical examiner system of inquest

trail and punishment if any are awarded by the judicial magistrate.
- This type of inquest is done in United Kingdom and some states of USA.
- This type of inquest was practiced in many parts of India during the British period; it is no more in practice in India now and was lastly withdrawn from Bombay in the year 1999.

Medical Examiner System of Inquest

- This is the type of inquest prevalent in most states of USA and also in many advanced countries. A medical examiner (forensic expert) is appointed to perform the functions of the coroner.
- On receipt of information of a death, the medical examiner visits the scene of crime and conducts the inquest. Thus he is able to gather first-hand evidence which is interpreted in proper perspective owing to his knowledge of medical science and he himself conducts the autopsy on the body and hence, better corroboration of evidences and thus better administration of justice.
- This is said to be **the most superior type of inquest**.

WHAT IS COGNIZABLE OFFENCE? (FM1.3)

- An **offence** means any act of commission or omission punishable by the law.
- Cognizable offence is an offence for which the police officer can arrest an individual without a warrant from the magistrate; e.g., rape, murder, dacoity, etc.
- The cases which come under cognizable offence are offences for which the punishment is more than 2 years.
- In these cases, the arrested person is sent to the doctor by the police for examination.

WHAT IS NONCOGNIZABLE OFFENCE? (FM1.3)

- In a noncognizable offence, the police officer cannot arrest the accused person without a warrant from the judicial magistrate. These offences are of those for which the punishment is less than 2 years.
- In a noncognizable offence, the individual may go direct to the doctor, or files an affidavit in court and then the magistrate sends the person to the doctor for examination (Section 41 CrPC).

DESCRIBE THE VARIOUS CRIMINAL COURTS OF INDIA AND ARE THEIR POWERS? (FM1.4)

- The **Supreme Court** situated in Delhi is the highest tribunal of the country. No cases of trail takes place in Supreme Court. It entertains only appeals from High Court, except in situations when a case decision is binding for the whole country no one can go to Supreme Court directly.
- The **High Court** is usually situated in the capital of the state. Some states do not have separate High Court, for example, the State of Pondicherry is annexed to Madras High Court. Some states have branch of High Court in some other city for easy access of the people, for example, the State of Tamil Nadu has established a branch of the Madras High Court at Madurai. The High Court also entertains only appeals from Sessions court, except when a decision is binding for whole of the state no one can directly go to the High Court.
- The **District Sessions Court** situated in the head of the district is the highest judicial power, it has equal power as that of high court except that when capital punishment is awarded in a case, it has to be confirmed by the High Court. District courts may have additional district sessions courts and

assistant district session courts according to the needs and case loads of the district. All the offences for which the punishment is more than 7 years the trial is conducted in the sessions courts directly. The district sessions court also entertains appeals from the magistrate courts.
- All these courts tabulated in **Table 2.2** and their hierarchy depicted in **Flowchart 2.1**.
- **Judicial Magistrate Courts (Table 2.3)** are usually situated at Taluk levels. All offences for which the punishment is less than 7 years the trail will be conducted in the magistrate courts.

Judges

- The **chief justice of India** is appointed by the **President of India** and usually, the senior most judge is appointed as the chief justice of India.

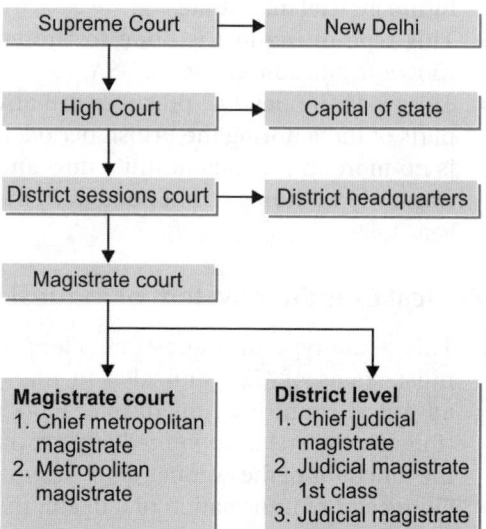

Flowchart 2.1: Criminal courts of India.

TABLE 2.2: Criminal courts of India (FM1.4).

Court	Location	Powers
Supreme Court	New Delhi	Highest Judicial Tribunal of the country. Can pass any sentence. Usually, considers only appeals from the High Court
High Court	State Capital	Highest Judicial Tribunal of the state. Can pass any sentence. Usually, considers only appeals from the lower courts
Session Court (District Sessions Court)	District Head Quarters	Highest Judicial Tribunal of the district. Can pass any sentence but death sentence has to be confirmed by the High Court

TABLE 2.3: Magistrate courts.

Court	Location	Powers
Chief Metropolitan Magistrate Chief Judicial Magistrate	Metropolitan areas District (not being a Metropolitan area)	Can pass a sentence of imprisonment up to 7 years Fine without limit
Metropolitan Magistrate Judicial Magistrate of First Class	Metropolitan area Subdivision of a district	Can pass a sentence of imprisonment up to 3 years: Fine up to ₹ 10,000/-
Judicial Magistrate of Second Class	Taluk level	Can pass a sentence of imprisonment up to 1 year: Fine up to ₹ 5,000/-

CHAPTER 2

The Indian Legal System

 KEY WORDS

Inquest, Police inquest, Magistrate inquest, Coroner's court, Criminal courts in India, cognizable offences, Supreme court, High court, Sessions court, Magistrate court, Labor court, Family court, summons, conduct money, court procedures, witness, exert witness, evidence, documentary evidence, medical evidence, dying declaration, compos mentis, dying deposition, perjury, hostile witness, leading question, Government standing orders for medicolegal cases.

FM1.3 Describe legal procedures including criminal procedure code, Indian Penal Code, Indian Evidence Act, civil and criminal cases, inquest (police inquest and Magistrate's inquest), Cognizable and noncognizable offences.

FM1.4 Describe courts in India and their powers: Supreme court, High court, Sessions court, Magistrate's court, Labor court, Family court, Executive magistrate court and Juvenile justice board.

FM1.5 Describe court procedures including issue of summons, conduct money, types of witnesses, recording of evidence oath, affirmation, examination in chief, cross-examination, re-examination and court questions, recording of evidence and conduct of doctor in witness box.

FM1.6 Describe offenses in court including perjury; court strictures vis-a-vis medical officer.

FM1.7 Describe dying declaration and dying deposition.

FM1.8 Describe the latest decisions/notifications/resolutions/circulars/standing orders related to medicolegal practice issued by Courts/Government authorities, etc.

INTRODUCTION

The legal system in India is governed by **(FM1.3).**

Indian Penal Code (IPC) Formed in the Year 1860 (FM1.3)

- It deals with substantial criminal laws of India. It defines various offences and prescribes punishment for all offences.
- Hence, when a case is booked under IPC the doctor who conducts any examination and issues certificate should remember that the case will come to court for trial and he has to go to court and depose evidence at later stage.

present days. Almost all the offences against the human body requires medical opinion in order to deliver an impeccable justice in the court of law. The primary interest is to provide the source of information about medical science to confine the needs of the law.
- Forensic medicine is mostly an exercise of common sense combined with the application of knowledge and experience acquired in other branches of medicine.
- Forensic medicine involves:
  i. Observation of facts,
  ii. Collection of evidence,
  iii. Interpretation of the scene of crime and
  iv. Reconstruction of the events based on medicolegal examination.
- In all cases of crime involving human body, e.g., homicide, suicide, assault, sexual offences, criminal abortion, traffic accidents, poisoning, etc., the help of the medical officer is sought by the investigative agency. In all such cases, the doctor will be required to appear in the court as an expert witness and depose evidence.
- In some cases, as in cases of sudden death, the authorities will have to depend completely on the medical witness in establishing the cause of death.
- A properly prepared physician often finds his court room experience educative. The physician must bear testimony within the limits of science. The attitude of the scientific witness should be the same whether he is called by the prosecution or by the defense.
- The sole obligation of the medical witness is to present the truth as he sees it, adding nothing, withholding nothing and distorting nothing. The doctor must be honest, unbiased and truthful, for the confidence is inspired by honesty and success depends on *confidence.*

WHAT ARE THE CIRCUMSTANCES A DOCTOR MAY BE CALLED TO THE COURT?

- A doctor may be called to the court to testify:
  i. As an ordinary witness who saw something happen.
  ii. As a medical practitioner who treated the patient.
  iii. As an expert witness to give opinion on matters of science.

MULTIPLE CHOICE QUESTIONS

1. **Medical jurisprudence means:**
   a. Knowledge of medicine required for lawyers
   b. Knowledge of law required for doctors for medical practice
   c. Knowledge of medicine required for doctors
   d. Knowledge of law required for legal practice
2. **"Medical etiquette" deals with:**
   a. The conventional laws of the courtesy observed between members of the medical profession
   b. Legal responsibilities of the physician
   c. The study and application of the effects of violence or unnatural disease in its various forms
   d. The moral principles which should guide members of the medical profession in their dealings

ANSWERS
1. b   2. a

- Medical jurisprudence deals with the laws which govern the practice of medicine hence any violation of the said law relating to medical practice will attract penal action and punishment against the doctor as per the provisions of the Indian Penal Code.

DEFINE MEDICAL ETHICS AND ETIQUETTE (FM1.1)

- **Medical ethics** deals with the moral principals which should guide the members of the medical profession in their dealings with each other, towards their patients and the State.
- **Medical etiquette** deals with the conventional laws of courtesy observed between the members of the medical profession.

DESCRIBE THE HISTORY OF FORENSIC MEDICINE (FM1.2)

Ancient Medical Texts

- Manu (3100 BC) was the first traditional king and lawgiver in India. His famous treatise "***Manusmriti***" lays down various laws prevailing in those days.
- The "***Atharva Veda***" gives details about remedies for various conditions. They were able to treat wounds, burns, poisoning, snake bite and insanity.
- Vedas prescribe rules and punishment for offences and physicians were recognized.

Medicolegal Work in Ancient India

- The first treatise on Indian medicine was the "***Agnivesa Charaka Samhita***" (700 BC). "Charaka Samhita" lays down an elaborate code regarding the training, duties, privileges and social status of the physicians. It also gives a detailed description of various poisons, signs and symptoms and treatment for various poisoning.
- This is considered as the origin of medical ethics; charaka samhita also prescribes punishment for the physicians who practice wrong treatment.

Kautilya's Arthashastra (460 to 377 BC)

- This is the oldest of Indian codes. It States that death can be caused by three ways:
  i. Stopping the breathing by four ways (strangling, hanging, asphyxiation or drowning)
  ii. Physical injuries in two ways (by beating or by throwing from a height)
  iii. Poisoning (poisons, snake or insect bite, or narcotic drugs)
- Kautilya's arthashastra describes the necessity of Autopsy in establishing the cause of death. It states that a postmortem shall be conducted on any case of sudden (unnatural) death, after smearing the body with oil to bring out bruises, swellings and other injuries.

Medicolegal Work in British India

- The earliest hospital was established by Sir Edward Winter in Chennai in 1664 for treatment of sick soldiers.
- The first medical school was established in 1822 at Calcutta and was later converted into medical college in 1835. The second oldest medical college in the country was the Madras Medical College, Chennai.
- The incidence of custodial death and its certification by medical practitioners was reported in Chennai in 1678.
- The earliest medical certificate was issued by Edward Bulkley and Samuel Browne, after examining Mr John Nicks on August 16th 1693.

WHAT IS THE SCOPE OF FORENSIC MEDICINE? (FM1.2)

- Forensic medicine deals almost entirely with crimes against human beings. In

CHAPTER 1

Introduction and Scope of Forensic Medicine

KEY WORDS

Forensic medicine, medical jurisprudence, medical ethics, medical etiquette, Atharva Veda, Agnivesa Charaka Samhita, Kautilya's Athashastra.

FM1.1	Demonstrate knowledge of basics of forensic medicine like definitions of forensic medicine, clinical forensic medicine, forensic pathology, state medicine, legal medicine and medical jurisprudence.
FM1.2	Describe history of forensic medicine.

DEFINE FORENSIC MEDICINE (FM1.1)

- Forensic medicine or legal medicine also called as state medicine.
- The word "Forensic" originates from the Greek which means "open forum" a public debating place (court of law).
- Forensic medicine is a branch of medical science which deals with the application of medical knowledge to help or aid in the administration of justice.
- It is a branch of medical science which bridges the law and medicine. In short, the subject deals with the **Medical Aspects of the Law**.
  Forensic medicine can be broadly divided into:
  - *Clinical forensic medicine:* Deals with the examination of the living individuals, such as cases of sexual offences, wound certificate, age estimation, medical leave certificate, etc.
  - *Forensic pathology:* Deals with interpretation of autopsy findings in the medicolegal investigation of death (Forensic Thanatology—study of death).

DEFINE MEDICAL JURISPRUDENCE (FM1.1)

- **Juris:** Law; Prudentia: Knowledge.
- Medical jurisprudence deals with the legal responsibilities of the physician with reference to those particularly arising from physician–patient relationship, such as medical negligence, consent, rights and duties of doctors, serious professional misconduct, etc. (in short, it deals with the **Legal Aspects of Practice of Medicine**).

- The judges of the Supreme Court are appointed by the President of India on the recommendations of the collegium system (a closed group of 4 members, the chief justice of India and top 3 senior most judges of the Supreme Court).
- The High Court judges are appointed by the President of India, with the consultation of the chief justice of India and respective Governors of the state.
- A person who has been for not less than 7 years as advocate or pleader, who is not in service of the union or the state are eligible for the post of district sessions judge. The posting and promotion of district judges is made by the Governor of the state in consultation with the High Court.
- The judicial magistrates are selected by the respective state government by conducting **State Judicial Service** Examination. Any individual who possess a graduate degree in law and aged more than 21 years and less than 35 years are eligible to appear in the examination.

DESCRIBE JUVENILE JUSTICE COURTS (FM1.4)

The Juvenile Justice (Care and Protection of Children) Act, 2000.
- As per the Act a 'Juvenile' means a person who has not completed 18 year of age.
- The aim is to provide care, protection, development and rehabilitation of the delinquent juveniles.
- 'Juvenile in conflict with the law' means: a juvenile who is alleged to have committed an offence.
- A juvenile cannot be retained in a place where there are no provisions for rehabilitation.
- Juvenile offender cannot not be trialed along with an adult, even though if he is involved in a crime along with an adult.
- Juvenile courts are preceded by 1st class women magistrates.

DESCRIBE ABOUT LABOR COURTS AND FAMILY COURTS (FM1.4)

Labor Courts

- In order to protect and safeguard the interests of the workers, the Ministry of Labor and Employment has established the labor courts, with due regard to create a healthy working environment.
- As per the Industrial Dispute Act, either of the parties the labor or the employee can approach the labor court in case of any dispute within them.
- Labor courts are Presided by judicial officers of cadre of district sessions judge.
- Labor courts handles cases which comes under:
    - Industrial Disputes Act
    - Workmen Compensation Act
    - Employees State Insurance Act
    - Indian Factories Act

Family Courts

- Family courts were established as per the Family Courts Act, 1984.
- Family courts were established with a view to promote concilation to secure speedy settlement of disputes relating to marriage and family affairs.
- Family courts manage and adjudicate disputes between parents and others with parental responsibility for children and young people, including living arrangements.
- These courts deals with cases related to marriage dissolution, parents, child custody and guardianship and protection of domestic violence against woman.

WHAT IS A SUMMONS CASE AND WARRANT CASE? (FM1.5)

- **Summons case:** Summons cases are noncognizable offences for which the punishment is less than 2 years.

- **Warrant case:** These are cognizable offences for which the punishment is death penalty, life imprisonment or imprisonment for more than 2 years.

WHAT IS THE PROCEDURE OF TRIAL IN THE COURT? (FM1.5)

- Any criminal trial, it is the duty of the prosecution to prove the crime beyond any reasonable doubt.
- After the witness enters the witness box, they have to take oath before recording the evidence.

Oath Taking

- "I swear in the name of God that the evidence I shall give to the court shall be the truth, the whole truth and nothing but the truth".
- After the witness takes the oath, recording of evidence commences.

Examination-in Chief

- Done by the side who has called him, usually by prosecution.
- The witness is allowed to reproduce all the facts concerned with the case, which are known to him. Then the prosecution is allowed to put forth any questions necessary to prove the crime. They are permitted to ask only direct questions.

Cross-examination

- It is done by the defense counsel to elicit points in his favor. The defense raises doubts and it is the duty of the prosecution to clarify those doubts logically. The defense is allowed to ask leading questions.
- Usually, after the cross-examination, the presiding officer puts forth his questions to the witness. But if the defence has introduced any new issues, then a re-examination is permitted.

Re-examination

By the prosecution to get more clarity, on the said matter and to rectify deviations if any. (Not in all cases)

Re-cross Examination

When a re-examination is allowed, then a re-cross examination is also permitted to cross the new points introduced if any by the prosecution.

Court Questions

At the end of the recording, the court questions are asked by the Presiding Officer (*Judge*) to clarify his mind regarding the whole presentation of evidence.

DESCRIBE ABOUT SUMMONS (FM1.5)

Summons is also Known as *Subpoena*

(Sub-Under; Poena-Penalty); Section 61 to 69 of CrPC deals with summons.

- Summons is a document compelling the attendance of a witness in a court of law **under penalty**, on a particular day, time and place, for the purpose of giving evidence.
- The witness is also required to bring with him any document under his control, which he is bound by the law to produce as evidence.
- Summons is issued to the witness by the court and usually served through the police.
- If the witness is a government servant, summons is sent to the head of the office where he is working and served through him to the witness.
- Usually, three copies are served and the witness signs in one copy and sends it to the court through the police who serves the summons, as an acknowledgement that he has received the summons.

- The person who has received a summons is bound to attend the court at the prescribed time and date without fail.
- If he is unable to obey the summons due to unavoidable and acceptable reasons, he has to intimate the court well in advance, about his inability to attend the court.
- If a person receives two summonses from different courts on the same day; he has to give priority to criminal courts over the civil court.
- If both the summonses are from criminal court, then priority is to be given to the higher court; if both the courts are of equal status, then he has to attend the court from which he received the summons first and inform the other court, that he may be summoned later.
- If the witness fails to obey the summons without informing the court, the court may issue a warrant to produce the witness in the court.

WHAT IS CONDUCT MONEY? (FM1.5)

The expert witness is paid money to meet his expenses for coming to the court from his residence and back; it is usually paid along with the summons or in the court after giving evidence. If the doctor feels it insufficient he can ask the court to get it enhanced; however no such money is paid in criminal cases as it is considered as a responsibility of the expert towards the state.

WHO IS A WITNESS? DESCRIBE THE TYPES OF WITNESSES (FM1.5)

Witness: Sections 118 to 134 of IEA deals with Witnesses
- Witnesses are individuals who testify under oath what he knows about the issue under dispute. All persons are competent to testify unless they are prevented from doing so.
- Hence, there is no age limit to be a witness, but the individual who gives evidence should have enough mental maturity to understand the court questions and answer them logically, or else it becomes easy for the defence to disqualify such witnesses. Hence, it is always preferable that the age of the witness is more than 12 years.
- People suffering from insanity and those under the influence of any drug or intoxication are prevented to be witnesses in the court of law.

Types of Witnesses

Witness can be a common witness or expert witness.

Common Witness

- Any individual who was present nearby or comes to know about any crime and has seen, heard or perceived any information regarding it, can be a common witness; and it is the social responsibility of every citizen to inform the police regarding any crime and also come forward to the court to give evidence regarding what he knows about that particular incident or crime.
- The common witness is not permitted to volunteer any statement in the court of law and is bound to answer only what it is being asked to him.

Firsthand Knowledge Rule

The common witness must possess the firsthand information regarding the matter under dispute.

WHO IS AN EXPERT WITNESS? (FM1.5)

Expert Witness

- Expert witness is a person who has been trained or skilled in technical or scientific subject, and is capable of drawing inferences, opinions and conclusions from

the facts observed either by himself or by others; e.g., doctor, firearm expert, finger print expert, chemical examiner, etc.
- An expert witness is expected to help the court to arrive at the near truth, by his special knowledge and skill.
- He is called to the court to clarify certain doubts, on that particular specialty and hence should restrict himself in clearing the doubts logically and scientifically; his answers must be direct wherever possible as he is there to help the court with his special knowledge.
- As far as possible he should not volunteer any statement; at the same time never hesitate to volunteer a statement, if he feels that there is a chance of miscarriage of justice due to failure of the court to elicit a particular issue.

WHAT ARE THE DIFFERENCES BETWEEN COMMON WITNESS AND EXPERT WITNESS? (FM1.5)

Common witness vs expert witness are depicted in **Table 2.4**.

CONDUCT OF A DOCTOR IN THE WITNESS BOX (FM1.5)

- Attend the court in time, neatly dressed and always with the white coat.
- Respect the court, approximate both hands together near the chest and bend forward as a token of respect before entering the court and also after entering the witness box.
- Go to the court well prepared and do not forget to take all the necessary documents relating to that particular case.
- Be frank and clear on the subject matter; speak audibly and clearly.
- Use simple language and avoid technical terms as far as possible.
- Give reasonable time in between for the stenographer to type your statement.
- Give direct answers wherever possible.
- If you don't know the answer to a particular question, be frank to admit it.
- Never volunteer a statement; but, don't hesitate to volunteer a statement if you feel that there is a chance of miscarriage of justice, because of failure of the court to elicit an important issue.

TABLE 2.4: Common witness vs expert witness.

Features	Common witness	Expert witness
Evidence	Gives evidence of what he seen or heard. Firsthand knowledge rule	Skill in a particular field of science and able to draw inferences and opinions from the facts observed
Volunteering a statement	Not allowed. The witness is allowed to answer only what is asked to him	Can volunteer a statement when he finds because of the failure of court to address an important issue, there is a chance of miscarriage of justice
Drawing inferences and opinions	Not allowed. The witness is allowed to talk only what he saw	As an expert, he has to draw inference and cannot abide from giving an opinion from the facts observed
Responsibility and reliability	Less	More because all the opinions drawn out of facts are scientific
Conduct money	Cannot claim conduct money	Can claim contact money in civil cases
Punishment for false evidence	Less	More severe punishment, as the court relies upon the expert witness to help the court arriving at the near truth

- In medical science, it is always difficult to separate fact from opinion; hence, the doctor attending the court as a scientific witness, has to express his opinion arising out of the facts observed by him.

In Cases of Medical Negligence

- It's hard to criticize a colleague, but never conceal what you know to be true. Since, the court or the complainant does not possess any knowledge on medical science; whereas the medical man has enough medical knowledge to defend himself; the very purpose of our evidence is to help the court in deciding what's right or wrong based on medical opinion and hence never hide anything which you saw or know.
- There is no perfect witness, but efforts must be made by everyone to be a perfect witness.
- Our evidence should in no way be inferior to anyone else and thus a reasonable standard has to be there, which can be achieved only by strong knowledge on medical science.
- Many a times, you may have to wait for a long time for your evidence to be recorded, but never lose patience. Wait for your turn and present the case clearly and nicely, thus win the respect of the court and I am sure that when you go to the same court next time, the judge will make every effort to record your evidence first.
- Due to the bitter experiences in the past the doctor, may feel hesitant to go to the court and many a times, there may not be even a single question raised by the defense; but don't care for those things in your mind, develop a positive thought inside you; feel it is our duty as a citizen to attend the court and give evidence whenever we are summoned, and be proud that since we have this special knowledge of medical science, we are being called by the court to assist it with our special knowledge.
- A medical witness by his honest, unbiased and straightforward opinion can win the confidence of both the prosecution and as well as the defense.

DEFINE EVIDENCE? WHAT ARE THE TYPES OF EVIDENCES? (FM1.6)

- **Evidence** means and includes all the statements which the court permits or requires to be made before it by the witnesses, in relation to the matter of fact under inquiry.
- For the evidence to be accepted by the courts, it must be properly identified as to what it is, where it was found and how it is related to the crime.

Chain of Custody

It is a method to verify the actual possession of an object from the time it was first identified, until it is offered as evidence in the court.

Types of Evidences

- **Direct evidence:** The witness testifies directly of his own knowledge as to the facts in dispute; only those witnesses who have seen heard or perceived can give direct evidence in the court of law—**First-hand knowledge rule**.
- **Circumstantial evidence (Presumptive evidence):** The circumstances tend to prove the ultimate fact in issue; it is the evidence derived from circumstances as distinguished from direct and positive proof.
- **Substantial evidence:** The evidence which a reasonable prudent man will accept as adequate for arriving at the decision in that case.
- **Corroborative evidence:** The evidence that concurs with another evidence. Generally, in the court of law the eye witness is considered as positive evidence and the medical witness or the expert witness is only corroborative in nature.

- **Hearsay evidence:**
  - It's the evidence of a person other than the actual witness. It is the evidence of a 3rd person, what was told to him by someone else. Such evidences are only useful only to ascertain whether the facts contained in the statement are true.
  - Individuals giving Hearsay evidence cannot be cross-examined as they are not actual witnesses.

DESCRIBE ABOUT ORAL EVIDENCE? WHAT ARE THE EXEMPTIONS TO ORAL EVIDENCE? (FM1.6)

Evidence presented in the court could be either oral or documentary.

Oral Evidence

In all cases oral evidence must be direct; it must be the evidence of a person who saw, heard or perceived. Hence, oral evidence is given more preference in the court of law. Oral evidence is the best type of evidence because it is subjected to **cross-examination**.

Exceptions to Oral Evidence

- Dying declaration
- Expert opinion expressed in a treatise (textbooks, journals, peer reviews)
- Evidence of a doctor recorded in a lower court
- Evidence of a witness given in a previous judicial proceedings, etc.

WHAT IS DOCUMENTARY EVIDENCE? GIVE EXAMPLES OF DOCUMENTARY EVIDENCE: DESCRIBE ABOUT MEDICAL EVIDENCE (FM1.6)

Documentary Evidence

- Document means any matter expressed by means of letters, figures or marks.
- Documentary evidence includes all the documents produced for the inspection of the court.
- Documentary evidences must conform to the matters in issue and are admitted by the count on the basis of relevance of the document to the matter in dispute.
  Examples: Medical leave certificate, medicolegal reports like: Age certificate, sexual offences certificate, dying declaration, postmortem certificate, etc.

Medical Evidence

- When any case is presented to a doctor for examination, he gives his opinion in the form of a certificate (Documentary evidence) which includes the findings observed by him and his opinion based on the observations; hence, all the evidences of any expert are given in the form of a document.
- The investigation team investigates the case on the basis of his opinion and in all situations, the doctor must come to the court, testify all his statements under oath and cross-examined by the defence, for his evidence to be accepted as a proof in the court of law.

WHAT IS PERJURY? WHO IS A HOSTILE WITNESS? (FM1.6)

Perjury

Section 191 IPC defines perjury as "willfully giving and/or fabricating false evidence under the oath". Perjury is breaking the oath and the witness is liable to be prosecuted under section 193 IPC (imprisonment which may extend up to 7 years).

Hostile Witness

- After making a particular statement in the court, the witness contradicts his own statement, and hence is supposed to have some interest or motive to conceal part of the truth or gives completely false

evidence, and then he is declared hostile by the court.
- When the witness is declared hostile, then he can be cross-examined by the side by which he has been called by; i.e., leading questions are permitted even in examination in chief.

WHAT ARE LEADING QUESTIONS AND THEIR IMPORTANCE IN THE TRIAL? (FM1.6)

Leading Question

The question which suggests an answer or caries a hidden answer inside is a leading question.
Example: In case of an injury:
- **Direct question:** Which weapon will cause the injury?
- **Leading question:** Can the injury be caused by a single edged knife?

Importance of Leading Questions
- Leading questions are allowed only in cross-examination, since the aim of the prosecution is to **prove the crime**, whereas the aim of the defense **is to weaken the witnesses**.
- Leading questions are not allowed in the examination in chief; but allowed when the witness turns **hostile** as per Section 154 of IEA.

DESCRIBE DYING DECLARATION, COMPOS MENTIS AND DYING DEPOSITION (FM1.7)

Dying Declaration: Section 32 IEA
- It's the statement oral or written made by a person who is in the verge of death, as a result of some unlawful act. The statement should relate to the cause of his death, or to the circumstances which has resulted in the present condition.
- Dying declarations are admissible in the court, and may provide useful information to the court and may help to obtain justice. In case of death of such a person, the dying declaration is accepted as evidence without any cross-examination.
- It's believed that any individual who is about die will speak only the truth, but in the present days, due to the change in the attitude of the human beings, these types of declarations have lost their values in the courts of law.
- If the individual survives after making such declaration, they are accepted as evidences, but only as corroborative evidence; and the individual has to come to the court, reproduce those statements under oath, get cross-examined by the defence before they are accepted as concrete evidences by the court.
- The statements should be recorded in the same language as narrated by the individual. The person recording the declaration should not ask any leading questions when the individual is giving the statement.
- No additions or deletions or any alterations should be made in the statement.

Duty of a doctor while recording dying declaration:
- Upon admission into the hospital, in such cases, the doctor should immediately inform the judicial magistrate about the condition of the patient for the purpose of recording the dying declaration.
- Dying declarations are usually recorded by the judicial magistrates; in the absence of the magistrate or when there could be a relative time delay for him to arrive then, it can be recorded by the police officer or any individual who is present by the side. Even the doctor himself can record such declarations when no one else is present or when there is no time to wait.

Compos Mentis
- Before recording the statement and also throughout the recording till the end, the doctor should certify that the person

is conscious and his mental faculties are normal.
- The doctor who certifies compos mentis cannot record the declaration even under emergency. Some other doctor can record it, if it is so much urgent.
- If the individual dies or becomes unconscious before completing his declaration, then the process of recording is stopped at that stage and signed by the doctor and by the person who was recording it and handed over to the court in a sealed cover.

Dying Deposition

This is superior to dying declaration and recorded only by the magistrate; while recording the deposition, the accused and his lawyer are allowed to be present. The statements made by the victim are then and there cross-examined by the defence, and hence carries equal value as that of a trial conducted in the court. This is not practiced in India.

DIFFERENCES BETWEEN DYING DECLARATION AND DYING DEPOSITION (FM1.7)

Dying declaration vs dying deposition are described in **Table 2.5**.

DESCRIBE THE LATEST DECISION MADE BY GOVERNMENT REGARDING MEDICO-LEGAL ISSUES (FM1.8)

Some significant developments and initiatives related to medical legal issues in India include:
- **Clinical Establishments (Registration and Regulation) Act 2010:** This act aims to regulate the registration and functioning of all clinical establishments in the country to ensure quality healthcare services and patient safety.
- **Mental Health Care Act 2017:** This act aims to provide legal framework for the protection of the rights of persons with mental illness. It decriminalizes suicide, ensures access to mental healthcare, and establishes mental health authorities at the central and state levels.
- **Medical Termination of Pregnancy (Amendment) Act:** In 2021 the Government of India amended the MTP Act to expand access to safe and legal abortions. The amendment increases the gestation limit for abortion from 20 weeks to 24 weeks in specific cases.
- **National Medical Commission (NMC) Act 2019:** This act aims to reform medical education and regulate the medical

TABLE 2.5: Dying declaration vs dying deposition.

Dying declaration	Dying deposition
Usually, recorded by the judicial magistrate but in emergency any one can record the declaration	Only the judicial magistrate should record the deposition
Only the person recording the declaration and the doctor are allowed to be present during the recording	The alleged accused and his lawyer must also be present during the deposition
Statements are recorded as such as narrated by the individual and no one is allowed to ask any questions in between the recording	Every statement made by the person are then and there cross-examined by the defense lawyer
Less value because the gravity of the statements not cross-examined	More value, equal to trail in the court of law
It is in routine practice in India	Not practiced in India

profession in India. The Act establishes the National Medical Commission to replace the Medical Council of India and introduces various changes aimed at improving medical education and ensuring ethical practice of medicine.

RESOLUTION MADE BY COURT REGARDING MEDICOLEGAL PRACTICE (FM1.8)

- **Verdict of guilty or not guilty:** In cases where a healthcare professional is accused of medical malpractice or negligence, the court may render a verdict of guilty if the evidence demonstrates that the professional failed to meet the standard of care expected and caused harm to the patient. Alternatively, if the evidence does not support the allegations, the court may issue a verdict of not guilty.
- **Monetary damages:** If a court finds a healthcare professional liable for medical malpractice or negligence, it may order the payment of monetary damages to the affected party. The damages could cover medical expenses, lost wages, pain and suffering, and other losses incurred as a result of the negligence.
- **License suspension or revocation** In serious cases of professional misconduct or repeated instances of medical malpractice, the court may order the suspension or revocation of the health care professional's license to practice medicine. This resolution aims to protect the public and maintain the standards of medical practice.
- **Remedial actions:** In some instances, the court may require the healthcare professional to undergo additional training or supervision, participation in ethics courses, or take specific remedial actions as a condition for maintaining their medical license.
- **Injunctions or restraining orders:** In certain cases, the court may issue injunctions or restraining orders to prevent a healthcare professional from engaging in specific activities or practicing medicine under certain circumstances. This resolution aims to protect potential patients from harm while the legal process unfolds.
- These actions are designed to ensure the professional competence and adherence to proper medical practices.

DISCUSS THE LATEST NOTIFICATIONS REGARDING POSTMORTEM EXAMINATION (FM1.8)

Effect of Decomposition

- The questions to be determined by a *post-mortem* examination vary in different cases, and the possibility of determining them effectually is not in every case equally dependent on the stage which the process of putrefaction has reached.
- Thus, in death from drowning, strangulation and various diseases, questions respecting the appearance of flesh tissues and the amount of blood in parts require to be considered, and these can only be determined soon after death and before putrefaction has made much progress.
- But it would be quite possible to determine the existence or absence of a wound or severe bruises of soft parts, even if decomposition were considerably advanced; and injuries of bones, pregnancy, presence of foreign bodies, metallic poisoning, and some profound organic diseases, are ascertainable long after death.

Duty of Medical Officer to conduct post-mortem examination when nothing is known about causes of death: In such circumstances, the discovery of the body, which are communicated by the police, will enable the Medical Officer to form an opinion as to whether it would be possible by a postmortem examination to throw any light on the cause of death; and whenever such possibility exists, or when ever nothing is known, it is his duty to make as full an examination as possible.

Exhumation of body when advisable for examination: These considerations should guide a Magistrate in determining on the propriety or otherwise of exerting the power given him by law of ordering the exhumation of the body. In case of doubt the Magistrate should, if possible, consult a Medical Officer before passing such an order.

Officer authorized to conduct postmortem examination: The following notification is issued regarding the Medical Officers authorized to conduct postmortem examinations,
- All Civil Surgeons
- All Medical Officers holding collateral civil charges
- All Staff Surgeons
- All Assistant Surgeons

MULTIPLE CHOICE QUESTIONS

1. Police inquest is not applicable in one of the following deaths:
    a. Hanging
    b. Rape and murder
    c. Murder
    d. Dowry related deaths
2. All are cognizable offences, *except*:
    a. Rape
    b. Murder
    c. Attempted suicide
    d. Upraise against the state
3. Following are true of corners court, *except*:
    a. Court of trial
    b. No power to impose fine
    c. Contempt of court punishable
    d. Accused need not be present
4. IPC is:
    a. Procedure for investigation
    b. Code for punishment
    c. Both
    d. None
5. 'Prima facia' means:
    a. Body of evidence
    b. First officer who faces the crime scene
    c. Primary substantial evidence of crime
    d. Primary substantial evidence to disprove the prosecution
6. Volunteering a statement can be done by:
    a. Eye witness
    b. Medical witness
    c. Hostile witness
    d. Investigation officer
7. If a person survives after making a dying declaration, then it stands as:
    a. Invalid
    b. Valid for 48 hours
    c. Corroborative evidence
    d. None of the above
8. The most important duty of a physician while recording a dying declaration is:
    a. To record the evidence, as he tells
    b. To maintain life
    c. To certify the Mental State of the individual
    d. To sign as a witness
9. Juvenile court is presided by:
    a. First class women magistrate
    b. Second class women magistrate
    c. First class magistrate of any sex
    d. Any of the above
10. Oral evidence carries more value than documentary evidence because:
    a. It is preferable to hear than to read
    b. It is easy to comprehend
    c. The witness can be cross-examined
    d. The witness cannot turn hostile
11. Evidence given to the court where the witness has not witnessed the act, but came to know about it through someone else is called:
    a. Secondary evidence
    b. Impersonal evidence
    c. Hearsay evidence
    d. Circumstantial evidence
12. Summons case is a case in which:
    a. The witness is summoned to the court
    b. Maximum punishment is 2 years

c. Maximum punishment is 7 years
d. A warrant cannot be issued
13. **True regarding dying deposition:**
    a. Statement recorded in the presence of the accused
    b. Can be recorded by the police officer
    c. Is inferior to dying deposition
    d. It is common practice in India
14. **Punishment can be awarded on failure to obey summons in:**
    a. All types of summons
    b. Only in civil cases
    c. Only in criminal cases
    d. Only in summons from the High Court
15. **An arrested person can request for medical examination to prove his innocence under:**
    a. 53 CrPC
    b. 54 CrPC
    c. 174 CrPC
    d. 176 CrPC
16. **Perjury means:**
    a. Breaking the oath
    b. Speaking only the truth
    c. Submitting a document
    d. Not attending the court
17. **Re-examination is done by:**
    a. Lawyer conducting the main examination
    b. Lawyer conducting cross-examination
    c. Presiding officer of the court
    d. None of the above
18. **Powers of 1st class judiciary magistrate:**
    a. Imprisonment up to 5 years and fine up to 1 lakh
    b. Imprisonment up to 3 years and fine up to ₹ 10,000
    c. Imprisonment up to 3 years and fine up to ₹ 5,000
    d. Imprisonment up to 1 years and fine up to ₹ 1,000
19. **Hostile witness is:**
    a. Willful utterance of falsehood under oath
    b. Contradicts his own statement, given in the court
    c. It is punishable under Section 193 IPC
    d. Conduct money is paid to the witnesses
20. **Oral evidence is an exception in all the following, *except*:**
    a. Chemical examiner's report
    b. Deposition of a doctor in a lower court
    c. Dying declaration
    d. Postmortem report
21. **Conduct money is paid to the witness along with the summons from:**
    a. Additional district magistrate court
    b. Principal sessions court
    c. Additional claims tribunal court
    d. Human rights court
22. **Leading questions are allowed in:**
    a. Chief examination
    b. Cross-examination
    c. Re-examination
    d. Court questions
23. **Consider the following statements:**
    i. In India every state has go a High Court
    ii. Judges of High Court are appointed by the governor of the state
    a. 1 is correct
    b. 2 is correct
    c. Both 1 and 2 correct
    d. Neither 1 nor 2 is correct
24. **Consider the following statements:**
    i. The consumer protection Act (CPA) applies to all goods, but not any services.
    ii. The CPA provides for establishing four-tier consumer dispute redressal machinery at the national, state, district and block levels.
    Which of the statements given above is/are correct?
    a. 1 only
    b. 2 only
    c. Both 1 and 2
    d. Neither 1 or 2
25. **Perjury is an offence punishable under:**
    a. 197 IPC
    b. 93 IPC
    c. 498A IPC
    d. 302 IPC
26. **Inquest which is carried out in India is:**
    a. Coroner's inquest
    b. Medical examiner system
    c. Procurator fiscal system
    d. Magistrate inquest
27. **A lady died due to unnatural death within seven years after her marriage. The inquest in this case will be done by:**
    a. Medical examiner
    b. Commissioner
    c. Sub-divisional magistrate
    d. Coroner

SECTION 1: Medical Jurisprudence

28. **Medical man in the witness box is:**
    a. Expert witness
    b. Common witness
    c. Both common and expert witness
    d. Voluntary witness
29. **Perjury is an offence committed when:**
    a. Police officer on duty at the police station tells lies
    b. A witness under oath tells lies
    c. Lawyer during examination of a witness tells lies
    d. A jury tells lies in the court
30. **Hostile witness is one who:**
    a. Threatens the judge
    b. Threatens the lawyer
    c. Refuses to answer questions
    d. Changes his own words

ANSWERS

1. d	2. c	3. a	4. b	5. c	6. b	7. c	8. c	9. a	10. c
11. c	12. b	13. a	14. a	15. b	16. a	17. a	18. b	19. b	20. d
21. c	22. b	23. d	24. d	25. b	26. d	27. c	28. c	29. b	30. d

CHAPTER 3

Medical Ethics and the Law

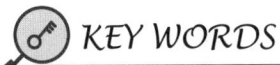 **KEY WORDS**

Medical ethics, etiquette, hippocratic oath, National Medical Commission, State Medical Council, professional misconduct, dichotomy, covering, penal erasure, Red Cross emblem, professional secrecy, privileged communication, rights and duties of a RMP, ethics and etiquette regulations by NMC, doctor and media, stem cell research, victims of domestic violence, euthanasia, bioethics, human experimentation, ethical committee, stress management, malingering.

FM4.1	Describe medical ethics and explain its historical emergence.
FM4.2	Describe the Code of Medical Ethics 2002 conduct, etiquette and ethics in medical practice and unethical practices and the dichotomy.
FM4.3	Describe the functions and role of National Medical Commission and State Medical Councils.
FM4.4	Describe the National Medical Commission Register.
FM4.5	Rights/privileges of a medical practitioner, penal erasure, infamous conduct, disciplinary Committee, disciplinary procedures, warning notice and penal erasure.
FM4.6	Describe the laws in relation to medical practice and the duties of a medical practitioner towards patients and society.
FM4.7	Describe and discuss the ethics related to HIV patients.
FM4.8	Describe the Consumer Protection Act-1986 (medical indemnity insurance, civil litigations and compensations), Workman's Compensation Act and ESI Act.
FM4.9	Describe the medico-legal issues in relation to family violence, violation of human rights, NHRC and doctors.
FM4.10	Describe communication between doctors, public and media.
FM4.11	Describe and discuss euthanasia.
FM4.12	Describe legal and ethical issues in relation to stem cell research.
FM4.13	Describe social aspects of medico-legal cases with respect to victims of assault, rape, attempted suicide, homicide, domestic violence, dowry-related cases.
FM4.14	Describe and discuss the challenges in managing medico-legal cases including development of skills in relationship management—human behavior, communication skills, conflict resolution techniques.

FM4.15 Describe the principles of handling pressure—definition, types, causes, sources and skills for managing the pressure while dealing with medico-legal cases by the doctor.

FM4.16 Describe and discuss bioethics.

FM4.17 Describe and discuss ethical principles: respect for autonomy, non-malfeasance, beneficence and justice.

FM4.23 Describe the modified declaration of Geneva and its relevance.

FM4.24 Enumerate rights, privileges and duties of a registered medical practitioner. Discuss doctor-patient relationship: professional secrecy and privileged communication.

FM4.25 Clinical research and ethics. Discuss human experimentation including clinical trials.

FM4.26 Discuss the constitution and functions of ethical committees.

FM4.27 Describe and discuss ethical guidelines for biomedical research on human subjects and animals.

FM4.28 Demonstrate respect to laws relating to medical practice and ethical code of conduct prescribed by Medical Council of India and rules and regulations prescribed by it from time to time.

FM4.29 Demonstrate ability to communicate appropriately with media, public and doctors.

FM4.30 Demonstrate ability to conduct research in pursuance to guidelines or research ethics.

DESCRIBE MEDICAL ETHICS (FM4.1)

- **Medical ethics** deals with the moral principles which should guide the members of the medical profession in their dealings with each other, their patients and towards the state.
- **Medical etiquette** deals with the conventional laws of courtesy observed between the members of the medical profession.
- Ethics reflects the **conduct**, **character** and **attitude** of a doctor; whereas, negligence is related to the **competence**, **knowledge** and **skill** of a doctor.
- Ethical violation is professional misconduct and the State Medical Council takes action.
- Code of ethics is different from the law, since non-adherence to the prevailing ethical standards may not be considered as an offence by the law and hence any doctor, who violates the ethical codes, cannot be punished by the law rather will attract an action for the infamous conduct by the State Medical Council.

Historical Emergence of Ethics (FM4.1)

- The word ethics is derived from Greek term "ethikos" which stands for rules of conduct that govern the natural deposition in human beings.
- Ethics is self imposed code of conduct assumed voluntarily by the medical profession.
- Code of ethics retains the moral guidelines and cannot run contrary to the society and the ethical codes must always be in conformity with the law of the land.
- The first basic code of medical ethics is universally known as "Hippocratic Oath" (around 500 BC) hippocrates was the father of western medicine lived in Greece.
- At the time of registration of a medical graduate has to sign a declaration which is the modern version of **Hippocratic Oath**

and is called as the Declaration of Geneva (1948).

THE DECLARATION OF GENEVA (1948) (FM4.23)

Modified Version of Hippocratic Oath

- I solemnly pledge to consecrate my life to the service of humanity.
- I will give my teachers the respect and gratitude which is their due.
- I will practice my profession with conscience and dignity.
- The health of my patients will be my first consideration.
- I will respect the secrets which are confined in me, even after the patient dies.
- I will maintain by all means and power, the honor and the noble traditions of the medical profession.
- I will consider my colleagues as my brothers.
- I will not permit considerations of religion, nationality, race, party politics or social standings to intervene between my duty and my patients.
- I will maintain the most respect for human life from the time of conception.
- Even under threat I will not use my medical knowledge contrary to the laws of humanity.
- I make these promises solemnly, freely and upon my honor.

DESCRIBE ABOUT THE MEDICAL ETHICS AND ETIQUETTE REGULATIONS 2002 (AMENDED IN 2010) (FM4.2)

Ethics and Etiquette Regulations 2002

Chapter 1

- Declaration
- Duties and responsibilities of the physician
- Character of the physician
- Maintain good medical practice—membership in societies
- *Maintenance of records:*
  - ♦ The doctor is bound to maintain all the records of his patients for a minimum of 3 years and if any of the cases goes for litigation then those records are to be maintained lifelong. All MLC records should be maintained lifelong there is no time limit for maintenance of MLC records.
  - ♦ When the patient or his authorized attendant asks for a copy of the records, the request should be obliged, and the doctor has to give the copy of all the records requested by the patient within 72 hours of receiving the request. Charges can be collected towards making xerox copies of the records.
- *Display of registration certificate:* The doctor should display a copy of his education qualification certificates and certificate of registration in State Medical Council.

Chapter 2

Duties of physician towards patient:
- Obligation to the sick
- Patience, delicacy and secrecy
- Prognosis: Covey the prognosis of the patient condition periodically to the patient as well as the authorized attendants.
- Patient should never be neglected
- **Obstetric case:** When a doctor has accepted to treat an obstetric case, he should be available to the patient's service at time and cannot say I will look after only during my consultation hours. In his absence he should depute as an alternative doctor to attend the patient during emergency.

Chapter 3

Duties of physician in consultations:
- Avoid unnecessary consultations.
- All consultation must be for the benefit of the patient.
- **Punctuality:** Stick on to your consultation timings displayed on the board as far as possible.
- **Statement to the patient:** Summarize all the disease problems, investigations done, treatment given, prognosis and the appointment for next consultation.
- **Reference to specialists:** Refer to the patient whenever he needs a specialist consultation but all such referrals and consultations must be for the benefit of the patient.
- **Fees and other charges:**
  - *Display the fees:* It is better to display the fees for consultation. Inform the patient regarding the fees and other charges for the services provided before starting the treatment and not after the treatment procedures are over.
  - *Prescription letter (drugs dispensed):* The prescription letter should contain all the medicines used/prescribed to the patient. If you have given some injections or dispensed some drugs from your clinic, it should be mentioned in the prescription letter.

Chapter 4

Responsibilities of physician to each other:
- **Conduct in consultation:** Maintain high standard of conduct during consultation of any patient.
- **Consult not to take over the case:** When a patient is referred to you for specialist opinion or sent to you to take care of the patient in his absence, treat the patient but do not take over the patient.
- **Appointment of substitutes in his absence:** Always appoint a substitute to take care of the patient in your absence.

Chapter 5

Duties to the public:
- **Physician as citizen:** A physician should be an example to the society as a best citizen of India.
- **Public and community health:** An Indian Medical Graduate (IMG) should be a person who cares for the society and the community health as a whole.
- **Pharmacist/nurses:** Good association and understanding is necessary with the pharmacist and paramedical staff and all should be only for the benefit of the patient.

Chapter 6

Unethical Acts
- **Advertising:** A doctor can advertise in the following circumstances:
  - On starting a medical practice
  - Change in type of practice
  - Change of address
  - On resuming to practice after a period of absence
  - Succeeding to another type of practice
- Patent and copyrights
- **Running a open shop:** A doctor should not run a open medical shop, but however he can prescribe and dispense drugs to his own patients.
- **Rebate and commission:** A doctor must never receive any commission in any form from anyone for prescribing or referring to another doctor or for any investigation to laboratory.
- **Secret remedies:** A doctor should never resort to secret remedies (magic remedies are drugs which does not contain the name of the ingredients present in the dispensed medicine), giving such medicines to your patient about which, you are unaware of the composition, mode of action and adverse effect of any such medicines.
- **Human rights:** Human rights must always be preserved as per the NHRC guidelines.
- **Euthanasia:** Should never resort to or help euthanasia.

Chapter 7

Professional misconduct: A physician should not be involved in any of the unethical acts.
- Violation of regulations of ethics will attract a charge of infamous conduct on the part of the doctor and will attract subsequent punishments by the State Medical Council.
- Adultery
- Conviction by court of law
- Sex determination tests

Chapter 8

Describes the procedure of disciplinary action and subsequent punishment if the doctor is proved to have committed some professional misconduct.

CONSTITUTION NATIONAL MEDICAL COMMISSION (NMC) (FM4.3)

- NMC was formed by the President of India and came into force on 5th September 2020; it replaced Indian Medical Council which was formed under the **Indian Medical Council Act 1956** and was dissolved by the President of India on 15th May 2010.
- NMC is a regulatory body which consists of 33 members which regulates medical education and medical professionals.

Constitution of the National Medical Commission (NMC)

- The NMC consists of 33 members including: **a Chairperson** (medical professionals only).
- 10 Officio Members
- The President of the Under-Graduate Medical Education Board.
- The President of the Post-Graduate Medical Education Board.
- The President of the Medical Assessment and Rating Board.
- The President of the Ethics and Medical Registration Board.
- The Director General of Health Services, Directorate General of Health Services, New Delhi.
- The Director General, Indian Council of Medical Research.
- Director of any of the All India Institutes of Medical Sciences.
- Two persons from amongst the Directors of Postgraduate Institute of Medical Education and Research, Jawaharlal Institute of Postgraduate Medical Education and Research, Tata Memorial Hospital, North Eastern Indira Gandhi Regional Institute of Health and Medical Sciences, and All India Institute of Hygiene and Public Health.
- One person to represent the Ministry of Health and Family Welfare.

Number of Part Time Members-22

- Three members appointed from amongst persons who have special knowledge and professional experience in such areas including management, law, medical ethics, health research, consumer or patient rights advocacy, science and technology and economics.
- Ten members appointed on rotational basis from amongst the nominees of the states/union territories in the Medical Advisory Council.
- Nine members appointed from amongst the nominees of the States and Union territories in the Medical Advisory Council.
- Of these at least 60% of the members must be medical practitioners.

WHAT ARE THE FUNCTIONS OF THE NATIONAL MEDICAL COMMISSION? (FM4.3)

Functions of the NMC Include

- **Laying down policies for regulating medical institutions and medical professionals:**

SECTION 1: Medical Jurisprudence

TABLE 3.1: Schedule of medical degrees.

First schedule	Second schedule	Third schedule part A	Third schedule part B
Medical degrees offered by different universities in India, which are recognized by the council	Medical degrees offered by different universities outside India, which are recognized by the council	Medical degrees conferred by Indian universities, which are not mentioned in the 1st schedule	Standard medical qualifications of foreign countries, which are not mentioned in 2nd schedule

- It regulates the standards of undergraduate and postgraduate medical education. This is one of the most important functions of the Indian Medical Council. The IMC maintains a uniform standard of medical education throughout the country.
- There are many medical colleges and universities in India and the teaching pattern and exam pattern varies from university to university, but the syllabus and number of years of study and period of hours of training at different levels and different subjects are maintained at a uniform standard by the Medical Council of India. It prescribes a minimum standard of education for undergraduate, postgraduate and super specialty courses.
• **Assess the requirements of human resources and infrastructure in healthcare and medicines.**
   - Ensuring compliance by the State Medical Councils with the regulations made under the bill.
   - Framing guidelines for determination of fee for up to 50% of the seats in the private medical institutions.
   - The NMC will make guidelines for a new cadre of non-MBBS mid-level health service providers such as nurse practitioners and pharmacists with limited rights to prescribe medicines.
   - *Common entrance examination:* For undergraduate and postgraduate medical courses and allied medical education courses.

• **Maintenance of medical register (FM4.5):** Maintains a Register containing the names, address and qualification of medical practitioners who have registered with any State Medical Council. The IMC has no direct role towards this function of maintenance of register.
• **Recognition of medical degrees:** All the medical degrees awarded inside as well as outside India are regulated and are to be recognized by the council if the individual is practicing medicine in India. The medical council maintains three schedules, described in **Table 3.1.**
• **Appellate tribunal:**
   - Appeal by either of the parties when some action is taken by the State Medical Council for any infamous conduct committed by the medical practitioner.

WHAT IS CONSTITUTION AND FUNCTIONS OF STATE MEDICAL COUNCIL? (FM4.4)

State Medical Council

- State Medical Council consists of members elected by the registered medical practitioners of the respective state and members nominated by the state government.
- The president and the vice-president are elected amongst themselves; a registrar is nominated to carry out the day to day works of the council.

Functions of SMC

- **Maintenance of medical register:** This is one of the most important functions of any State Medical Council.
  - Every medical graduate, upon passing his final year exams, has to get his name temporarily registered in the SMC to pursue his internship; upon completion of 1 year internship he has to get permanently registered himself in the respective SMC and a permanent registration number is allotted to him.
  - He needs to specify the registration number wherever necessary. A doctor cannot start his medical practice before he gets himself permanently registered in any SMC.
- **Disciplinary action and control:** Disciplinary action is purely the function of the SMC. Enquiry and action for any infamous conduct is carried out by the State Medical Council only.
- **Issue warning notice periodically:** (**Warning notice** is a list of offences which comprises of infamous conduct; it is not a complete list and not intended to be complete also)

DEFINE INFAMOUS CONDUCT?

Discuss the Acts Which Amounts to Professional Misconduct? (FM4.3)

Definition

- Infamous conduct is any act done by a Registered Medical Practitioner which is considered disgraceful and dishonorable by his professional colleagues of good repute.
- When a complaint is filed against a doctor for in the State Medical Council, appropriate enquiry and action (punishment) is taken by the SMC.

- There are various actions of a doctor labeled as infamous conduct and are listed in the warning notice. Some of those acts which amounts to professional misconduct are:
  - *Abortion:* Bye passing any of the provisions of the Medical Termination of Pregnancy (MTP) Act 1971, amounts to criminal abortion and the doctor is directly punished by the law, as per the provisions of the act and will simultaneously attract a charge of infamous conduct against the doctor.
  - *Adultery:* A doctor must maintain the highest degree of professional integrity. He using his professional status develops any intimate relationship with any of the patients, patient attendants or relatives is adultery and will attract a charge of infamous conduct against him.
  - *Alcoholism:* A doctor is not supposed to examine or treat any patient under the influence of alcohol.
  - *Addiction:* A doctor has access to many of the drugs of abuse by virtue of his professional status; if he is addicted to any of the drugs of abuse will attract a charge of infamous conduct against the doctor.
  - *Advertising:* The view of advertisement is changing in many ways in the recent past. A doctor is entitled to advertise the facilities of the hospital and the types of services offered to the patients. However, he should not advertise the individual capability of a person as superior to all others of the same specialty.
  - *Association:* A doctor should not associate with unqualified people and procure patients using touts and agents.

- *Dichotomy:* **"Fee Splitting"** getting commission/monetary benefits for referring a patient to another doctor, investigation, prescribing drugs of a particular company or sending prescription to a particular retail shop, etc.
- *Covering:* Assisting/associating with unqualified people to carry out the work of a qualified medical professional. Appointing unqualified paramedical staff to render qualified service to the patients under his cover, thus protecting them and promoting them to do the work of qualified staff is "Covering" and it amounts to infamous conduct.
- Violation of any of the provisions of any of the acts which is in force from time to time which governs the medical profession.
- *Issuing false certificates:* Issuing false certificate in any regard is an infamous conduct.

  It is in common practice to issue medical leave certificates to people working in Government and private sectors; issuing false medical certificates without valid grounds amounts to professional misconduct.
  - As far as possible issue medical certificate only when you have treated the patient.
  - At any one time do not issue sickness certificate for more than 15 days.
  - When you have treated the person as outpatient, specify in the certificate itself that you have treated him as outpatient only.
  - Do not issue certificates to unknown persons; be sure that the individual comes in person and signs in front you in the prescribed place in the leave certificate.
- *Death certificate:* Make efforts to examine the dead body physically before issuing the death certificate; do not attempt to issue the certificate by going through the old treatment records, statement from the relatives or hearsay information. Issue death certificate when you were the only treating doctor in the recent past.
- Notification of birth, death, infectious diseases, etc., in interest of the community and public, the doctor is bound to notify these to the concerned authorities. Failure to notify such diseases amounts to professional misconduct.
- Withholding information about notifiable diseases to public authorities; It is the duty of the doctor towards the community/state to inform the authorities about any notifiable diseases he comes across.
- Refusal to treatment on religious or social grounds.
- *Disclosure of professional secrecy:* Never disclose the secrets of your patients to anyone, even to the close relatives without the consent of the patient.

DEFINE PROFESSIONAL SECRECY; WHEN IT CAN BE REVEALED? (FM4.23)

Explain Privileged Communication with Suitable Examples?

- The doctor in the course of the treatment of his patients will come to know certain information about the patient. The doctor is obliged to keep all the information provided by the patient about his condition or any information he comes to know concerning the patient as secret;

and he should not divulge the information about the patient to anyone **without the consent** of the patient. He should not divulge such information to anyone **even after the death** of the patient.
- However, there exists no professional secrecy when a person subjects himself voluntarily for examination as in cases of insurance or examination for issuing driving license and also in medico-legal cases. The doctor is bound to reveal all information regarding the patient to the concerned authorities in such circumstances. The consent for divulging the information is implied as he subjects himself voluntarily for such examination. Also, it becomes the duty as a physician to reveal all the findings of the examination is such circumstances.
- Breach of professional secrecy is infamous conduct except, when it is required by the law to be revealed. The only exception to professional secrecy is privileged communication.

Privileged Communication

- It is a statement made **bonafide upon** any subject matter by a doctor to the concerned authorities, due to his duty to protect the interests of the community or of the state.
- To be privileged, the communication must be made only to a person having interest in it, or in reference of which he has a duty.
- The doctor should first persuade the patient, obtain his consent before notifying the proper authority. The doctrine of privileged communication fails, if the information is revealed to more than one person.

Examples:
- **Infectious diseases:**
    - A patient suffering from communicable disease like gastroenteritis, enteric fever, etc., working in a common eating place like hotel; in these situations, the patient should be persuaded to stay away from the job till he becomes non-infectious; if the patient refuses, then the doctor can inform the employer about illness of the patient.
    - A teacher or children's nurse suffering from tuberculosis or other easily contactable infectious diseases. The patient is advised that she is unfit for the job till you become non-infectious; if the patient does not obey and continues to do the same work; now the doctor can inform the employer (parents of the child) about the disease condition of the patient and not to employ her till she becomes noninfectious.
- A person suffering from venereal disease (syphilis or gonorrhea) is about to marry. First the patient is advised to postpone the marriage or use condoms to prevent the spread of the disease to his partner, till he becomes non-infectious; if he refuses to obey the advice then the doctor can make a privileged communication to the concerned person.
- **Servant and employees:** An engine driver, bus driver or ship's employee suffering from epilepsy, high blood pressure, drug addiction or color blindness. The doctor should advice them to quit the job, if the patient fails to obey; then the doctor can inform the concerned authorities in the interest of the community.

PROCEDURE OF INITIATION OF ACTION FOR INFAMOUS CONDUCT AGAINST A DOCTOR?

What are the Punishments that could be Given for Professional Misconduct? (FM4.5)

- Infamous conduct is an ethical violation and hence no legal action can be taken

- against a doctor for such conduct, unless his act falls into any of the punishable provisions of the penal code.
- Only the patient or the legal relatives of the patient can initiate an action for the infamous conduct committed by the doctor in the State Medical Council.
- On receipt of the information of the complaint against a doctor, the executive committee analyses such a complaint and if it finds there is prima facie evidence, then the SMC sends intimation to the concerned doctor, asking for explanation regarding the alleged complaint.
- The reply of the doctor if found satisfactory, then the petition of the complainant is dismissed at that stage itself; if the council is not satisfied with the explanation given by the doctor and feels that the doctor is guilty of committing an infamous conduct, then the SMC forms an executive committee, from amongst its members consisting of 5, 7, or 9 members depending as the situation warrants.
- The executive committee summons the doctor for a personal enquiry, where the doctor is asked to be present before the committee on a particular date and time with the relevant documents to prove his innocence.
- The doctor may appear in person or can also send a representative, with authorization to represent him for the enquiry. The complainant is also summoned to be present during the phase of the enquiry.
- The complaint is first read, and the doctor is given chance to defend himself against the complaint with necessary relevant documents if any; after hearing the statement of both the parties the executive committee takes the action after following the due process of the law. Depending on the outcome, the doctor is either found guilty or innocent; if he is found guilty, there are three types of punishments meted out to the doctor.
  - *Warning:* For simple and minor issues, where the doctor is warned not to repeat such acts, and a severe punishment will be awarded if he continues to involve himself in such a type of infamous acts.
  - *Temporary erasure:* The name of the doctor may be temporarily removed from the medical register, for a variable period which may extend from 2 months to 5 years. Upon completion of the suspension, his name will be re-instated.
  - *Permanent erasure:*

Penal Erasure

Penal erasure is otherwise called as **"professional death sentence"**. The name of the doctor may be permanently removed from the medical register. His degree is withdrawn and is not allowed to practice medicine profession anymore.

This type of permanent erasure are done when the doctor commits some serious professional misconduct and also done when the doctor dies, or if he is convicted by the court of law for any serious offences committed by him like rape, murder, etc.

WHAT IS WARNING AND WHAT IS A WARNING NOTICE?

Warning and Warning Notice

Most students often confuse with the terms warning and warning notice.

Warning

- Warning is the minimum punishment for a doctor who is proved to have committed an infamous conduct. That is, giving a warning to the doctor with advice not to get involved in any such misconduct in future and if he indulges himself in such repeated misconducts it would attract a more severe punishment like temporary erasure.

Warning Notice

- Warning notice is not related to any punishment; it is a list of offences which are considered as professional misconduct and any doctor committing any of those acts listed in warning notice will attract a charge of infamous conduct and subsequent enquiry and appropriate punishment by the State Medical Council will be undertaken.
- The list is not complete and not intended to be complete; any new type of infamous acts are done by a doctor in future, then those professional misconducts would be added in the subsequent warning notice.
- At the time of registration with the State Medical Council the warning notice is given to the registered medical practitioner not to involve in any such acts.
- The IMC as well the SMC issues updated warning notices periodically to maintain adequate standard of ethical practice amongst the medical practitioners.

MENTION A FEW IMPORTANT ACTS WHICH GOVERN THE MEDICAL PROFESSION? (FM4.6)

- An act is a body of law, which lays down certain guidelines for carrying out some activity and also prescribes punishment if that activity is not carried out in accordance with the law.
- The doctor practicing medicine should be aware of the important Acts which are in force. Some of those Acts which are related to medical profession are:
- The Indian Medical Councils Act 1956.
- The Drugs and Cosmetics Act 1940; The Drugs and Cosmetics Rules 1945.
- The Drugs and Magic Remedies (objectionable advertisement) Act 1954.
- Narcotic Drugs and Psychotropic Substances (NDPS) Act 1985.
- Birth and Death Registration Act 1969.
- Medical Termination of Pregnancy (MTP) Act 1971.
- Preconception and Prenatal Diagnostic Techniques (prohibition of sex selection) Act 1994.
- The Mental Health Act 1987.
- The Consumer Protection Act 1986.
- The Transplantation of Human Organs Act 1994 (THOA).

WHAT IS THE STATUS OF USING RED CROSS EMBLEM BY DOCTORS?

Red Cross Emblem

- Section 12 of the Geneva Convention Act, prohibits the use of the Red Cross and allied emblems, for any purpose without approval by the Government of India.
- Section 13 lays down penalty of ₹ 500 for unauthorized use of such emblems and also forfeits the goods upon which the emblem is used.

WHAT ARE THE RIGHT AND PRIVILEGES OF A RMP? (FM4.6)

- **Right to choose your patient:** Except in emergency, the doctor has the right to choose his patients.
- **Rights to add titles and qualifications:** The doctor can add his qualifications and titles which are given by recognized universities.
- Right for appointment into authorized hospitals.
- **Right to treat patients in accordance with the law:** Strictly adhere to the legal provisions and responsibilities of a doctor.
- In circumstances of Medico-Legal Cases (MLC), the relatives and attendants of the

patient themselves may request not to register a case as MLC case. The doctor should not oblige the request, he has to register as an MLC and make a police intimation.
- **Right to prescribe and dispense drugs:** The doctor has the right to prescribe drugs to the patient whatever is necessary. He can also dispense drugs to his patients.
- **Right to receive the consultation charges:** The doctor is entitled to receive his professional charges. The doctor should intimate the patient his charges before rendering the professional service to the patient and not after the procedure or treatment is over. It is advisable to display the consultation fees in the clinic.
- **Rights to issue certificates:** The doctor can and has to issue certificates where ever necessary and when he has treated the patient.
- Right to be an expert witness.
- **Right for exemption from serving as a jury:** When many other witnesses are available the doctor can request for exemption from serving as a jury. The time and service of the doctor are more needed by the community rather than wasting his time by serving as a jury; thereby he may have to attend frequent enquires by the investigation officer of the case and subsequently attend the court as a witness. But when no other witness is available in that particular case, the doctor has to oblige the request of the I.O as the doctor should be a more responsible citizen than others.

DEFINE AND DESCRIBE EUTHANASIA (FM4.11)

- The word "Euthanasia" was derived from the Greek word which means 'good death.'
- Euthanasia is mercy killing, assisted suicide or aid in dying.

Definition

Euthanasia refers to infliction of a painless form of death on an individual suffering from severe, incurable diseases, resulting in intractable pain and suffering to the patient.

Various Forms of Euthanasia

- **Voluntary:** The patient gives consent to end his sufferings.
- **Nonvoluntary:** The patient is not in a position to give consent, e.g., comatose patients.
- **Involuntary (compulsory):** Decision by the society to terminate the life of an individual; it is done against the will and consent of the individual. It is decided by the relatives/health authorities depending on the severity of the case. Example: An individual having a deadly dangerous disease with high risk of spreading the disease to the society. This is a very rare situation, but these types of new diseases keep on changing from time to time.

Classification of Euthanasia

- **Active:** Inflicting death by an act of commission, e.g., injecting lethal dose of morphine.
- **Passive:** By an act of omission, e.g., withdrawing life saving supports in comatose patient.
- **Pediatric:** To the seriously sick or deformed infants, e.g., severe congenital anomalies.
- **Geriatric:** Seriously sick, bed ridden aged individuals.
- **Battlefield:** Severely wounded or handicapped individual in the war field, to end his sufferings and also to prevent him from getting caught and tortured by the enemy.

Legal Status of Euthanasia in India

- Euthanasia is not legalized in India and hence any doctor practices or helps in

euthanasia will be charged of causing murder/manslaughter or abatement of suicide, respectively.
- **Article 21** of the basic Constitution of India gives right to live but not right to die.
- **As per the supreme court view: Passive voluntary euthanasia** can be visualized as a fundamental right protected under **Article 21 of the constitution**, which assures right to privacy; it gives the patient a right to refuse lifesaving medical treatment.
- The right to personal liberty includes the freedom to die with dignity.
- Active euthanasia though viewed as a crime, no convictions have been made so far against any individual for commission of such offence in our country, since most of the cases are not reported or undisclosed and concealed.
- No doctor in any situation encourage such act, even on humanitarian grounds. Even though it may be the only better option for the patient, it is against the law, and it should not be practiced.

WHAT IS MALINGERING? NAME SOME DISEASES WHICH ARE COMMONLY FEIGNED AND HOW WILL YOU DIAGNOSE SUCH CASES?

Malingering (Shamming)

Malingering means planned feigning or pretending a disease for the sake of gain.

Reasons

- By soldiers or policemen to evade duties
- Prisoners to avoid hard work
- Businessmen to avoid a business contract
- Workmen to claim compensation
- Criminals to avoid legal responsibilities
- **Diseases that are usually feigned are:** (i) Ophthalmia; (ii) Dyspepsia; (iii) Intestinal (abdominal) colic; (iv) Sciatica (back pain); (v) Epilepsy; (vi) Insanity and (vii) Artificial bruise.
- The individual may do some **act of commission** to sham a disease, examples:
    - He may injure the nasopharynx with sharp instrument, swallow the blood and regurgitate in front of the doctor to mimic hematemesis.
    - Excessive intake of digitalis may simulate a heart disease
    - Eating large amount of carrot, produce carotenemia and may simulate jaundice.

Diagnosis

- In most cases detection is easy, but in some cases it may be difficult.
- History is taken from the patient, relatives and friends, and any inconsistencies in the description of the symptoms are noted.
- Usually, the signs and symptoms will not confirm (fix into) any known disease.
- Malingering can be diagnosed by keeping the patient under observation and watching him without his knowledge. Rarely an anesthetic may be given to detect malingering.

WRITE SHORT NOTES ON TORTURE AND MEDICAL PROFESSION?

- Doctors are often called inside the team to torture an individual to extract information from the arrested person.
- The World Medical Association adopted some specific guidelines for the medical professionals concerning torture and other cruel inhuman or degrading treatment in relation to detention and imprisonment (**The Declaration of Tokyo 1975**).
- **Accordingly:**
    - The doctor should not countenance or participate in the practice of torture (physical or mental) whatever be the offence of the prisoner under all situations, including armed services.

- The doctor should not provide any premises, instruments, substances, or knowledge to facilitate the practice of torture.
- The doctor shall not be present during any procedure of torture and other inhuman activities.
- The must have complete clinical independence in deciding about the health of the patient/prisoner.
- If the prisoner refuses nourishment and is capable of forming rational decisions about the consequences, the doctor should not feed him artificially.

DESCRIBE AND DISCUSS ETHICAL PRINCIPLES: RESPECT FOR AUTONOMY, NON-MALFEASANCE, BENEFICENCE AND JUSTICE (FM4.17)

Basic principles of medical ethics:

Patient's Autonomy

- It is the right of the patient to make decisions about his medical care,
- Patient autonomy does allow the healthcare provider to educate the patient but does not allow to make decision for the patient.
- Exercising patient autonomy empowers him to feel more confident in his ability to take healthcare decisions and to choose the right doctor.
- Application of the principle of respect for autonomy:
  - Tell the truth
  - Respect the privacy of others
  - Protect confidential information
  - Obtain consent for interventions with patients

Beneficence

- Beneficence is doing what is in the best interest of the patient throughout the process of diagnosis and treatment.
- A physician's intent to beneficence conflicts most often with patient autonomy.
- When disagreement arises between healthcare provider and the patient, the healthcare provider must explain the reasons for his recommendations, allowing the patient to make a more informed decision.

Non-maleficence (Do no harm)

- Complementary to beneficence, non-maleficence seeks to ensure the patient, no worse will happen (physically, mentally or otherwise) after the treatment than before.
- The principle of nonmaleficence supports the following rules:
  - Do not kill
  - Do not cause pain or suffering
  - Do not incapacitate
  - Do not cause offense

Justice

- Patient should get the justice; only right thing should be done to the patient.
- The principle of justice obliges us to equitably distribute benefits, risks, costs, and resources. The following arguments (rules) are supported by the principle of justice:
  - To each person an equal share
  - To each person according to need
  - To each person according to effort
  - To each person according to contribution
  - To each person according to merit

Privacy and Confidentiality

A Patient's privacy is related to the body and confidentiality is related to the mind.

Privacy

It's the inner fear of the patient that he/she is not being seen or under surveillance by anyone and/or by any mode; either directly or indirectly.

Confidentiality

The patient trusts that the physician will not allow anyone to know the particulars of his illness.

DEMONSTRATE ABILITY TO CONDUCT RESEARCH IN PURSUANCE TO GUIDELINES OR RESEARCH ETHICS (FM4.30)

- **Medical research:** A medical practitioner may carry out, participate in work in research projects funded by pharmaceutical and allied healthcare industries.
- A medical practitioner is obliged to know that the full-fillment of the following:
    - Ensure that the particular research proposal(s) has the due permission from the competent concerned authorities;
    - Ensure that such a research project(s) has the clearance of national/state/institutional ethics committee/bodies;
    - Ensure that it full-fills all the legal requirements prescribed for medical research;
    - Ensure that the source and amount of funding is publicly disclosed at the beginning itself;
    - Ensure that proper care and facilities are provided to human volunteers, if they are necessary for the research projects;
    - Ensure that undue animal experimentations are not done, and when these are necessary they are done in a scientific and a humane way;
    - Ensure that while accepting such an assignment, a medical practitioner shall have the freedom to publish the results of the research in the greater interest of the society by inserting such a clause in the MoU or any other document/agreement for any such assignment.

Declaration of Helsinki (1964)

Adopted by the 18th WMA General Assembly held at Helsinki, Finland in **June 1964** and amended in 1975, 1983, 1989, 1996, 2000, 2002 and 2004. Prescribes ethical principles for **Human Experimentation.**

CHALLENGES IN DEVELOPMENT OF SKILLS IN RELATIONSHIP MANAGEMENT-HUMAN BEHAVIOR, COMMUNICATION SKILLS, CONFLICT RESOLUTION TECHNIQUES (FM4.14)

Conflict with patient or relatives can be best avoided with collaboration which require open communication, often requires assertiveness and creative problem solving.

- Remain calm and composed.
- Create a calm atmosphere to be in a position to talk to the relatives.
- Do not let conflict situations faster; do something about the situation.
- Do not react without thinking the situation through.
- Maintain respect throughout. Do not personalize the dispute.
- Be aware of the sorts of issues that can turn into conflict.
- Choose an appropriate time where the other party is more amenable to listening and there are no time pressures.
- Discuss the matter in a neutral location away from the patient.
- Begin the discussion on a broader level by asking open questions and answering them clearly and precisely.
- Focus on the issues and listen respectfully to their viewpoint.
- Respect on both sides is likely to improve the chance of a positive outcome.

- If there is any chance of escalation of conflict or fear of threat to life or injury initiate code purple.

DESCRIBE THE PRINCIPLES OF HANDLING PRESSURE WHILE DEALING WITH MEDICO-LEGAL CASES BY THE DOCTOR (FM4.15)

Stress in Doctors

- Stress is the psychological and physical state that results when the resources of the individual are not sufficient to cope with the demands and pressures of the situation.
- Situations that are likely to cause stress are those that are unpredictable, uncontrollable, uncertain, ambiguous, non-familiar, involving conflict, loss or performance expectations and misunderstanding.
- Doctors are increasingly reporting emotional burnout. Mental stress and acute physical exhaustion due to long working hours and increasing patient load are reasons.
- It is the product of interaction between the demanding nature of work and insufficient rewards and subjective lack of control. The pressure and responsibility can be very hard to handle.
- Mild mental stress is beneficial, as it is shown to increase the work efficiency. If it exceeds a critical level the person goes to depression and exhaustion. Stress, if unmanaged or poorly managed, can carry severe consequences for physicians.
- Doctors have high rates of divorce, substance abuse and highest suicide rates among professionals.

Management of Stress

- Keep a regular exercise schedule
- Eat a well balanced diet
- Getting enough sleep at night
- Meditation
- Take a vacation
- Reading books of your own interest
- Music, dance, art and drawings 8. Talk to someone. Talk to your colleagues, your family and friends.

Professional colleague may be suffering from burnout. You may not be able to practically do anything but can share and be a good listener.

Stress in Handling Medico-legal Cases

- Stress may be caused by time limited events, such as apprehension of dealing with police, the pressure of avoiding errors or fear of attending courts.
- Stress can be avoided by professional competence, avoiding confrontation, enhancing communication skills and constant up gradation of the knowledge.

DESCRIBE AND DISCUSS ETHICAL GUIDELINES FOR BIOMEDICAL RESEARCH ON HUMAN SUBJECTS AND ANIMALS (FM4.27)

Human Experimentation

- Human subjects (living individuals) are used for research and clinical trials.
- Research involving human subject is the clinical trial. Human subjects are subjected to novel vaccines, drugs, dietary choices, dietary supplements and medical devices.
- Health Authority/Ethics committee approval is mandatory to start the research.
- In order to protect the rights, dignity and safety of the participant in all biomedical researches the four basic principles—autonomy, beneficences, nonmaleficence and justice should be kept.

Ethical Guidelines in Human Experimentation

Human research subject is a living individual about whom the investigator obtains data. So the rights of the individual should be protected. National institute of Justice in U.S. published **the rights of the human subjects in clinical researches:**
- Voluntary and informed consent
- Respect of human subject Right to end the participation in research at any time
- Right to safeguard integrity
- Protection from physical, mental and emotional harm
- Access to information regarding research
- Protection of privacy and wellbeing.

Ethical Guidelines Set by International Communities

- Common rules published in 1991 by office of human research protection in US. It gives a set of guidelines for the institutional review boards in obtaining informed consent and assurance of compliance for human subject participants in research studies.
- Nurenberg code in 1949: It prevents the research on prisoners including prisoners of war and patients.
- Declaration of Helsinki was established in 1964 to regulate international research. Declaration of Helsinki is regarded as cornerstone document on human research ethics.
- Belmont report in 1978 was created to protect the human subjects of biomedical and behavioral research. Privacy, confidentiality and informed consent were the key concerns.

Unethical Human Experimentations

Unethical human experimentations violate the principles of medical ethics. It has been performed by countries including Nazi Germany, Imperial Japan, North Korea, US and Soviet Union. Nazi Germany performed human experimentation on large numbers of prisoners in its concentration camps.

DESCRIBE "DECLARATION OF HELSINKI"

- The world medical association framed a code of ethics (**Declaration of Helsinki**) on human experimentation in 1964 and revised in 1975.
- Biomedical research should be based on scientifically established facts by animal and laboratory experiments.
- The clinical research study must be combined with high quality of professional care. The doctor should be free to use new therapeutic measures which are likely to save the patient's life and should be done with proper informed written consent of the patient and the legal guardian.
- Human experimentation may be:
    - *Therapeutic:* The human experimentation is primarily aimed at improving the condition of the patient from the disease or condition he is suffering from.
    - *Research:* The experimentation is by using human subjects as a means of expanding scientific knowledge for the benefit of humanity.
    - *Innovative:* Using human participants for therapeutic procedures that are not in practice yet and to be newly introduced in medical practice.

ICMR Guidelines for Human Experimentation

ICMR has laid down guidelines on human research which should necessarily ensure that:
- The purpose of the research should be directed towards increasing knowledge

about human condition in relation to social and environmental conditions.
- The human subjects taking part in the study must be dealt with in a manner conductive to and with dignity and wellbeing.
- Research should be subjected to evaluation at all stages.

DISCUSS THE CONSTITUTION AND FUNCTIONS OF ETHICAL COMMITTEE (FM4.26)

The composition should be as follows:
- Chairperson (not-affiliated to SGPGI)
- Member secretary (SGPGI faculty member)
- Two faculty members of SGPGI
- Dean, SGPGI
- One to two clinicians (not affiliated to SGPGI)
- Basic medical scientists
- Clinical pharmacologist
- One legal expert or retired judge or medico-legal expert
- One social scientist/representative of non-governmental voluntary agency
- One philosopher/ethicist/theologian
- Lay person from the community
  - The Ethics Committee division deals with the applications seeking registration, re-registration and post approval changes of Institutional Ethics Committee. No Ethics Committee shall review and accord its approval to a clinical trial protocol without prior registration with the Licensing Authority.
  - An application for registration of Ethics Committee shall be made to the Licensing Authority in accordance with the requirements as specified in the Appendix VIII of Schedule Y.
  - The Licensing Authority after being satisfied that the requirements have been complied with, may grant registration to the Ethics Committee subject to such conditions as may be stated therein.
  - The registration of Ethics Committees is valid for a period of three years. The re-registration applications need to be made within 3 months before the expiry of registration. Registration remains deemed continued unless otherwise orders are passed or until the registration is suspended or cancelled. Accordingly, applicant shall apply to CDSCO for re-registration as per checklist.

DESCRIBE THE CONSTITUTION AND FUNCTIONS OF INSTITUTIONAL ETHICAL COMMITTEES (IEC) (FM4.26)

Constitution
- It will have members from various disciplines like medicine, law, social science, political science, theology etc. The Internal Ethics Committee (IEC) is headed by a chairperson and supported by other members.
- **The purpose** of the IEC is to protect human subjects by ensuring high ethical standards and conduct in all researches. According to the ICMR guidelines in 2006, the basic responsibility of the IEC is "**to ensure a competent review of all ethical aspects of the project proposal received by it in an objective manner.**"
- The IEC is to protect and promote, dignity, rights, and wellbeing of research participants.
- Ethical committee clearance should be obtained from legally formed EC to start medical researches.

Functions of IEC
- According to New Drugs and Clinical Trials Rules, 2019, Institutional Ethical

- Committees are entrusted with the responsibility to undertake the ethical review of research proposals prior to initiation.
- They have continuing responsibility to regularly monitor the approved research to ensure ethical compliance during the conduct of research and clinical trials using human participants.

DESCRIBE AND DISCUSS BIOETHICS (FM4.16)

- Bioethics is concerned with the ethical questions that arise in the relationships among life sciences, biotechnology, medicine and medical ethics, politics, law, theology and philosophy. The term Bioethics (Greek, bios-life, Ethos-behavior) was coined by Fritz Jahr in 1926 while addressing the use of animals and plants in scientific research.
- Now the field of bioethics address human enquiry on wide range of issues like, drug experimentations, abortion, euthanasia, surrogacy, organ donation, healthcare rationing, right to refuse medical care for religious or cultural reasons, gene therapy, stem cell research, human cloning etc.
- Some bioethics would narrow ethical evaluation only to the morality of medical treatments or technological innovations and the timing of medical treatment of humans.
- One of the first areas addressed by modern bioethicists was that of human experimentation. National Commission for the protection of Human Subjects of Biomedical and Behavioral Research was established in 1974 to identify the basic Ethical principles that should be underlined in the conduct of biomedical and behavioral research involving human subjects.
- Fundamental principles announced were respect of persons, beneficence and justice.
- Later nonmaleficence, human dignity and sanctity of life were added to the cardinal values. Bioethicists come from a wide variety of backgrounds and have training in diverse array of disciplines.
- The field contains individuals trained in philosophy, medically trained clinical ethicists, lawyers, political scientists, social scientists, religious scholars and theologians.
- Many bioethicists, especially medical scholars, accord the highest priority to autonomy.
- Gene therapy involves ethics because scientists are making changes in the genes which are making building blocks of the human body. There is also controversy because in gene therapy genes in a sperm or egg can be edited to prevent genetic disorder in the future generation. It is unknown how this type of gene therapy affects long term human development. It is important of medical college to teaches bioethics so that students can gain a biomedical ethics and use the knowledge to provide better patient care.

DESCRIBE AND DISCUSS THE ETHICAL ISSUES RELATED TO HIV PATIENT (FM4.7)

Ethics plays a paramount role in a complex condition like HIV. The ethical spectrum around a patient positive for HIV includes a number of important things which includes confidentiality, informed consent, access to care, etc.

- **Confidentiality:** Maintaining a patient's confidentiality is the fundamental of HIV care. Healthcare professionals are obliged to protect the privacy and confidentiality of their patients. This ensures trust between

patient and the healthcare provider thus encouraging promptness for treatment.
- **Informed consent:** Throughout the treatment, it's mandatory to have informed consent of the HIV patient. The patient should be accurately informed of the nature of the disease, type of treatment, potential side effects, benefits, etc. This promotes active participation of patients in their treatment.
- **Stigma and discrimination:** Though it's a serious challenge, the health care professionals need to overcome these issues through nonjudgmental and compassionate care to the patients. Creating an inclusive and supporting environment is important for the overall wellbeing of the HIV patient.
- **Access to care:** Providing proper access to prevention, testing, treatment and supportive care irrespective of geographical and social barrier.
- **Research:** Research is always promoted but with maintaining the secrecy of the patient. Researchers must take informed consent of the patient to proceed with their experiments. The research should be conducted by qualified professionals only. There shouldn't be any conflict of interest from the researcher's part both financial and nonfinancial.
- **Community** level participation can be promoted through proper ethical questionnaire.
- If a **blood donor** is diagnosed as positive for HIV, the information is kept away from that person as per as GOI.
- **Doctors** are obliged to treat any HIV patient referred to them and also need to inform the status of the patient to the associated healthcare professionals.
- A **HIV positive female** is advised against pregnancy due to chances of transmission to fetus. A HIV positive mother is advised not to breastfeed because of possible risk to her baby. Also, the spouse of an HIV positive patient is confidentially informed about the condition.

A known case of AIDS getting married and spreading the infection to the spouse is booked under **Section 269 IPC and 270 IPC** (6 months and 2 years of imprisonment respectively).

ETHICAL AND LEGAL ISSUES OF STEM CELL RESEARCH

- The advancement in science and technology has been incredible in the past few decades.
- Unimagined doors stand open to us, mainly in the spheres of biomedicine and biotechnology.
- Stem cell research is one of the latest aspects that have come to light in the field of biotechnology.
- With this new development it promises to cure even neuro-degenerative diseases like spinal cord injuries, parkinson's disease, alzheimer's disease and regeneration of damaged organs.
- Some of the research being carried out include embryonic stem cell research, adult stem cell research etc.
- Human embryonic stem cell research has always been a debatable issue, because of its potential ramifications as a violation of human rights. The issue of whether it is an act of morality, to kill an unfertilized embryo in order to possibly save many is the biggest question.

Ethical issues in relation to stem cell research includes:
- Duty of care.
- Protection of the people.
- Nonabandonment.
- Confidentiality except justified legal breach.
- Informed consent.

MEDICO LEGAL ISSUES IN RELATION TO FAMILY VIOLENCE, VIOLATION OF HUMAN RIGHTS, NHRC AND DOCTORS (FM4.9)

- Family violence is a major issue affecting several families all across the globe. These include physical, mental and sexual abuse. Often these cases goes unreported making its medico-legal aspects very complicated.
- Violation of human rights has victimized several people across the globe. The duty of the forensic doctor and National Human Rights Commission (NHRC) are:
  - Identification and documentation of injury to be done carefully for the legal proceedings and evidence in court.
  - Confidentiality may be breached by the doctor to report family violence to prevent any further harm to the victim.
  - Informed consent has to be taken by doctor from the victim and if unable to take so the doctor must follow proper guidelines to protect the victim's rights.
  - Mandatory reporting under special conditions to the responsible authorities.
  - Testifying in the court about cause and severity of the injuries accurately and truthfully.
  - Forensic examination of blood, hair, semen, etc.

DEMONSTRATE ABILITY TO COMMUNICATE APPROPRIATELY WITH MEDIA, PUBLIC AND DOCTORS (FM4.10 AND 4.29)

- Media being the bridge between authorities and the audience, it has a major importance in spreading awareness and information related to health. The doctors can capitalize this to spread mass awareness. This can be achieved by:
  - Voluntary service to media in the form of news article, television panel or as radio broadcast.
  - Contribute medical writings and blogs.
  - Organize medical camps, blood camps, etc., and allowing media coverage.
- Doctor have benefits and risks when using social media platforms such as Twitter, Instagram, Facebook or You tube for patient care or discussing patients.

Benefits

- Can engage people in public health and policy discussions.
- Help to establish national and international professional networks.
- Can facilitate patients' access to information about health and services.

Risks

Professional boundary: It will become difficult to maintain a professional boundary between doctor and patients. Doctor cannot mix social and professional relationships and should direct his patients to his professional profile.

Breach of Confidentiality

When communicating publicly, including speaking to or writing in the media, you must maintain patient confidentiality. You must not use publicly accessible social media to discuss individual patients or their care.

Medical Etiquette

Criticizing and expressing controversial opinions between doctors on social media may create confusion to patients and public. You must not bully, harass, or make unsustainable comments about your colleagues.

Anonymity

If you are identified as a doctor in social media, you should not make anonymous opinions. Contents uploaded anonymously can be traced back and create problems.

Advertising

Doctor should not use the public media for advertising himself or his firm or institution.

Medico-legal Issues

- It is always better for doctors not to make posts commenting on medico-legal issues in public media. That case may be under investigation and your comments on public media as a professional may create confusion.
- The concerned doctor can discuss with the investigation team and communicate his observations to help the investigation in that particular case. If such issues are discussed in the public media that may cause harm to the investigation process.

DESCRIBE THE SOCIAL ASPECT OF ML CASES IN CASE WITH VICTIMS OF ASSAULT, RAPE, ATTEMPTED SUICIDE, HOMICIDE, DOMESTIC VIOLENCE AND DOWRY RELATED CAUSES (FM4.3)

Assault

- **Support system:** The victims often rely on family, friends and community organizations for social support.
- **Stigma and shame:** The victims are prone to feeling of guilt, shame and self blame. This compromises their willingness to disclose and seek for help.
- Social reaction of family, friends and the community significantly influence their healing process. Under supportive condition, they tend to heal faster.
- Seeking legal help is at times not done due to complexity of the process and the influence of the society. Giving quick and smooth justice is mandatory for overall wellbeing of the victim.
- Impact on relationship may be there. Post assault, where the victims fail to maintain a healthy connection with the people around them.
- Community awareness and prevention along with providing supportive network.
- Post assault recovery support to be given to the victim.

Rape

In addition to the above as in cases of assault

- Disclosure and reporting of such cases are often compromised due to fear of retaliation and insult resulting in reduced legal involvement.
- Psychological impact can be long lasting, even till the rest of life. This can impact their personal relation.

Attempted Suicide

In addition to the above

- Self blame stigma and shame are some of the factors that create barriers for recovery of the person.
- Counseling to help them empower their life.

Attempted Homicide

In addition to the above

- Trauma informed care to be given to the victim which includes psychological and emotional support
- Post traumatic growth and reintegration into the society.

Domestic Violence

- At times domestic violence goes under reported. It includes physical, mental and emotional trauma from within the family causing shame and stigma to the victim.

- Support system from community, friend and organization such as child welfare. By promoting independence of the abused can help them grow.

Dowry

Dowry related assaults can be avoided by proper support from the community and spreading of awareness; empowerment to be given for the victims. Legal process can be at times overwhelming for the victim thus ensuring smoother process helps in wellbeing of the victim.

MULTIPLE CHOICE QUESTIONS

1. **The oldest code of medical ethics is:**
   a. Declaration of Geneva
   b. Declaration of Helsinki
   c. Hippocratic Oath
   d. Declaration of Sydney
2. **The following are the functions of IMC, except:**
   a. Regulation of medical education
   b. Recognition of medical degrees
   c. Maintains the medical register
   d. Disciplinary action
3. **Disclosure of illness to the following amounts to violation of professional secrecy:**
   a. Recruiting authorities of uniformed services
   b. Licensing authority for driving
   c. Life Insurance Company
   d. Prison authority
4. **The following are certain rights of the RMP, except:**
   a. Choose their patient
   b. Use of red cross emblem
   c. Prescribe and dispense drugs
   d. Use title and qualification
5. **"Professional Death Sentence" is a term which denotes:**
   a. Capital punishment (Judicial hanging)
   b. Rigorous punishment
   c. Severe warning
   d. Permanent removal of name from the medical register
6. **In India, Euthanasia has got:**
   a. Legal status
   b. No legal sanction
   c. Legal sanction in some special conditions
   d. Legal sanction only in cancer
7. **Infamous conduct comprises of all, except:**
   a. Adultery
   b. Advertising
   c. Procuring criminal abortion
   d. Examination of a patient without consent
8. **Privileged communication is between:**
   a. Doctor and patient
   b. Doctor and medical council
   c. Doctor and court
   d. Doctor and police
9. **A person voluntarily acting like having a disease is said to be:**
   a. Hypochondriac
   b. Masochist
   c. Munchason syndrome
   d. Malingerer
10. **In a comatose patient, removal of life support is:**
    a. Active euthanasia
    b. Passive euthanasia
    c. Voluntary euthanasia
    d. Involuntary euthanasia
11. **Falanga is:**
    a. Sitting in abnormal position
    b. Hitting the feet with stick
    c. Electric current for torture
    d. Pulling of hair
12. **Dichotomy refers to:**
    a. Fee splitting
    b. Study of structure of plants
    c. A branch of anatomy
    d. An ultramicroscopic study of tissues
13. **Schedule that recognize medical qualifications awarded by institutions in India:**
    a. Schedule I
    b. Schedule II
    c. Schedule III Part I
    d. Schedule III Part II
14. **Declaration of Helsinki is about:**
    a. Organ transplantation
    b. Torture
    c. Human experimentation
    d. Code of ethics

SECTION 1: Medical Jurisprudence

15. Prohibition of participation in torture by a doctor comes under:
    a. Declaration of Tokyo
    b. Declaration of Helsinki
    c. Declaration of Oslo
    d. Declaration of Geneva

16. Declaration of Oslo' is related to which among the following:
    a. Torture
    b. Medical termination of pregnancy
    c. Capital punishment
    d. Human experimentation

ANSWERS

| 1. c | 2. d | 3. d | 4. b | 5. d | 6. b | 7. d | 8. c | 9. c | 10. b |
| 11. b | 12. a | 13. a | 14. c | 15. a | 16. b | | | | |

CHAPTER 4

Consent and Medical Negligence

KEY WORDS

Consent, informed consent, rules of consent, loco parentis, professional negligence, Section 304-A IPC, res ipsa loquitor, calculated risk doctrine, novus actus interveniens, vicarious liability, therapeutic misadventure, corporate negligence, products liability, contributory negligence, CPA, professional indemnity policy, Workmen's Compensation Act, ESI Act.

FM4.18	Describe and discuss medical negligence including civil and criminal negligence, contributory negligence, corporate negligence, vicarious liability, res Ipsa loquitor, prevention of medical negligence and defenses in medical negligence litigations.
FM4.19	Define consent. Describe different types of consent and ingredients of informed consent. Describe the rules of consent and importance of consent in relation to age, emergency situation, mental illness and alcohol intoxication.
FM4.20	Describe therapeutic privilege, malingering, therapeutic misadventure, professional secrecy, human experimentation.
FM4.21	Describe products liability and medical indemnity insurance.
FM4.8	Describe the Consumer Protection Act-1986 (medical indemnity insurance, civil litigations and compensations), workmen's, Compensation Act and ESI Act.

INTRODUCTION

Negligence

- Diligence means due care and skill; negligence is the opposite of diligence.
- In negligence, the degree of skill and care exhibited by a doctor while performing the procedure was below the prescribed standard.

DEFINE CONSENT? (FM4.19)

Definition

- Consent is defined as "voluntary agreement, compliance, permission or accepting for the act proposed by another" and is valid only for that specified act or purpose.
- Indian Contracts Act, Section 13 states that "two or more persons are said to consent

when they agree upon the same thing in the same sense".
- To be legally valid, the consent given must be intelligent and informed.
- The doctor examining or treating a patient without the consent amounts to the offence of assault.

WHAT ARE THE TYPES OF CONSENT? (FM4.19)

Types of Consent

There are two types of consent: (i) Implied consent, and (ii) Expressed consent.
- **Implied consent:** The behavior or the act of patient or the individual, itself indicates that he has consented for the act; you can take it for granted that he/she has given the consent. This is applicable only for minor procedure of medical practice like general physical examination, checking the pulse, blood pressure or giving injection, etc.
- **Expressed consent:** The doctor has to ask for the consent and obtain it before any procedure or treatment. Expressed consent is of two types: (i) oral consent, and (ii) written consent.
  i. *Oral consent:* Is of equal value as that of written consent, but when a dispute arises between the two parties then, it becomes difficult for the doctor to prove that he has obtained a proper consent. Hence, oral consent holds good only for simple procedures like per abdominal examination, giving IV fluids or testing the blood, etc.
  ii. *Written consent:* It's always better to go for written consent whenever the procedure is a slightly complicated or prolonged procedure like a suturing for an injury, an incision and drainage for an abscess, etc.

WHAT ARE THE INGREDIENTS OF INFORMED CONSENT? (FM4.19)

Informed Written Consent (The Corner Stone of Medical Practice)

This is the most superior form of consent in medical practice. Informed consent is called as the "**doctrine of full disclosure**". The law believes that the patient alone is the best person to care for himself and he has the right to choose what is good or bad for him and what is needed to be done on him to get cured of his disease or the problem he is suffering from.

Informed Written Consent in Medical Practice

- A doctor after examining the patient must explain to the patient and/or the relatives:
  - What's the disease or problem he is suffering from?
  - What is his proposed treatment plan, for that disease or condition?
  - What are the other standard alternate treatments/procedures available for that particular disease or condition?
  - What are the advantage and disadvantage of his proposed treatment; and why he prefers to follow that particular treatment option?
  - What are the advantage and disadvantage of the alternative line of treatment?
- The information provided to the patient should be in writing in simple language and in the language in which the patient is familiar. Then allow the patient to choose what type of treatment he needs and to be done for him.
- In important situations like surgery, it is always better to explain all these to the

patient and to the close relatives of the patient and get it signed by the patient as well as the legal guardian. Since, if suppose the patient dies the relatives are the people who are going to file the case if any and hence they should be convinced that the doctor did everything which is good for the patient and death was unavoidable.
- **Informed refusal:** When the doctor feels that, a particular type of treatment will be the best for the patient and if the patient does not accept for the proposed treatment plan, there are many chances that it could result in some other life threatening complications at later stage; in spite of explaining all these in detail, the patient still refuses for the doctor's proposed treatment plan, then the doctor has to bring all in writing and get it signed by the patient; this is called as "informed refusal".

Consent in medico-legal cases: Informed written consent should be obtained in all medico-legal examinations. It should be informed to the individual that, the opinion you are going to arrive after the examination, will be issued in the form a certificate; which may go in favor of him or against him in the court of law; but, if he refuses to give consent for examination then it will definitely (100%) go against the him in the court.

WHAT ARE THE RULES OF OBTAINING CONSENT? (FM4.19)

Rules of Obtaining Consent

- Consent is a mandatory for every medical examination and treatment.
- Oral consent should be obtained in the presence of disinterested third party.
- Written consent is not necessary in all situations, but when a dispute arises it becomes difficult for the doctor to prove that he obtained a valid consent. Hence, any procedure beyond routine physical examination such as blood transfusion, collection of blood, etc, expressed consent, preferably written consent is necessary.
- In major procedures such as surgery, written informed consent is necessary and is mandatory.
- The doctor should explain the objective of his examination and also inform the patient that he has the right to refuse consent.
- When the person subjects himself voluntarily for examination, such as insurance or for issuing driving license, no consent is necessary and also there exists no professional secrecy.
- **In criminal cases**, the victim cannot be examined without informed consent; but the accused of a crime can be examined using reasonable amount of force without consent, under the request of police not below the rank of Sub-Inspector **(Section 53 CrPC)**.
- As per Section 54 CrPC, an accused person can request for medical examination to prove his innocence.
- **Consent in alcohol intoxication cases:** In cases of drunkenness or under the influence of any drug, the individual may be unconscious or not in a state to understand and give consent. In such situations the doctor can examine the patient without consent if requested by the investigating officer, withhold the results of examination and hand it over to the authorities after the individual becomes fit to give consent. But if he refuses to hand over the report at this stage, it has to be obliged; but not in criminal cases (Section 53 CrPC, if he is accused of a crime) the doctor can hand over the results without the consent.
- A prisoner can be treated forcefully in the interest of the society. Same way an individual starving himself to death can be treated forcefully without consent, since no individual has the right to die.

- Consent given for committing a crime or illegal act such as criminal abortion is not valid.
- Consent given by an individual under fear or intoxication or by an insane is invalid.
- In case of emergency, when no relatives are available or no time to wait for their arrival, the doctor can proceed on with the treatment even without consent.
- When a treatment is made compulsory by the law, then no consent necessary (Example: Vaccination, where the Govt. gives the consent).
- In treatment or surgery, which is expected to involve his sexual capacity or fertility, the consent of both the husband and the wife are necessary.
- If any person has consented or given willingness for donation of any organ or body after his death; the consent of the legal heirs is mandatory to harvest the organs, after death of the individual (no individual has any right over his body after his death).

CONSENT IN RELATION TO AGE; WHAT IS LOCO PARENTIS? (FM4.19)

- An individual under 18 years cannot give consent to suffer any harm **(Section 87 IPC)**.
- An individual above 18 years can give valid consent to suffer any harm which may result from an act, done in good faith, not known or intended to cause death. **(Section 88 IPC)**.
- An adult individual cannot be detained inside the hospital without his consent, he has to be discharged under 'against medical advice'.

What is Loco Parentis (Local Parent)?

- An individual <12 years of age cannot give consent to suffer any harm, done in good faith and for his benefit. The consent has to be obtained from the parents or guardian, if they refuse to give consent, the doctor cannot treat the patient even to save the life **(Section 89 IPC)**.
- In an emergency involving children when the parents or guardian is not available, the person in-charge can give consent (e.g., teacher in a school).

PROFESSIONAL NEGLIGENCE (MEDICAL MALPRACTICE) (FM4.18)

Define Professional Negligence: What are the Components to be Established in a Case of Negligence Against a Doctor?

Definition

- Professional negligence is defined as "omission to do something which a reasonable competent man would do or doing something which a prudent reasonable man would not do, either of these results in direct damage or death of the patient".
- Medical negligence arises when the standard of care exhibited by the doctor while doing a procedure or treatment was below the prescribed standard.
- Negligence results either from the doctor's lack of knowledge and skill or failure to excise reasonable degree of care and skills while performing the procedure/act.
- When a patient dies during the treatment due to alleged medical negligence, the doctor is booked under Section 304 (A) of IPC.

Section 304 (A) IPC

- Whoever causes death of any person by rash and negligent act, not amounting to culpable homicide, shall be punished with imprisonment for a term which may extent to 2 years, with or without fine.

Components of a Negligence Suit

- For the charge of negligence to be established against a doctor, the following components have to be proved beyond any reasonable doubt:
  - Existence of a duty of care
  - Dereliction of such duty
  - Damage
  - *Direct cause:* The resultant damage should be a direct effect of such dereliction. Also, it has to be proved that the resultant damage was reasonably foreseeable (commonly expected).
- Even if it is proved that the doctor was negligent but such an act did not cause any damage to the patient, then the doctor cannot be held liable for any compensation.

Ordinary degree of professional skill is a must:

- The doctor is not expected to give the best available treatment; he is only expected to give the reasonable degree of care. Hence, average degree of professional skill is the minimum requirement from any doctor.
- His act will be compared with that of another doctor possessing the same qualification and practicing medicine under the same circumstances. The care given by a doctor in a rural set up cannot be compared with that of a doctor practicing medicine at a corporate hospital in a city.

Error in judgment either in diagnosis or treatment is not negligence:

- The doctor cannot be held liable for the error in investigations and if his treatment was based on the results.
- If he has treated the patient presuming a diagnosis and later found by investigations that his diagnosis was wrong, even then the doctor cannot be held liable but he has to clarify clearly what was the basis on which he arrived at that diagnosis.

DIFFERENCES BETWEEN CIVIL AND CRIMINAL NEGLIGENCE (FM4.18)

Civil vs criminal negligence are described in **Table 4.1**.

WHAT IS NOVUS ACTUS INTERVENIENS?

An unrelated act intervening: this arises rarely when some new unrelated act interferes;

TABLE 4.1: Civil vs criminal negligence.

Features	Civil negligence	Criminal negligence
Offence	No specific and clear violation	There is specific violation of a particular of law criminal law in question
Negligence	Simple absence of care and skill	Gross negligence, inattention or lack of competency
Conduct of physician	Compared to a generally accepted standard of professional conduct	Not compared to a any single test
Consent for act	Good defense in court of law cannot recover damages	Not a defense; can be prosecuted
Trial	Civil court	Criminal court
Evidence	Strong evidence is sufficient	Guilt should be proved beyond reasonable doubt
Punishment	Damages to be paid	Imprisonment

Example: Some accidental injuries sustained in the course of the treatment by a doctor which added to the damage/precipitated death. In these circumstances the doctor can prove that death was due to unrelated act which happened in between.

DESCRIBE RES IPSA LOQUITOR (FM4.18)

- Res ipsa loquitor means "**the evidence speaks for itself**".
- It is also called as "**doctrine of common knowledge**".
- In any case of negligence the burden of proof rests on the patient and he has to prove by evidence and witnesses that the doctor was negligent and the damage has been caused directly by his negligent act.
- In res ipsa loquitor, it is clearly evident that the damage was a direct result of the negligent act of the doctor act and hence the burden of proof is shifted to the doctor's side and he has to prove his innocence and that the resulted damage was not due to his act.
- Examples: Leaving surgical instruments or any foreign body like gauze or blade inside the abdomen during an abdominal surgery; operating on the wrong limb or operating on a wrong patient, etc. In these circumstances it is proved that the doctor was negligent; hence the burden of proof shifts to the doctors side.
- When res ipsa loquitor is filed, the burden can only be shifted as someone else's negligence is the direct cause for the damage. When the burden is shifted on someone, then he has to pay the compensation for the damage.

DISCUSS COMPOSITE NEGLIGENCE?

- Composite negligence refers to the negligence on the part of two or more persons. Where a person is injured as a result of negligence on the part of two or more wrong doers, it is said that the person was injured on account of the composite negligence of those wrong-doers.
- In such a case, each wrong doer is jointly and severally liable to the injured for payment of the compensation for the entire damages and the injured person has the choice of proceeding against all or any of them.
- In such a case, the injured need not establish the extent of responsibility of each wrong-doer separately, nor is it necessary for the court to determine the extent of liability of each wrong-doer separately.

WHAT ARE THE DEFENSES AVAILABLE FOR A DOCTOR IN CASES OF MEDICAL NEGLIGENCE? (FM4.18)

Consent

- Is a very good defense in any charge of negligence, provided it has been obtained following the rules of consent in a proper format.
- Most of the charges of negligence against a doctor are due to failure in obtaining a proper informed written consent. A proper consent saves the doctor in almost 99% cases of negligence. Since, most of the treating doctors are not much aware of the legal provisions and anyone cannot judge the outcome of the case at that moment of time, and no one can guess which case will go wrong and which patient may file a case at a later time. But doctors should note that consent is a defense only in civil cases.

Contributory Negligence

- The doctor was already negligent and the patient also has added to the resultant damage; the doctor has to prove that the patient by his negligent actions has added to the damages caused. Then the amount of compensation may be reduced.

Examples:
- A doctor has advised the patient to keep the wound clean; come and change the dressing everyday in his clinic; the patient fails to follow the instructions and advice, which resulted in severe infection and results in some damage.
- Failure of the patient to take medicines as advised by the doctor can all be brought forward as a defense, but the doctor has to prove it.

Corporate Negligence

In corporate hospitals, the management is responsible for the negligent act of any individual doctor or paramedical staffs. The case is filed against the hospital in most cases and the hospital has to give the compensation. May be the hospital authorities can recover the amount from the doctor or may terminate his service as they feel correct.

Products Liability (FM4.21)

- The burden of proof rests on the doctor; he has to prove that the resultant damage was due to faulty machine, instrument or drug.
- Here again, the instrument has to be maintained as per the norms of the manufacturer; faulty handling of the instruments, not servicing the instrument at the proper interval of time or not checking the functional status of the instrument before commencing the procedure are the duty of the doctor. If the damage is due to faulty usage of the machine, then the manufacturer will not be held liable for the resultant damage.

Therapeutic Misadventure (Medical Maloccurance) (FM4.20)

- This is a very good defense for the doctor, if he has excised reasonable degree of skill and care while doing that procedure or a line of treatment.
- This is applicable in situations where the treatment procedure carries inherent risk of complications. The doctor was reasonably good and has taken proper care and precautions while giving treatment, and in spite of doing everything correctly, unfortunately the patient suffers some damage or dies.
- This is mainly due to individual variation in response of different patients to different procedures or drugs, which is totally unexpected.
- Here again, the burden of proof rests on the doctor and he has to prove that he had followed standard guidelines and taken enough precautions to avoid the expected adverse effects, and in spite of this the death or damage had resulted.
- **Examples:**
  - Breaking of a needle while giving intramuscular injection;
  - Damage to recurrent laryngeal nerve during thyroidectomy;
  - When a seriously ill patient is under treatment of a doctor and later the patient dies, it is enough if the doctor brings forth evidences to prove that he had taken all necessary measures to save the life of the patient, but death was inevitable.

Calculated Risk Doctrine

Every medical procedure, how small it may be has got some inherent risk, hence the percentage of the expected risk is important in any case of negligence and again the same has to be well informed to the patient at the time of obtaining the consent. If the risk percentage/the expected mortality rate is high, then the doctor can defend himself that death was inevitable.

Vicarious Liability: (Respondent Superior) "Let the Master Answer"

- For any act done by the employee the employer is responsible. The chief doctor

is responsible for the entire negligence act done by his assistants and paramedical staffs.
- This doctrine can be enforced only in cases of civil negligence involving monitory compensations.

ENUMERATE THE STEPS TO BE TAKEN BY A DOCTOR TO PREVENT MEDICAL NEGLIGENCE? (FM4.18)

- Always take valid consent, how small the procedure may be.
- Employ fully qualified staffs and associates.
- Attend the patient in time; in cases of emergencies treatment has to be done even if the patient does not pay the fees at that moment.
- Update your knowledge as far as possible, especially on the commonest issues and on those types of cases which you are seeing frequently.
- Maintain accurate and complete medical records about all the patients, for a minimum period of 3 years; general practitioners at the periphery can at least make a note of all the patients in the diary, which is difficult to be manipulated at a later date and hence the court will have better belief on the doctor.
- Reasonable degree of care and skill is a must, at least be thorough in what you do.
- Do not criticize another doctor, even though the other doctor may be wrong or may not have been right.
- **Guard against therapeutic hazards:** Even if you don't do good to the patient, be sure you don't harm him and cause any damage due to improper treatment procedures.

WHAT IS PATERNALISM?

- Paternalism is acting upon one's own idea of what is best for another person without consulting that other person. Among doctors it is a practice, where the doctor in the best interests s of the patient, forcibly treats him against his wishes.
- **Example:** Removing a malignant organ like a carcinomatous breast or amputation of leg because of osteosarcoma.
- **MLI:** Paternalism (in a conscious, mentally sound, adult patient), although done in the patient's best interests, is illegal. The doctor may be sued U/S 350 IPC.

DESCRIBE CONSUMER PROTECTION ACT 1986: CPA/COPRA (FM4.8)

- Enacted originally in 1986, the Consumer Protection Act was amended in 1991 and 1993 to make it more consumer friendly.
- The Consumer Protection Act 2019 was notified on August 9th 2019, came into effect from July 20th 2020.
- According to the **Consumer Protection Act 2019,** a **consumer** is a person who buys any goods or avails any services for a consideration, which has been paid or promised to pay or partly paid or partly promised or under any scheme of deferred payment. A consumer also includes a person who is using the goods or beneficiary of service with the approval of the buyer and applies to both online and offline transactions through electronic means of teleshopping or direct selling or multilevel marketing.
- The 2019 Act varies from the 1986 in multiple ways viz. widening the scope by dealing with three more unfair trade practices, E-commerce, product liability, unfair contracts, by introducing a new regulatory body named Central Consumer Protection Authority and by making the already existing penalties more stricter.
- The six consumer rights are defined under the Section 2(9) of the Consumer Protection Act, 2019:
  i. The right to be protected
  ii. The right to be informed
  iii. The right to be assured

iv. The right to be heard
v. The right to seek redressal
vi. The right to consumer awareness.
- The Act specifies the parameters for direct selling and e-commerce. The Consumer Protection Act of 2019 includes provisions for mediation and other forms of alternative dispute resolution to allow the parties to comfortably resolve their issue without the hassle of court proceedings.
- The new updated Consumer Protection Act of 2019 provides consumers with a wide range of benefits and rights to safeguard them from unfair business practices, false or misleading advertising, etc.
- The complaint has to be lodged within 2 years from the date of purchase or service rendered, with relevant documents to support the allegation and the amount of compensation he is claiming.
- No court fee is charged in such cases and once the cases are taken up, compensations if any are awarded within a reasonable period of time.
- Doctors are also covered under the Act (Supreme court judgment, 13th November 1995) as the doctor provides a service to the patient and for which he is being paid. Government hospitals and those who provide free treatment to all the patients at all times, are not covered under this Act.
- A bench of Justices DY Chandrachud and Hima Kohli affirmed the Bombay High Court verdict which held that doctors and healthcare service providers are covered under the ambit of the Consumer Protection Act. Supreme Court said healthcare services are not excluded from the consumer protection ACT.
- Three-Tier Grievances Machinery under the Consumer Protection Act are:

District Commission

- A district commission includes a president (who can be a working or retired judge of the District Court) and two other members. They are appointed by the state government. One can file a complaint for goods and services of up to 1 crore or less in this agency.
- For the complaints filed, if the district commission feels a requirement, it sends the goods to the laboratory for testing and gives its decision based on the laboratory report and facts.
- If the aggrieved party is not happy with the jurisdiction of the district commission, then they can appeal against the judgment of this agency in the State Commission within 45 days.

State Commission

- A state commission includes a president (who must be a working or retired judge of the High Court) and at least two other members. They are appointed by the state government. One can file a complaint of goods and services worth >1 crore and <10 crores in this agency.
- After receiving a complaint from the aggrieved party, the State Commission contacts the party against whom the complaint has been filed. Also, for the complaints filed, if the State Commission feels a requirement, it sends the goods to the laboratory for testing.
- If the aggrieved party is not happy with the jurisdiction of the State Commission, then they can appeal against the judgment of this agency in the National Commission within 30 days by depositing 50% of the fine money.

National Commission

- A National Commission includes a president and four other members one of whom shall be a woman, and Central Government appoints them.
- One can file a complaint of goods and services worth more than 10 crores in this agency.
- After receiving a complaint from the aggrieved party, the National Commission

informs the party against whom the complaint has been filed. Also, for the complaints filed, if the National Commission feels a requirement, it sends the goods to the laboratory for testing, and then gives judgment based on the reports.
- If the aggrieved party is not happy with the jurisdiction of the National Commission, then they can appeal against the judgment of this agency in the Supreme Court within 30 days by depositing 50% of the fine money.

WHAT IS PROFESSIONAL INDEMNITY POLICY? (FM4.8)

- The doctors can ensure their professional practice by way of taking professional indemnity policy. In the event of compensation if any to be paid in medical negligence cases the insurance company which provides the service will pay the compensations to the patient.
- The professional indemnity service is also provided by the respective Indian Medical Association at the state level branches.
- Depending on their clinical set up and the types of patients they handle, the doctors can take policies up to their convenience and necessity, and make their own options in payment of premium money.
- In such cases, the case itself is taken over by the insurance company and the compensation is also paid by them directly to the patient, within the limits of their insurance amount.
- Hence, it is advisable that every doctor should protect his practice by taking a professional insurance cover before they start up their medical practice, since no one can say when things may go wrong and at what moment of time litigations may arise during their professional practice.

DESCRIBE WORKMEN COMPENSATION ACT (1923) (FM4.8)

- This act provides for the payment of compensation to the employee for the injuries sustained by accident, in the course of his work or employment at his work place.
- If the workman dies, then the dependents are entitled to receive the compensation.
- If he contracts any diseases, as an occupational disease related to that particular employment, it is deemed to be an injury by accident for the purpose of compensation.
- The amount of compensation depends upon whether the injury has caused death, permanent total disablement or permanent partial disablement.
- Any medical sequence which connects the disability or death with the event at work is legally adequate for awarding compensation.
- The workman is not eligible for compensation if at the time of sustaining the injuries he was under the influence of alcohol or drugs.
- In all industrial diseases and injuries medical evidence is mandatory; hence the doctor must keep all relevant treatment records and is also bound to opine the relationship between the injury and death or acceleration of a pre-existing natural disease by the injury.
- The medical certificate issued in all such cases must be accurate and without any influence or ambiguity.

ESI (EMPLOYEES STATE INSURANCE) ACT 1948 (FM4.8)

- ESI Act aims to provide certain benefits to the employees in case of sickness, maternity and employment injury and to make provision for certain other matters in relation thereto.
- The ESI Corporation is headed by the Union Minister of Labor, as its Chairman, whereas the Director General, appointed by the Central Government functions as its Chief Executive Officer.
- Every insurable employee under the Act gets medical benefits the day he becomes

an employee. This benefit extends to his family members as well. This medical benefit has no ceiling in terms of expenditure on healthcare. Hence, the ESI Corporation takes care of all treatment expenses as per its rules.
- The ESI scheme is applicable to all factories and other establishments as defined in the Act with 10 or more persons employed in such establishment and the beneficiaries monthly wage does not exceed ₹ 21,000.
- The ESIC has fixed the contribution rate of the employees at 0.75% of their wages and the employer's contribution at 3.25% of the wages for financial year 2023–24. Employees earning daily average wage up to ₹ 176 are exempted from ESIC contribution.
- **Maternity benefit:** For pregnancy is payable for 26 weeks, which can be extended up to 1 month on medical advice.
- ESI registration provides social security to employees and their dependents in case of contingencies.

MULTIPLE CHOICE QUESTIONS

1. **Consent is not a must in:**
    a. Examination of victim of sodomy
    b. Examination of a drunken person
    c. Examination of an accused of dacoity
    d. Testing blood for malaria
2. **In case of an unconscious person requiring emergency surgery, there are no relatives to give consent then, the doctor should:**
    a. Operate without consent
    b. Operate with the consent of the police
    c. Wait for the relatives to come
    d. Operate with the consent of medical superintendent of the hospital
3. **Which of the following is the best form of consent obtained for an operation?**
    a. Verbal consent
    b. Implied consent
    c. Guardian informed consent
    d. Written informed consent
4. **A doctor while examining the patient without consent in an emergency is protected under:**
    a. Section 87 IPC
    b. Section 89 IPC
    c. Section 90 IPC
    d. Section 92 IPC
5. **When a patient dies due to some unintentional act during treatment by a doctor or agent of a doctor in the hospital?**
    a. Therapeutic privilege
    b. Therapeutic misadventure
    c. Vicarious liability
    d. Error of judgment
6. **All are true regarding criminal negligence, except:**
    a. Trial is by criminal court
    b. Can be imprisoned
    c. Consent for the act is a good defense
    d. Guilt should be proved beyond doubt
7. **All the following are examples of res ipsa loquitor, except:**
    a. Death on the operation table
    b. A forceps left over in the abdomen during surgery
    c. Twenty barbiturate tablets found in the stomach at autopsy
    d. Operation on the wrong limb
8. **Novus actus interveniens is:**
    a. An unrelated action intervening
    b. The thing speaks for itself
    c. Calculated risk doctrine
    d. Assisting unqualified persons in the treatment of patients
9. **Under Consumer Protection Act complaints has to be filled within:**
    a. 3 months
    b. 6 months
    c. 1 year
    d. 2 years
10. **A plaintiff is a person who:**
    a. Files the complaint
    b. He's the assailant
    c. He's the defendant
    d. Is the public prosecutor
11. **The burden of proof lies with the doctor in cases of:**
    a. Mens rea
    b. Res judicata
    c. Res ipsa loquitor
    d. Respondent superior

12. **Contributory negligence is related to:**
    a. Eggshell rule
    b. Master-servant rule
    c. Common knowledge rule
    d. Avoidable consequences rule
13. **Doctrine of common knowledge is a variant of:**
    a. Medical maloccurrence
    b. Novus actus interveniens
    c. Res ispa loquitor
    d. Calculated risk doctrine
14. **Vicarious responsibility pertains to:**
    a. Patient's contribution towards negligence
    b. Hospitals contribution towards patient's damage
    c. Responsibility for action of a colleague
    d. Responsibility of senior for actions of junior
15. **If death of a patient occurs during surgery due to the negligence of the surgeon, then he can be charged under:**
    a. 299 IPC
    b. 300 C IPC
    c. 304 A IPC
    d. 304 B IPC
16. **In civil negligence cases against the doctor, the onus of the proof lies with:**
    a. Doctor
    b. Patient
    c. Defense lawyer
    d. Police not below the rank of sub-inspector
17. **Burden to prove lies with the doctor in case of:**
    a. Mens rea
    b. Res ipsa loquitor
    c. Res judicata
    d. Respondent superior
18. **During an operation, if a pair of scissors is left in abdomen, the doctrine applicable is:**
    a. Res indicata
    b. Res judicata
    c. Res gestae
    d. Res ipsa loquitor
19. **Apex body dealing with medical negligence cases under Consumer Protection Act:**
    a. National Medical Commission
    b. High Court
    c. Supreme Court
    d. National Consumer Commission
20. **Maximum amount that can be received under the Consumer Protection Act:**
    a. 25 lakhs
    b. 50 lakhs
    c. 75 lakhs
    d. More than 100 lakhs
21. **Doctor liable to get sued by patient till what time limit from alleged negligence:**
    a. 1 year
    b. 2 years
    c. 3 years
    d. 4 years
22. **According to recent SC judgment, doctor can be charged for medical negligence under 304-A, IPC only if:**
    a. He is from corporate hospital
    b. Negligence is from inadvertent error
    c. Therapeutic misadventure
    d. Gross negligence
23. **Liability for wrong limb amputation can be considered under:**
    a. Criminal negligence
    b. Civil negligence
    c. Both civil and criminal
    d. Contributory negligence
24. **The punishment for criminal negligence may be:**
    a. Fine
    b. Imprisonment
    c. Erasure of the name from medical register
    d. All in combination

ANSWERS

1. c	2. a	3. d	4. d	5. b	6. c	7. a	8. a	9. d	10. a
11. c	12. d	13. c	14. d	15. c	16. b	17. b	18. d	19. d	20. d
21. b	22. d	23. c	24. d						

SECTION 2

Personal Identity

SECTION OUTLINE

Chapter 5: Identification of the Living and Dead
Chapter 6: Trace Evidences and Forensic Science Laboratory

CHAPTER 5

Identification of the Living and Dead

> ## 🔑 KEY WORDS
>
> Identity, corpus delicti, race, cephalic index, age, medicolegal importance of age, Gustafson's method, sex, barr bodies, Davidson's body, concealed sex, intersex, Klinefelter's syndrome, Turner's syndrome, Krogman's accuracy, Hasee's rule, age, mixed dentition, stature, bite marks, forensic odontology, dactylography, cheiloscopy, dermatoglyphics, scars, tattoo marks, superimposition.

FM3.1	Define and describe corpus delicti, establishment of identity of living persons including race, sex, religion, complexion, stature, age determination using morphology, teeth-eruption, decay, bite marks, bones-ossification centers, medicolegal aspects of age.
FM3.2	Describe and discuss identification of criminals, unknown persons, dead bodies from the remains-hairs, fibers, teeth, anthropometry, dactylography, foot prints, scars, tattoos, poroscopy and superimposition.

INTRODUCTION

- **Identification** is defined as the determination of individuality of a person based on certain physical characteristics; i.e., fixation of the personality.
- Identification of an individual may be complete or partial.
    - *Complete (Absolute) identification:* The absolute fixation of individuality of a person.
    - *Incomplete (Partial) identification:* Ascertainment of only some facts about the identity of an individual; while others remains still unknown. Adding on the data will help in establishment of absolute identity at later stage of time.
- Identification of the living is usually carried out by the police; but in the identification of the dead, the doctor has a great role to play.
- Many a time's medical men are called for elucidation of disputed facts in the process of fixing the identification.

DISCUSS THE MEDICOLEGAL ASPECTS OF IDENTITY?

- The question of identity may arise, both in civil and criminal cases.
- Absolute identity is required in civil courts in cases of (i) Insurance, (ii) Inheritance claims, (iii) Pension, (iv) Marriage, (v) Disputed sex, (vi) Passport, (vii) Missing persons, etc.

- Identity an essential components in many criminal cases like:
  - Absolute identification of both the accused and the victim is mandatory in cases of assault, rape, murder, etc.
  - Interchange of newborn in hospital.
  - Impersonation (one person going in the place of other).
  - In deaths due to fire, explosion, travel accidents and other mishaps (mass disasters).
  - When an unknown dead body is found somewhere.
  - In decomposed or mutilated bodies and skeletal remains.

WHAT IS CORPUS DELICTI? (FM3.1)

- Corpus delicti refers to the body of offence or the essence of crime; corpus delicti refers to the fact of any criminal offence.
- **Example:** In cases of murder, corpus delicti is the fact that a person died due to some unlawful act. It includes positive identification of the dead body of the victim and the other facts which are conclusive of death due to foul play; such as a bullet or broken knife found in the body or at the scene of crime and which is responsible for death. It also includes any trace evidences present in the scene of crime, like blood stains, hair, etc.
- Accurate identification of the dead body and proof of corpus delicti is mandatory before a sentence is passed in homicidal deaths.
- There are recorded cases where unclaimed dead bodies, decomposed bodies, portions of a dead body or bones are brought to the doctor to support a false charge. However, there are circumstances where punishment was awarded even when the body was not found or was not identified.

WHAT ARE THE VARIOUS DATA USEFUL FOR IDENTIFICATION?

- Race
- Religion
- Sex
- Age
- General development and stature
- Complexion and other features
- External peculiarities such as moles, birth marks, deformities, malformation, scars, tattoo marks, occupational marks, etc.
- Anthropometric measurements
- Finger prints (dactylography)
- Foot prints (dermatoglyphics)
- Lip prints (cheiloscopy)
- Teeth
- Clothes and personal articles (pocket contents, jewels, etc.)
- DNA profile

In the living: In addition to the above, the following data are also useful.

- Hand writing
- Speech and Voice
- Gait, tricks, manner and habits
- Memory and education

DESCRIBE RACES OF HUMAN POPULATION? (FM3.1)

Race

Human beings are broadly divided into three broad races namely, caucasoid, negroid and mongoloid. The features of race are well evident in the skull and it is based on the cephalic index. Features useful to find out the race are described in **Table 5.1.**

WHAT IS CEPHALIC INDEX? (FM3.1)

$$\text{Cephalic index} = \frac{\text{Maximum breath of the skull}}{\text{Maximum length of the skull}} \times 100$$

TABLE 5.1: Features useful to find out the race.

Features	Indians	Europeans	Negroes
Complexion (limited value)	Brown	Fair	Black
Eyes	Dark eyes, a few have brown eyes	Blue or grey eyes	Black
Hair	Black, thin and wavy hair	Fair, light brown or reddish hair	Black, wooly hair (arranged in tight spirals)

TABLE 5.2: Cephalic index and race.

Types of skull	Cephalic index	Race
Dolichocephalic (long headed)	70 to 75	Negroes and pure aryans
Mesaticephalic (medium head)	75 to 80	Europeans
Brachycephalic (short headed)	80 to 85	Mongolians

- The length (frontal eminence to occipital protuberance) and the breath (bi-parietal) are measured using osteometric board.
- The race of an individual can be identified by calculating the cephalic index. Based on the cephalic index the skulls are grouped into three major categories of races, tabulated in **Table 5.2**.

APPLICATION OF RELIGION IN FIXING THE IDENTIFICATION (FM3.1)

- Some of the features may help in finding out the religion of an individual.
- Muslim males are circumcised and the females wear full covered black dress.
- Hindu males may have some religious markings on the forehead depending on the customs of their sub-division. Hindu married females may have vermillion mark on their forehead.
- All these are of less value in finding out the religion and hence the religion of a person has less value in determination of identity of an individual.

DESCRIBE HOW TO DETERMINE THE SEX OF AN INDIVIDUAL? (FM3.1)

- Sex plays a major role in establishing the identification, as all the individual fall into any one of the two sexes.
- Determination of sex becomes necessary in cases relating to legal heir disputes, marriage, divorce, legitimacy, impotence, rape, etc.

Sex of a person can be determined from:
- Physical morphology
- Microscopic study of sex chromatin
- Gonadal biopsy

Table 5.3 describes presumptive evidence of sex. **Table 5.4** outlines highly probable evidence of sex. **Table 5.5** details positive evidence of sex.

TABLE 5.3: Presumptive evidence of sex.

Features	Male	Female
General built	Muscular, strong and stout	Less muscular, delicate and slender
Scalp hair	Short and coarse	Long and fine
Eye brows	Coarse and thick	Fine and thin
Beard and mustache	Present	Absent
Pubic hair	Coarse, and thick extends upwards with apex at umbilicus	Thin, fine does not extend upwards. Triangular in distribution

TABLE 5.4: Highly probable evidence of sex.

Features	Male	Female
Breast	Not developed, nipple and areola small	Well developed after puberty
Distribution of SC fat	Absent	Present
Vagina and cervix	Absent	Present
Penis	Present	Absent

TABLE 5.5: Positive evidence of sex.

Features	Male	Female
Ovaries, fallopian tubes and uterus	Absent	Present
Scrotum with testis, prostrate and seminal vesicle	Present	Absent

Sex Chromatin

- The demonstration of Barr bodies and Davidson's bodies are used in sex determination.
- Out of 46 chromosomes present in each cell of our body, 44 (22 pairs) are autosomes and 2 (1 pair) are sex chromosomes.
- In males, the patterns of sex chromosomes are XY and in females it's XX.
- In 1949, Barr and Bertram noticed a nodule in the nuclei of some cells of female cats.
- Later, investigations revealed that this nodule was found in a percentage of all normal women's cells (chromatin positive).

Barr Bodies

- Microscopically, this nodule is seen as a condensed material towards the nuclear membrane inside the nucleus of the cell. This is called the **sex chromatin** or **Barr body**.
- The Barr bodies are best demonstrated in the cells of **buccal mucosa**, skin and cartilages.
- In the buccal smear, sex chromatin is demonstrable as a small plano convex mass, lying near the nuclear membrane inside the nucleus (Intranuclear inclusion bodies); which are present in 20 to 30% in female cells and only in 0 to 4% of male cells.

Davidson Body

- In neutrophilic leucocytes (WBC), the sex chromatin is often present in the form of nuclear lobes, resembling a drumstick. This is known as Davidson body.
- To differentiate sex by demonstration of Davidson's bodies, the peripheral smear must show these bodies in at least 6% cells, to identifying the individual as female.

Gonadal Biopsy

Confirmatory method of determining the sex is by Gonadal biopsy. In all the cases of disputes in sexual identity, Biopsy from the primary gonads is called for.

WHAT IS CONCEALED SEX?

- Criminals may try to conceal their sex to avoid detection by the police by wearing costume of the opposite sex.
- Simple undressing may be rewarding in many cases, other investigations may be necessary in some cases to reach a satisfactory conclusion in the identification of sex.

WHAT IS INTERSEX? HOW DO WE CLASSIFY INTERSEX? (FM3.1)

Intersex: Intersex is due to disorders of sexual differentiation.

- Whole of the world population will fall into either of the two sexes, there are individuals

who are neither male nor female and they are categorized as intersex.
- Intersex is an intermingling of sexual characters of both the sexes in a single individual to a varying degree including, physical forms, reproductive organs and sex behaviors.
- Sexual differentiation is a sequential and ordered process. Chromosomal sex, established at the moment of fertilization determines the Gonadal sex, which in turn causes the development of phenotypic sex. Defects in any of the stages sex differentiation process results in intersex.

Classification of Intersex

- Disorders of chromosomal sex:
  - Klinefelter's syndrome in males, and
  - Turner's syndrome in females
- Disorders of Gonadal sex:
  - Pure gonadal dysgenesis
  - Gonadal agenesis (absent testis syndrome)
- Disorders of phenotypic sex (hermaphroditism)
  - True hermaphroditism
  - Pseudohermaphroditism: Male and female.

DESCRIBE KLINEFELTER'S SYNDROME AND TURNER'S SYNDROME? (FM3.1)

Disorders of Chromosomal Sex

Klinefelter Syndrome

- It is male hypogonadism and the chromosomal pattern is 47 XXY; the incidence is 1 in 850 male live births. It is the commonest cause of hypogonadism in males.
- The characteristic features include eunuch body habits and behaviors, abnormally long legs and upper limbs.
- Small atrophic testis often associated with small penis, lack of some secondary sexual characteristics such as deep voice, beard, mustache and male pattern of distribution of pubic hair.
- Gynecomastia is a usual finding, associated with varying degree of mental retardation.
- It is the principal cause of male infertility.

Turner Syndrome

- Female hypogonadism and the chromosomal pattern is 45 XO.
- Most common sex chromosomal abnormality in females.
- The characteristic features are short stature, low posterior hairline, webbing of neck, broad chest with widely spaced nipples, cubitus valgus, pigmented naevi, and peripheral lymph edema.
- Coarctation of aorta is a common finding.
- It is the most important cause of primary amenorrhea.

Disorders of Gonadal Sex

- **Pure gonadal dysgenesis:** There is defective and improper development of gonads.
- **Gonadal agenesis (absent testis syndrome):** In this condition, there is complete absence of both the testis.

DISCUSS ABOUT TRUE HERMAPHRODITISM?

Disorders of Phenotypic Sex

Hermaphroditism: Means co-existence of sexual characteristics of both males and females, to a varying degree in the same individual.

True Hermaphroditism

- True hermaphroditism implies the presence of both ovaries and testis in the same individual.
- It's extremely rare. In some cases, there may be a testis on one side and an ovary on the other side. Whereas in some

cases, there may be combined ovarian and testicular tissue known as ovotestis; karyotype is 46 XX in 50% of cases, and 46 XY in 25% of cases.

MALE AND FEMALE PSEUDOHERMAPHRODITISM

Female Pseudohermaphroditism (Fig. 5.1)

- In this, the chromosomal sex pattern is 46 XX in all cases.
- The development of Gonads (ovaries) and internal genitalia are normal.
- Only the external genitalia are ambiguous or virilized.
- The basis of this disorder is excessive and inappropriate exposure to androgenic steroids during early fetal life.

Male Pseudohermaphroditism

- In this, the chromosomal sex pattern is 46 XY in all cases.
- But the external genitalia are either ambiguous or of completely feminine.
- Commonest cause is defective virilization of male embryo, which usually results from genetically determined defects in androgen synthesis or activity or both.

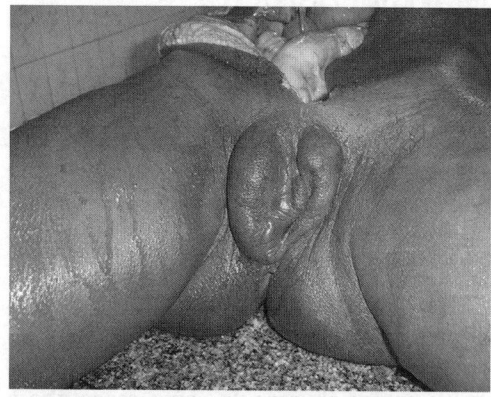

Fig. 5.1: Female pseudohermaphroditism *(For color version see Plate 1).*

HOW TO DETERMINE THE SEX IN THE DEAD/DECOMPOSED/ SKELETAL REMAINS? (FM1.3)

In a Decomposed Body

- Make a search for the cervix, fallopian tubes and ovaries.
- Uterus is the last internal organs to putrefy in a female and prostrate in males.
- When the primary sex organs are totally unidentifiable, one has to look for sexual characteristics in the skeleton.

Sex from Skeletal Remains

- For a trained Forensic Pathologist, it seldom poses a problem to determine the sex from skeletal remains.
- The accuracy of estimating the sex from skeletal remains depends upon the number of bones available.

WHAT IS KROGMAN'S ACCURACY?

Krogman's degree of accuracy is a method to identify the sex from skeletal remains. The degree of accuracy depends on the total number of bones available and the type of bone available for examination.

- When the entire skeleton is available the accuracy is 100%.
- When pelvis alone is available it is 95%.
- When skull alone is available the accuracy is 90%.
- When both pelvis and skull are available, the accuracy is 98%.
- Sex differentiating features are prominent only after puberty.
- The pelvis is the best suited bone for determining the sex even before attainment of puberty, since by nature the pelvic bone in females is designed for delivery of a fetus.
- Greater sciatic notch is small, narrow, deep and V shaped in males and large, wide, shallow and U shaped in females.

(Sciatic notch index = Width of the sciatic notch/Depth × 100)
- Preauricular sulcus present near the attachment of anterior sacroilliac ligament. In female pelvis, this will be broad, deep and frequently seen.
- Sex differences in the morphology of skull and mandible are quite reliable.
- Long bones, sternum and ribs were all tried for determination of sex; but, they are used only when skull, pelvis and mandible are not available.

WHAT IS MEDULLARY INDEX?

Sex of a long bone can be determined by the medullary index. Sex differentiating features are identifiable only on the ends of the long bones and are useful only when the whole intact long bone is available. When a fragment of bone or only the shaft is available, then medullary index is useful in determining the sex.

$$\text{Medullary index} = \frac{\text{Diameter of the medulla}}{\text{Diameter of the whole bone}} \times 100$$

WHAT IS ANTHROPOMETRY? (FM3.1)

Anthropometry is the method of identification of a person using the study of measurements of various body parts. It was a widely used method for identification of the living mainly missing or escaped prisoners and in mass disasters. But, after the invention of dactylography and DNA fingerprinting this method of identification has lost its importance.

WHAT IS STATURE? HOW DO WE ESTIMATE THE STATURE OF AN INDIVIDUAL FROM LONG BONES? (FM3.1)

- Estimation of stature or height of a person is subject to variations during life due to muscular relaxation and elasticity of intervertebral discs, but still is valuable.
- Height of an individual is mainly based on genetic factors and nutritional status.
- Growth of the long bones determines the height of an individual, which is by appearance and fusion of various secondary ossification centers of the long bones, which in turn are directly proportional to the nutritional status of the individual.
- All the bones fuse by about 18 to 21 years and hence the height of an individual does not increase after 21 years; and the height decreases after 35 years due to degenerative changes in the bones.
- In the examination of skeletal remains, stature of an individual is estimated using the length of the long bones; the length of the long bones is measured using Hepburn's Osteometric Board.

Stature: The approximate height of an individual will be:

2 × length of an arm + 30 cm + 4 cm
2 × length from vertex to symphysis pubis
8 × height of the skull with the mandible

HOW DO WE ESTIMATE THE AGE OF INDIVIDUAL? (FM3.1)

- **Estimation of age of an individual is based on:**
  - General physical development
  - Teeth (eruption of deciduous and permanent teeth)
  - Appearance and fusion of various secondary ossification centers of the bones
  - Secondary sexual characteristics
  - Age related changes (degenerative changes, after 25 years of age)
- **Age in intrauterine life:** It is assessed by the developmental morphology, appearance of primary ossification centers in the bones and germination of teeth.

- The intrauterine age of a fetus is calculated by applying the Rule of Hasee:
- **Hasee's rule:** This is a method to determine the age of the fetus in the intrauterine life. Length of the fetus (crown-heel length) is measured; if the length is less 25 cm, then the square root gives the approximate age of the fetus in months; when the length is more than 25 cm, then the length divided by 5, which gives the approximate age of fetus in months. For example, if length is 9 cm, then the age is 3 months; if length is 35 cm, age is 7 months.

AGE ESTIMATION IN CHILDREN AND ADULTS UNDER 25 YEARS

This is the crucial period of age, where the court refers the individual to the doctor for the estimation of age; even if there are reliable records like birth certificate, school certificate, or any other documents which specifies the correct age, the court relies on the opinion of the doctor is estimation of age based on scientific medical facts.

The various data useful to estimate the age below 25 years are:
- Physical examination and secondary sexual characteristics.
- **Dental examination:** Eruption and completion of root formation.
- **Radiological examination:** Appearance and fusion of various secondary ossification centers

Physical Examination and Secondary Sexual Characteristics (Table 5.6)

The external appearance including the height, general built, etc., will indicate the approximate age of an individual. In addition to this, presence or absence of secondary sexual characters like beard and mustache in males, development of breast in females, axillary and pubic hair in both the sexes are helpful in estimation of age of the individual.

APPLICATION OF ERUPTION OF TEETH IN ESTIMATION OF AGE (FM3.1)

Dentition

- Every individual has two sets of teeth in his/her life time. They are temporary teeth and permanent teeth.
- Temporary teeth or deciduous teeth or milk teeth, are 20 in number.
- Permanent teeth 32 in number. Those teeth which erupt in the place of a temporary teeth are called "successive teeth" (20 in number) and all the three the permanent molars which erupts behind the successive teeth are called '**super added teeth**" (12 in number).
- The eruption of both temporary and permanent teeth follows a chronological order, this is useful for estimation of age of an individual; root formation gets

TABLE 5.6: Growth of hair in male and female.

Features	Male	Female
Pubic hair	13–15 years	13–14 years
Axillary hair	14–16 years	14–15 years
Beard and mush	15–17 years	Absent
Hair on other parts	17–20 years	Sparse
Graying of hair	Scalp: 40 years (not reliable) Pubic hair: 55 years (reliable)	Scalp: 40 Pubic hair: 55 years
Baldness	After 40 years (not reliable)	Rare

completed after 2 to 3 years of eruption of the teeth in the oral cavity.
- At birth, there are 44 germ tooth present inside the jaw of a full term baby (20 + 24).
- These germ teeth develop and erupt outside into the oral cavity, and then the root formation takes place.
- By 3 years, there are totally 20 teeth all are temporary.
- By 6 to 7 years, there are 24 teeth (20 temporary and 4 permanent).
- From 6 to 12 years total number of teeth remains as 24 (mixed dentition).

WHAT IS MIXED DENTITION?

- The period of time when both temporary teeth and permanent teeth are present inside the oral cavity; i.e., from the eruption of 1st permanent molar to the time of eruption of last permanent canine (6 to 12 years).
- By the end of 12 years, the total number of teeth remains 24, but all are permanent.
- By 14 years, there are 28 teeth.
- Third molar erupts by 17 to 25 years (wide range) and not useful in estimation of age. It may not erupt at all or may get impacted, depending upon the length of the mandible.

- The root formation take 2 more years after the eruption of the teeth in the oral cavity and is 3 years for the 3rd molar for completion of formation of the root. Hence, while examination of radiological picture of teeth for age estimation, the root of the last erupted teeth and the crown of the next to erupt teeth is considered to arrive at a more accurate age.

HOW TO DIFFERENCE TEMPORARY TEETH FROM PERMANENT TEETH?

See **Table 5.7**.

APPLICATION OF RADIOLOGY IN ESTIMATION OF AGE (FM3.1)

- Estimation of age is based on the appearance and fusion of various secondary ossification centers in the body.
- The bones of human body develop from a number of ossification centers.
- At 11–12th week of intrauterine life, there are 806 centers of ossification.
- At birth there are about 450 centers.
- The adult human skeleton carries only 206 bones.
- After birth, the growth of the bone is by formation of various secondary

TABLE 5.7: Differences between temporary teeth and permanent teeth.

Features	Temporary teeth	Permanent teeth
Size	Small, light and narrow	Large, heavy and broad
Color	Milky white	Ivory white
Edges	Smooth cutting edges	Irregular cutting edges
Neck	Neck is constricted	Not constricted
Inclination	Vertically placed	Inclined forward
Ridge	Thick ridge is present at the junction of crown and root	No such ridge is present
Roots of molar teeth	Roots of the molar teeth are small and more divergent	Roots of the molars are big and less divergent
X-Ray/OPG	Germ toot of permanent teeth present	Germ tooth are not seen

ossification centers. The bone growth gets completed by fusion of the shaft with the ossification center.
- The appearance and fusion of various secondary ossification centers have a sequence and time period; this chronological sequence is used for determination of age.
  (Please Note: The appearance and fusion of various ossification centers are discussed in practical exercise—You need to write the tables in exams)

DESCRIBE GUSTAFSON'S METHOD?

- It is a method useful to estimate the age of an individual after 25 years, by the degenerative changes occurring in the teeth; it's used only for dead individuals and not for the living. Only attrition can be made out in living individuals, which is a least reliable data.
- The various criteria taken into consideration are (APSRTC):
  - *Attrition:* Wear and tear seen over the occlusal surface.
  - *Paradentosis:* The gum margins become retracted and there is loosening of teeth.
  - *Secondary dentin:* Deposition of dentin (secondarily) within the pulp cavity.
  - *Root resorption:* Root resorption due to ageing and tooth may fall off at varying ages.
  - *Transparency of root:* It is the transparency of the dentin at the root level.
  - *Cementum apposition:* Apposition of cementum at and around the root of the teeth.
- Among the above said criteria, the transparency of the root is most reliable indicator for the estimation of age. In addition to this, the incremental lines on cross-section of the teeth are also used for estimating the age of an individual.

- After 25 years, the estimation of age becomes more uncertain. It's difficult to achieve an accuracy of even 5 years.
- The closure of skull sutures is considered reasonably reliable up to 45 years.
- The changes occurring on the articular surface of symphysis pubis are considered as a reliable index for ageing beyond 25 years of age. But this indicator cannot be used for age estimation in living individuals.

WRITE SHORT NOTES ON FORENSIC ODONTOLOGY

- Forensic odontology is a branch of dental medicine applicable in resolving issues pertaining to law.
- It's a separate super specialty in advanced countries; in India, this branch is attached to oral medicine department. The applicability is for identification, comparison and examination of bite marks.
- As like finger prints, the teeth pattern of any individual is unique; no two individual may have the same teeth pattern and hence useful when previous records are available and helps to fix or exclude a subject by comparison of both the data.
- Useful in identification, especially in mass disasters; when the antemortem records are available. This can be easily compared to fix the absolute identity.
- In criminal cases, the pattern can be compared with that of the accused person, thus helps to conclude or exclude a particular individual.

While documenting a data regarding a tooth, charting should be with reference to:
- Extractions of teeth (fresh or old)
- Tooth filling
- Missing tooth
- Artificial teeth (implanted or metal tooth—gold tooth)
- Broken tooth
- Crowned tooth

- Pathological conditions and congenital defects.
- Artificial dentures are also used for identification.

DISCUSS THE METHODS OF CHARTING OF TEETH?

- There are various methods of charting teeth they are (i) Universal system, (ii) Palmar notation, (iii) Haderup system and (iv) FDI system. Among these palmar notation and FDI system are conventionally followed.
- **Palmer's notation:** The oral cavity is divided into four quadrants; right and left are marked. Each tooth is given a number from 1 to 8, starting from the incisors to the 3rd molar. For temporary teeth it's marked as "T" and for permanent teeth as "P" above the respective teeth.

Right															Left
8|7|6|5|4|3|2|1|1|2|3|4|5|6|7|8
8|7|6|5|4|3|2|1|1|2|3|4|5|6|7|8

Federation dentaire internationale (FDI) system:
- It's similar to palmer's notation but one number in added in front of the tooth number, which indicates the quadrant in which the tooth is located. Each tooth is identified by a two digit number in which, the proximal digit indicates the quadrant and the distal digit indicates the actual tooth. While numbering the permanent teeth, the quadrants 1, 2, 3, 4 are used for designating right upper, left upper, left lower and right lower quadrants respectively. Whereas 5, 6, 7, 8 are used for the corresponding temporary teeth.

DESCRIBE ON BITE MARKS? (FM3.1) (FIGS. 5.2 AND 5.3)

- Bite marks can be present on a living individual, dead body or any remnants of food, etc.
- Human bite marks are elucidated by using a hand lens to examine the bite mark.
- Since the teeth pattern is individualistic, bite marks present on the victim or the accused in cases of serious crimes like murder or sexual assault are useful for identification.
- A bite mark cast is prepared from the surface of the bite mark and compared with that of the subject, thus helps to include or exclude a particular individual.
- Bite marks on remnant food materials, such as on an apple or cheese can also be used to fix the identity.

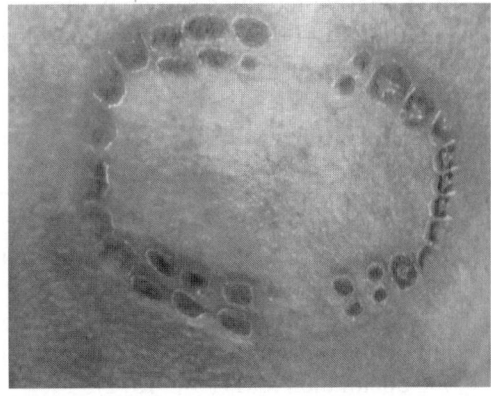

Fig. 5.2: Human bite mark showing the impression of all the 32 teeth *(For color version see Plate 1)*.

Permanent teeth

18	17	16	15	14	13	12	11	21	22	23	24	25	26	27	28
48	47	46	45	44	43	42	41	31	32	33	34	35	36	37	38

Temporary teeth

			55	54	53	52	51	61	62	63	64	65			
			85	84	83	82	81	71	72	73	74	75			

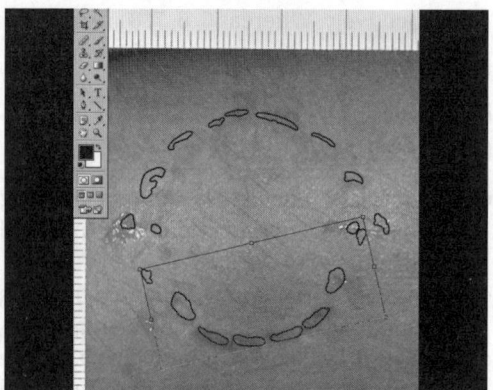

Fig. 5.3: Marking the bite marks and measuring the various dimensions for positive identification of the assailant *(For color version see Plate 1).*

- Bite marks may also give a clue to the motive of the offence by the site over which it is present. For example, over the breast and thighs in cases of sexual assault.
- While examining bite in dead bodies, the bite marks are dissected and bruising of the underlying tissues can be made out. The extent of bruising also gives an idea about the intensity of the bite.

DISCUSS THE MEDICOLEGAL IMPORTANCE OF AGE? (FM3.1)

- Within about a week of fertilization, the ovum gets impregnated in the uterus and it is termed as embryo.
- **3 lunar months (12 weeks):** Pregnancy can be terminated under the decision of one doctor alone (MTP Act 1971)
- **20 weeks:** The opinion of two doctors is necessary for termination of pregnancy.
- **210 days (7 calendar months):** The fetus becomes viable; viability is the ability of a fetus to have a separate existence of its own out of the mother's womb.
- **Ten lunar months:** Full term fetus.
- **1 year:** Up to 1 year of age after birth, the baby is called as an "Infant"; killing of the baby up to this age amounts to infanticide (Section 318 IPC).
- **5 years:** Above this age, a child becomes responsible for his act leading to wreckage of a train (according to Indian Railway Act).
- **7 years (minimum age of criminal responsibility):** Below this age a child is not criminally responsible (Section 82 IPC).
- **7 to 12 years:** A child is criminally responsible, if the child has attained sufficient mental maturity to understand the nature and consequences of his act (Section 83 IPC).
- **10 years:** Kidnapping a child with the intention of taking away dishonestly any movable property (Section 369 IPC).
- **12 years:**
  - Age of criminal liability; every individual above 12 years is criminally responsible for all the acts committed by him.
  - Consent can be given for simple procedures which are not known to cause any harm.
- **14 years:** Below this age a person (child) cannot be employed into any work and will amount to child labour: According to Indian Factories Act.
- **15 years:**
  - Below the age of 15 years, sexual intercourse with a woman, even if she is his own wife, amounts to Rape.
  - A person above this age can be employed in a factory like an adult.
- **18 years:**
  - A female can give valid consent for sexual intercourse.
  - *Majority:* Up to 18 years an individual is considered as a juvenile.
  - *Kidnapping:* Taking away an individual of less than 18 years from the legal guardian amounts to the offence of kidnapping.
  - *Marriage:* Minimum permissible age of marriage for girls, as per the Hindu Marriage Act.
  - *Consent:* A person above this age can give valid consent to suffer any

harm done in good faith; e.g., consent for surgery, blood donation, organ donation, etc.
- *Vote:* Age for voting and for obtaining driving license.
- *Will:* A person can make a valid will (testamentary capacity), if he is mentally sound (compos mentis).
- **21 years:**
  - A person who is under the guidance of the court attains majority.
  - Minimum age of marriage for boys.
  - Up to this age, a juvenile offender can stay in a borstal school.
  - Importing a girl below this age from outside the country for the purpose of forcing or seducing her to illicit intercourse amounts to kidnapping.
- **25 years:** Minimum age for contesting in elections.
- **35 years:** Minimum age for appointment as President/Vice-President of India or Governor of a state.
- **60 years:** Senior citizen, age of retirement.

DESCRIBE DACTYLOGRAPHY (GALTON SYSTEM)? (FM3.2)

- Dactylography is a system of identification of an individual based on fingerprints.
- This system was first discovered by Sir William J Herschel, he introduced this system in Hooghly District of Bengal in 1877.
- It was later systematically put into practice in 1892 by Sir Francis Galton, an English Anthropologist.
- The 1st case where finger printing was used for identification was in Argentina in the year 1892.

Principle

- The skin covering the ball of the thumb and other fingers is made up of characteristic epidermal ridges.
- These ridges are present both in the dermis and epidermis.
- The arrangement and distribution of these ridges are formed during intrauterine life and remain constant and persists throughout the lifetime.
- Fingerprints are highly individualistic. They are not similar even in monozygotic twins.

Classification

There are four types of fingerprints, they are:
1. Loops (radial or ulnar)—most common about 67%
2. Whorls (concentric or spiral)—25%
3. Arches (plain or tented)—6–7%
4. Composites (central pocket loops, double loops or accidentals)—1–2%

Identification is based on:
- Counting the ridges between the core and delta, where core is the central portion and the peripheral components are called the delta region.
- Minute details of the ridges like ridge ending, bifurcation, spur formation, dots, lake formation, broken ridge, short ridge, etc., are compared with the existing available data base of the fingerprints.
- 16 to 20 points of similarity are necessary to establish positive identity.
- Now a computed automatic system (soft ware) is used, where it analyses nearly 100 points of comparison and it takes very less time to confirm or rule out a suspect.

Fingerprints in Decomposed Bodies

- In advanced putrefaction and cases of drowning, the skin is frequently found loose like a glove, which can be removed, preserved in formalin and used for taking impressions.
- If epidermis is lost due to decomposition, still prints can be obtained from the dermis.

WHAT IS POROSCOPY? (FM3.2)

- Papillary ridges of the epidermis are studded with minute Pores, which contain sweat glands through which sweat exudes out.
- The number, size, shape and the site of a pore in a given length of a ridge vary from person to person and are unique for an individual.
- This method of studying the pores and used for identification is called "**Poroscopy**". This method was introduced by Edmond Locard.
- Combination of dactylography and poroscopy helps to fix better accuracy of identity.

DISCUSS THE METHODS OF REMOVAL OF FINGERPRINTS?

- Criminals may attempt to mutilate the finger print pattern by inflicting injuries or burns on the bulb of their fingers but there still exist definite delineation unless the true skin is destroyed. The injuries or burns produce a new different pattern which is unique to that particular individual.
- In mummified bodies where the tip of the finger shrunken formalin is injected into the tip of the finger to restore its original size and shape. Then the finger prints are obtained.

DESCRIBE THE TYPES OF FINGER-PRINTS IN THE SCENE OF CRIME?

There are three types of prints left over/ obtained from the crime scene and they are:
1. **Visible prints:** Prints which are contaminated with blood, paint, dirt, dyes etc. These prints are recorded by photography with suitable light and filters.
2. **Plastic prints:** These are impressions made on a soft substance like soap, cheese, wax, clay, etc.
3. **Latent prints:** Impressions due to deposition of sebaceous and sweat gland secretions. These are made visible by suitable reagent powders and recorded by a process called "**lifting**".

WHAT IS DERMATOGLYPHICS? (FM3.2)

- Study of footprints is called dermatoglyphics.
- Impressions of human feet on various substrates have been studied and found to be quite reliable and individualistic.
- Dermatoglyphics (the ridge pattern) if clearly visible is a positive factor for identification.
- In the absence of ridge pattern (prints on soil, sand etc.) measurement of length and width of foot toes and toe pads, arch pattern, the angle of inclination are used for comparison.

WHAT IS CHEILOSCOPY? (FM3.2)

- Cheiloscopy is the study lip prints; the furrows and grooves present on human lips are analyzed for a positive identification.
- The patterns of the furrows are unique and individualistic and are useful for identification.
- Lip print of a suspect can be obtained from wine glasses or other utensils.
- They are classified into four types. They are:
  1. Linear
  2. Bifurcate
  3. Reticular
  4. Undetermined
- Identification is based on analyzing the different appearances in a given length of the print.

DISCUSS THE OTHER UNIQUE FEATURES OF IDENTITY OF AN INDIVIDUAL?

- **Palatoprints:** The anterior part of the palate, structural details like rugae are

unique, specific and permanent in an individual. Hence, palatoprint is useful for positive identification as like fingerprints.
- **Ear print:** Based on the shape of the ears oval, round, rectangular or triangular. These prints are usually recovered from the doors, windows, etc., where the person leans or falls on these surfaces leaving a print. Which are made visible as like fingerprints. These ear prints are used to compare with the suspect.
- **Nose prints:** The lines on the nose and the shape of tip of the nose may also be helpful in positive identification. As like ear prints the impression of the nose may be isolated from doors, walls, etc.
- **Retina and iris:** The retinal pattern is unique to any individual. It is different even in monozygotic identical twin. The pattern is specific, reliable and remains unchanged from birth to death. Today the retinal pattern is used as most reliable biometric. The retina is scanned using low energy infrared rays. The result of the scanning are converted into computer code and stored in a database and used as best biometric tool.

WHAT IS A SCAR? WHAT ARE THE MEDICOLEGAL IMPORTANCE OF SCAR? (FM3.2) (FIGS. 5.4 TO 5.6)

- Scar is an acquired defect on the skin, widely accepted as a marker of identification.
- Scar is the result of repair mechanism to an injury involving the epidermis. It is covered by epithelium and is devoid of pigmentation, sweat glands and hair follicles.
- The size, shape and location of a scar can aid in positive identification.
- Peculiar scars like surgical scars, keloid formations, scars from burns and injuries, contracture due to acid burns, are reliable features to fix the identity of a person.

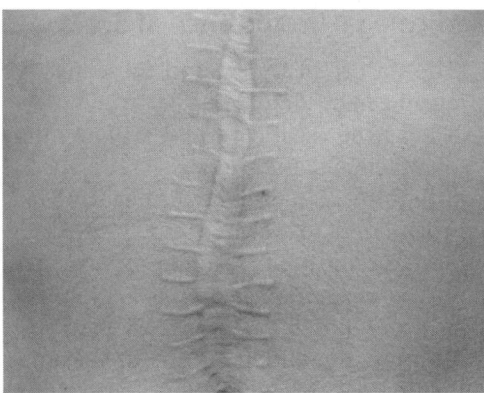

Fig. 5.4: Surgical incised wound scar of laparotomy, an unique feature of identification *(For color version see Plate 1).*

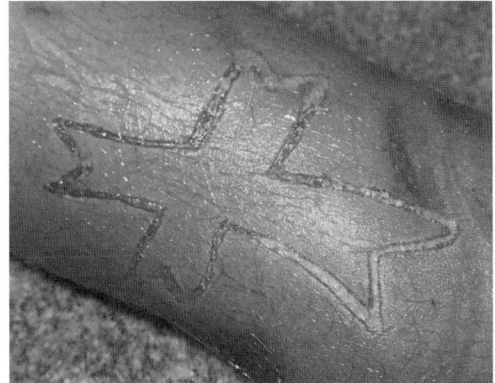

Fig. 5.5: Unique scar bearing the symbol of a cross, mode of infliction is suicidal *(For color version see Plate 1).*

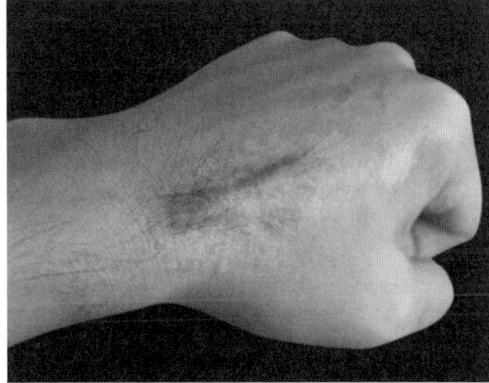

Fig. 5.6: Keloid formation on a pre-existing scar *(For color version see Plate 1).*

Medicolegal Importance of Scars

- The nature of injury and the causative agent can be identified.
- The age of a scar correlates with the time of infliction of the injury.
- Scar forming injuries on the head and face will amount to grievous hurt.
- Scars around a joint resulting in permanent restriction of movements also amounts to grievous hurt.
- Scars on the abdomen due to caesarian section or linea albicantes are indicative of delivery.

DESCRIBE TATTOO MARKS? (FM3.2) (FIGS. 5.7 AND 5.8)

- **Tattoo marks** are designs or patterns imprinted on the skin surface by multiple small punctured wounds with the help of needles dipped in coloring material (dye).
- The commonly used dyes are:
  - Carbon (black), Cinnabar
  - Vermillion (red)
  - Ochre (brown)
  - Chromic oxide (green)
  - Prussian blue (blue)
- The permanent nature of the tattoo mark depends on the type of dye used and the depth of penetration into the skin.
- Stable pigments such as carbon (black) or Prussian blue, impregnated into the deeper layers of skin last for a longer period of time.
- **Latent tattoo marks** can be revealed or made visible by use of ultraviolet light.
- Faint or disappeared tattoo marks can be made out by histological study of the regional lymph nodes.
- In decomposed bodies, they are made visible by treating the area with 3% hydrogen peroxide. When the epidermis is lost, the tattoo can be well appreciated as they are present on the dermis also.
- Tattoo marks can be removed by surgical method or use of laser beams, without leaving any permanent mark.
- A tattoo mark can be altered or superimposed over another subsequently, for the purpose of concealment of identity.

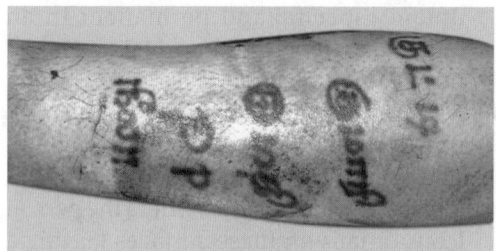

Fig. 5.8: Tattoo mark, especially useful for identification of decomposed bodies; well visible after skin slippage *(For color version see Plate 2).*

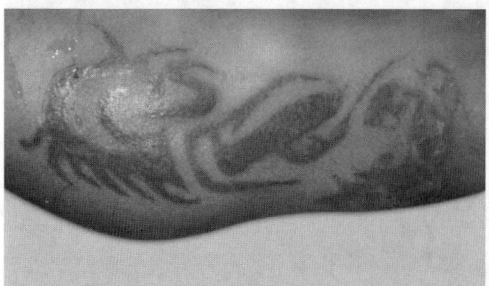

Fig. 5.7: Tattoo mark a unique tool of identification *(For color version see Plate 2).*

Complications of Tattoo Mark

- Septic inflammation
- Erysipelas
- Abscess
- Gangrene
- Syphilis and AIDS

Removal of Tattoo Mark (Erasure)

Tattoo mark can be erased by the following methods:

- Application of carbon dioxide snow.
- Application of caustic substances, e.g., mixture of papain in glycerin, Zn, Cl and tannic acid.

- Surgical method: Complete excision and skin grafting.
- Electrolysis.
- Laser beam.

Medicolegal Importance

- Tattoo marks are especially useful in decomposed bodies.
- Apart from identification, tattoo marks also provide additional information regarding: (1) Race (2) Religion (3) Nationality (4) Language (5) Mental makeup (6) Social status (7) Sex behaviors, etc.
- The name tattooed could be that of him or of a person associated or related to him.
- Drug addicts often imprint tattoos over areas of multiple injection mark, in order to conceal them.

DESCRIBE THE METHOD OF SUPERIMPOSITION OF SKULL? (FM3.2)

- Superimposition is a technique applied to determine whether the skull is that of the person in the photograph or not.
- An unknown skull with mandible and a photo of the missing person are required to perform superimposition.
- All the soft tissues attached to the skull are removed.
- The skull along with the mandible is fixed in a stand.
- The photograph is enlarged to "life size".
- The skull is adjusted to the same inclination and orientation as in the photograph.
- The negative of the photograph and the skull are superimposed over one another, by aligning the characteristic points in the negative.
- The anatomical landmarks are compared for a positive match.
- Recently, a computer graphic superimposition technique utilizing a laser scanner and indigenous computer software has been developed in India, which is being successfully employed in practice, which has got greater accuracy of matching.
- Performa based methodical approach can greatly improve the results and minimize errors.
- In superimposition, negative results are of more significance rather than a positive match. Since, the possibility of two individuals having the same morphologically similar skull pattern is possible. But in case of a mismatch, it can be conclusively said that the skull does not belong to the person in the photograph.

MEDICOLEGAL IMPORTANCE OF EYES

- It is useful for the purpose of identification; e.g., artificial eyes, color of iris, squint, cataract, etc.
- In certain poisoning cases findings in the eye plays an important role, e.g.
  - *Dilated pupil:* Datura, atropine, cannabis, cocaine, alcohol, etc.
  - *Contracted pupil:* Opium, Phenol, OPC compounds, pilocarpine, barbiturates, etc.
- **Arcus senilis:** It is circular, grey opaque ring like appearance surrounding the margins of the cornea. It is seen in old age individuals.
- **Mercurialentis:** Accumulation of mercury vapors on the anterior lens capsule in chronic mercury poisoning.

MULTIPLE CHOICE QUESTIONS

1. **The most reliable part of an inanimate bone to identify the sex of an individual is:**
   a. Obturator foramen
   b. Preauricular sulcus
   c. Greater sciatic notch
   d. Ischial tuberosity
2. **Cephalic index is used to determine:**
   a. Age
   b. Race
   c. Sex
   d. Stature

SECTION 2: Personal Identity

3. The total number of germ tooth present in a full term fetus is:
   a. 20
   b. 28
   c. 44
   d. 48
4. Karl Pearson's formula is to find out:
   a. Age
   b. Race
   c. Sex
   d. Stature
5. Barr body is seen in:
   a. Cornea
   b. Buccal epithelium
   c. Red blood cells
   d. White blood cells
6. Mixed dentition usually exists between:
   a. 3–5 years
   b. 5–10 years
   c. 6–12 years
   d. 7–14 years
7. 100% accuracy in personal identity can be done with:
   a. DNA finger printing
   b. Superimposition
   c. Photograph
   d. Dactylography
8. "XXY" pattern of sex chromosome is seen in:
   a. Hermaphrodites
   b. Pseudohermaphrodites
   c. Turner's syndrome
   d. Klinefelter's syndrome
9. Davidson's body is seen in:
   a. Neural epithelium
   b. RBC
   c. WBC
   d. Buccal epithelium
10. Medullary index is to find out the:
    a. Age
    b. Stature
    c. Race
    d. Sex
11. Age estimation by Gustafson's method is done more reliably with:
    a. Attrition
    b. Secondary dentin
    c. Transparency of root
    d. Cementum apposition
12. The basisphenoid unites with the basiocciput at the age of:
    a. 12 years
    b. 20 years
    c. 35 years
    d. 55 years
13. Corpus delicti means:
    a. Postmortem certificate
    b. Body of evidence
    c. Viscera report
    d. Inquest report
14. Minimum age for criminal responsibility is:
    a. 7 months
    b. 5 years
    c. 7 years
    d. 12 years
15. An obliterated tattoo mark can best be detected by:
    a. Treating the area with 0.1% HNO_3
    b. Histological study of regional lymph nodes
    c. Treating the area with 2% hydrogen peroxide
    d. All of the above
16. Trichology is the study of:
    a. Hair
    b. Tattoo
    c. Scars
    d. Complexion
17. The fingerprint pattern may be impaired permanently in cases of:
    a. Eczema
    b. Scalds
    c. Scabies
    d. Leprosy
18. Sample for DNA finger printing are all, *except*:
    a. Body tissues
    b. Blood
    c. Hair
    d. Nail
19. Tattoo mark help in identification of:
    a. Living individuals
    b. Death due to burns
    c. Death from electrical burns
    d. Decomposed bodies
20. Rule of Hasee is meant for:
    a. Estimation of age
    b. Estimation of gestational age
    c. Estimation of height of an individual
    d. Determination of sex
21. The most reliable test for blood:
    a. Benzidine test
    b. Phenolphthalein test

c. Spectroscopy
d. Kastle mayor test
22. Fingerprints at scene of crime can be found up to_____ after a crime if not disturbed.
a. 6 weeks
b. 6 months
c. 1 year
d. 3–6 years
23. Barr body is NOT seen in:
a. Turner syndrome
b. Klinefelter syndrome
c. Down's syndrome
d. Marfan's syndrome
24. A 19 year old female with short stature, wide spaced nipples and primary amenorrhea. Most likely she has a karyotype of:
a. 47 XY
b. 46 XXY
c. 47 XXY
d. 45 XO
25. Most common cause of congenital adrenal hyperplasia:
a. 21- Hydroxylase deficiency
b. 11- Hydroxylase deficiency
c. 17-α-Hydroxylase deficiency
d. 3-β-Hydroxylase dehydrogenase deficiency
26. All are true about permanent teeth, *except:*
a. Ridge is present between neck and body
b. Anterior teeth are inclined forward
c. Roots of molars are larger
d. They are ivory white in color
27. The most frequent tooth to be impacted:
a. Lower third molar
b. Upper third molar
c. Lower canine
d. Upper premolar
28. In males, first pubertal sign is:
a. Testicular enlargement
b. Hoarseness of voice
c. Pubic hair development
d. Penis enlargement
29. Species identification is best done by:
a. Neutron activation analysis
b. Acid dilution test.
c. Haemin crystal test
d. Precipitin test
30. The cephalic index of Indian population is between:
a. 70 to 75
b. 75 to 80
c. 80 to 85
d. 85 to 90
31. Commonest cause of female pseudohermaphroditism is:
a. Virilizing ovarian tumor
b. Ovarian dysgenesis
c. Exogenous androgen
d. Congenital adrenal hyperplasia
32. First permanent tooth to arise:
a. Incisors
b. Canine
c. Premolar
d. Molar
33. The percentage of sex chromatin in female blood leucocyte may be:
a. 0.02
b. 0.06
c. 0.1
d. 0.25
34. According to Factory Act, a person cannot be employed in factory or mines not attending the age of:
a. 12 years
b. 14 years
c. 18 years
d. 21 years
35. When the minor is under the guardianship of the court, he becomes major by the age of:
a. 18 years
b. 21 years
c. 25 years
d. 30 years
36. Crown-heel length of five month mature fetus would be:
a. 9 cm
b. 6 cm
c. 25 cm
d. 35 cm
37. A child has permanent teeth 20 and temporary teeth 4, the age of the child is:
a. 9 years
b. 10 years
c. 11 years
d. 14 years
38. Bertillon system is employed based on:
a. Measurements of skull
b. Measurements of long bones
c. Measurements of body parts
d. Measurements of pelvis

39. Most common type of fingerprint is:
    a. Arch
    b. Radial loop
    c. Ulnar loop
    d. Whorl
40. Cheiloscopy is the study of:
    a. Fingerprint
    b. Hair
    c. Palate pattern
    d. Lip print
41. A convict whose family or relations was not known and no biological sample was available with jail authorities, escaped from the jail. A dead body resembling the convict was found in nearby forest, but due to mutilation of face, identity could not be established. The positive identity that he is the same convict who escaped from jail can be established by:
    a. Blood grouping
    b. DNA profile
    c. Anthropometry
    d. HLA typing
42. Identification of face using skull X-ray called as:
    a. Gustafson's technique
    b. Odontology
    c. Radio imaging
    d. Superimposition
43. Dental numbering is done by all, *except*:
    a. FDI two digit system
    b. Anatomic and diagrammatic charting
    c. Palmer notation
    d. Universal system
44. Palatoprint is commonly taken from which part of palate:
    a. Anterior part
    b. Lateral wall
    c. Medial wall
    d. Posterior part
45. Primary dentition is complete by:
    a. 1.5 years
    b. 2.5 years
    c. 3.5 years
    d. 4.5 years
46. All true about pisiform, *except*:
    a. Last carpal bone to ossify
    b. Attached to flexor carpi ulnaris
    c. Can be seen on newborn X-ray
    d. It is a sesamoid bone

ANSWERS

1. c	2. b	3. c	4. d	5. b	6. c	7. d	8. d	9. c	10. d
11. c	12. b	13. b	14. c	15. b	16. a	17. d	18. d	19. d	20. b
21. c	22. d	23. a	24. d	25. a	26. a	27. a	28. a	29. d	30. b
31. d	32. d	33. d	34. b	35. b	36. c	37. c	38. c	39. c	40. d
41. c	42. d	43. b	44. a	45. b	46. c				

CHAPTER 6

Trace Evidences and Forensic Science Laboratory

KEY WORDS

Biological trace evidences hair, blood and semen, forensic science laboratory, analytical toxicology, polygraph, narcoanalysis, brain mapping, DNA profile, truth serum, word association, hypnosis.

FM2.18	Crime scene investigation—describe and discuss the objectives of crime scene visit, the duties and responsibilities of doctors on crime scene and the reconstruction of sequence of events after crime scene investigation.
FM3.2	Describe and discuss identification of biological trace evidences–hairs and fibers.
FM3.15	Describe and discuss preservation and despatch of trace evidences.

INTRODUCTION

Each state has a central forensic science laboratory and many regional forensic science laboratories at the district level or region level covering a few districts. The main function of FSL is to analyze trace evidences.

WHAT ARE TRACE EVIDENCES? (FM3.2)

What is Locard's Principle of Exchange?

Trace evidences are materials or substances which connects the crime scene with the perpetrator of the crime. They are most important in any crime scene investigations. There are basically four biological trace evidences, namely: hair, blood, semen and other body fluids.

Locard's Principle of Exchange

- It states that "when two objects come into contact with each other, there is always transfer of some material between them", This is helpful in crime investigations, especially in sexual offences.
- Any person during the commission of a crime will almost always leave something and take away something from the scene of crime. This is the theory of interchange.
- It is a well settled hypothesis that there is almost zero percentage of chances to commit a crime without any exchange of material. But there exist limitations of science in finding out those transferred materials.

WRITE SHORT NOTES ON HAIR AS TRACE EVIDENCE? (FM3.2)

What are the Medico-Legal Importance of Hair?

Hair as Trace Evidence

- Hair is one of the very important biological trace evidences which could be present in the scene of crime, either in the process of struggle or the hair falling off by itself.
- The average rate of hair fall per day is 50 to 100/day. Hence, there are chances that when a person just moves his hair with the hand or when the victim tries to holds the hair of the assailant, the hair may fall of by itself and also the victim may tightly hold the hair and forcefully pulled off. But it is very unfortunate that due to poor knowledge of the investigation team, it's always missed.
- In the examination of hair recovered from the scene of crime as trace evidence efforts must be made to answer some important questions regarding it.
    1. Whether they are actually hair or some other fiber.
        - Hair consists of a root (or pulp) and a shaft; whereas fibers do not contain a root or pulp. Hair consists of: (i) Cuticle, (ii) Cortex and (iii) Medulla, which can be made out by microscopic examination.
    2. If it is hair, whether they are of human or animal origin, which can be concluded by morphology and microscopy.
        - It should also be compared with the hair of common types of animals present in that area, which could have gained access into the scene, if they are animal hair.
        - Human hair will be fine and thin, cortex is thick, well striated and 4 to 10 times as broad as medulla; whereas animal hair is coarse and thick, cortex is thin less than twice as broad as that of medulla.
    3. If found to be human hair, then from which part of the body it is derived from?
        - Hair from the scalp will be thin and wavy; whereas axillary and pubic hairs are curly, thick, coarse and curly.
    4. Sex of the person can also be determined from the hair, by the demonstration of Barr bodies.
    5. Age of the individual could be grossly assessed from the hair.
        - Hair root of the children will dissolve readily in a solution of caustic potash, but that of the older people resist such treatment; this is due to the presence of abundant keratin in the old aged people.
    6. Blood Groups (ABO) of the individual can be determined from a single hair of any part of the body by modified absorption-elution technique with 100% accuracy.
    7. Hair has to be examined for evidence of dyeing, bleaching, disease or poisons like arsenic.
    8. Is the hair identical with that of the victim or the suspect?
        - This can be made out by careful comparison under a comparison microscope.
    9. Did it fall naturally or was it forcibly removed?
        - Made out by the ruptured root sheath since considerable force is required to pluck out a healthy hair from scalp and still higher force is required to pull out a hair from other parts of the body.

Medico-Legal Importance of Hair

- Used for identification in cases of assaults and accidents.

- It plays an important role in identification of the offender in sexual offence cases.
- In cases of injury to the hair, nature of weapon can be made out by microscopic examination of the severed end of the hair.
- Singeing of hair helps to differentiate burns from scalds and also in the interpretation of firearm injuries (contact range and close range).
- Time since death can be estimated from the length of hair on face, as the average rate of hair growth on the face is 0.4 mm/day.
- Age of a person can be determined from hair growth on different parts of the body (secondary sexual characteristics and graying of hair).
- Sex can be differentiated from distribution of hair on different parts of the body, texture and identification of Barr bodies.
- In chronic heavy metal poisoning, traces of the metal gets deposited on the hair and can be detected by chemical analysis, especially arsenic.

WHAT ARE THE DIFFERENCES BETWEEN HUMAN HAIR AND ANIMAL HAIR? (FM3.2)

Table 6.1 is depicted the differences human hair and animal hair.

Medullary index of hair:

$$\frac{\text{Diameter of the medulla}}{\text{Diameter of the whole hair (Shaft)}}$$

WRITE SHORT NOTES ON BLOOD AS TRACE EVIDENCE? (FM3.2)

What is Precipitin Test?

- The following questions are to be answered, by subjecting the blood stains present in the crime scene to physical and chemical examination:
  1. **Whether the stain is blood or not:**
     (a) Benzidine test (b) Phenolphthalein test (**Kastle-Meyer test**)
     - These chemical tests are based upon the presence of the enzyme peroxidase present in the red blood cells.
     - Haemin crystal test (Teichmann's test) and Hemochromogen crystal test (**Takayama test**) are also useful to identify blood stains.
     - Electrophoresis and immune-electrophoresis can positively identify blood stains.
     - Spectrometry is most useful and reliable test for detection of blood stains, even with <0.1 mL of blood and especially useful for old stains.
     - Confirmation is by subjecting the sample to microscopic examination of red blood cells (not useful for old stains)
  2. If it is blood, then **whether human or animal origin**: can be confirmed by

TABLE 6.1: Human hair vs animal hair.

Features	Human hair	Animal hair
General appearance	Fine and thin	Coarse and thick
Cuticular scales	Short, thin and irregularly annular	Large, thick and wavy in appearance
Cortex	Thick and 4 to 10 times broader than medulla	Thin and only 2 times broader than medulla
Medulla	Narrow and fragmented	Wide and continuous
Pigmentation	Evenly distributed	Present only in medulla
Precipitin test	Specific for humans	Specific for different animals
Medullary index	Less than 0.3	More than 0.5

serological testing of blood (precipitin test) and by microscopy.

Precipitin test:
- Human serum containing proteins is injected into an animal like horses (H type) and rabbits (R type), the animals are sensitized against these proteins and antibodies to human blood develop in the animal.
- When human serum is brought into contact with the serum extracted from these sensitized animals, it reacts with the proteins of human serum and forms a precipitate. This is a confirmatory test for identifying the human origin of any biological substance.

3. Note the color, shape, size and direction of the stain.
4. Whether the blood is of **arterial or venous origin:**
   - Arterial blood is bright red and venous blood is dark red in color.
   - There will be spurting blood if it is of arterial origin, whereas venous blood stains will be circular, due to dribbling perpendicularly onto the surface.
5. **Age of the stain:**
   - Fresh stains look bright red in color, which turns reddish brown in 24 hours. After 24 hours it turns dark brown and then finally turns black when the duration is longer.
6. **Whether antemortem or postmortem in nature:**
   - Antemortem bleeding cause coagulation and the clot can be taken out en mass and the area after removal of the clot retains the impression of the fibrinous network owing to the process of clot formation.
   - Postmortem bleeding occurs without proper coagulation and the clot will be brittle and easily friable due to absence of fibrinous network.
- **Spectrometry** is the best test to analyze blood stains. However for old and minute trace blood stains **absorption and elution** is a good method for old stains.

WRITE SHORT NOTES ON SEMINAL STAINS? (FM3.2)

- **Physical examination:** Seminal stains on white fabric appear yellow with borders appearing darker than the center. When examined under ultraviolet light seminal stains exhibit strong bluish white fluorescence.
- **Chemical examination: Florence test and Barberio's test:** These tests will demonstrate the presence of choline and spermine crystals respectively. These can be detected by thin layer chromatography (TLC).
- **Acid phosphatase test:** The normal amount of acid phosphatase in the seminal fluid is 350 bodansky units. The acid phosphatase test can be done for all old stains and in the vaginal washings in cases of rape (can be detected even after 36 hours). This a specific test for detection of seminal stains. However, confirmation of seminal stain is by demonstration of the presence of spermatozoa, under microscopy.

WHAT ARE THE BASIC FACILITIES REQUIRED FOR A FORENSIC SCIENCE LABORATORY?

- This is a very vast area of analysis, which needs a co-ordination of work by a number of experts from various fields of science, mainly:
- Biophysics, biochemistry, histo-chemistry, microbiology, analytical toxicology, etc.

- Any material evidence must be analyzed as to what it is? From where it was recovered? And how it is related to or involved in the crime. A chain of custody is maintained at every step of transfer of evidence.
- A basic analytical center or laboratory should consist of facilities to analyze,
    i. *Biological trace evidences:*
       Blood: Grouping, detection of stains, analysis of the source, DNA etc. Semen, hair and saliva.
    ii. *Analytical toxicology:* Detection and estimation of various poisons including drugs and medicines. This is done by using various instruments and methods like, automated solvent extractor, chromatography: UV spectrometry, gas spectrometry and Mass spectrometry.
    iii. Computed automated system for: Fingerprinting and superimposition.
    iv. Hand writing comparison experts.
    v. Firearms: Ballistics experts.
- A doctor is not expected to know the functions and techniques involved in each division, but he is bound to know the basics of all the branches and their modes of operation.
- Those which are related to medical science are discussed briefly.

WRITE SHORT NOTES ON POLYGRAPH (LIE DETECTOR)?

- Polygraph makes a continuous record of pulse, blood pressure, respiration and electro-dermal reactive changes in response to particular stimuli in the form of questions.
- It is based on the principle that when an individual tells a lie, there is fear in his mind that he could be detected and by the emotions caused by the fear there is stimulation of the sympathetic nervous system and results in certain physiological changes, some of which can be easily recorded.
- In pretest interview the questions are framed with the mutual consent of the subject and the examiner, that they are adequate to serve the purpose of the particular examination.
- The questions are framed in such a manner that the individual is easily able to understand it and give 'yes' or 'no' as the answer.
- Relevant and irrelevant questions are mixed up; and control questions are inserted to reduce the natural nervousness.
- A question is asked every 20–25 seconds and the polygraph chart recorded in 3–4 minutes.
- Usually, the same test is repeated twice or thrice to check for any possible error.
- An experienced and competent polygraph examiner can detect truth or lie in about 80 to 90% of cases. A few errors do occur in deceptive subjects.
- Offenders, suspects, complainant, witnesses and informants are examined by this method, to test the truth of their statement.

WHAT IS NARCOANALYSIS? WHAT IS TRUTH SERUM?

- Based on the principle that at a point close to unconsciousness, an individual will be mentally incapable of resistance to questions, and is incapable of inventing the falsehood that he has used to conceal his guilt.
- The following drugs are commonly used to extract information which the individual wants to conceal. These drugs will remove his inhibitions and he may not be able to tell lie and maintain his false statements to conceal the information regarding the

crime. Hence these drugs are also called as **"Truth Serum"**. The methods used are:
i. Injection Scopolamine 0.5 mg SC, followed by 0.25 mg every 20 minutes, for an average of 3 to 6 injections, until the subject reaches proper stage of questioning.
ii. Sodium amytal or sodium pentothal 2.5 to 5% IV, at 1 mg/min, until proper stage is induced.
iii. Injection sodium seconal 0.1 gm, 15 mg morphine sulphate and 0.5 mg scopolamine IV.

- A large number of false negative results are common in this method because the individual goes into hallucinatory phase due to the effects of the drugs and there are chances that he may fabricate new imaginary stories during the test. Many a times the courts do not accept these tests. One main use is if the individual has revealed a new information which he intended to hide, it will be helpful if the police are able to bring forth evidences supporting the statements he has revealed during the test.

Word Association

- Change in the reaction time of the subject's reply to word stimuli, either visual or auditory or by stereotype of answers are used.
- **Hypnosis** is the other methods used for lie detection, but very less application as the level of hypnosis that could be obtained on an individual widely varies.

WRITE SHORT NOTES ON BRAIN MAPPING (BRAIN FINGERPRINTING)?

- It is based on the information stored in the brain and cognitive brain response; they are not affected by emotional responses and hence said to be more accurate than polygraph.
- The basis is that the suspect's reaction to the details of an event or activity will reflect if he had prior knowledge of the event or activity.
- The technique measures the recognition of familiar stimuli by measuring the electrical brain wave response to words, phrases, or pictures that are presented on a computer screen.
- This technique uses multidisciplinary approach involving brain imaging, neurophysiology, computer science and bioinstrumentation.
- An equipment called 'electro cap' is fixed on the suspect's head; and he is questioned about the crime and also shown visuals of the crime scene (victim, weapon, how the crime was committed, etc); to stimulate his brain and encourage a reaction on computer monitor.
- Apart from verbal replies, another computer records his neuronal impulses emitted (brain waves and chemical response) when the visual is shown.
- The intensity of the brain wave shoots up whenever a question or visual stimuli matches the information stored in the brain.

WHAT IS FORENSIC DNA TYPING?

What are the Applications of DNA Fingerprinting?

- The first application of DNA typing in forensic science was done by Dr Alec Jeffries (USA) in 1985.
- DNA is extracted from a biological sample and processed to generate a pattern for each individual called 'DNA profile'.
- DNA is found in the chromosomes which are present only in the **nucleus** of a cell;

the average length of a DNA molecule in a nucleus is 180 cm.
- **Mitochondrial DNA:** Abundant sample of DNA, but inherited only from the mother (especially useful, when a fallen hair is available at the crime scene, without the root).

Gene and chromosomes:
- A chromosome contains two complementary strands of deoxyribonucleic acid (DNA) each consisting of phosphate, deoxyribose and one of the four bases: adenine, thymine, guanine and cytosine. They always forms pair (A-T and C-G); the two strands are antiparallel and run in opposite direction.

Genetic polymorphism:
- Within a species, one chromosome of a given type is similar to another, but at some places (loci) there may be some variability; detectable variations occurring at a single genetic locus are called 'alleles'.
- 'Genetic marker' applies to any observable variation at a single genetic locus.
- This may be serological marker ABO blood group or a DNA marker.

The four main types of DNA markers are:
- RFLPs: Restricted fragment length polymorphisms
- VNTRs: Variable number of tandem repeats
- STRs: Short tandem repeats
- SNPs: Single nucleotide polymorphisms.

Basis of DNA typing:
- Some chromosomal regions contain repeating units of the same type of DNA; the numbers of repeating units vary from individual to individual. Hence, chromosomal regions with short tandem repeating DNA units are used for human identification.

Method:
- DNA is isolated from the biological samples
- The purified DNA is cut into fragments using restriction enzymes and the pattern is taken
- *Example:*
  GCGCATGTTGCGCAAGAGCGC—repeated three times
  GCGCATTGAATGCAAGTAGCGC—repeated two times
- The restriction enzyme will cut between first G and first C. The result will be fragments either small fragment or large fragment.
- Restriction fragments are negatively charged and can be separated by '**gel electrophoresis**' which separates the DNA based on their sizes.
- The samples of DNA are allowed to run on a slab of electrophoretic gel, across which a positive charged probe is placed; the smaller fragments running faster, thus separating the DNA samples into distinct bands, which are visualized using luminescent dyes.
- Quite large amount of biological material is needed to get reasonable accurate results.
- *Polymerase chain reaction (PCR) technique:* This requires only trace amount of DNA and hence useful, when only limited sample is available, as like the crime scene.

Application of DNA Typing

- Paternity disputes (accounts for 50% cases of DNA typing done in India)
- Maternity resolutions
- Detection of cases of child swapping
- Identification of the culprit in rape cases and gang rapes
- Identification of mutilated remains

- Identification in exhumed bodies and partially burnt bodies.

DISCUSS AND DESCRIBE THE OBJECTIVES DUTIES, RESPONSIBILITIES, OF DOCTOR IN RECONSTRUCTION OF GRIME SCENE? (FM2.18)

Investigation of the Scene of Death

- **Basic rules:** The basic rules for investigation of any scene of crime are:
  - Verify that a crime has been committed.
  - Look for signs of how it was committed.
  - Recover and preserve evidence that might lead to the arrest and conviction of the guilty.

The Objectives in a Crime Scene are to Find Out

- Who is the victim? (Identification).
- When the death and injuries occurred? (Time of death and injuries).
- Where the death occurred? (Scene and circumstances of death).
- What injuries are present? (Description of injuries).
- Which injuries are significant? (Major, minor, true, artefacts, postmortem injuries).
- Why and how injuries were produced? (Mechanism and manner of death, i.e., natural, accidental, suicidal or homicidal). If unnatural, determine the means or agent causing death, e.g., knife, firearm, poison, etc., and if homicide assist in identifying the person responsible for death.

Conduct and Duties of the Doctor at the Scene of Crime

- Crime scene investigation aids in identification of suspects or victims.
- Prove or disprove alibi and identify a modus operandi.
- Establish the corpus delicti and establish associations among victim, suspect, scene and evidence.
- It is the responsibility of the police to preserve and protect the scene of crime. The doctor can ask police to arrange his visit to the scene of crime. The doctor should carry with him a hand lens, measuring tape and ruler, gloves, slides, swabs, chemical thermometer and envelopes if possible.
- Complete and accurate recording of the scene as it was found is very important. This can be done by accurate diagrams, notes and photography. The scene may show evidence of struggle and on the body vital trace evidence may be present.
- The examination at the scene should be limited to a search for such evidence which might be dislodged or possibly lost during the transfer of the body to the mortuary. If a doctor sees the dead body for the first time in the autopsy room, he may form incorrect opinions about the origin of various injuries. Seeing the body at the scene of crime with the various surrounding objects, helps to avoid such mistakes.
- The visit to the scene of death is more valuable if the body shows a patterned injury, the origin of which is in doubt. Even a retrospective visit to the scene enables the doctor to have a true appreciation of the nature of the surroundings, which are usually found to differ from the impression formed from the descriptions by other persons, and will be of help in interpretation of the findings on the victim.
- The scene of a violent death usually shows significant findings for understanding, reconstructing and solving problems. The finding of a dead body together with evidence of burglary indicates murder.

Disturbance of furniture may be seen sometimes, if a person dying suddenly and naturally falls down and injures himself.
- The sequence of events preceding death must be reconstructed logically to support or contradict inferences from other areas of investigation.
- The fatal injuries should be evaluated to find out how much purposeful action and walking, the victim could have carried out before he became disabled and died.
- In every case, priority must be given to the injured, and to any action designed to prevent further casualties. Evidence to connect victim, suspect and location of the murder may be found at the scene of the incident, on the clothing or bodies of victim and suspect, or some other place to which the body was transported.
  - The doctor must make sure that death has occurred.
  - If the victim of an assault is living when first seen, the doctor must do everything to save the life.
  - If death is about to occur, he should obtain a dying declaration, for otherwise valuable information will be lost, e.g., in criminal abortion.
  - He must obtain all possible information regarding the crime.
  - If he suspects foul play, the police should be informed.
  - He should retain any material which is relevant, e.g., in cases of suspected poisoning, he must look for and retain any specimens, such as vomit, leftover poison, or drinking utensils.
  - He must identify the body, which should also be identified by the relatives and the police.
  - He must enquire whether the body has been moved at all before he first saw it.
  - Never touch, change, or alter anything until identified, measured and photographed. He should ask the investigating officer before moving anything. Photograph the scene from several angles. He should follow but not lead the police around the scene.
- He should not give opinions without proper thought.

Basic Rules for Preservation of Medico-legal Evidence (FM3.15)

For evidence to be legally accepted by the Courts: (1) It must be obtained in a legal manner. (2) It must be relevant to the issue. (3) The chain of custody of the item must be intact and known. (4) It must be evaluated by qualified experts.

Collection of Evidence

- Collect every article even remotely likely to be helpful in the investigation. Note the source and the relative location of the exhibits at the time they were recovered.
- Collect any item likely to carry fingerprints.
- Use separate container for each item.
- Every article collected must bear identifying marks. Two marking methods are commonly used. (i) Direct, in which marks are put on the item of evidence itself. (ii) Indirect, in which notations of identification are placed on a container in which the evidence is placed. The container should be labeled. The data to be recorded on the label are: case number, location and description of the recovered evidence, a specific number, person who recovered the evidence, date of recovery and initials. The disadvantage of attaching a tag is, it can be accidentally torn off or intentionally removed as the evidence is handled or examined forensically.
- Exhibits must be protected against mutilation, alteration, or contamination. If any alteration has been made between the

time the exhibit was recovered and the time it was offered in evidence, this must be justified by the laboratory technician.

Preservation of Physical Evidence (FM3.15)

- **Always use:** (1) Card board "pillbox" type of containers. (2) Envelopes. (3) The pharmacist fold using paper. (4) Film containers (35 mm). (5) Plastic vials and jars are useful for small samples, e.g., hair, bullets, blood and organs. (6) Airtight, leak proof, unbreakable containers for liquids and volatile substances. (7) Plastic bags for organs, clothing and larger articles, and to cover the hands or other parts of the body. (8) Larger plastic bags may be used for bodies.
- Avoid excessive handling of the evidence that is gathered, as it may use contamination or loss of transitory materials.

MULTIPLE CHOICE QUESTIONS

1. **When one object touches another, part of the energy gets transferred to the other is known as?**
   a. Locard's exchange principle
   b. Magnan's principle
   c. Koch's principle
   d. Mc Naughten principle
2. **Study of hair is called:**
   a. Hairlegraphy
   b. Trichology
   c. Thanatology
   d. Dactylography
3. **DNA finger printing done by:**
   a. Sequence in nuclear DNA
   b. Nonsequence in nuclear DNA
   c. Sequence in nuclear RNA
   d. Nonsequence in nuclear RNA
4. **Fingerprint Bureau was first established in:**
   a. England
   b. China
   c. India
   d. Singapore
5. **In humans, cortex of hair is usually:**
   a. Double that of medulla
   b. Same as medulla
   c. 4–10 times broader than the medulla
   d. Thin in comparison to medulla
6. **In a charred body, which of the following means is useful in its identification?**
   a. Stature
   b. Comparison of dental records
   c. Scar marks
   d. Skeletal features

ANSWERS

1. a   2. b   3. a   4. c   5. c   6. b

SECTION 3

Forensic Pathology

SECTION OUTLINE

- **Chapter 7:** Medico-Legal Autopsy
- **Chapter 8:** Thanatology: Death and its Causes
- **Chapter 9:** Postmortem Changes
- **Chapter 10:** Violent Asphyxial Deaths
- **Chapter 11:** Death due to Starvation

CHAPTER 7

Medico-Legal Autopsy

KEY WORDS

Autopsy, aims and objectives of medico-legal autopsy, dissection methods, blood less dissection, preservation of viscera, artefacts, NHRC guidelines for custodial death, mutilated bodies or fragments, charred bones, bundle of bones, obscure autopsy, embalming, exhumation, second autopsy, air embolism.

FM2.11	Define and discuss autopsy procedures including postmortem examination, different types of autopsies, aims and objectives of postmortem examination.
FM2.12	Describe the legal requirements to conduct postmortem examination and procedures to conduct medico-legal postmortem examination.
FM2.13	Describe and discuss obscure autopsy.
FM2.14	Describe and discuss examination of clothing, preservation of viscera on postmortem examination for chemical analysis and other medico-legal purposes, postmortem artefacts.
FM2.15	Describe special protocols for conduction of medico-legal autopsies in cases of death in custody or following violation of human rights as per National Human Rights Commission guidelines.
FM2.16	Describe and discuss examination of mutilated bodies or fragments, charred bones and bundle of bone.
FM2.17	Describe and discuss exhumation.

DEFINE AUTOPSY; WHAT ARE THE TYPES OF AUTOPSIES? (FM2.11)

- Autopsy is defined as "Scientific Dissection of the Dead Body".
- There are two types of autopsies in practice they are:
  i. Pathological autopsy;
  ii. Medico-legal autopsy.

Pathological Autopsy

- Pathological autopsy is also called as academic or clinical autopsy. It is done by the clinicians who were treating the patient with the association of the clinical pathologist. Consent of the legal heir is mandatory. Pathological autopsy can be done only in cases of natural death where the cause of death is already confirmed. Academic autopsies are done to acquire knowledge which will be useful for the clinician while treating similar patients in future.

Medico-Legal Autopsy

Medico-legal autopsy can better be defined as "investigative scientific dissection of a dead body".
- Medico-legal autopsies are done under an authorization of the police (not below the rank of sub-inspector) or the executive magistrate (officers of the revenue department, appointed by the state government, usually not below the rank of Tahsildar).
- There is no need for consent of the relatives, since it's done under an authorization and it will be done even if the relatives object for the postmortem examination. Medico-legal autopsies are done in all Unnatural and sudden deaths.
- There are two other types of autopsies which does not involve dissection of the dead body and they are:

Psychological Autopsy
- A procedure for investigating a person's death by reconstructing what the person thought, felt, and did before death, based on the information gathered from his personal documents, police reports, medical and other available records.
- Face to face interviews with family members, friends and others who had contact with the person before the death.
- It can help address the ambiguity of establishing whether death was as a result of natural cause, suicide, accident or murder.

Verbal Autopsy

Done in infant deaths for data on infant mortality rate.

DIFFERENCE BETWEEN MEDICO-LEGAL AUTOPSY AND CLINICAL AUTOPSY (FM2.11)

Medico-legal autopsy vs clinical or pathological autopsy are described in **Table 7.1**.

TABLE 7.1: Medico-legal autopsy vs clinical or pathological autopsy.

Criteria	Medico-legal autopsy	Clinical autopsy
Conducted in	Unnatural, sudden and suspicious death	Only in natural death, where cause of death is confirmed and the clinician issues a cause of death certificate
Inquest	Mandatory an autopsy is conducted only when the IO gives requisition to conduct autopsy along with a copy of inquest report	No inquest is necessary as the cause of death is already confirmed as natural death
Consent of legal heirs	Not necessary and autopsy will be done even the legal heir objects	Consent of the legal heirs is mandatory
Complete dissection	Mandatory; all the body cavities must be opened and examined even if not necessary as the cause of death, could be evident during examination as like crush injury of the head	Need not be complete; the clinician/pathologist who conducts autopsy has the choice to dissect and examine whatever he feels necessary to know about that particular case
Autopsy conducted by	Authorized medical officer/forensic pathologist	The clinician who treated the patient with the help of the pathologist if he feels necessary

WHAT ARE THE AIMS AND OBJECTIVES OF A MEDICO-LEGAL AUTOPSY? (FM2.11)

To Find Out the Cause of Death

- Finding out the medical cause of death is one of the prime objectives of conducting an autopsy. Certifying the cause of death can be done only by an allopathic physician. He also has to assess whether the death is natural or unnatural.
  - *Natural death:* Implies that death is purely due to disease and the pathological process of the disease must be demonstrated at autopsy.
  - *Unnatural death:* Can be accidental, suicidal or homicidal.

To Estimate the Time Since Death

Assess the probable time interval between which death could have occurred, by the changes which take place in a dead body after death.

Documentation

- One of the most crucial and critical part of conducting a medico-legal autopsy is documentation. The autopsy surgeon should give foremost importance to documentation. A proper documentation as observed by him will aid anyone to arrive at a logical conclusion. But it's very unfortunate that most of the doctors doing autopsy have a very poor documentation style and many of the questions of the cross examination goes unanswered in the courts of law due to the deficiency in the skill of the doctor in documentation while conducting postmortems and all these benefits of doubts goes to the accused.
- Documentation should be with reference to postmortem changes, the pathological process of any disease and the injuries present on the body.
- All the injuries present on the body must be documented. How small an injury may be, must be documented clearly; since, that could be the only evidence of struggle. Injuries must be documented with reference to the type of injury (naming the injury correctly), exact dimension (size), shape and location of the injury.
- The autopsy surgeon also has to assess the mode of infliction of the injuries; time of infliction of the injury, the probable weapon used/involved in causation of the injury and the relative position of the victim and the assailant at the time of infliction of the injuries.
- To fix the **identity** of the individual when not known.
- To preserve relevant tissues and organs for analysis: HPE and chemical analysis.
- In **new born** to find out whether the baby was a dead born, stillborn or live born.

WHO IS AUTHORIZED TO CONDUCT MEDICO-LEGAL AUTOPSY?

What are the Documents Produced to the Doctor to Conduct an Autopsy? (FM2.12)

- Medico-legal autopsies can be done only by allopathic physicians. Any doctor with MBBS degree working in an authorized autopsy center can perform medico-legal autopsies.
- **Note:** *In Tamil Nadu, there is MD degree in Siddha Forensic Medicine, offered by The Tamil Nadu Dr MGR Medical University; but they are not permitted to undertake any medico-legal work including medico-legal autopsies, since they lack the basic MBBS degree.*
- Hence, every allopathic physician should be proud and bear in mind that it's our honorable duty to perform medico-legal autopsies, as well as appear in the court as an expert medical witness and help the court in matters of any dispute in medical science.

- Requisition for conducting medico-legal autopsy is submitted by the investigating officer along with the following documents:
  - Two copies of the request letter to conduct autopsy
  - Two copies of the history of the case
  - *Two copies of Inquest Report:* Which consists of details regarding the dead body, identification marks, and clothes on the body; injuries present on the body and apparent conclusion regarding the cause of death as judged by the IO
  - One copy of FIR (first information report), and
  - One copy of AR (accident register) copy.
  - Any other relevant documents like treatment records, investigation reports, hospital case sheets, death certificate, etc.
- The medical officer must carefully go through the inquest report and gain as much information as possible regarding the case before commencing the autopsy.

WHAT ARE PROCEDURES OF EXTERNAL AND INTERNAL EXAMINATION IN AN AUTOPSY? (FM2.12)

External Examination

- Clothes on the body; with special reference to stains and tears.
- The clothing should be dried packed without any preservative and sealed and sent to forensic science laboratory.
- Take necessary photographs of the clothing with any stains present on the body.
- Wash the body thoroughly before commencing the autopsy.
- Check the identification marks.
- Look for any discoloration and postmortem changes like postmortem hypostasis, Rigor mortis, putrefaction changes, etc.
- **Document the injuries:** From head to toe, with reference to the type of injury (abrasion, laceration, cut wound, stab wound, etc.), exact dimension and location with reference to prominent anatomical landmarks wherever necessary.
- Take necessary photographs of all the injuries, before commencing the dissection. In present days, this is an easy task as mobile cameras are available with almost every doctor.

DISSECTION OF INTERNAL ORGANS

Dissection of internal organs during autopsy are shown in **Figure 7.1**.

Dissection Methods

- Open the head by an incision from one mastoid process to another, along the vertex. Any contusion or bruise on the scalp tissue is noted, documented and photographed (at least using a mobile camera) and examine the temporalis muscle.

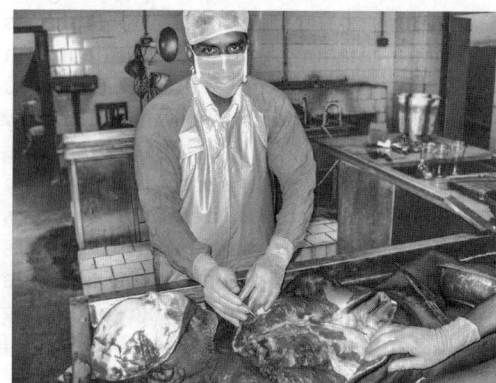

Fig. 7.1: Dissection of internal organs during autopsy *(For color version see Plate 2).*

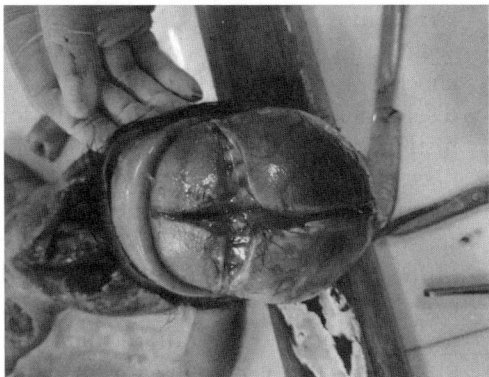

Fig. 7.2: Fetal skull dissection *(For color version see Plate 2).*

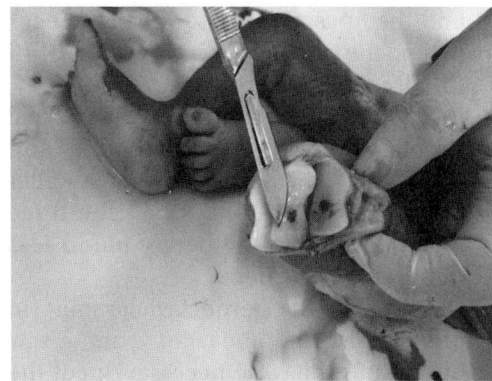

Fig. 7.3: Demonstration of ossification center in femur during autopsy–full term fetus *(For color version see Plate 2).*

- Look for any fractures on the skull (**Figs. 7.2 and 7.3**); fissured, comminuted, depressed, or cut fracture.

Open the calvarium: Look for any intracranial hemorrhages:
- **Extra-dural hemorrhage:** Seen on the membranes, as soon as we remove the vault of the skull. It may be a thin film or even a large hematoma, usually present on the same side of the external injury (coup injury).
- **Remove the meninges:** Look for subdural hemorrhage, which appears as a thin or rarely a thick film on the brain surface; wash the brain thoroughly under flowing water, SDH is easily washed out. If still any more hemorrhage is present on the surface of the brain is subarachnoid hemorrhage, which cannot be washed off since they lie beneath the arachnoid matter.
- Dissect the arteries of the circle of Willis, for evidence of disease (atheromatous plaques, aneurysm, or spontaneous rupture).
- Brain tissues are then sliced into multiple pieces by linear incisions using a brain knife; any hemorrhages present inside the brain matter are intracerebral hemorrhages.
- Pons and cerebellum are also examined for any abnormality and hemorrhages.

Basic skin incisions:
There are three types of skin incisions to open the major cavities.
1. "I" incision
2. "Y" incision
3. Modified "Y" incision

"I" Incision

- Open the thoracoabdominal cavity by making an **"I" shaped incision** extending from the chin to the symphysis pubis with a curvilinear deviating either to the right or left near the umbilicus.

"Y" Incision

- Extends from Acromion process runs down below the breast on both sides of the chest to the xiphoid process. From there the incision is carried downwards to the symphysis pubis.

Modified "Y" Incision

- The incision starts from the suprasternal notch to the symphysis pubis. The incision extends from the suprasternal notch over the middle of the clavicle on both sides

and then passes upwards over the neck behind the ears.
- In cases of suspected neck pathology, incision is made from the suprasternal notch to the symphysis pubis and dissection of the neck is done at last after removing the contents of all the three major cavities of the body—**blood less dissection of the neck.**
- Disarticulate the sternoclaviclar joint (in individuals aged above 40 years, a saw or rib cutter may be necessary); cut the ribs along the costochondral junction; reflect the sternum by releasing all the attachments; release the floor of the tongue, close to the border of the mandible and pull out all the organs enmass from the tongue to the rectum, after releasing the diaphragm and retroperitoneal attachments. Then examine and dissect the individual organs separately.

Lungs

- Examine the surface after washing the lung; check for petechial hemorrhages on the surface of both the lungs; presence of petechial hemorrhages is a sign of asphyxia; multiple petechio-ecchymotic hemorrhages more on the upper lobes of the lung in cases of aspiration; more concentrated towards the inter-lobar surfaces in death due to electrocution and sometimes larger areas of sub-pleural hemorrhages (paultaf's hemorrhages) in drowning.

  It's preferable to dissect along the lumen of trachea and the bronchus, especially in cases of drowning, burns and aspiration; (froth, water and mud particles in drowning, soot particles in burns and stomach contents in aspiration) these must be present on the mucosal surface of larynx, trachea, primary and the secondary bronchioles to confirm it as antemortem findings. Make multiple sections in all the lobes of both lungs to check for macroscopic findings relating to disease or pathology; take bits of tissues for histopathological examination whenever necessary.
- **Esophagus and stomach:** Pass the scissors into the esophagus from the floor of the tongue, cut open the lumen and examine for any erosions, hemorrhage, discoloration and ulceration (mainly in poisoning and especially in corrosive poisoning). Stomach is first cut out from the lower end of esophagus to the duodenum; stomach opened by passing a scissors along the lesser curvature; the stomach contents are measured and described with reference to the consistency, color and odor of the contents; distinct visible particles if any present must be noted and isolated and sent separately for chemical analysis in a separate container. The stomach along with the other stomach contents can be sent in a separate container.

Liver

Surface is examined for evidence of discoloration and nodularity; multiple parallel linear incisions are made and examined layer by layer for any abnormality.

Kidneys

- Surface of the kidneys examined for petechiae; examine the adrenals for any evidence of hemorrhage and inflammation (especially in anaphylactic deaths). Longitudinal sections of the kidneys is made and expose the cut surface; usually the cortex and medulla are distinctly visible but in cases of degenerative diseases, nephritis and in some poisons (mercury) the cortico-medullary differentiation is poor. Look for any calculi or renal cyst. If there is any visible pathology, preserve the tissues for microscopic examination.

Spleen

Examine the size, shape and surface, then make serial sections and look for any visible pathology.

Female Genital Tract

Examine the external surface of the uterus, both anterior and posterior surface; examine the fallopian tubes and ovaries for any obvious pathology. Make a longitudinal incision and examine the uterine cavity and its contents if any (like products of conception, fibroids, endometrium, etc). If any fetus is present measure the crown heal length and the circumference of the head. Examine the various ossification centers of sternum, lower end of femur, talus and calcaneum; also examine whether sex differentiation is possible.

METHOD OF DISSECTION OF HEART

Heart

- Examine the pericardial fluid and wash the surface of heart thoroughly; the surface of heart is inspected for any evidence of pericarditis (which may appear as white or pale areas of discoloration). Weigh the heart; look for sub-epicardial petechio-ecchymotic hemorrhages (more on the left ventricle in death due to electrocution, in any asphyxial death) and these petechiae may also be present on the root of aorta.
- Dissection of the heart is **along the way of blood flow**; identify superior and inferior vena cava; pass the scissors through them and open the right atrium; extend the dissection till the right auricle, to expose the whole of right atrium; examine the valves and cut open the right ventricle along the right border of the heart and come out through the pulmonaries; enter the left atrium through the pulmonary veins, extend the dissection to the left auricle; examine the valves and open the left ventricle along the left border of the heart; examine the endocardium and look for any hemorrhages.
- Thickness of the left ventricle is measured 1 cm below the atrio-ventricular septum.
- **Dissection of the coronary arteries:** Identify the right and left coronary ostia; dissect the coronaries by passing a small curved coronary scissors into the lumen of the coronaries, through the ostia. Pass the scissors along the entire course of the vessel and their branches; expose the lumen and examine in bright light and check for atheromatous plaques, thickening and narrowing of the lumen of the coronaries; any hemorrhage or clot found inside the lumen is washed thoroughly and examine the underlying lumen surface for plaques and any rupture from the plaques.
- Another way of examining the coronaries is by making serial sections on the epicardial surface, along the course of the vessel at 3 mm intervals. This technique is useful to examine sequential narrowing of the lumen of the coronary arteries. Most common site of obstruction is the anterior one third of the descending left coronary artery 1 cm from the coronary ostia.

WHAT ARE THE METHODS OF RECONSTRUCTION OF THE DEAD BODY?

- After complete examination, any organs or tissues to be subjected for analysis are retained and all other examined organs and tissues including brain are put back into the thoracoabdominal cavity, packed with cotton, place the sternum in its position and sutured using strong thread by continuous sutures. The skull cavity is packed with cotton, the cap in laid in its position and sutured by continuous sutures. Then the body is washed, whipped and the legs are tied together and the hands tied together by placing the hands on the abdomen. Then packed by two layer packing material; using polythene sheet and then white cotton cloth. All the body parts should be covered *except* the face.

- **Note:** If any fetus is present, it's also put back into the abdominal cavity after thorough examination of the fetus. There could be request from the relatives of the deceased to hand over the fetus separately, especially when the fetus is near term. But we are not supposed to hand over the fetus separately, as we receive requisition to conduct autopsy on one body and we are supposed to hand over only one body.

WHAT IS AN OBSCURE AUTOPSY/ NEGATIVE AUTOPSY? (FM2.13)

- After a thorough complete autopsy, chemical examination of all relevant internal organs, necessary histopathological and biochemical analysis, if no definite cause of death could be found or made out. Then it is termed as negative autopsy.
- The commonest situations of negative autopsy are:
  - The most common situation occurs in decomposed bodies. Decomposition is always a challenge to the autopsy surgeons. The outcome percentage also depends upon the magnitude of decomposition.
  - Many natural causes of death may not leave any specific autopsy findings or will be difficult to elicit at autopsy, especially: Vagal inhibition, anaphylaxis, metabolic causes like uremia and cerebral concussion.
  - Cardiac lesions: In blunt force injury to heart, it may stop functioning without any visible signs. Cardiac arrest can occur during or immediately following heavy exercise in which there is increase in heart rate and systolic pressure with progressive ischemia and cardiac arrest. Cardiac arrythmias which, may be precipitated by emotional excitement can cause physiological asystole and may lead to death.
  - In deaths due to some rare poisons: Nonavailability of proper detection methods.
  - Difficulties may also arise in cases of death due to snake bite, electrocution, etc., where the bite marks or the electrical entry wound is not be visible.
  - Inadequate, false or misleading history may sometimes lead to a negative autopsy.
- The incidence of negative autopsy is 2 to 5% of the cases as per many studies, but in India the incidence is much higher, due to poor standard of the mortuaries, improper/inadequate training of doctors in conducting autopsies and lack of development in scientific crime detection methods.

PRESERVATION HERE TISSUES ARE PRESERVED FOR HPE AND CHEMICAL ANALYSIS? (FM2.14)

Sending the tissues or organs for analysis:
- **Histopathology:** The tissues are preserved using formalin as preservative (10% formaldehyde). Labeled and sent to the

pathology lab, with description of autopsy findings concerned with that particular organ.
- **Chemical analysis:** In many situations, the doctor may have to preserve the viscera for chemical analysis; it is mandatory to preserve the viscera in the following situations:
  - All cases of poisoning brought dead or treated.
  - In all murder cases to detect any poison and alcohol.
  - In road traffic accidents to detect alcohol.
  - In all cases of magistrate inquest.
  - In all suspicious and sudden deaths.

WHAT ARE ARTEFACTS? WHAT ARE TYPES OF ARTEFACTS? (FM2.14)

The word artefact is derived from Latin '**arte**' using art; '**factum**' something made.

Definition

- Artefacts are changes caused or features introduced in the body and those which are likely to be misinterpreted at autopsy as an antemortem finding are called as artefacts. (The possibilities of misinterpretation of many findings are discussed then and there in the relevant texts).
- These changes could have been introduced in the body just before death or at the time of death or after death and they can be therapeutic, agonal, or postmortem artefacts.

Therapeutic Artefacts

- These are changes introduced in the body during the attempt to resuscitate the patient in the terminal stage of death. Examples:
  - Cardiac defibrillators used may produce findings simulating bruising of chest wall.
  - Vigorous cardio-pulmonary resuscitations during terminal phase of life may cause fracture of ribs at the costochondral junction, sometimes the fractured end of the ribs may piece into the lung and may cause lung collapse and may pierce the heart causing hemopericardium.
  - Shape and size of a wound could be altered by surgical intervention during treatment (Kennedy phenomenon).
  - Any major surgery done for serious injuries may alter the autopsy findings (hence, before autopsy verify relevant medical records and understand what therapeutic procedure has been done).

Agonal Artefacts

- These are changes introduced in the agonal phase of death of a person. Examples:
  - Aspiration of gastric contents as an agonal terminal event (especially when unconsciousness precedes death and in alcoholism) or during resuscitation measures, or while handling the dead body after death (primary flaccidity allows the contents of stomach to escape into the respiratory tract).
  - Careful dissection of the bronchial tree would show, these contents present only up to the level of primary bronchus. Absence of these materials in the bronchioles will help to confirm that these are not antemortem findings.
  - In cases of injuries when death was so rapid, there may not be visible hemorrhage or extravasation in the surrounding soft tissues to conclude the antemortem nature of injuries; similarly, an individual may collapse and die on the roadside and subsequently run over by a vehicle resulting in collection of blood in the cavities, which should not be mistaken as antemortem injuries as the cause of death.

Postmortem Artefacts

- These kinds of artefacts would result due to handling, transportation and storage of dead body like drag marks, cold stiffening, etc.
- Artefacts introduced by predators or deliberate mutilation.
- Decomposition changes like marbling or postmortem purge are likely to be misinterpreted at autopsy, especially when the doctor is less experienced.
- Adopting improper autopsy techniques may result in false interpretation of the findings during autopsy.

AUTOPSIES IN CASES OF DEATH IN CUSTODY OR FOLLOWING VIOLATION OF HUMAN RIGHTS AS PER NHRC GUIDELINES (FM2.15)

- As per the NRHC, a set of protocols has to be followed for any cases of death in police custody, police firing or in prison.
- The report for such cases has to be sent to the commission in 24 hours.
- At the time of post mortem examination, photographs to be taken and the entire examination has to be video filmed.

The aim of the photographic and the videographic recording is to:
- Detailed findings and presence of injury marks (denoting torture).
- Rule out any undue influence or suppression on findings.
- For an independent review in later stages of the investigation.

The protocol for the videography and photography are:
- Voice of the doctor to be recorded throughout the examinations. The doctor narrates his prima facie observation conducting the postmortem examination.
- Total 20 to 25 color photographs of the victim's whole body has to be taken, some of which without removing the clothes.

The photographs should include:
- Profile photo face front, right lateral, left lateral, back of face.
- Front of body (chest and abdomen) and the back.
- Upper extremity: front and back.
- Lower extremity: front and back.
- Focusing on each injury, zoomed after proper numbering of the injury.
- Photographs to be taken after incorporating post mortem number, date of exam, scale of dimension of photograph, etc.
- While taking photographs, the camera to be held at right angle to the object being photographed.
- To be done by someone trained in forensic photography and videography, using a camera which should be at least 10X megapixel with 10X zoom lens.
- Both hands of the deceased should be wrapped in white paper bags before transportation.
- Clothing should not be removed by the police or any other person. Only the doctor performing the forensic test can remove, preserve and examine the clothes.
- For suspected firearm deaths radiological examination of the body to be done.
- The forensic report, the photos and the videos to be sent to the commission within 2 months of the incident. For special cases viscera can be removed and the viscera report should be sent to the commission.

DESCRIBE AND DISCUSS EXAMINATION OF MUTILATED BODIES OR FRAGMENTS, CHARRED BONES AND BUNDLE OF BONES? (FM2.16)

- Mutilated bodies are those which are extensively disfigured, or in which a limb or a part is lost but the soft tissues, muscles and skin are attached to the bones. Sometimes, only a part of the body, such as head, trunk or a limb may be found. The scene should be photographed before anything is disturbed. The body parts should be arranged in anatomic order. Appropriate specimens should be obtained for toxicological analysis and DNA profiling, such as muscle, a piece of long bone, plucked hair.

- **Human or animal:** Recognition may be made by shape, structure and weight of the objects. This is easy if the head, trunk or limbs are available, but when pieces of muscle only are available without attached skin or viscera, it is very difficult. In such cases, definite opinion can be given by performing precipitin test, or antiglobulin inhibition test using blood, or any other soft tissue, if the tissue is not severely decomposed.
- **One or more bodies:** This is determined by fitting together all separate parts. If there is no disparity or reduplication, and if the color of the skin is same in all parts, they belong to one body. Testing for similarity of blood groups and hemoglobin from different parts is helpful.
- **Sex:** It can be determined if the head or trunk is available, from the presence and distribution or absence of hair, characters of the pelvis, skull, etc. It can also be determined from the recognition of prostatic or uterine tissue under a microscope which resist putrefaction and are found even in advanced state of putrefaction.
- **Age:** Age can be determined from general development, skull, teeth and ossification of bones. Calcification of cartilages, changes in sacrum, symphysial surface of pubic bone, changes in joints, color of hair.
- **Stature:** It can be determined from the measurement of long bones.
- **Identity:** It can be determined from fingerprints, tattoo, marks, scars, moles, hair, teeth, deformities, any disease, absence of any internal organ, etc., articles of clothing and superimposition technique.
- **Race:** It can be determined from hair, skin and skull.
- **Manner of separation of parts:** This is determined by examining the margins of the parts, whether they had been cleanly cut, sawn, hacked, lacerated, disarticulated at the joints or gnawed through by animals.
- **Time since death:** Time since death may be inferred from the progressive changes in the body after death and entomology of cadaver.
- **Cause of death:** The cause of death can be made out if there is evidence of fatal injury to some vital organ or large blood vessel, or marks of burning or deep cuts or fractures of bones, especially of the skull or the cervical vertebrae, hyoid bone or of several ribs.
- **Antemortem or postmortem:** This may be determined by examining the margins of parts for evidence of vital reaction. In decomposing bodies, hemorrhage along the wound track on dissection indicates antemortem nature.

WHAT IS EXHUMATION? DESCRIBE THE PROCEDURE OF EXHUMATION? (FM2.17)

- Exhumation (**Fig. 7.4**) is digging out the already buried dead body legally. Order for exhumation can be issued only the concerned executive magistrate. There is no time limit for exhumation in India.
- Autopsy on exhumed bodies are performed when any suspicion is raised after burying the dead body or when any unnatural death such as suicide, accident or murder has been concealed and the body has been buried.

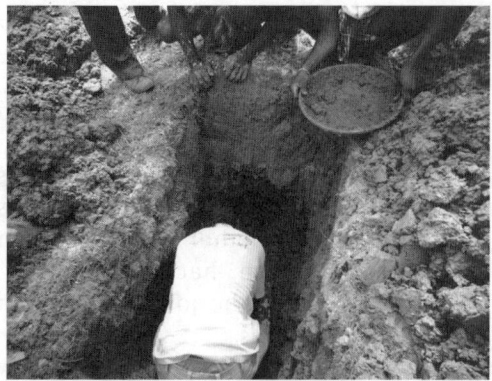

Fig. 7.4: Exhumation
(For color version see Plate 2).

- The body is exhumed under the supervision of the medical officer, executive magistrate, the police and whenever possible the executive magistrate should inform the relatives and request their presence throughout the procedure.
- Exhumation is conducted only in daytime **(Fig. 7.5)**. Positive identification of the grave site such grave plot number, distance of the grave from permanent objects such as trees, rocks, fence road, etc., are noted.
- The grave site is completely covered for 10 to 15 meters as no public has access to witness the procedures. The clothing at the time of burial is noted and checked.

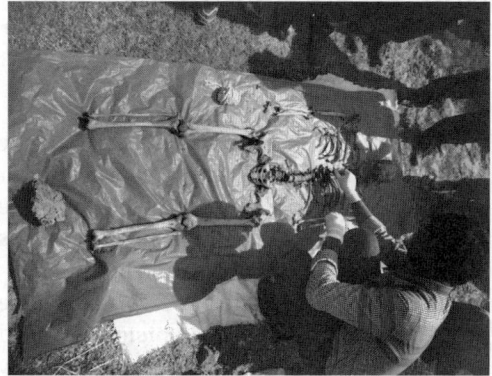

Fig. 7.5: Reconstruction of the body after exhumation with the recovered skeletal remains *(For color version see Plate 3).*

Document the condition of the body and check the clothing.
- Autopsy is done as per the usual procedures. If there needs to be detailed dissection of the body, then it is always advisable to take the body to the mortuary and perform the autopsy procedures. If the exhumation procedure was done for some confirmation of identity or take samples for investigation, then the procedures can be done there itself and the body can be buried in the same place immediately.
- All the viscera should be preserved for chemical analysis. No disinfectants should be sprayed on the body which may interfere with the results of chemical analysis.
- All the possible artefacts should be considered while interpreting any finding. If the body is reduced to skeleton, then all the bones have to be sent for expert opinion.

WHAT IS SECOND AUTOPSY? (FM2.17)

- Autopsy performed on a body for the second time when there is an allegation on the part of the first autopsy doctor or on the investigation team. This is always done under the court order only. If the body is already buried, then the executive magistrate must issue necessary orders for exhumation and it follows the usual procedures of exhumation.
- The doctor performing second autopsy must go through all the necessary documents like FIR, previous autopsy report, autopsy photographs, hospital records or any other valuable document like histopathology report and chemical analysis report.
- If possible, the doctor who performed the first autopsy can be requested to be present during the second autopsy, but if there is any allegation against the first

autopsy doctor then it is better to avoid his presence, rather any correlation of findings or doubts can be clarified from him through phone.
- Interpretation of findings on a previously autopsied exhumed body is very difficult due to progressive decomposition. Attempts are to be made to verify the findings of the first autopsy report and should make attempts to solve the issue of allegation for which the second autopsy was done.
- Even though no new information could be obtained in a second autopsy, the findings of the first autopsy report can be verified and the allegations for which the second autopsy was ordered by the court can keep an end to the rumors.

WHAT IS EMBALMING?

- Embalming is a method of preserving the dead body using chemicals.
- The embalming solution contains 10% formaldehyde and glycerin. When the body tissues come into contact with the solution, the proteins are coagulated, tissues are fixed, and internal organs are hardened.
- The decomposition process is completely arrested if embalming is done shortly after death; if done sometimes later then the body would be preserved at that stage and further decomposition is arrested.
- Embalming usually does not alter the appearance of the body tissues and organs, but slight difficulty may be encountered while we interpret any disease or injury.
- Due to fixation of the tissues by the embalming fluid, poisonous substances if present cannot be extracted from the embalmed body for toxicological analysis.
- **Method of embalming:** The embalming fluid is injected into the body with the aid of a hand or foot pump and bulb syringe. The solution is pushed inside the body through the cut down of an artery (usually femoral artery). Another cut down is made on the opposite side blood vessel (vein, usually femoral vein) to let out the blood and the excess embalming fluid, either intermittently or continuously. The injected embalming fluid is allowed to stay in the body for a reasonable duration of time to facilitate perfusion into the capillaries and permeation into the organs.
- **Embalming a body after autopsy:** All the internal organs are taken out, cut into smaller pieces as possible and soaked into embalming solution for some period of time (30 min or more depending upon the time available) and these organs are put back into the thoracoabdominal cavity and covered by cotton dipped in the embalming fluid. The stomach and the intestinal contents are squeezed out before they are put back into the body. The external body surface is embalmed by injecting the solution using syringe. The solution can be injected into the eyeballs and all parts of the face to prevent decomposition as the face is an important part to be preserved.
- The embalmed body if left to dry will turn into a mummy due to shriveling and dehydration.
- **Note:** When the body has been kept in cold storage, then the body has to be brought back to atmospheric temperature before embalming, if pressure pumps are to be used.

WHAT ARE THE METHODS OF PRESERVATION OF DEAD BODY?

Embalming Fluid

- Embalming is the best method of reservation of dead bodies; other methods of preservation of a dead body are:
  - *Freezing:* If the dead body is refrigerated at 4 degree, then it can

be preserved as long required. When the body is brought back to normal temperature, then the usual process of decomposition will start.
- *Antiseptics:* Bodies which are in water or soil containing antiseptic substances may be preserved and do not decompose.
- *Heavy metals:* By injecting solution containing arsenic, lead sulfide and potassium carbonate into the femoral vein or heart and bodies could be preserved for the purpose of dissection.
- *Mummification and adipocere formation:* These are modified forms of putrefaction, and the bodies are preserved for long.

WHAT IS AIR EMBOLISM? WHAT ARE THE CAUSES AND AUTOPSY FINDINGS IN A CASE OF DEATH DUE TO AIR EMBOLISM?

- Air embolism comprises of an interruption of the circulatory system by air bubbles (or other gas) that gain access to the circulation, usually through the venous route. The air entering the venous side gets sucked towards the right heart through pulmonary trunk and arteries, rarely emerging on the pulmonary vein side.

Causes

- Entry of air into the circulation is usually resulted from trauma, surgical or therapeutic, barotraumas, tubal insufflation, pneumoencephalography, instrumental interference of pregnancy or criminal abortion.
- Accidents may occur during transfusion or infusion and may form the basis of negligence. Injuries to veins of the neck or chest can also lead to air embolism wherein the air gets sucked in due to negative pressure.

Autopsy

External Examination

- The body should be examined while still clothed and equipped (where possible) or such information may be collected from those who have the same.
- A close observation of the evidence of trauma or hypothermia (hypothermia is sometimes an associated hazard of diving) should be carried out.
- Minor lesions, including abrasions and/or bruises, may correspond in location and pattern to parts of the diving apparatus, giving an insight into the idea of their origin from excessive pressure or forceful movement at the time of the incident. Subcutaneous emphysema in the face, neck and upper chest, probably is indicative of pulmonary barotrauma.
- Otoscopic examination is needed for assessment of barotrauma of the ears.
- Radiological examination prior to dissection is advised. A view taken in the lateral decubitus position may be helpful in demonstrating pneumothorax. The examination must cover the head, neck, chest and abdomen. Radiography or computed axial tomography (CAT) can assist in diagnosing extra-alveolar air in the pleural or pericardial cavities or intravascular locations more easily than the standard postmortem examination.

Internal Examination

- Evaluation of presence of air in the heart by dissecting the heart under water; opening of ventricles by incising across the apex with the heart in situ.
- The brain and spinal cord need be preserved for detailed study in cases where neurological dysfunction was recorded antemortem.

MULTIPLE CHOICE QUESTIONS

1. At autopsy, heart should be opened under water to:
   a. Confirm fat embolism
   b. Confirm air embolism
   c. Confirm myocardial infarction
   d. Confirm constrictive pericarditis
2. Postmortem in a newborn baby is done by opening first:
   a. The skull
   b. The chest cavity
   c. The abdominal cavity
   d. Any of the above
3. Time limit for exhumation in India:
   a. 10 years
   b. 20 years
   c. 30 years
   d. No limit
4. Exhumation is requested by:
   a. Inspector of Police
   b. Superintendent of Police
   c. Judicial Magistrate
   d. Tahsildar
5. Brain is preserved in all the following, *except*:
   a. OPC poisoning
   b. Alkaloid poisoning
   c. Heavy metal poisoning
   d. Volatile organic poisoning
6. Best tissue sample for DNA analysis is:
   a. 10 mL of blood in EDTA
   b. Hair
   c. Femur with its bone marrow without preservative
   d. Nail
7. Commonest site of coronary atherosclerosis:
   a. Anterior 1/3rd of descending branch of left coronary artery
   b. Middle 1/3rd of left coronary artery
   c. Middle 1/3rd of right coronary artery
   d. Circumflex branch of left coronary artery
8. Transmission rate of HIV by needle slick injury in health professionals is:
   a. 0.3%
   b. 1%
   c. 5%
   d. 9%
9. Microscopically and macroscopically, there will be no change to the heart in cases of MI deaths up to:
   a. 10 hours
   b. 6 hours
   c. 8 hours
   d. 3 hours
10. Before doing postmortem examination, body identification should be completed by:
    a. Relative
    b. Policeman
    c. Medical officer
    d. Legal heir
11. Last part to be dissected during autopsy in asphyxia death:
    a. Neck
    b. Head
    c. Abdomen
    d. Thorax
12. Viscera are preserved in rectified spirit after:
    a. Death from anesthesia
    b. Corrosive poisoning
    c. Alcohol poisoning
    d. Paraldehyde poisoning
13. Saturated solution of common salt is not used as preservative in:
    a. Corrosive poisoning
    b. Organophosphorus poisoning
    c. Arsenic poisoning
    d. Lead poisoning
14. Minimum quantity of blood required to be preserved for chemical examination is:
    a. 2 mL
    b. 10 mL
    c. 25 mL
    d. 50 mL
15. To preserve specimens, formalin is used in concentration:
    a. 1%
    b. 10%
    c. 40%
    d. 50%
16. The following do not require any preservative, *except*:
    a. Long bones
    b. Hairs
    c. Nails
    d. Uterus

17. Method of autopsy in which various systems organs are removed en masse:
    a. Rokitansky
    b. Virchow
    c. Ghon
    d. Lettulle
18. Virchow method of organ removal is:
    a. Organs removed en masse
    b. Organs removed one by one
    c. In situ dissection
    d. Organs removed en bloc
19. True about subendocardial hemorrhages are all, *except*:
    a. May be seen after head injury
    b. Involves the right ventricular wall
    c. Continuous pattern
    d. Flame shaped hemorrhages
20. Best site for blood collection for toxicology sampling:
    a. Abdominal aorta
    b. Femoral vein
    c. Carotid artery
    d. Heart
21. Specimens for toxicological studies are preserved in:
    a. 10% of formaldehyde
    b. Alcohol
    c. Saturated solution of common salt
    d. Normal saline
22. Ideal time to start exhumation:
    a. Mid night
    b. Late evening
    c. Afternoon in proper light
    d. Early morning
23. CSF sample is preserved for which poisoning:
    a. Heavy metal
    b. Alphos
    c. Organophosphates
    d. Alcohol
24. Fluoride, used in the collection of blood samples, inhibits the enzyme:
    a. Glucokinase
    b. Hexokinase
    c. Enolase
    d. Glucose-6-phosphatase

ANSWERS

1. b	2. c	3. d	4. d	5. c	6. c	7. a	8. a	9. c	10. b
11. a	12. b	13. a	14. b	15. b	16. d	17. d	18. b	19. b	20. b
21. C	22. d	23. d	24. c						

8

CHAPTER

Thanatology: Death and its Causes

 KEY WORDS

Death, suspended animation, brain death, apnea test, brain stem reflexes, THOA 1994, cadaveric donation, anoxic time, anoxia, somatic death, molecular death, coma, syncope, vagal inhibition, asphyxia, sudden natural death, Winslow's test, Magnus's test, Icard test.

FM2.1	Define, describe and discuss death and its types including somatic/clinical/cellular, molecular and brain-death, cortical death and brain stem death.
FM2.2	Describe and discuss natural and unnatural deaths.
FM2.3	Describe and discuss issues related to sudden natural deaths.
FM2.4	Describe salient features of the organ transplantation and the human organ transplant (Amendment Act 2011) and discuss ethical issues regarding organ donation.
FM2.5	Discuss moment of death, modes of death—coma, asphyxia and syncope.
FM2.6	Discuss presumption of death and survivorship.
FM2.7	Describe and discuss suspended animation.

DEFINE DEATH? (FM2.1)

- Death is defined as the "complete and irreversible cessation of circulation, respiration and brain functions".
- As long as oxygenated blood is maintained to the brain stem, life continues to exist.
- Section 46 IPC denotes death as death of human being unless the contrary appears from the context.
- Birth and Death Registrations Act 1969, Section 2(b) defines death as "permanent disappearance of all evidence of life at any time after live birth has taken place".

WHAT IS SUSPENDED ANIMATION? (FM2.7)

- Suspended animation is a condition in which the vital functions of the body come down to a minimum level, just compatible with that of life. The person appears apparently dead but life is still present. This is a rare occurrence, usually involuntary and encountered in many cases; the most commonest situations in order of priority are:
  - Newborn
  - Electrocution

- Drowning
- Hypothermia
- *Drugs:* Mainly morphine, barbiturates and alcohol.
- Induced voluntarily by practice (yoga): Voluntary suspended animation.
* Medico-legally suspended animation is very important as a person under suspended animation can be easily resuscitated by artificial means.
* Suspended animation has to be ruled out to avoid a premature certification of death.
* Especially important in newborn, timely resuscitation measures should be attempted before declaring the baby as still born.

WHAT IS PERSISTENT VEGETATIVE STATE?

* Persistent vegetative state occurs in conditions where there are damages to the higher centers of the brain, but the brain stem is intact. The individual breaths spontaneously and a stable circulation is present, but is unaware of self and the environment.
* This condition occurs in diffuse bilateral cerebral hemisphere disturbance, with an intact brain stem.

WHAT IS BRAIN STEM DEATH? WHAT ARE TESTS FOR BRAIN STEM DEATH? (FM2.1)

* Brain stem death is a condition in which the patient is irreversibly unconscious and irreversibly apneic (damage to the respiratory center) due to compression/damage to the brain stem **(Flowchart 8.1)**.
* The tests include test for brain stem reflexes and apnea test.

Test for Brain Stem Functions

* Pupillary reflex (afferent 2nd and efferent 3rd cranial nerves).
* Corneal reflex (afferent 5th and efferent 7th cranial nerves).
* Reflex to grimace (afferent 5th and efferent 7th cranial nerves).
* Vestibulo-ocular reflex (afferent 8th and efferent 3rd and 6th cranial nerves).
* Gag or cough reflex (afferent 9th and efferent 10th cranial nerves).

Apnea Test

* The aim of the test is to prove that the patient is incapable of spontaneous breathing and there are no cells alive in the brain stem, which can trigger respiration.
* **Method:** 100% oxygen is given for 10 minutes, followed by 95% oxygen (high oxygen) and 5% carbon dioxide (high CO_2, since brain stem is triggered more by increased levels of CO_2, rather than reduced O_2 levels) and the ventilator is disconnected; if there are any cells alive in the brain stem, then the patient will breathe spontaneously.

TRANSPLANTATION OF HUMAN ORGANS ACT 1994 (THOA)

(Cadaveric donation: Warm anoxic time/beating heart donor; Harvard's criteria of diagnosing brain stem death)

* TOHA was passed in 1994 and it deals with the regulation of:
  - Removal and storage of human organs.
  - Transplantation of human organs for therapeutic purposes.
  - Prevention of commercial trade in human organs.
* THOA defines human organ as any part of the human body, which if wholly removed cannot be replicated by the body.

CHAPTER 8: Thanatology: Death and its Causes

Flowchart 8.1: Procedure of brain death certification and organ retrieval.

```
                    ┌─────────────────────┐
                    │  Brain stem death   │
                    └──────────┬──────────┘
                               ▼
         ┌────────────────────────────────────────┐
         │ Brain stem death test–GOMs No. 75 and  │
         │          Form 8 THO Act                │
         └──────────────────┬─────────────────────┘
                            ▼
         ┌────────────────────────────────────────┐
         │   Near relative consent–Form 6 THO Act │
         └──────────────────┬─────────────────────┘
                            ▼
         ┌────────────────────────────────────────┐
         │ Hospital request to investigating      │
         │ officer (IO) to do inquest Form 1      │
         │ (GOMs No. 259)                         │
         └──────┬──────────────────────┬──────────┘
                ▼                      ▼
    ┌──────────────────────┐  ┌──────────────────────────┐
    │ 2nd brain stem death │  │ IO conducts inquest Form │
    │ test–GOMs No. 75     │  │ 6 and 8 of THO Act       │
    │                      │  │ should be with IO        │
    └──────────┬───────────┘  └──────────┬───────────────┘
               ▼                         ▼
    ┌──────────────────────────┐  ┌──────────────────────────────┐
    │ If postmortem (PM) not   │  │ If PM required               │
    │ required–IO to inform    │  │ a. Requisition for PM        │
    │ near relatives and organ │  │ b. Form II Organ Functional  │
    │ retrieval takes place    │  │    ↓Status Certificate       │
    │                          │  │    (GOMs No. 259 now         │
    │                          │  │    amended in this GO)       │
    │                          │  │ c. Form 6 and 8 to be given  │
    │                          │  │    to medical officer doing  │
    │                          │  │    PM                        │
    └──────────────────────────┘  └──────────────┬───────────────┘
                                                 ▼
                                   ┌──────────────────────────┐
                                   │   PM by medical officer  │
                                   └──────────────┬───────────┘
                                                  ▼
                                   ┌─────────────────────────────┐
                                   │ MO doing PM shall authorise │
                                   │ organ retrieval–Form III    │
                                   │ (GOMs No. 259)              │
                                   └──────────────┬──────────────┘
                                                  ▼
                                   ┌──────────────────────────┐
                                   │      Organ retrieval     │
                                   └──────────────┬───────────┘
                                                  ▼
                                   ┌──────────────────────────┐
                                   │ PM to be conducted by MO │
                                   └──────────────┬───────────┘
                                                  ▼
                                   ┌──────────────────────────────┐
                                   │ Body handed over to police   │
                                   │ for final handing over to    │
                                   │ near relatives               │
                                   └──────────────────────────────┘
```

- The only organ which can be donated during life is kidney.
- The donor must be above 18 years of age.

Board of doctors to certify brain stem death:
- Registered medical practitioner (RMP) treating the patient.

- RMP in charge of the hospital.
- Neurologist/neurosurgeon nominated from the panel of names approved by the appropriate authority (the director of medical services is the appropriate authority).
- An independent medical specialist (MD in general medicine) nominated from the panel of names approved by the appropriate authority.
- None of the member certifying brain stem death should be associated with the transplantation team.
- THOA 1994 aims to put an end to unrelated live donation and transplantation. This act also prescribes punishment for unauthorized removal of human organs and commercial dealings in retrieval and transplantation. Punishment ranges from temporary erasure of the name of the doctor from SMC for 2 years for the first offence and penal erasure for subsequent offences, and imprisonment with fine, depending on the gravity of the offence.

Cadaveric Donation

- Brain stem death certification by the team of doctors is mandatory for transplantation.
- RMP certifying death should not be a part of the transplantation team.
- Organs are removed when the donor heart is still beating: "**Beating Heart Donor**".
- Success of transplant depends on the functional status of the donated organs, which again depends on the "*warm anoxic time*" (time interval between cessation of arterial oxygen supply and the refrigeration of isolated organs) and in cadaveric donation the warm anoxic time is almost reduced to zero.
- Kidneys are removed within 30 to 60 minutes and generally not stored for more than 12 hours.
- The period of viability of other organs are as follows: Cornea: 6 hours; skin: 24 hours; bone: 48 hours; and blood vessels: 72 hours, after death.

Diagnosis of Brain Stem Death

- **British code or harvard criteria:**
    - *Preconditions:*
        - Comatose patient on a ventilator
        - Positive diagnosis of cause of coma: There should be irreversible/irremediable structural damage to the brain, making the patient unresponsive and comatose.
    - *Exclusion:* Before the certification of brain stem death (i) hypothermia, (ii) coma due to drugs and (iii) metabolic and endocrine causes of coma should be ruled out.
    - *Tests:* (i) Tests for brain stem reflexes, and (ii) Apnea test.

Types of Transplant

- **Homologous donation:** Grafting of cells from one part of the body to another in the same patient. Example: Skin grafting, bone grafting, blood vessels, etc.
- **Heterologous donation (live donation):** Blood, bone marrow and other organs from one individual to the other after proper tissue matching and HLA compatibility.

WHAT ARE STAGES/TYPES OF DEATH? (FM2.1)

There are two stages of death: Clinical death and cellular death.
1. **Somatic or clinical death:** It's the moment of death; it is the time at which circulation, respiration and brain functions irreversibly ceased.
2. **Molecular or cellular death:** Death of the cells and tissues individually, which follows somatic death.

WHAT IS NATURAL AND UNNATURAL DEATH? (FM2.2)

According to Causative Agent death may be classified as:
- **Natural:** Death is purely due to disease. A person suffering for long time from any disease dies directly due to the effects of the disease. Example: Chronic pulmonary tuberculosis, chronic renal failure, congestive cardiac failure, etc., wherein the disease process he is suffering from is not compatible with normal life.
- If the person dies suddenly due to any natural causes, then the pathological process of the disease must be demonstrated at autopsy.
- **Unnatural:** It could be homicidal, suicidal or accidental. Example: Fall from height, road traffic accidents, accidental drowning, suicide by hanging or poisoning, assault by some other person(murder), etc.
  In all unnatural deaths, an inquest is conducted and the body is subjected to postmortem examination,

WHAT IS MODE OF DEATH? (FM2.5)

Mode of death depends on which of the three major life supporting system failed first; there are three modes of death and they are: (i) Coma, (ii) Syncope, and (iii) Asphyxia.

Coma

- Coma is defined as Insensibility of the individual due to damage to the brainstem. Coma is clinical condition and not a cause of death or diagnosis; it occurs in:
  - Compression of brain
  - Drugs induced: Opium, cocaine, alcohol.
  - Metabolic causes: Uremia, diabetes.
  - Infection: Pneumonia, infectious fever, etc.
  - Others: Thrombosis and Embolism, epilepsy, hysteria, etc.

Syncope

- Syncope is sudden stoppage of the function of Heart. This is due to vasovagal attack resulting from reflex parasympathetic stimulation.
- In this condition blood pressure falls suddenly, causing cerebral anaemia and rapid unconsciousness.
  Causes:
  - *Anemia:* Sudden blood loss
  - *Deficient power of heart:* Myocardial infarction, poisons, fatty degeneration
  - *Vagal inhibition:* Reflex inhibition of the heart
  - Exhausting conditions like dehydration and cholera.

Asphyxia

Interference with respiration due to any cause, or lack of oxygen in respired air, due to which the organs and tissues are deprived of oxygen (together with failure to eliminate carbon dioxide) leading to unconsciousness and death.

WHAT IS ANOXIA? WHAT ARE THE TYPES OF ANOXIA?

Anoxia (Hypoxia: Lack of Oxygen)

- Gordon and his co-workers in 1994 claimed that the only mode of death is Anoxia. Let any of three life supporting systems fail first, the end result is tissue anoxia.
- There are four types of anoxia:
  1. *Anoxic anoxia:* Deficient oxygenation in the lungs; from mechanical interference as in hanging and breathing in a contaminated atmosphere.
  2. *Anaemic anoxia:* Due to sudden reduction in blood volume, in this condition the oxygen carrying capacity of the blood is reduced. Example: Injuries resulting in heavy blood loss.

3. *Stagnant anoxia:* Due to impaired circulation, oxygen delivery to the tissues is reduced. Example: Vagal inhibition, myocardial infarction.
4. *Histotoxic anoxia:* There is enough oxygen in the blood whereas the tissues are unable to take up or utilize oxygen. Example: Cyanide poisoning.

WRITE SHORT NOTES ON VAGAL INHIBITION/SYNCOPE (FM2.5)

- Sudden deaths occurring within seconds or minutes due to minor trivial trauma or relatively simple and harmless peripheral stimulation are caused by VAGAL inhibition.
- Pressure on the baroreceptors situated in the carotid sinuses, carotid sheath and carotid body causes an increase in BP, slowing of the heart rate, leading to dilatation of blood vessels with resultant fall in BP. Afferent impulses from the carotid body pass through the glossopharyngeal nerve to the 10th nucleus in the brainstem, and efferent returns through the vagus nerve.
- Some individuals show marked hypersensitivity to stimulation of the carotid sinuses, characterized by bradycardia and cardiac arrhythmias ranging from ventricular arrhythmia to cardiac arrest.

These types of vagal inhibition (syncope) may occur in:
- Pressure over the neck as in hanging, strangulation and compressive pressure on the neck.
- Sudden blows to larynx, chest, epigastrium and genital organs.
- Sudden distension of hollow muscular organs, e.g., during attempts at criminal abortion, when some fluid, gas or instruments are passed into the uterus.

WHAT IS SUDDEN DEATH? WHAT ARE THE DUTIES OF A DOCTOR IN SUCH CASES OF SUDDEN DEATH? WHAT ARE THE COMMONEST CAUSES OF SUDDEN NATURAL DEATH? (FM2.3)

Natural Death
Death occurring due to some natural disease or pathological condition, old age or debility. Death is not intended or attempted.

Sudden Death
- Death is said to be sudden or unexpected when a person not known to have been suffering from any disease, injury or poisoning dies with in 24 hours after the onset of terminal illness.
- The doctor treating the patient should not issue a death certificate in any case of sudden death, even if he has diagnosed the case as death due to natural cause. This is because some other unknown events could have interfered in causing death of the individual, especially involvement of some poisons (many of the signs and symptoms of such poisoning will mimic a natural disease).
- Hence, if death of a patient occurs within 24 hours after the onset of terminal illness, the case has to be considered as sudden death. All such cases should be made as medico-legal case and all such cases must be referred for autopsy after intimating the concerned police station.
- The association of disease with trauma has to be assessed and may involve compensation benefits for the relatives.
- Situations may arise where trauma per se is not fatal and the pathological lesion found at autopsy may have been compatible with continued life, e.g., chronic heart disease. In these situations the effects of trauma on

the existing disease in causing death has to be assessed and evaluated to arrive at a right decision.
- Most of the sudden and unexpected deaths are due to diseases of the Cardio Vascular system. Diseases of the CVS account for nearly 40 to 50% of all sudden deaths.

The **common causes of sudden natural death** are classified according to the system involved as follows:

Cardiovascular System

- **Coronary occlusion: (atheroma, thrombus, embolism): Localization of atheroma:** Left anterior descending artery (45 to 64%), right coronary artery (24 to 46%), left circumflex artery (3 to 10%), and left main coronary (0 to 10%).
- Coronary atherosclerosis with thrombosis **(Fig. 8.1)**.
- Coronary artery embolism
- Cardiac tamponade
- Angina pectoris
- Rupture of aneurysm and dissecting aortic aneurysm
- **Cardio myopathies:** Especially hypertrophic obstructive cardiomyopathy.
- Lesions of conducting system.

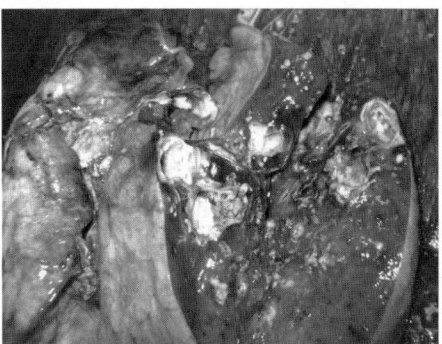

Fig. 8.2: Cross section of the lung, showing multiple cavities filled with pus interspersed with firm yellowish septum—a case of chronic pulmonary tuberculosis *(For color version see Plate 3)*.

Respiratory System

- Air embolism, pulmonary thromboembolism.
- Pneumothorax, bronchopneumonia.
- Status asthmaticus, TB **(Fig. 8.2)**.
- Acute edema of glottis.
- Foreign body impaction in the airway (aspiration and choking).

CNS

- Intra cranial Hemorrhage: Cerebral, cerebellar, pontine hemorrhages.
- Brain tumors, meningitis and encephalitis.
- Cerebral thrombosis and embolism.
- Status epilepticus.
- Rupture of berry aneurysm.

WHAT IS PRESUMPTION OF DEATH? (FM2.6)

- Arises in connection with civil cases.
- A person is presumed to be alive, if there is nothing to suggest the probability of his death within 30 years. But, if proof is produced that the same person is not been heard of for 7 years by his relatives and friends, whom should have heard of him

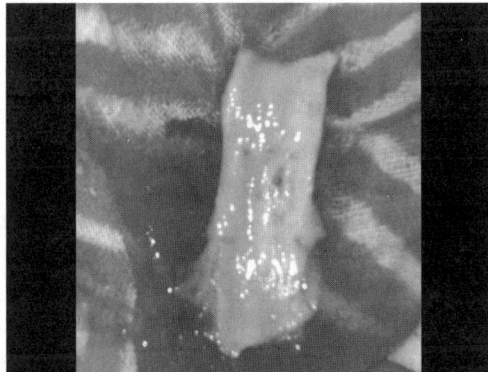

Fig. 8.1: Dissection of lumen of left coronary artery, showing thrombosis *(For color version see Plate 3)*.

if he would have been alive; then death is presumed.

WHAT IS PRESUMPTION OF SURVIVORSHIP? (FM2.6)

- Arises in connection with inheritance of property.
- When two or more persons die in a common disaster. Example: earth quake, plane crash, etc. The question arises who survived longer. The case is decided on facts and evidences available. In the absence of such evidence, age, sex, built, Nature and Severity of injuries and the mode of death are taken into consideration, in deciding the survivorship.

WHAT ARE THE TESTS FOR STOPPAGE OF CIRCULATION, RESPIRATION AND BRAIN STEM FUNCTION?

Tests for Stoppage of Circulation

- **Auscultation:** Absence of heart and breath sounds.
- **Icard's test:** 1% alkaline solution of fluorescein is injected subcutaneously, if there is minute capillary circulation then, the dye will gradually spread with a greenish hue.
- **Ligature test:** A ligature is tied around the root of a finger, if there is little amount of circulation present, the finger will become swollen and red, and the proximal part of the ligature will become pale (blanched).
- **Magnus's test:** A light is placed between webs of the fingers if there is capillary circulation still present there will be a reddish-glow. If there is no circulation, the light will have a yellow and waxy hue.
- **Finger nail test:** When the nail of a finger is pressed firmly, the nail becomes pale; when pressure is released the original red color reappears, if circulation is present.
- **Arterial spurting test:** A small artery if nicked the arterial blood will spurt, if there is little circulation still present (this test is usually not attempted).
- **Heat test:** When heat is applied momentarily over the skin, there will be formation of a blister, with redness and congestion at that place, if there is slightest circulation still present.
- **ECG:** Continued flat wave in all the leads, for a continuous period of 5 minutes signifies stoppage of heart (iso-electric line).

Tests for Stoppage of Respiration

- **Feather test:** Feather of a bird is placed in front of the nose, to check whether it moves; if slight respiration is present, the feather will move. This test has got limitations due to influence from external factors.
- **Mirror test:** A mirror is placed in front of the mouth and if there is slight respiration, then there is deposition of droplets of vapor on the surface of the mirror (useful test).
- **Winslow's test:** A pot containing water or mercury is placed over the chest and a beam of light is focused on it from a fixed source. The reflected image seen on the opposite side is focused on a screen. If there is slightest movement of the chest, there will be gross deflection of the reflected image on the screen.

Tests for Stoppage of Brain Function

- Absence of motor and sensory functions.
- Testing brain stem reflexes.
- Persistent flat EEG.

MULTIPLE CHOICE QUESTIONS

1. **All are involved in brain stem death certification under the Transplantation of Human Organ Act:**
   a. Doctor in-charge of the hospital where brain stem death has taken place
   b. A neurologist or a neurosurgeon appointed from the panel

c. Chief doctor of the transplantation team
d. The doctor treating the patient who's brain stem death has taken place

2. Pick out the odd one:
a. In medico-legal autopsies consent is not required
b. A victim of rape cannot be examined without written consent
c. A person above 18 years can give valid consent to suffer any harm
d. If any person has consented for donating his eyes after death, the eyes can be removed without the consent of legal heirs

3. Suspended animation is seen in the following, *except*:
a. Head injury
b. Electrocution
c. Drowning
d. Barbiturate poisoning

4. One of the following can give consent for harvesting organs from a cadaver when the next kin could not be traced in reasonable time:
a. Dean
b. Medical superintendent
c. The physician who treated the deceased
d. RMO

5. Suspended animation is seen in all, *except*:
a. Newborn
b. Drowning
c. Cholera
d. Partial hanging

6. Find the wrong match:
a. Winslow's test: Respiration
b. Icard's test: Circulation
c. Diaphanous test: Finger webs
d. Magnus test: Respiration

7. A woman with infertility receives an ovary transplant from her sister who is an identical twin. Type of graft is:
a. Xenograft
b. Autograft
c. Allograft
d. Isograft

8. An old lady with mitral stenosis underwent hysterectomy for uterine fibroid and died after developing pulmonary edema. The order of cause of death in international certificate is:
a. Mitral stenosis, pulmonary edema, hysterectomy
b. Pulmonary edema, mitral stenosis, hysterectomy
c. Pulmonary edema, hysterectomy, mitral stenosis
d. Hysterectomy, pulmonary edema, mitral stenosis

9. Cyanides poisoning causes:
a. Histotoxic anoxia
b. Anoxic anoxia
c. Anemic anoxia
d. Stagnant anoxia

10. True about somatic death are all, *except*:
a. Cooling of the body
b. Cessation of spontaneous respiration
c. Cessation of circulation
d. Flat isoelectric EEG

11. All the following are found in brain dead patients, *except*:
a. Absent pupillary reflexes
b. Complete apnea
c. Heart unresponsive to atropine
d. Decreased deep tendon reflex

12. Xenograft is transplantation of tissue:
a. From a different species
b. From genetically identical twins
c. From same species
d. From one part of body to another

13. Molecular death is:
a. Complete and irreversible cessation of brain, heart and lungs function
b. Total loss of EEG activity, but heart is functioning
c. Death of individual tissues and cells after somatic death
d. Vitals functions are at low pitch that cannot be detected by clinical examination

14. Agonal period is the duration between:
a. Traumatic event and information given to the relatives
b. Traumatic event and starting of the operation
c. Lethal trauma up to death
d. Death and postmortem examination

15. Diffusion of oxygen at the tissue level is affected in all the following poisonings, *except*:
a. Carbon monoxide
b. Phosgene
c. Cyanides
d. Curare

16. **Gordon's clarification of death signifies:**
    a. Mechanism of death
    b. Causes of death
    c. Modes of death
    d. Manner of death
17. **All the statements regarding atherosclerosis are true, *except*:**
    a. Naked eye changes are not visible for the first 12 hours
    b. Triphenyl tetrazolium chloride can help in detecting infracted area
    c. Most commonly involves the left coronary artery
    d. Common site is the anterior wall of right ventricle
18. **Immediate sign of death is:**
    a. Decrease in body temperature
    b. Changes in skin
    c. Dilatation of pupil
    d. Cessation of respiration and circulation
19. **Suspended animation may be seen in:**
    a. Electrocution
    b. Hanging
    c. Lightening
    d. Burns
20. **All are tests associated with cessation of circulation, *except*:**
    a. Winslow's test
    b. Magnus test
    c. I-card's test
    d. Diaphanous test

ANSWERS

| 1. c | 2. d | 3. a | 4. d | 5. d | 6. d | 7. d | 8. c | 9. a | 10. a |
| 11. d | 12. a | 13. c | 14. c | 15. d | 16. c | 17. d | 18. d | 19. a | 20. a |

CHAPTER 9

Postmortem Changes

KEY WORDS

Postmortem changes, time since death, changes in the eye, Tache Noire, Kevorkian's sign, algor mortis, postmortem caloricity, livor mortis, contact flattening, primary flaccidity, rigor mortis, cadaveric spasm, heat rigor, cold stiffening, gas stiffening, autolysis, putrefaction, honeycomb liver, marbling, postmortem purge, coagulative putrefaction, Casper's dictum, mummification, adipocere, carbon dating, forensic entomology, presumption of death, presumption of survivorship.

FM2.8	Describe and discuss postmortem changes including signs of death, cooling of body, postmortem lividity, rigor mortis cadaveric spasm, cold stiffening and heat stiffening.
FM2.9	Describe putrefaction, mummification, adipocere and maceration.
FM2.10	Discuss estimation of time since death.

INTRODUCTION

- The changes that take place in the dead body after death are called as **postmortem changes**.
- They are classified into three stages; all these changes commence simultaneously after death, but evident to our eyes only when time advances.
  - *Immediate changes:* Few minutes after death to maximum 30 minutes.
  - *Early changes:* 30 minutes to 36 hours.
  - *Late changes:* After 36 hours.

WHAT ARE THE IMMEDIATE CHANGES AFTER DEATH? (FM2.8)

- These are changes which take place immediately or at the moment of death and are important for the clinicians to confirm death and issue a death certificate.
  - Complete and irreversible cessation of functions of brain, heart and lungs.
  - Muscles of the body become flaccid. (primary flaccidity).
  - Corneal and pupillary reflexes are abolished.
  - *Insensibility and primary flaccidity of the muscles:* This is one the earliest sign of death and very much concurrent with the moment of death (somatic death), but cannot be considered positive because it is also seen in cases of deep coma, narcosis and suspended animation.
  - *Permanent stoppage of circulation:* Stoppage of circulation for more than

5 minutes, but in certain conditions, even after stoppage of respiration, heart may continue to beat for more than 10 minutes as in cases of hanging (idio-synchrotic rythm).

WHAT ARE THE EARLY CHANGES AFTER DEATH? (FM2.8)

- Changes in the skin
- Changes in the eyes
- Algor mortis (cooling of the body)
- Livor mortis (postmortem hypostasis)
- Rigor mortis (cadaveric rigidity)

DESCRIBE THE CHANGES IN THE SKIN AND EYE AFTER DEATH? (FM2.8)

Changes in the Skin

Skin loses its elasticity immediately after death. Skin which was translucent during life becomes pale and ashy-white.

Changes in the Eyes

- **Pupils:** Dilated and fixed (no reaction to light), later becomes constricted (with onset of rigor mortis).
- **Cornea:** Looses its luster, becomes dull, hazy, and finally opaque and wrinkled.

Tache Noire Sclerotica (Fig. 9.1)

- A thin film of cell debris and mucus forms two yellow triangles of desiccated discoloration on the sclera each at the side of the iris; which becomes brown and then black, due to continuous exposure to the atmospheric air when the eyelids are open.
- **Intraocular pressure:** Normal intra ocular tension is 14 mm Hg. After death it falls so rapidly that by 1 hour its 3 mm Hg and by 2 hours, the intra ocular pressure is nearly zero. Eye balls appear sunken.
- **Changes in retina:** Fragmentation or segmentation of blood columns appears

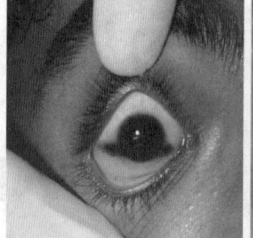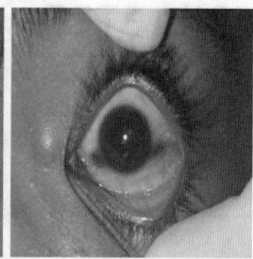

Fig. 9.1: Tache Noire sclerotica
(For color version see Plate 3).

within minutes after death called as *"Trucking"* (**Kevorkian sign**). Retina is Pale for the 1st two hrs. Then at about 6 hours after death the disc outline is hazy. It becomes totally blurred in 7 to 10 hours. These changes in the retina can be appreciated only by using an ophthalmoscope, and interpreted by an expert ophthalmologist.

- **Chemical changes in vitreous humor:** Vitreous humor is the only body fluid which is reliable indicator to assess the time since death. There will be a gradual raise in the potassium level after death up to 4 or 5 days.

DESCRIBE ALGOR MORTIS (COOLING OF THE BODY)? (FM2.8)

- During life there is a constant balance between heat production and heat lost. After death heat production is lost, hence the body starts cooling.
- The body looses heat by conduction, convection and radiation.
- Body surface starts loosing heat rapidly, but the inner body core temperature does not alter until a gradient is established between the core body temperature and the environmental temperature.
- There is no significant change in the core body temperature up to 2 hours from the time of death. Once the gradient is established, the body starts losing heat at a constant rate.

- The rate of cooling is proportional to the difference in temperature between the body and the surface (Newton's Law).
- Temperature is measured by using a chemical thermometer graduated from 1 to 50 degrees centigrade, inserted 10 cm into the rectum. When there is history of suspected sexual assault, then the temperature is measured from the undersurface of the liver by making a slit opening on the upper part of right side of the abdomen (sub-hepatic temperature).
- Time since death = $\dfrac{\text{Normal body temp} - \text{Rectal temp/sub-hepatic temp}}{\text{Rate of fall of temp/hour}}$
- **Example:** $\dfrac{37 \text{ (Normal temp)} - 35.5 \text{ (measured)}}{1.5 \text{ (constant)}} = 1 \text{ hour}.$
- Factors affecting the rate of cooling
  - The environmental temperature has a direct proportional effect on cooling of the body.
  - Coverings on or around the body; clothing prevent heat loss from the body.
  - Built of the cadaver:
    - Heat loss is proportional to the surface area of the body; ultimately, the body of children and old people cool rapidly.
    - Fat is a bad conductor of heat; hence females and obese bodies cool slowly.

WHAT IS POSTMORTEM CALORICITY? (FM2.8)

Usually after death the body starts cooling. But in certain circumstances, there is an increase in the body temperature for the first few hours after death, it is called postmortem caloricity. The mechanism and conditions of this phenomenon are as follows:
- When the heat regulatory mechanism has been severely disturbed before death: For example, sun stroke and pontine hemorrhage.
- When there is increased heat production in the muscles of the body before death due to convulsions: For example, tetanus, strychnine poisoning and epilepsy.
- Excessive bacterial activity during life: For example, Septicemic deaths, cholera and other infections.

DESCRIBE LIVOR MORTIS? (FM2.8) (POSTMORTEM STAINING/ POSTMORTEM LIVIDITY/ POSTMORTEM HYPOSTASIS)

- Purplish red discoloration of the skin which takes place on the dependent parts of the body after death is called postmortem staining. After stoppage of circulation, the blood which is fluid in nature, gradually settles down in the toneless capillaries on the dependent parts of the body by 2 to 3 hours after death.
- Those parts of the body which is in actual contact with the surface do not show this staining, as the capillaries are firmly pressed by weight of the body, and this is known as areas of "**contact flattening**". When the body is supine position, the occipital region, shoulder blades, the both buttock, back of this, back of legs and the heel do not show the postmortem staining. These are areas of contact flattening. But when the body is tilted then soon staining develops in these areas, if the staining has not yet been fixed.

Time of Appearance (Figs. 9.2 and 9.3)

- Postmortem lividity begins as mottled patches ranging from 1 to 2 cm in diameter in 2 to 3 hours after death. These patches

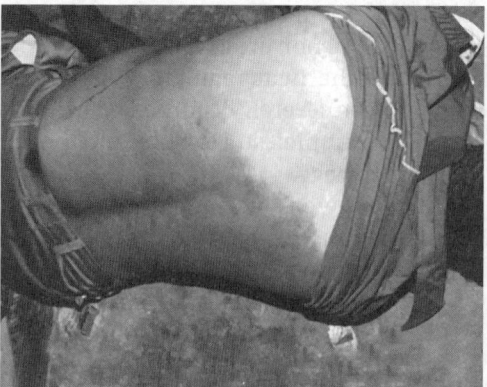 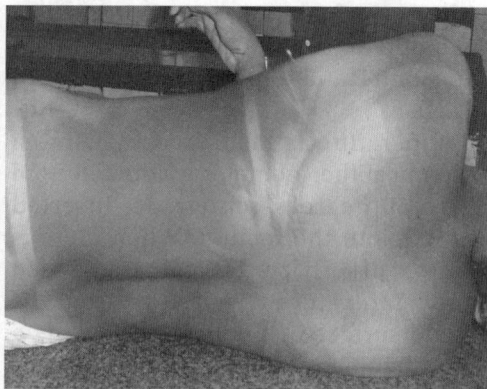

Figs. 9.2 and 9.3: Fixed postmortem staining with areas of contact flattening time since death is more than 6 hours *(For color version see Plate 3).*

gradually increase in size and coalesce with each other to form a uniform area of staining in 4 to 6 hours.
- If the position of the body is altered within a few hours of death, then these patches gradually disappear, and reappear in the new dependent parts.
- Fixation of postmortem staining takes place in 6 to 8 hours. When we apply pressure on the skin using our thumb, the staining disappears at the point of application of force and that area become pale (blanching) and the staining reappear when the pressure is released. Which means postmortem staining is not fixed. If it is fixed, then blanching will not be there when we apply pressure and postmortem staining will remain as such.
- PMS does not disappear and are present as such, but they are masked with the onset of color changes of putrefaction. During putrefaction the skin color changes to greenish black and hence postmortem staining cannot be appreciated.
- PMS may not develop at all, if the body is tossed and turned continuously as seen in fast flowing water in rivers.
- PMS cannot be appreciated properly in dark colored individuals.
- PMS may not be appreciated even in fair skinned bodies if they have bled profusely before death or were severely anemic at the time of death.
- PMS has to be differentiated from contusion.

Medico-legal Importance

- It is a sign of death.
- It helps in estimating the time since death.
- Indicates the posture of the body at the time of death; it also indicates any alteration/deliberate disturbance in the position of the body after death.
- The color of postmortem staining gives a clue to the poison involved in causing death, described in **Table 9.1.**

TABLE 9.1: Color of PMS and poison.

Poison	Color
Carbon monoxide	Cherry red
Cyanide	Bright red
Hydrogen sulfide	Greenish blue
Phosphorus	Brown
Nitrobenzene, potassium chloride	Brownish red
Aniline	Blue or bluish brown

DESCRIBE RIGOR MORTIS? DISCUSS THE CONDITIONS ALTERING THE APPEARANCE OF RIGOR MORTIS? (FM2.8)

Rigor mortis is also called "**cadaveric rigidity**"
- Rigor mortis is a state of stiffening of the body due to rigidity with relative shortening of the muscle fibers. At the moment of death, the muscles go into primary flaccidity and rigor mortis sets in the muscles with passage of time. The muscles go in for secondary relaxation after rigor mortis passes off.
- It indicates the molecular death of the muscles and the muscles do not react to electrical stimulus after rigor mortis has set in.
- Rigor mortis appears in all the muscles of the body, skeletal and smooth muscles; voluntary and involuntary muscles.
- Rigor mortis is a chemical process and is not dependent upon blood supply or nerve supply. It is an internal process within the muscles and hence appears even in an amputated limb.
- **Mechanism (ATP depletion):** The muscle fibers are made of two contractile units namely, actin and myosin filaments. When the muscles are contracted as when walking, lifting some objects or doing any kind of work the actin and myosin filaments come close to each other; later gets relaxed. Energy required for this process of relaxation is derived from the ATP and the ATP gets reduced to ADP.
- During life ATP is constantly synthesized in the body. After death there is no synthesis of ATP, but the muscles fibers have some amount of ATP in store. As long as there is ATP storage in the muscles the fibers remains relaxed. Once the stored ATP is exhausted the muscle fibers goes in a far a permanent state of contraction called Rigor mortis.
- **Order of appearance: Proximo-distal spread**—rigor mortis starts first in the eyelids then it gradually spreads to the muscles of the face, jaw, neck, upper limbs, chest, abdomen and lastly the lower limbs, this is called proximo-distal spread of rigor mortis.
- **Time of appearance (Rule of twelve):**
  - Starts in 3 to 6 hours
  - Takes 12 hours to complete
  - Stays for another 12 hours
  - Passes off in the next 12 hours.
- Rigor mortis passes off in the same order of appearance.

Conditions Altering the Onset and Duration of Rigor Mortis

- **Age:** Rigor mortis does not occur in a fetus of less than 7 months of intra-uterine age. This is because the myofibrils are formed completely only by seven months of intra-uterine life. Thus, helps to find out whether the fetus is viable or not (age of the fetus) In healthy adult it develops slowly but well pronounced and passes off late. Whereas, in children and old it is feeble and rapid; appears early, stays for a short duration and passes off early.
- **Muscular state at the time of death:** Onset of rigor mortis slow and duration is long in cases where muscles are at rest and healthy before death. Appears early and passes of early if the individual dies after great exhaustion.
- **Nature of death:** In deaths from diseases causing great exhaustion and wasting, the onset is early and duration is short.
- **Atmospheric condition:**
  - Onset is slow and duration is long in cold winter
  - Onset is fast and duration is short in hot weather

Medico Legal Importance

- Rigor mortis a sign of death
- Helps in estimation of time since death; in India, we depend more on rigor mortis to assess the time since death.

- Indicates the position of the body at the time of death (to some extent and not always). For example, an individual dies while sitting on a chair. Sometimes, the body may slip down to the floor during the phase of primary flaccidity.

WHAT ARE THE CONDITIONS SIMULATING RIGOR MORTIS? WHAT IS CADAVERIC SPASM? (FM2.8)

Conditions which look like rigor mortis are:
- Cadaveric spasm
- **Heat stiffening:** Due to coagulation of muscle protein, e.g., death due to burns.
- **Cold stiffening:** Due to solidification of subcutaneous fat and water content of the body, for example, bodies subjected to extreme cold temperature, as in high altitudes and when stored in refrigerators in mortuaries.
- **Gas stiffening:** Due to gas accumulation under the skin and subcutaneous tissues in the process of putrefaction.

Cadaveric Spasm or Instantaneous Rigor

- A group of voluntary muscles which were at strenuous work during life (at the time of death) goes into a sudden state of contraction without passing through the stage of primary flaccidity, is called as cadaveric spasm. It is of great medico legal importance:
- Occurs especially in cases of sudden death, death due to exhaustion and fear, etc.
- It reflects the last action of the individual at the time of death. For example, firearm in the hands of victims in suicidal gunshot injuries, plants and weeds in the hands of victims in cases of drowning, the weapon in the hands of victims in cut throat injuries, etc.
- Cadaveric spasm cannot be mimicked.
- With the onset of rigor mortis the whole body goes in for stiffening (cadaveric spasm merges with rigor mortis); when rigor mortis passes off cadaveric spasm also passes off. Difference between Rigor mortis and Cadaveric spasm tabulated in **Table 9.2**.

DISCUSS THE PROCESS DECOMPOSITION OF A DEAD BODY? (FM2.9)

Short Notes: Color Changes of Decomposition; Colliquative Putrefaction

Marbling; Honey-comb Liver

Late change: Decomposition of the body.
- It is a process of gradual destruction of body tissues by combined effects of enzymes and destructive action of microorganism, after death.
- It occurs in 2 ways: (1) **Autolysis**: Enzyme action, and (2) **Putrefaction**: Bacterial Action.

TABLE 9.2: Difference between Rigor mortis and Cadaveric spasm.

Rigor mortis	Cadaveric spasm
Occurs in all the muscles of the body	Occurs only in a group of voluntary muscles
Follows primary flaccidity (starts 3 to 6 hours after death)	Occurs immediately at the time of death
Postmortem finding	Antemortem finding
Helps to estimate the time since death	Not useful to find the time of death
Does not reflect the last act	Reflects the last act of the individual

1. **Autolysis:**
   - Cells become permeable after death with release of cytoplasm containing enzymes.
   - The proteolytic enzymes cause chemical digestion and disintegration of the organs.
   - Autolysis is increased by heat and stopped by freezing.
   - Autolysis is an aseptic process which results in maceration of dead fetus in the uterus.
   - Auto disintegration occurs in: (i) brain (liquefaction) (ii) stomach and GIT (iii) pancreas.
2. **Putrefaction:** The process of putrefaction is divided into three stages for easy understanding, However, all the changes starts occurring from the time of death and are evident to our eyes as time advances.
   - Color changes,
   - Production of foul smelling gases,
   - Liquefaction of tissues.

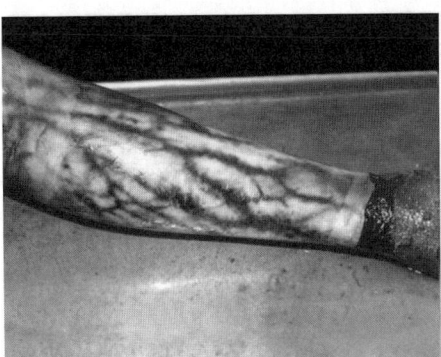

Fig. 9.4: Marbling of veins
(For color version see Plate 4).

Color Change

- 1st external sign of decomposition is the Greenish discoloration in the right lilac fossa; which become evident in 12–24 hours in summer and 1 to 3 days in winter.
- The color change first occurs in the right iliac fossa because of the presence of caecum, where there are more colonic bacteria and normal bacterial flora of the gut. The bacterial colonies produces hydrogen sulfide, which combines with hemoglobin to form sulphmethaemoglobin, which responsible for the greenish discoloration.
- This color change spreads to the entire abdomen, and extends further to the chest, neck, face and last to the limbs.
- Color gradually changes to dark green then finally black.

- The putrefaction bacteria spread easily in the body fluid and colonize in the venous system. The superficial veins of the limbs, chest, abdomen and neck are stained greenish blue due to hemolysis of red cells and stain the walls of the vessels. This condition is called as "**Marbling**" (**Fig. 9.4**) which occur 36 to 48 hrs after death, in summer and 2 to 3 days in winter. Marbling has to be differentiated from filigree burns, which is due to lightening. Marbling is well appreciated after the peeling of cuticle, due to rupture of subcutaneous gas blebs.

Evolution of Foul Smelling Gases (Fig. 9.5)

- The main gases are ammonia, carbon dioxide, hydrogen sulfide, phosphorated hydrogen and methane.
- In early stages, these gases are non-inflammable; later on with the formation of enough hydrogen sulfide the gases become inflammable.
- Due to continued accumulation of gases, there is distention of breast in females, penis and scrotum in males.
- Abdomen gets distended due to accumulation of gases in the intestines. Diaphragm is pushed up compressing the lungs and heart. Due to the increased

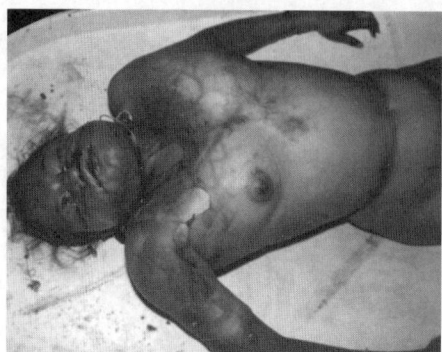

Fig. 9.5: Postmortem purge with gas stiffening *(For color version see Plate 4).*

intra-abdominal pressure, blood stained frothy fluid exudes from the mouth and nostrils, which is called "*postmortem purge*". This can be mistaken for antemortem findings of pulmonary oedema or drowning.
- Involuntary urination, defecation, seminal ejaculation and delivery of dead fetus occur at this stage.
- Gas bubbles accumulate in all the tissues; subcutaneous tissues become emphysematous.
- Eyes bulge out from their sockets; tongue is forced out between the swollen lips.
- Due to the formation of gas blebs, blisters appear **(Fig. 9.6)** between the epidermis and dermis all over the body.
- Epidermis becomes loosened (skin slippage) producing large, fragile sacs of clear or pink red serous fluid. These blisters gradually enlarge, join together and rupture, exposing large areas of slimy pink dermis **(Fig. 9.7)**.
- By three days the face becomes discolored, bloated and distorted that identification becomes very difficult.
- The muscles become soft, loose and are converted into a thick semisolid pinkish mass and are gradually separated from the bones by around 2 weeks.
- The cartilages and ligaments are softened in the final stage of decomposition.

Liquefaction of Tissues (Colliquative Putrefaction)

- Colliquative putrefaction begins from 5 to 10 days.
- The abdomen bursts and contents of abdomen comes out of the cavity.
- The omental, mesenteric and peritoneal fat liquefy into a translucent, yellow fluid filling the body cavities between the organs.
- All encapsulated internal organs are converted into bags of putrid fluid and subsequently burst open into the thoraco-abdominal cavity

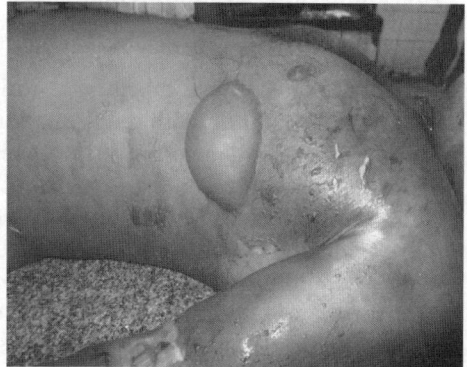

Fig. 9.6: Postmortem blister formation *(For color version see Plate 4).*

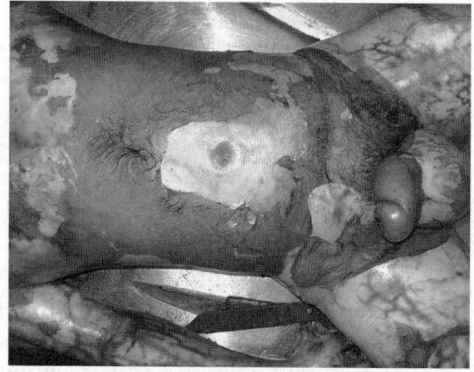

Fig. 9.7: Postmortem peeling of cuticle of skin with gas stiffening *(For color version see Plate 4).*

- The rate of putrefaction of the individual organs depend on the enzyme content, water content and blood supply of the organs. Adrenals and pancreas are the first organs to undergo putrefaction; followed by stomach and intestines; next, the spleen and liver (due to more blood present inside them); then the lungs and later the heart undergoes putrefaction.
- Liver becomes softened and flabby in 24 hours. During the phase of accumulation of gases, multiple blisters appear in the liver, which on cut section appears as yellowish-gray, dendritic figures in the parenchyma in 2 to 3 days; which is called "**foamy**" liver or "**honeycombed**" liver.
- Kidneys and urinary bladder putrefy relatively late.
- Prostrate in males and uterus in females are the last internal organs to undergo putrefaction due to presence of large amount of fibrous tissues.

Skeletonization

- In an exposed body flies, maggots, ants, cockroaches, rats, dogs, vultures, etc., may reduce the body to skeleton in a few days.
- When the body is in water it may be attacked by fishes, crabs, etc., and the body is skeletonized within a few days.
- Unconfined body buried in a shallow grave there is moderate delay of putrefaction.
- If deeply buried, due to low temperature and lack of air circulation, the process of putrefaction gets delayed.
- The main factors affecting Skeletonization are seasonal and climatic variations, moisture content of the soil, presence and absence of air circulation and PH of soil.
- In India, an unconfined buried body is reduced to skeleton within one year.
- Bodies placed in airtight coffins, decomposition may not occur for several decades.

WHAT ARE THE CONDITIONS AFFECTING THE RATE OF PUTREFACTION?

Short Notes: Casper's Dictum (FM2.9)

External Factors
- Temperature
- Moisture
- Air
- Clothing
- Manner of burial
- **Temperature:** Even though putrefaction begins to set in above 10°C, the optimum temperature is between 21°C to 38°C; putrefaction is completely is arrested if the temperature is below 0°C and above 48°C.
- **Moisture:** Moisture is necessary for putrefaction

  Bodies recovered from water, if left in the air decompose rapidly. Organs which contain more water decompose readily than the dry ones.
- **Air:** Free movement of air hastens putrefaction.
- **Clothing:** Initially clothing's enhances putrefaction by maintaining body temperature. But later on the clothing delay putrefaction by preventing the access of airborne organisms, flies and insects. Putrefaction is delayed under tight garments (belts, socks, undergarments, boots, etc.) which drives out the blood from that part of the body and there by prevent the entry of bacterial organisms.
- **Manner of burial:**
  - *Putrefaction is delayed:* (i) When the bodies are buried soon after death; (ii) If buried in dry, sandy soil or in a grave deeper than 2 meters; (iii) In coffined bodies (exclusion of air, water and access for insects); (iv) Salt and lime markedly delay putrefaction
  - *Putrefaction is rapid:* (i) In a body buried in a damp, marshy or shallow grave; (ii) In porous sandy soil, than

in soils with excess of clay; (iii) More rapid if changes of decomposition are already present at the time of burial; (iv) In acidic soils even the bones may be destroyed.

Internal Factors

- **Age:** Bodies of children putrefy early than the old people. Bodies of new born that have not been fed decompose slowly; if fed before death or if there are any injuries on the body then the process of decomposition is rapid.
- **Sex:** No significant difference in the rate of putrefaction between male and female. But females due to their high fat content may retain the body heat for long time (fat is a bad conductor of heat and hence may prevent the body from cooling) thus favoring the process of putrefaction.
- **Condition of the body:** Fat bodies putrefy quickly than lean bodies, due to larger amount of fluid, excess fat and greater retention of heat.
- **Cause of death:**
  - Putrefaction is rapid in persons dying from Septicemia, Peritonitis, Inflammatory and septic conditions and asphyxia (abnormal fluidity of blood helps the spread of bacteria).
  - Putrefaction is rapid in infection due to Cl. Welchii for example acute intestinal obstruction, Abortion and Gas gangrene.
  - Putrefaction is delayed if death is due to: (i) Wasting diseases, Anemia and Debility (less blood prevents spread of the bacteria) (ii) Poisoning by phenol, zinc chloride, strychnine and chronic heavy metal poisoning (arsenic, lead, mercury)
- **Mutilation:** Bodies with wounds putrefy rapidly, as it allows easy access of bacteria and flies. In dismemberment, the limbs putrefy slowly and the trunk putrefies rapidly.

- In advanced putrefaction, no opinion can be given as to the cause of death, except in cases of poisoning, fractures, fire arm injuries, etc.

Putrefaction in Water

Putrefaction is delayed when a body is lying deep in water and covered by clothing.

Casper Dictum

$$1 : 2 : 8$$
$$\text{Air} : \text{Water} : \text{Earth}$$

- Rate of putrefaction is low in water than in air; rapid in warm fresh water than in cold salt water; still lower when buried under the earth.
- This is casper dictum, putrefaction in air is 2 times faster than in water and it is 8 times slower when the body buried in the earth.

WHAT ARE THE MODIFIED FORMS OF PUTREFACTION? (FM2.9)

Short Notes on Adipocere and Mummification

Adipocere and Mummification, are the two modified forms of putrefaction. These modified putrefaction occurs when the condition favors them.

Adipocere (Saponification)

- This is a modified form of putrefaction.
- The fatty tissues of the body change into a substance similar to soaps, known as adipocere.
- Commonly seen in bodies immersed in water or in damp warm environment.

Mechanism

- Gradual hydrolysis and hydrogenation of preexisting fats, such as olein, into higher fatty acids, which combine with calcium and ammonium ions to form insoluble soaps.

- These soaps being acidic in nature inhibit the putrefactive bacteria.
- The body fat is converted into palmitic, oleic, stearic and hydroxystearic acid by the fat splitting enzyme lecithinase, produced by clostridia group of organisms, mainly clostridium perfringens.
- The water required for hydrolysis is obtained mainly from the body tissues.
- If the body is in water, this fluid contributes to the hydrolysis of the subcutaneous fat. Water also helps to remove glycerin which is formed during hydrolysis of fat.
- Both moisture and heat are important for the formation of adipocere.

Properties

- Adipocere has a distinct offensive or sweetish odor. In the early stages, a penetrating ammoniacal odor is noticed.
- Fresh adipocere is soft, moist, whitish, translucent, greasy and resembles pale rancid butter.
- After some years it becomes dry, hard cracked, yellowish and brittle.
- It is inflammable and burns with a faint yellow flame.
- Floats in water and dissolves in alcohol and ether.

Distribution

- It can occur at any site, where fatty tissue is present.
- First subcutaneous fat gets converted into adipocere. Adipocere change is usually partial affecting face, buttocks, breast and abdomen. Occasionally the whole body may be affected. The epidermis disappears as the process of adipocere formation advances.
- Initially, it appears as multiple whitish grey rounded outgrowths varying from 1 to 10 cm in diameter. It joins with each other to cover the entire body at a later stage.
- In adipocere the liver looks prominent and retains its shape.
- The gross features and histological appearance of the organs can sometimes be appreciated.

Time required for adipocere formation

- The minimum time required is 3 weeks in summer.
- Process of stiffening, hardening and swelling of fat occurs over a period of months.
- In most cases the change is partial and irregular.
- Complete conversion in an adult limb requires at least 3 to 6 months.
- Obese individuals with more fat content and mature new born form adipocere rapidly.
- Nonviable fetus do not show this change.
- Adipocere may persist for years or decades.

Medico-legal Importance

- The morphological features are well preserved and help to establish the identity of the individual.
- Cause of death can be made out as the injuries are usually well preserved.
- Time since death can be assessed based on the stage and extent of adipocere.

Mummification

- It is a modified form of putrefaction which produces dehydration, drying and desiccation, and shriveling of the cadaver. Occurs due to evaporation of water content in the body.
- It begins in exposed parts of the body like face or limbs, and then extends to the entire body including the internal organs.
- Skin is shrunken and contracted, dry, brittle, leathery and rusty brown in color and Stretched tightly over the bony prominences such as cheek, chin, ribs, hip and adheres to the bone.
- Mummification may be partial in some cases, with only head or limb being affected.

- Internal organs become black, shrunken, hard, and become a single mass.
- Body loses weight, becomes thin, stiff and brittle.
- Mummified bodies if protected can be preserved for years; Mummified bodies are practically odorless.
- Marked dehydration before death favors mummification.
- It takes 3 months to 1 year for the entire body to be mummified.
- Absence of moisture, continuous action of dry warm air is necessary for this process. **Example:** The mummies in Egypt.
- Mummification of new born may occur if left in a trunk or cupboard.
- Mummification occurs in bodies buried in shallow graves in dry sandy soils.
- Chronic arsenic and antimony poisoning favors the process of mummification.
- Occasionally some parts of the body shows mummification and some parts may undergo putrefaction or even adipocere formation (especially when part of the body is in water).

Medico-legal Importance

- Features are well preserved, and help to establish the identity.
- Cause of death can be made out as the injuries are preserved.
- Time since death can be assessed, based on the extent of mummification.

DISCUSS ENTOMOLOGY OF CADAVER?

- Flies lay eggs on the fresh corpse, in the moist areas of the body, for example, eyelids, nostrils, angle of mouth, etc., soon after death.
- Once skin decomposition begins, eggs are laid down anywhere on the body
- Larvae and Maggots are produced from the eggs in 8 to 12 hours.

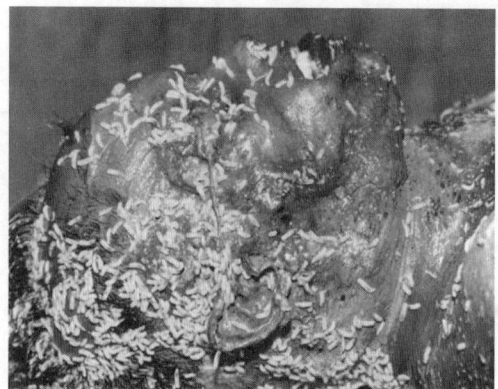

Fig. 9.8: Fully grown maggots crawling over the face *(For color version see Plate 4).*

- These maggots crawl into the interior of the body and Produce powerful Proteolytic enzymes and destroy the soft tissues
- Maggots become pupae in 4 to 5 days. They become adult flies in another 3 to 5 days shown in **Figure 9.8.**

Medico-legal Importance

- To estimate the time since death based on the stage of development of the insect.
- To identify the cause of death, in certain poisoning cases.
- To corroborate the scene of crime, by identifying the species of the insect.

WHAT IS TIME SINCE DEATH? (FM2.10)

Enumerate the Various Factors Useful in Estimating the Time Since Death

- The time interval between the time of Death and the time of conducting Autopsy is called the Time Since Death. Postmortem changes and the approximate TSD tabulated in **Table 9.3**
- The exact time of death cannot be fixed in any case, but a range of time between which death was presumed to have taken place, can be estimated. It is more of a

TABLE 9.3: Postmortem changes and the approximate TSD (hot climate).

	Postmortem changes	Time in hours
1.	Body warm, transparent cornea	Within 1 hour
2.	Postmortem lividity in patches	2 to 3 hours
3.	Body cold, uniform PMS and fixed; RM in upper parts of body	6 to 8 hours
4.	Rigor mortis all over the body	Around 12 hours
5.	Body cold and stiff, eggs and flies; greenish discoloration in the right iliac fossa	12 to 24 hours
6.	Rigor mortis passing off and abdominal distension	24 to 36 hours
7.	Greenish discoloration on abdomen and chest, marbling; distension of abdomen and thorax; PM blisters and maggots	36 to 48 hours
8.	Whole body bloated, face unrecognizable; nails and hairs easily pulled off; grown maggots/pupae all over body	3 to 5 days
9.	Colliquative putrefaction, internal organs are reduced to black unrecognizable pultaceous mass; most of the soft tissues disappeared; prostrate and non-gravid uterus recognizable	2 weeks
10.	Skeleton exposed bare	1 to 3 months

scientific guess, rather than a precise opinion.
- The longer the Postmortem interval, less accurate is the estimated Time Since Death.
- Determination of TSD is an indispensable component of corpus delicti.

Estimating the Time Since Death is Important as

- To know when the crime has been committed.
- A starting point for the Police in the investigation of the crime.
- Exclude some subjects and to search for the likely culprit.
- To check on a subject's statement.

To Give Opinion on Time of Death

- Go through all the available history.
- Local physical and environmental factors at the scene of crime (e.g., fire, open windows, environmental temp, etc.) should be considered before giving an opinion regarding the time since death.

External Examination

The body thoroughly examined for:
- Algor mortis (cooling of the body)
- Livor mortis (postmortem staining)
- Rigor mortis (cadaveric rigidity)
- Decomposition and/or its modifications
- Entomology of cadaver (maggots).

On Internal Examination of the Body

- **Stomach emptying time:**
  - Stomach starts emptying with in 10 minutes.
  - Bulk of the food is emptied in 2 hours
  - Light meal in 2 hours; Medium meal in 3 to 4 hours; and Heavy meal in 5 to 6 hours.
  - Digestion is delayed in sleep and suspended in coma.
  - Emotional disturbances cause hyper motility and can result in rapid emptying
  - Diet rich in carbohydrate empties faster than proteins, which is faster than fat.
  - Head of the meal reaches hepatic flexure in 6 hours; splenic flexure in 9

to 12 hours; and pelvic colon in 12 to 18 hours.
- If stomach is full and contains undigested food, the time since death would be approximately 2 to 4 hours.
- **Urinary bladder: bladder emptying time:**
  - Average urine volume of a healthy adult is 1.5 liters/day half of urine production occurs at night.
  - Depending upon the volume of urine in the bladder a rough estimate of time of death can be made out. The rate of formation of urine in an adult is 1 mL/min; the amount of urine present in the bladder will indicate the approximate time of death, if the previous bladder emptying time is known.
  - Since its customary with most people to evacuate the bladder before going to bed; if the bladder is full it can be said that the individual has lived for a reasonable period of time after going to bed. If the bladder contains only a few mL, then we can say the individual died shortly after going to bed.

Other useful indicators which can be assessed only by laboratory techniques are:
- **Cerebrospinal fluid:**
  - Lactic acid concentration raises from 15 mg % to 200 mg % in 15 hours;
  - Nonprotein nitrogen shows steady raise 15 mg % to 40 mgs % in 15 hours;
  - Amino acid evenly raises from 1 mg % to 12 mg % in 15 hours.

  Depending upon the rate of increase the approximate time of death can be assesses.
- **Blood:**
  - Potassium, phosphorus, magnesium—increase after death
  - Sodium and chloride—decrease after death
  - Other compounds the concentration of which increases after death are: Nonprotein nitrogen, amino acid nitrogen, lactic acid and bilirubin.
  - Certain enzymes like acid phosphatase, alkaline phosphatase, amylase, lactic dehydrogenase also increases after death.
- **Bone marrow:**
  - During life up to 40% of cells are neutrophils.
  - After death, within 1 hour the nuclei begin to swell; becomes round in 4 hours; formation of vacuoles in the cytoplasm, cell outline becomes obscure in about 10 hours.
- **Vitreous humor:**
  - Gradual increase in potassium and reduction in sodium occurs for the first 85 hours (3 to 4 days) after death.
  - The level of glucose and pyruvic acid decreases and lactic acid increases after death.
- **Hair growth:** During life hair grows at the rate of 0.4 mm/day. After death hair and nails stops growing. If the time of last shave is known, then an approximate interval of the time of survival can be made out.
- **Non-scientific data:** Examination of scene of crime for time since death
  - Certain scene markers like news papers, dates on a postal mail, the degree of coagulation of milk, state of food on a table will indicate the approximate time since death.
  - If the body lies on growing grass, underlying grass and vegetations soon dries and turns yellow or brown. This will indicate how long the body was lying at the scene.
- **Carbon dating:** (radio active carbon)
  - C14 content of the bone are steadily maintained during life.
  - After death Radioactivity of C14 gradually weakens with the half life being 5,600 years.

    Radioactive carbon dating is useful only for cases which date back to several centuries; it is not useful, for the bones which are less than a century old.

MULTIPLE CHOICE QUESTIONS

1. **Ideal site to measure the temperature of dead body, in suspected case of sexual abuse:**
   a. Mouth
   b. Axilla
   c. Rectum
   d. Sub-hepatic
2. **One of the following is more reliable in estimating the time since death in India:**
   a. Algor mortis
   b. Rigor mortis
   c. Livor mortis
   d. Putrefaction
3. **The following are the most common significance of rigor mortis, except:**
   a. Sign of death
   b. Time of death
   c. Position of death
   d. Age of fetus
4. **The following are the similarities of rigor mortis and cadaveric spasm, except:**
   a. Reflects the last act
   b. ATP depletion
   c. Stiffness of muscles
   d. Disappears with decomposition
5. **The color of hypostasis is characteristically seen in death due to:**
   a. Cyanide poisoning
   b. Nitrobenzene poisoning
   c. Potassium chlorate poisoning
   d. Carbon monoxide poisoning
6. **The earliest sign of decomposition:**
   a. Putrid purging
   b. Greenish blue hue over abdomen
   c. Skin slippage
   d. Marbling
7. **Livor mortis occurs prior to death in one of the following conditions:**
   a. Violent asphyxiation
   b. Cyanide poisoning
   c. Cardiac failure
   d. CO poisoning
8. **The best body fluid for estimation of time since death is:**
   a. CSF
   b. Serous fluid
   c. Pericardial fluid
   d. Vitreous humor
9. **The surest sign of death:**
   a. Absence of corneal reflex
   b. Absence of breathing
   c. Discoloration of right iliac fossa
   d. Absence of heart beat
10. **Unequal pupil is seen in the following; except:**
    a. Atropinized eye
    b. Cadaver pupil
    c. Hutchison's pupil
    d. Argyll Robertson's pupil
11. **The most important significance of hypostasis:**
    a. To estimate the time since death
    b. To assess the mode of death
    c. To ascertain the cause of death
    d. To confirm deliberate disturbance of the body after death
12. **One of the following aid adipocere formation:**
    a. Candida albicans
    b. Streptococci
    c. E. coli
    d. Clostridium welchii
13. **Postmortem caloricity is seen in the following, except:**
    a. Tetanus
    b. Strychnine poisoning
    c. Pontine hemorrhage
    d. Trench foot
14. **Which one of the tissues putrefies late:**
    a. Brain
    b. Prostate
    c. Liver
    d. Stomach
15. **False about cadaveric rigidity:**
    a. Appears in all the muscles, both voluntary and involuntary
    b. Does not appear in an amputated limb
    c. Proximo-distal spread
    d. Application of force results in braking of rigidity
16. **Tache noir sclerotica occur in open eyes after _____ hours after death.**
    a. 1–2 hours
    b. 2–3 hours
    c. 3–4 hours
    d. 4–5 hours
17. **Maceration means:**
    a. Septic autolysis
    b. Aseptic autolysis
    c. Putrefaction
    d. None

18. The following are true about postmortem staining, *except*:
    a. Irregular and occurs on dependent parts
    b. Mucus membrane appears dull
    c. Inflammatory exudates may be present
    d. Stomach and intestines when stretched show alternate stained and unstained areas
19. Postmortem staining is commonly confused with:
    a. Abrasion
    b. Flee bite
    c. Contusion
    d. Nappy rash
20. The best method for testing rigor mortis:
    a. Pulling the lower jaw downwards
    b. Dropping the legs down from a height
    c. Flexing the thighs or legs
    d. Flexing the forearms over the elbow
21. Appearance of "maggots" on dead body indicates:
    a. Cause of death
    b. Place of death
    c. Time since death
    d. Type of death
22. According to Casper's dictum—putrefaction in air, water, and earth occurs in the ratio of:
    a. 1:2:8
    b. 1:4:8
    c. 1:2:4
    d. 1:1:2
23. The following type of poisoning retards the decomposition of the body:
    a. Arsenic
    b. Copper
    c. Mercury
    d. Nux vomica
24. Tache noire is:
    a. Postmortem caloricity
    b. Postmortem lividity
    c. Change in eye after death
    d. None of the above
25. The ideal place to record body temperature in dead body is:
    a. Rectum
    b. Groin
    c. Mouth
    d. Axilla
26. Which of the following is outside the purview of Transplantation of Human Organs Act?
    a. Uterus
    b. Eardrums
    c. Ear bones
    d. Bone marrow
27. Minimum age to give consent for organ donation for therapeutic purposes:
    a. 12 years
    b. 18 years
    c. 21 years
    d. 14 years
28. According to Transplantation of Human Organs Act, 1994, punishment for doctor if found guilty:
    a. 2 years
    b. 5 years
    c. 7 years
    d. 2–5 years
29. What is matched before organ transplantation?
    a. mDNA
    b. HLA
    c. RNA
    d. Blood group
30. Which of the following organs obtained from cadaver is not used for transplant?
    a. Blood vessels
    b. Lung
    c. Liver
    d. Urinary bladder

ANSWERS

1. d	2. b	3. c	4. a	5. d	6. b	7. c	8. d	9. c	10. b
11. d	12. d	13. d	14. b	15. b	16. b	17. b	18. c	19. c	20. a
21. c	22. a	23. a	24. c	25. a	26. d	27. b	28. b	29. b	30. d

10
CHAPTER

Violent Asphyxial Deaths

 KEY WORDS

Asphyxia, asphyxial triad, hanging, lynching, strangulation, throttling, drowning, dry drowning, hydrocution, burking, bansdola, mugging, garroting, choking, suffocation, smothering, traumatic asphyxia, autoerotic asphyxia.

FM2.20	Define, classify and describe asphyxia and medico-legal interpretation of postmortem findings in asphyxial deaths.
FM2.21	Describe and discuss different types of hanging and strangulation including clinical findings, causes of death, postmortem findings and medico-legal aspects of death due to hanging and strangulation including examination, preservation and dispatch of ligature material.
FM2.22	Describe and discuss pathophysiology, clinical features, postmortem findings and medico-legal aspects of traumatic asphyxia, obstruction of nose and mouth, suffocation and sexual asphyxia.
FM2.23	Describe and discuss types, pathophysiology, clinical features, postmortem findings and medico-legal aspects of drowning, diatom test and gettler's test.

DEFINE ASPHYXIA? WHAT ARE THE CAUSES OF MECHANICAL ASPHYXIA? (FM2.20)

How do We Classify Mechanical Asphyxial Deaths?

- Asphyxia is the interference of respiration due to any cause mechanical, environmental or toxic, resulting in failure of intake of oxygen by the tissues together with failure to elimination carbon dioxide.
- Asphyxia literally means pulselessness. But in forensic context and everywhere in medical science, asphyxia means lack of oxygen.

Causes of Asphyxia

- There are various ways which results in asphyxia; they are grouped according to their mode of causation.
    - Closure of external orifices: Smothering.
    - Compression of neck: Hanging, strangulation, throttling, bansdola, mugging and autoerotic asphyxia.

- Occlusion of air passage from within: Gagging, choking and café coronary.
- Lack of oxygen in the atmosphere, or inhalation of irrespirable gases: Suffocation.
- Restriction of movement of the chest or abdomen: Traumatic asphyxia, burking and overlaying.
- Prevention of gas exchange in the lung by fluids: Drowning.
- Inability to utilize oxygen by peripheral tissues: Cyanide poisoning.

Mechanical Asphyxia

- Asphyxia due to mechanical force. The causes of mechanical asphyxia are classified into:
  - *Obstructive causes:* Smothering, gagging, choking and café coronary.
  - *Constrictive causes:* Hanging, strangulation, throttling, lynching, bansdola, mugging and garroting.
  - *Restrictive causes:* Traumatic asphyxia, burking and overlaying.
  - *Replacement causes:* Drowning.
- **Chemical asphyxiants:** Carbon monoxide and cyanide poisoning: even though these poisons cause death by asphyxia, they are discussed under toxicology and only death due mechanical asphyxia would be discussed in this chapter.

WHAT ARE THE CLASSICAL SIGNS OF ASPHYXIA? (ASPHYXIAL TRIAD) (FM2.20)

Classical Signs of Asphyxia

- Any way be the causation of asphyxia, it leaves certain signs on the body. They are not specific to asphyxial deaths alone, but invariably present is most cases of asphyxia and are hence called as the classical signs of asphyxia. They are also commonly referred to as "**asphyxial triad**" and they are:
  - Cyanosis
  - Congestion of organs
  - Petechial hemorrhages

Nonspecific signs:
- Abnormal fluidity of blood
- Dilatation of right chambers of heart

Specific sign:
- Specific sign indicates the exact way in which the fatal chains of events were initiated.

Example:
- Ligature mark on the neck in hanging and ligature strangulation.
- Finger nails abrasions on the neck in manual strangulation (throttling)
- Fluid in the air passage in drowning.
- Food bolus in the larynx in café coronary, etc.

Classical Signs of Asphyxia

Cyanosis (Fig. 10.1)

- The color of oxygenated blood is scarlet red. When the hemoglobin is not fully saturated with oxygen, then it's said to be reduced and the blood assumes a blue color, which is termed as "cyanosis".

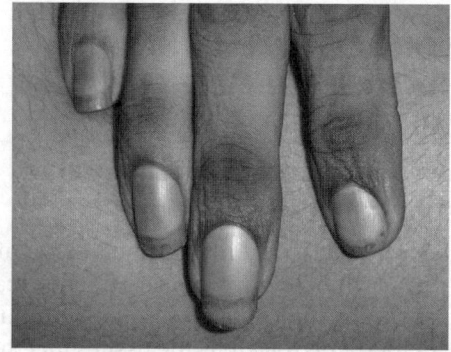

Fig. 10.1: Cyanosis of finger nails
(For color version see Plate 4).

CHAPTER 10: Violent Asphyxial Deaths

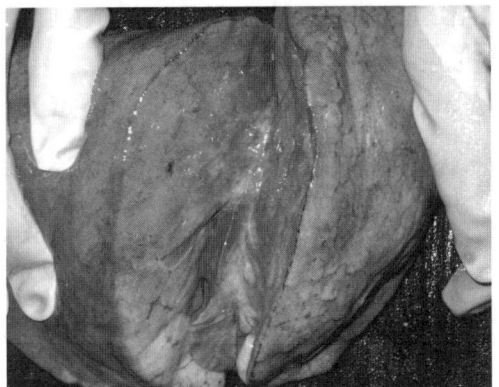

Fig. 10.2: Congestion of lungs
(For color version see Plate 5).

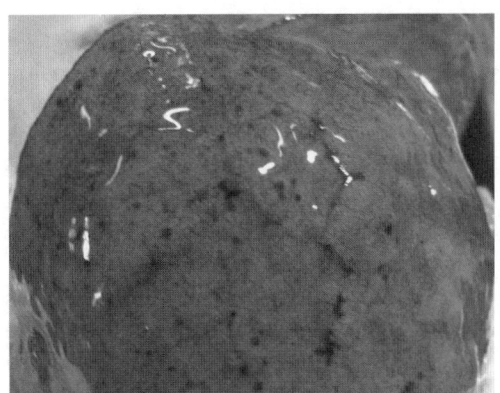

Fig. 10.3: Petechial hemorrhage
(For color version see Plate 5).

- For cyanosis to be evident externally there should be at least 5 grams of reduced hemoglobin per 100 mL of blood. Cyanosis is well appreciated in the peripheries like fingernails, lips and tongue and hence it's common use to say "peripheral cyanosis".

Congestion (Fig. 10.2)

- Collection and stasis of blood due to obstruction of venous return is called as congestion. When the neck is compressed as in hanging, due to defective venous return there is congestion of the face, as well as in all the internal organs.
- Congestion is associated with tissue swelling, if there is continued venous obstruction. Prolonged congestion leads to edema of the visceral organs.
- When circulation stops completely, the walls of the capillaries become permeable resulting in exudation of fluid from the capillaries into the neighboring tissues leading to edema.

PETECHIAL HEMORRHAGES (FIG. 10.3)

- Progressive increase in the venous pressure will lead to rupture of post-capillary venules. This leads to escape of blood producing small bleeding points, varying from pinpoint to pinhead size. They are called as petechial hemorrhages.
- They are readily appreciated on the serous membranes such as sclera, conjunctiva, pleura and the pericardium.

DEFINE HANGING? WHAT ARE THE TYPES OF HANGING? (FM2.21)

Definition

- **Hanging** is a form of asphyxia caused by suspension of the body by a ligature around the neck. The constricting force being his own body weight.
- Hanging is the preferred method of choice for committing suicide and is said to be a relatively painless form of death. **Hanging is almost always suicidal, unless proved otherwise.**
- **Note:** Suicide note is present in many situations and in some female cases, a note regarding the reason for committing suicide and details of individuals who were responsible in forcing her to commit suicide may be present in the suicidal note and hidden inside the inner garments and are recovered during autopsy. If any such documents are recovered they are handed over to the police with acknowledgement after retaining a copy of those recovered documents.

Types of Hanging

- Depending on the degree of suspension hanging is divided into:
  - *Complete hanging:* The entire body is suspended and no part of the body touches the ground. Hence, the whole of the body weight acts as the constricting force.
  - *Partial hanging:* The whole body is not suspended and some part of the body is in contact with the ground and the constricting force is only part of the body weight. Example: The feet are in contact with the ground; the individual is in kneeling position or in lying position with only the head hanging out.
- Depending on the position of the knot it is divided into typical and atypical hanging.

Typical Hanging

- The ligature passes symmetrically on both sides of the neck towards the point of suspension and the knot is at the nape of the neck. The head will be flexed and bent forward.
- The maximum pressure exerted by the ligature is directly opposite to the point of suspension and death is presumed to be purely due to asphyxia, and hence called as typical hanging.

Atypical Hanging

- When the knot is at any other place other than the nape of the neck: i.e., below the ears, below the chin, behind the mastoid process, etc.
- The position of the head is tilted toward one side, opposite to the point of suspension.
- Death may not be due to asphyxia; it could be due to compression of jugular, carotids or trachea only on one side, whereas, on other side may blood may continue to flow.

CAUSES OF DEATH IN HANGING (FM2.21)

- **Asphyxia:** Due to constriction of the trachea.
- **Venous congestion:** Due to occlusion of jugular veins.
- **Combined asphyxia and venous congestion:** Combination of the above two. Combined asphyxia and venous congestion is the cause of death in 90% cases.
- **Cerebral anemia:** Due constriction of carotid and vertebral arteries.
- **Reflux vagal inhibition:** When the ligature material rubs over the carotid sheath, there is stimulation of carotid body, which leads to reflux vagal inhibition, resulting in sudden stoppage of heart.
- **Fracture dislocation of cervical vertebra:** Occurs only in judicial hanging or hanging accompanied with a long drop (6 to 8 meters) and the knot is below the chin. Here the maximum pressure is exerted on the cervical vertebrae as a result of sudden drop accompanied by the weight of the body. This leads to dislocation and instantaneous fracture at the level of C2, C3 cervical vertebrae, with corresponding injury to the spinal column. In this condition death is instantaneous.

Delayed Deaths in Hanging

- When hanging attempt is foiled by timely intervention and resuscitation, the hypoxic and ischemic effects to the brain and brain stem, will lead to delayed deaths of the individual. In such cases death is due to:
  - Infection
  - Edema of larynx and lungs
  - Hypoxic ischemic encephalopathy
  - Infarction of brain
  - Brain abscess
  - Cerebral softening and liquefaction.

DESCRIBE THE POSTMORTEM FINDINGS IN A CASE OF DEATH DUE TO HANGING? (FM2.21)

Postmortem Appearance

All the classical signs of asphyxia namely, peripheral cyanosis, visceral congestion and petechial hemorrhages are present in most of the cases of death due to asphyxia.

Ligature Mark (Figs. 10.4 and 10.5)

- The compressing force of the ligature material results in the production of an injury around the neck in the form of a pressure abrasion.
- The ligature leaves a furrow of its own width and pattern. It develops due to the pressure exerted by the ligature material on the skin surface.
- The bed of the ligature mark is Pale and dry; pressure exerted by the ligature material, pushes the blood from the underneath skin surface and the tissues become pale. Later on with the passage of time, it becomes parchmentized due to the effect of drying.
- The edges are abraded (reddish-brown): Due to the frictional force between the skin

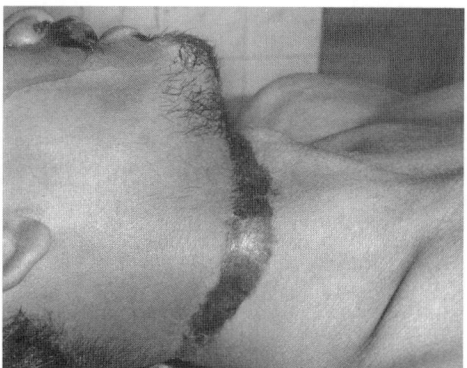

Fig. 10.5: Ligature abrasion of hanging *(For color version see Plate 5).*

and the ligature material. Ecchymosis and congestion of adjacent skin may be seen.
- The pattern of the ligature material often gets imprinted on the skin surface as a pressure abrasion/imprint abrasion. shown in **Figures 10.6 and 10.7**.
- The ligature mark is usually situated at the upper border of the neck, above the thyroid cartilage, just below the chin. It runs obliquely upwards and backwards, symmetrically on both sides of the neck, towards the point of suspension/the knot.
- **Microscopically,** the ligature mark displays the usual characteristics of abrasion, showing desquamation and flattening of cells of the epidermis.

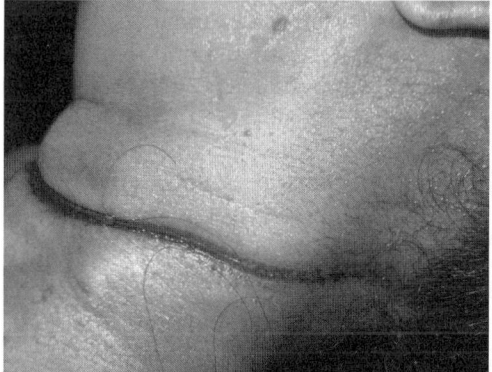

Fig. 10.4: Oblique ligature abrasion of hanging caused by a string *(For color version see Plate 5).*

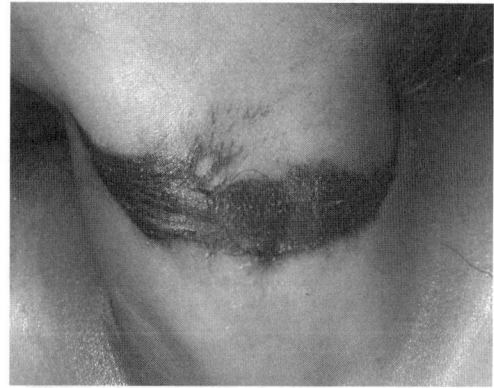

Fig. 10.6: Broad ligature abrasion of hanging caused by twisted clothing. Note the color of the abrasion—antemortem ligature abrasion of hanging *(For color version see Plate 5).*

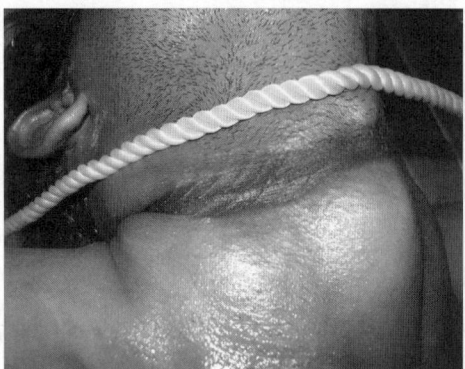

Fig. 10.7: Ligature abrasion of hanging caused by nylon rope. The material can be compared with abrasion—imprint ligature abrasion *(For color version see Plate 5).*

- If death has occurred quickly, evidence of vital reactions at the margins of the ligature mark may be difficult to demonstrate even by microscopy.

Other External Findings

- Face is congested, with cyanosis of lips and nail beds.
- Postmortem staining **(Fig. 10.8)** will be seen over the distal part of both upper and lower limbs of the body. This can be appreciated only if the body was in the suspended position for a minimum period of 4 to 6 hours. This type of distribution of postmortem staining is called "***glove and stockings fashion***" of postmortem hypostasis. Petechiae in the lower limbs, if the body is suspended for a long time (8 to 12 hours).
- Neck is elongated and the head is tilted towards one side away from the knot.
- Tongue may be protruded and bitten.
- **Salivary stains** at the angle of mouth: Diagnostic of antemortem hanging and could be present in 40 to 60% cases. When the ligature material rubs over the sub-mandibular salivary glands, there is increased salivary secretion, which could be found dribbled and dried along the angle of mouth of one side, when the head is tilted opposite to the point of suspension.
- In my postgraduate dissertation study and further experience (nearly 1000 cases of hanging) the salivary stains were present in nearly 40% cases. I have seen many cases where there were ants crawling along a line on the front of chest, after washing the body we could notice the underlying dried salivary stains, dribbled from the angle of mouth. Hence, a careful search for this finding of dried salivary stains will help to confirm a large number of cases as antemortem hanging.
- **Le facie sympathique:** If the knot presses on the cervical sympathetic ganglia, the eye on that side may remain open and the pupil dilated; the eyes on the other side will remain partially open or closed. This is very rare and observed in <1% cases, but if present it is also a surest antemortem sign of hanging.

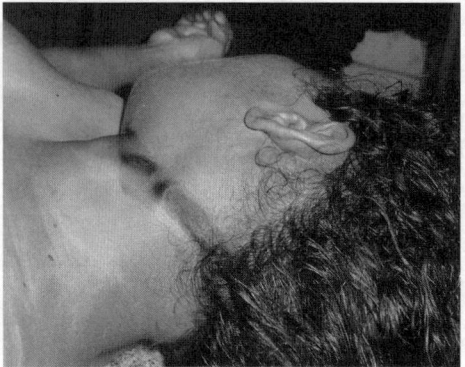

Fig. 10.8: Oblique ligature abrasion–note the postmortem staining above the ligature mark *(For color version see Plate 6).*

Neck Dissection

- Neck is examined after removal of the brain, thoracic and abdominal contents (blood less field of dissection).
- Superficial incisions of the ligature grooves may show small hemorrhages in the underlying layers of the skin, caused by direct trauma.

- Extravasation and bruising of the muscles of the neck may be present, especially over the sternocleidomastoid and platysma. The intima of the carotid arteries may show transverse tears (splits) with extravasation of blood in their walls. These changes are due to the traction effect of the body with the ligature material.
- The subcutaneous tissues immediately above and below the ligature mark are congested.
- The tissues underneath the ligature mark are pale and parchment like.
- The lymph nodes of the neck above and below the ligature mark, shows evidence of congestion, stasis and hemorrhage. This is also a useful finding of antemortem hanging.

Hyoid Bone

- The relevance of fracture of the hyoid bone in hanging is minimal. It only signifies that there was external compression over the hyoid bone.
- Hyoid bone is a highly compressible bone and hence fracture occurs only occasionally; fracture is more common above the age of 40 years as the bone gets calcified in old age and the flexibility is restricted.
- The commonest pattern of fracture is outward fracture (abduction fracture) which is due to antero-posterior compression. The broken piece of bone has an outward angulation.

Effects of Decomposition on Ligature Mark

- In any case, decomposition alters the findings, mainly the external injuries; but though ligature abrasion is a superficial injury fortunately resists putrefaction for a reasonable period of time. During the process of compression of the neck, the blood underneath the ligature abrasion is pushed away from those areas and hence putrefaction is markedly delayed on the ligature abrasion.

DESCRIBE LYNCHING AND POSTMORTEM HANGING?

Lynching

- Homicidal hanging of a person by the mob in the public is called as lynching.
- The person who is suspected to be involved in heinous crimes like dacoity, murder, or sexual assault (especially on the white people) is over powered by the mob, and hanged forcefully in the public to raise fear among the public. This was in practice in the ancient period and the aim of committing lynching is to raise fear among the public and as a deterrent to the society in committing such grave crimes.

Postmortem Hanging (Postmortem Suspension)

- Occasionally, after a victim has been murdered by some other means the body may be suspended to simulate suicidal hanging.
- Findings of asphyxia will not be evident and the actual cause of death may be easily made out during autopsy. Postmortem nature of ligature abrasion has to be differentiated and confirmed by the presence of vital reactions and HPE if necessary.
- When the victim is killed by throttling or ligature strangulation and then suspended; signs of asphyxia will be present and hence difficulties do arise. But a careful observation may reveal fingernail abrasions in throttling and horizontal complete encircling ligature abrasion in cases of ligature strangulation. Also, internal neck dissection (blood less field)

will be highly rewarding and most cases could be solved on the autopsy table itself.

Fibers of Ligature Material

- Presence of fibers of ligature material in the hands of the victim indicates that that the victim has handled the material either while committing suicide or by struggle to get rid of the constricting force during the process of death in hanging or strangulation. Absence of such fibers in the hands of the victim indicates that the victim has not touched the material at all, thus indicating postmortem hanging (especially when the material is a rope or clothing).
- In case of postmortem suspension, examination of the upper surface of the branch of the tree or beam (point of suspension) will indicate the direction of traction force. In such situation, the ligature material is first tied around the neck and is pulled from the opposite side to suspend the body. The direction of markings made by the fibers of the ligature material at the point of suspension will be away from the body (anti-clockwise). Whereas, if it is a case of suicidal hanging the markings will be in clockwise direction. This finding may occasionally be helpful in postmortem hanging.

WRITE SHORT NOTES ON JUDICIAL HANGING?

- Hanging is the form of capital punishment in India. Some countries adopt methods like electrical chair, lethal dose of drugs (morphine) and many countries have abolished death penalty. However, in India capital punishment is awarded even though rare under some circumstances and the method of execution is by hanging.
- Whenever a death sentence is awarded in a sessions court it has to be confirmed by the high court.
- The individual is made to stand on a movable platform the depth of the pit is abound 10 meters. The face is covered with a black mask. Then the ligature material is applied around the neck with point of knot below the chin. The length of the ligature material is around 6 to 7 meters.
- The platform is withdrawn and the body is allowed to fall which is restricted by the length of the ligature material. The body stops falling by a jerk; this results in sudden fracture dislocation of C2–C3 cervical vertebrae (Hangman's fracture) which results instantaneous loss of consciousness.
- The heart may continue to beat for 10 to 15 minutes and respiratory movements also continue for some minutes till complete anoxia causes arrest of all the systems.
- The body is allowed to hang for more than 20 minutes to ensure death. In proper judicial hanging signs of asphyxia would be usually absent.

WHAT IS STRANGULATION? DISCUSS ABOUT LIGATURE STRANGULATION? (FM2.21)

- It is a form of violent asphyxial death accomplished by application of external force to constrict the neck, either by hands (**manual strangulation/throttling**) or by a ligature material (**ligature strangulation**) or by any other means shown in **Figure 10.9**.
- There is no suspension of the body in strangulation and hence the constricting force is not the victim's own body weight rather external compression by an assailant.
- Ligature strangulation (**Fig. 10.10**) is mostly homicidal, occasionally accidental

CHAPTER 10: Violent Asphyxial Deaths

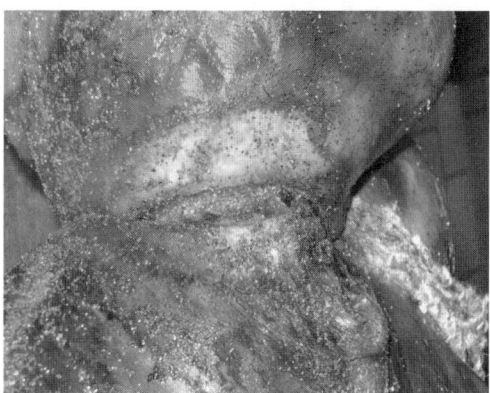

Fig. 10.9: Horizontal ligature abrasion of strangulation. Note: Even when the body has under gone reasonable degree of decomposition still the ligature mark is visible *(For color version see Plate 6)*.

and rarely suicidal (but a person cannot successfully commit suicide by throttling).
- Sometimes, death may occur due to sudden vagal inhibition without leaving any signs of asphyxia on the body.

Symptoms of Ligature Strangulation

- There is complete occlusion of air passage due to sudden compression of the neck. Unconsciousness develops very quickly and instant death is common, since the victim is overpowered by the perpetrator and evidence of struggle may or may not be present.
- In incomplete occlusion for a longer duration there will be intense cyanosis and congestion of the face, bleeding from the mouth, nostrils and ears may be seen.

Causes of Death

- Asphyxia
- Cerebral ischemia
- **Vagal inhibition:** If death is death is due to vagal inhibition, evidence of asphyxia will not be present on the body.

Postmortem Appearance in Ligature Strangulation

External Appearance

Ligature mark:

- The ligature mark is well defined and grooved. The intensity and the pattern depend on the amount of force exerted by external compression and the ligature material used.
- It is usually situated at or below the level of the thyroid cartilage.
- It completely encircles the neck, without any discontinuity.
- The direction of the ligature is horizontal or horizontally oblique, with crossing over to the opposite side. In some cases, the ligature material will be encircling the neck several times producing more number of markings and many a times there may be evidence of more than one knot.
- The direction of the ligature mark depends on the relative position of the assailant and the victim at that time of strangulation. (i) It will be horizontally oblique, if the victim was in lying position; (ii) horizontal, when both the victim and the assailant are in standing posture; and (iii) **oblique** if the victim was sitting and the assailant

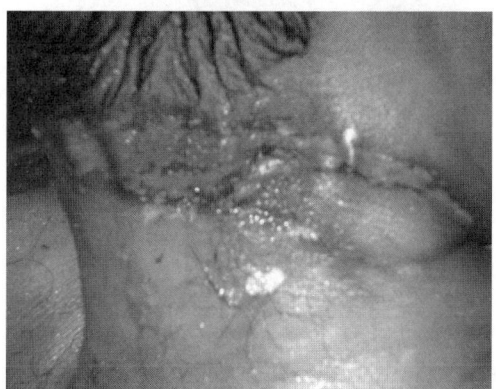

Fig. 10.10: Ligature strangulation–completely encircling ligature mark around the neck *(For color version see Plate 6)*.

standing behind and also when the victim is dragged from behind.
- The margins of the ligature mark will be reddish, ecchymosed and the base will be pale. With passage of time the ligature abrasion becomes dry, hard, parchment like.
- The pressure exerted on the neck by the ligature material produces an imprint abrasion.
- Abrasions and ecchymosis of adjacent skin will be more evident than in hanging.
- If the ligature material is soft and yielding or if it is removed soon after death, then the ligature mark may not be visible over the skin surface. In such situations, a second examination of the neck after several hours may show the presence of a faint pressure abrasion.
- If the ligature material is not present in situ and recovered later, the presence or absence of fibers from the ligature material over the ligature mark can be identified by application of adhesive cello tape and examination under the microscope for comparison.
- **Accidental ligature strangulation:** A scarf or dupatta may be caught in a moving fan, vehicle, machinery belt, etc., and can result in severe constriction of the neck and produce instantaneous death by ligature strangulation.

Asphyxial Signs

- All the classical signs of asphyxia will be more marked than in hanging.
- Eye balls may be open, prominent and congested with dilated pupils.
- Discharge of blood stained fluid may be seen over the mouth and nostrils.
- Intense congestion of face is usually present and multiple petechial hemorrhages over the forehead are a common finding.
- Tongue will be protruding, bitten by teeth, bruised, swollen and deeply cyanosed.
- Hands may be clenched. While the victim attempts to defend him by inserting his fingers in between the neck and the ligature material, nail scratch marks in the form of linear or crescentic abrasions can be seen over the neck and rarely cadaveric spasm may occur instantaneously at that moment.

Internal Appearance

- Excluding the neck, all the body cavities and visceral organs are examined first in order to get a bloodless neck field. This will also avoid introduction of artefacts in the neck field and the resultant misinterpretations.
- In case of ligature strangulation (**Fig. 10.11**) evidence of bruising will be present on all the underlying layers of tissues; namely, the subcutaneous layer, muscles of the neck, tracheal rings and also on the posterior pharyngeal wall.
- Since the pressure exerted by the ligature material is over the surface of the thyroid cartilage, fracture of the superior cornua

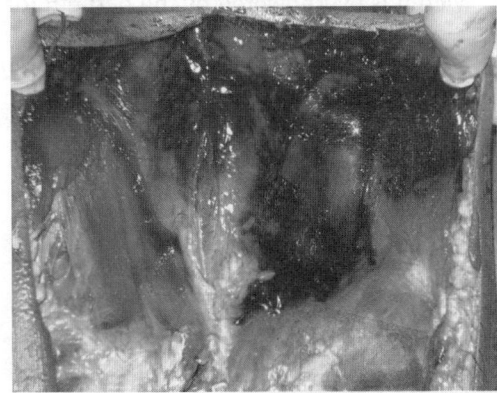

Fig. 10.11: Neck dissection in ligature strangulation. Note, the extensive extravasation of blood in the neck muscles trachea *(For color version see Plate 6).*

of thyroid cartilage is relatively common in strangulation, with extravasation of blood in the surrounding soft tissues.
- Other internal organs like larynx and trachea shows intense congestion, with frothy mucus and also petechial hemorrhages.
- Lungs show multiple hemorrhagic patches and petechiae over the surface, with marked congestion and emphysematous bullae. Presence of emphysematous bullae associated with congestion and petechiae indicates the agonal struggle of the victim.
- All the other internal organs will be congested and petechiae may be present.
- Involuntary discharge of urine and fecal matter may be seen in many cases.
- Since, ligature abrasion resists decomposition for relative period of time cases of ligature strangulation can be positively solved even if the bodies are recovered a few days later.

DIFFERENTIATE LIGATURE ABRASION OF HANGING FROM STRANGULATION?

Table 10.1 is depicted the differences between ligature mark of hanging and strangulation.

WHAT IS THROTTLING? DISCUSS THE POSTMORTEM FINDINGS IN CASE OF THROTTLING? (FM2.21)

Throttling (manual strangulation) **(Fig. 10.12)** is a form of violent asphyxial death, in which the assailant uses his hands to produce compression of the neck of the victim.

TABLE 10.1: Difference between ligature mark of hanging and strangulation.

Features	Hanging	Strangulation
Level	At or above the level of thyroid cartilage, but mostly slips to the upper end of neck. The mark is usually absent at the back of the neck, as it merges with the hairline	In the middle part of neck, at or below the level of thyroid cartilage. The hairline is usually not involved and the ligature mark is always at a lower level
Direction	Symmetrically oblique, runs towards the point of suspension	Horizontal or horizontally oblique
Knot	A point of knot is present at the upper most point of the mark and sometimes the impression of the knot is present on the skin	Knot is not always present, there may be crossing over of the mark, or twisting or sometime times multiple knots
Discontinuity	There is always a length of discontinuity even in cases of noose knots, due to the pulling down effect of the body weight	There is no point of discontinuity (if there is a discontinuity then there can be no effective compression). There is crossing over at any one point or a firm knot is present
Multiplicity	Usually there is no multiplicity, even if present all these marks may not compress the neck and there is a good length of discontinuity at the point of suspension	Many a times there are multiple twist of the ligature material around the neck and all these completely encircle the neck

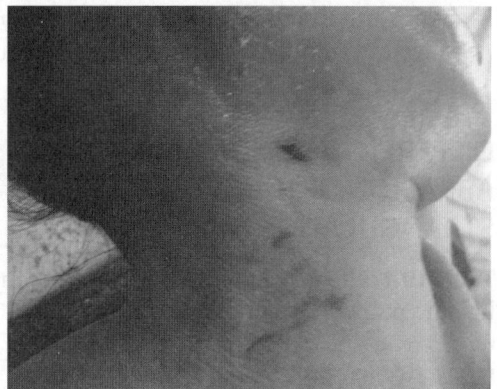

Fig. 10.12: Throttling–pressure abrasion and nail marks around the neck in case of throttling *(For color version see Plate 6)*.

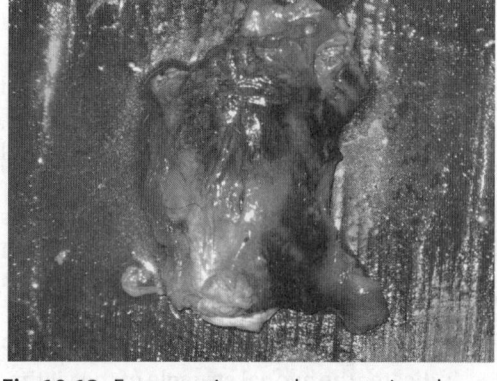

Fig 10.13: Extravasation on the posterior pharyngeal wall—a cased of throttling *(For color version see Plate 6)*.

Autopsy Findings

- All the classical signs of asphyxia will be markedly evident.
- Petechial hemorrhages on the forehead are a frequent finding, indicative of more severe forms of violent asphyxia than hanging.
- Multiple pressure spots of bruising will be seen over the neck due to assailant gripping the neck with fingers.
- The finger nails of the assailant produce crescentic and linear abrasions on both sides of the neck. The victim also produces certain nail marks by himself during the attempt of struggle to relieve the assailant's hands from causing compression.
- **Bruises:** Usually circular, dark red or purple in color 1–2 cm size, resembling the shape of the fingertips. If fingers slide over neck then it can produce elongated bruises.
- In case of throttling by one hand: There will be bruise mark by thumb on one side and bruise marks of four fingertips on the other side. These bruise marks which are red or purple in the beginning may turn brown later on. This way of using one hand is common when the victim is an infant.
- When both hands used for throttling: Corresponding thumb mark of one hand and four fingers of the other hand will be seen on either side of the neck.

Internal Findings

Very important to do a blood-less field of dissection.
- On dissection of neck, evidence of bruising on the underlying subcutaneous soft tissues and neck muscles are seen, which corresponds to the pressure abrasions present on the external skin surface (specific finding of death due to throttling).
- Signs of extravasation and bruising **(Fig. 10.13)** will be present over the tracheal rings and also on the posterior pharyngeal wall (as the posterior pharyngeal wall gets compressed over the hard vertebral column).

Hyoid Bone

Hyoid bone fracture is relatively more common in throttling. There is inward compression fracture (adduction fracture) and the broken fragment of bone has an inward angulation, with extravasation of blood into the surrounding soft tissues.

DIFFICULTIES ENCOUNTERED BY THE AUTOPSY SURGEON IF SOME SOFT INTERVENING MATERIAL IS USED

When Some Intervening Soft Material is Used between the Hands and the Neck?

- External signs such as fingernail scratches and pressure abrasion exerted by the bulb of the fingers would be absent. Even then, signs of asphyxia would help to group the death as asphyxial death, followed by dissection of the skin and subcutaneous tissues layer by layer will reveal bruising of underlying layers of skin and bruising of the neck muscles. Also, fracture of hyoid bone and contusion of tracheal rings and posterior pharyngeal wall would be present to confirm death was due to throttling.
- Evidence of struggle in the form of abrasions and bruises may be seen over the mouth, nose, cheeks and forehead, lower Jaw, back of shoulders or any other part of the body.
- Sometimes fracture of the ribs and injuries to organs inside the chest and abdomen may be present, when assailant kneels or sits over chest.

WHAT ARE THE TYPES OF HYOID BONE FRACTURES?

Hyoid bone may get fractured in any case of death due to compression of neck. Fracture hyoid bone is common in throttling compared to hanging.

Adduction Fracture

It occurs in throttling; the broken fragment has an inward angulation due to the force exerted by the fingers of the assailant.

Abduction Fracture

- In cases of hanging and ligature strangulation there is outward angulation fracture (abduction fracture) of the hyoid bone.
- This is due to antero-posterior compression exerted by the ligature material.
- The broken piece of bone has an outward angulation.

Antemortem Nature of Fracture

- In any case of hyoid bone fracture, the antemortem nature of the fracture is confirmed by the extravasation of blood at the fractured site and into the surrounding soft tissues.
- It can be confirmed by benzidine test. Histopathology may also be useful.
- Case studies have shown that, the incidence of hyoid bone fracture is relatively high when (i) the ligature material is a hard material like rope or string; (ii) the ligature material should directly compress the hyoid bone, and (iii) the longer the period of suspension of the body, the chances of fracture is increased. From this it is evident that the hyoid bone fracture should not be given much importance, it only indicates that there has been some pressure over the hyoid bone and no information regarding whether death is due to hanging could be made out from the fracture of hyoid bone. But the fracture of hyoid bone is more common in throttling, as there is direct pressure over the hyoid bone. In any fracture the antemortem nature should be checked; extravasation of blood and if necessary benzidine test and histopathology.

WRITE SHORT NOTES ON SMOTHERING? (FM2.22)

- Smothering (**Fig. 10.14**) is closure of the external orifices of respiration, namely

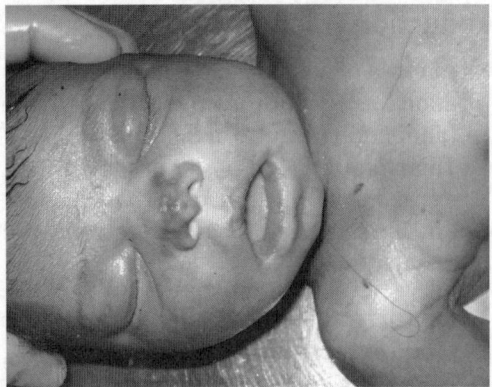

Fig. 10.14: Pressure abrasion and contusion around the mouth and nostrils—a case of smothering *(For color version see Plate 7).*

the mouth and the nostrils with the help of hands or other objects like pillows, bed sheets and soft materials, etc., resulting in death due to asphyxia. The victim is usually an infant or intoxicated individual.

Autopsy Findings

- If bare hands are used for smothering, an area of paleness around the mouth and the tip of the nose will be present, with scratch abrasions on the nose and mouth. Evidence of nail markings can also be made out around the site of compression.
- These external signs may be absent, if soft intervening materials such as a cloth or pillow is used to cause smothering. However, the internal findings of asphyxia will be evident irrespective of the method of smothering.
- All the classical signs of asphyxia like congestion, cyanosis and petechial hemorrhages will be present.
- In addition to these external signs, examination of the oral cavity will reveal bruising and lacerations on the inner surface of the lips, even if soft intervening materials were used. These injuries are a result of the counter pressure exerted by the teeth. Bleeding gums, bruising of the gingival surface and injury to the tongue are commonly encountered.

SHORT NOTE ON BURKING (FM2.22)

- Burking is a form of homicidal asphyxial death brought about by combination of smothering and traumatic asphyxia.
- It is named after William Burke and Hare, who used to murder the beggars by this method to supply dead bodies to the department of anatomy in a medical school.
- **Method:** In a grossly intoxicated individual, one will sit on the chest and hold the hands tightly by the side, while the other will firmly press over the mouth and nostrils and the result would be rapid asphyxia. Death is due to combined effects of traumatic asphyxia and smothering.

Autopsy Findings

- Signs of asphyxia namely cyanosis, congestion and petechial hemorrhages are present.
- Evidence of smothering mainly, bruising on inner surface of lips with lacerations due to counter pressure offered by the teeth will be evident.
- There may be fracture of ribs caused by the weight of the person sitting on the chest.
- Signs of resistance are minimal and drag marks in the form of abrasions over the back of shoulders and bony prominences may be present.

WHAT IS MUGGING?

Mugging is a homicidal form asphyxia brought about by compression of the neck by the angle of the elbow or the knee, also by the pressure exerted by the foot of the assailant on the neck. At autopsy, more pronounced asphyxial signs would be evident. The neck findings vary depending on whether angle of elbow or knees is used or if foot is used to compress the neck. There would be extensive bruising on the neck structures.

WHAT IS BANSDOLA?

It is a method of homicide, using bamboo sticks to bring about asphyxia. Two bamboo sticks are placed, one on the front of neck and the other on the back; one end is fixed by tying the two bamboo sticks together and the other end is slowly tightened with a rope, resulting in effective compression of the neck.

WHAT IS GARROTING?

- Garroting is homicidal form of asphyxia by applying a ligature around the neck, from behind the victim, when he is unaware.
- Hence, the victim is stunned followed by imminent loss of consciousness due to twisting the material quickly from behind.
- Since the victim is unaware, there is no evidence of any struggle as all the event unfolds so quickly.
- By this way it is possible to overpower even a healthy strong individual and kill him. Unfortunately, in these cases if the material is removed soon after death, then the ligature abrasion is faint that it may not be visible at all. Even then, the internal neck findings will be definitely helpful in finding out the cause of death as homicidal compression of neck.

WHAT ARE THE ACCIDENTAL FORMS OF DEATH DUE TO ASPHYXIA?

Short notes on: Suffocation; café coronary; traumatic asphyxia; sexual asphyxia; choking.

Suffocation (FM2.22)

- Is a form of asphyxia which produced by inhalation of irrespirable gases. The common gases involved are hydrogen sulfide, methane, carbon monoxide, carbon dioxide, etc.
- Suffocation can also occur in high altitudes and decompression sickness.
- In suffocation the respired air contains very low concentration of oxygen, resulting in breathlessness and asphyxia.

Café Coronary

- It is a misnomer; a grossly intoxicated individual while trying to eat a big bolus of food (meat) tries to speak or laugh and suddenly becomes pale, followed by unconscious and death.
- Due to gross intoxication there is absence of gag reflux resulting in failure to swallow or cough out the bolus of food and the result is choking.
- It appears as if the person died due to sudden cardiac arrest and hence the name "café coronary".

Autopsy Findings

The coronaries will be patent; signs of asphyxia will be evident and the bolus of food will be found impacted on the larynx resulting in choking of the respiratory passage.

Traumatic Asphyxia (FM2.22)

- Asphyxia produced as a result of restriction of movements of the chest and abdomen, as consequence of trauma is called as traumatic asphyxia. Trauma as such is not fatal. The traumatic episode results in compression of chest and/or abdomen resulting in restriction of movement of the thoracic cage leading to asphyxia and death.

- Examples of such incidence of traumatic asphyxia are:
  - *Steering wheel impact in road traffic accidents:* The steering wheel may get impacted over the abdomen, resulting in inability of movement of abdomen and chest. There is pronounced congestion above the level of impact and paleness below the level.
  - *Stampede:* In this, the individual gets trapped in a crowded place or falls down and the crowd of people stamps him, where it becomes improbable for the individual to breath with the weight of these individuals.
  - *Fallen masonry:* Falling of heavy objects like bricks, concrete slabs and other construction material on the chest and abdomen.
  - Falling of sand/rice bags on an individual.
  - Individual trapped in between two hard objects like heavy vehicles, heavy weight objects or machineries and in cases of collapsed buildings, where the individual gets trapped in between the two hard objects, which prevent the movement of chest and abdomen.
  - An intoxicated well built adult over lies on an infant during sleep (**overlaying**).
  - In all these circumstances, there is restricted respiratory movement due to external compression on the chest and abdomen.
  - Signs of asphyxia will be markedly evident.
  - There will be intense congestion mainly above the level of compression, cyanosis and multiple petechial hemorrhages seen both externally and internally.
  - Injuries may or may not be noticeable.

Sexual Asphyxia: Auto-erotic Asphyxia (FM2.22)

- It's presumed that the lowering of consciousness due to any cause such as drugs or partial compression of neck results in increased sexual pleasure by prolonging the time orgasm.
- People with perverted sexual behavior (masochist) partially asphyxiate themselves by compression of the neck, usually by hanging to go in for a transient period of unconsciousness to accomplish their aim of increased sexual pleasure by prolonging the time period of erection.

Method

- In this method, a thick soft material is used as a pad to protect the neck. Then a ligature is applied over the pad, around the neck in the form of running noose, with one free end tied to the limb (elbow, wrist or ankle) after passing through some mechanical device like a pulley.
- The noose can be tightened by extending the arms or legs, and when consciousness is lost, the relaxation of the limb releases the pressure on the neck and the individual regains consciousness after a brief period of time.
- Occasionally the constriction may not get relieved; due to faulty function of the mechanical device or the noose getting entangled. In such situation death results due to asphyxia as a result of accidental hanging.
- Death is unintentional as indicated by the scene and the devices used.
- The diagnosis of sexual asphyxia can be made by examination of the scene of crime, which will show the presence of pornographic materials or literature near

the body. The dead body may be partly or fully naked with female garments and costumes found nearby.
- The person may blindfold himself or stand in front of a mirror to watch the events. There may be evidence of recent seminal ejaculation.
- Old scars around the neck may be present, as evidence of previous episodes.
- These cases may be misdiagnosed as cases of suicidal hanging. Examination of the scene will reveal evidence of abnormal sexual behavior and evidence of such act practiced previously like grooves in rafter or doors.
- Findings consistent with suicidal hanging will be totally absent.

Gagging

- It is caused **when some pad or any piece of cloth is thrust into the mouth**. It is usually resorted to prevent the victim from shouting for help, and death is usually not intended.
- The gag not only blocks the mouth but also prevents the entry of air which comes through the back of throat from the nostrils.
- The cloth gets moistened with saliva and mucus fluid, and gets further sucked with inspiration, thus progressively leading to complete obstruction. Death in such cases is more likely to be due to pharyngeal obstruction.
- The victim's hands and legs may be found tied to prevent him from removing the gag and walking for help.
- Rarely, it may be homicidal, particularly when victims are infants or individuals incapacitated by alcohol or drug, old, infirm, etc.

DEFINE DROWNING? WHAT ARE THE TYPES OF DROWNING? (FM2.23)

Discuss the Mechanism of Death in Fresh Water and Sea Water Drowning?

What is Hydrocution?

Definition:
- **Drowning** is a form of asphyxial death in which there is replacement of air passages by any fluid usually water, resulting in displacement of air from the lungs.
- For drowning to occur, complete submersion of the body is not necessary. If the mouth and nose are submerged, it can cause drowning and result in death.
- A person, who doesn't know swimming when enters into water, sinks in water as the specific gravity of the body is higher than that of water.
- He raises up on to the surface of water due to buoyancy of the body, air trapped inside the clothing and by the struggling movements made by him.
- When the mouth and nose comes above the water level, he expire the air from the lungs to inhale fresh air, during this process he inhales more of water than air, and also swallows some amount of water. This process may continue two or three times and he finally sinks into water once he has inhaled enough of water.

Types of Drowning

- Drowning is classified into three types:
  1. Wet drowning
  2. Dry drowning
  3. Hydrocution (immersion syndrome): Death is due to vagal inhibition.
- With respect to presence or absence of water in the lungs, drowning is divided

into **wet drowning** and **dry drowning** respectively.
- **Wet drowning** is further subdivided into two types, according to the type of water:
  1. Fresh water drowning
  2. Sea or saltwater drowning
- According to the period of survival drowning may be labeled as:
  - Immediate drowning
  - *Near drowning:* Rescued but died within 24 hours
  - *Secondary drowning:* Death after 24 hours due to complications of drowning like infections, encephalopathy, hypoxia, etc.

Wet Drowning

Water enters into the lungs and the air present in the air passages is displaced. This water mixes with the residual air present in the lungs and forms a fine white froth, which is evident by dissection of the bronchioles during autopsy.

Mechanism of Death (Flowchart 10.1)

- The mechanism of death in drowning and the patho-physiology involved in the process of drowning depends on whether the medium of drowning is fresh water or salt water.
- Fresh water drowning:

Flowchart 10.1: Pathophysiology of fresh water drowning.

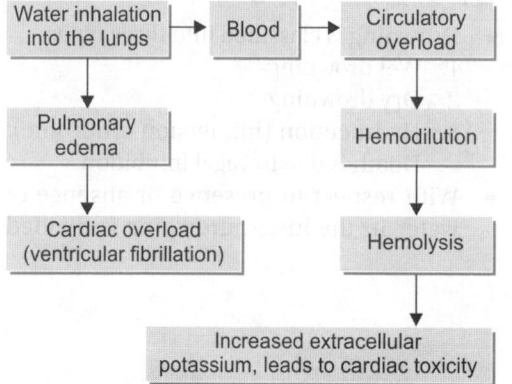

Flowchart 10.2: Pathophysiology of sea water drowning.

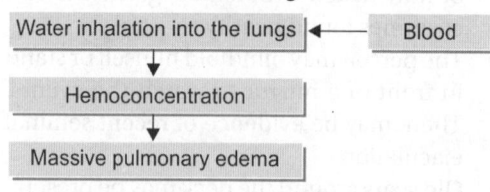

- Once water enters into the lungs, it gets absorbed into the circulation, resulting in hemodilution. This in turn leads to cardiac overload and acute pulmonary edema. During this process, there is lysis of the RBCs and release of potassium, leading to ventricular fibrillation. Death may take place in 5 to 8 minutes.
- Sea water drowning (**Flowchart 10.2**).
- When water with high salinity (sea water) enters into the lungs, water is imbibed from the circulation into the lungs, resulting in hemoconcentration and death is due to massive pulmonary edema. The individual may survive for 8 to 12 minutes in sea water drowning.

Dry Drowning

- In this type of drowning, water does not enter into the respiratory passages at all.
- When the person drowns, he may to try to withhold his breath to prevent water entering into the lungs, which results in intense **acute laryngeal spasm**.
- This intense laryngeal spasm prevents neither water nor air to enter into the respiratory tract; and the result is death by asphyxia due to drowning.

Hydrocution/Immersion Syndrome

- In some cases, when the cold water strikes over the epigastrium, it may result in vagal inhibition leading to reflex cardiac arrest.
- Even in people who know swimming, while they dive into the water, hyper stimulation of nerve endings all over the body by cold water leads to "hydrocution" and ventricular fibrillation.

- This form of drowning is very difficult to diagnose at autopsy, since the victim knows swimming. There is absence of any signs of asphyxia, no pathological evidence of any fatal disease and the chemical analysis report is negative.
- Arriving at the cause death is by ruling out, since vagal inhibition does not leave any specific autopsy findings. Hydrocution is one of the causes of negative autopsy.
- Opinion is based on the circumstantial evidences.
- Other causes of death in drowning:
  - Injuries sustained by the victim, by hitting over some hard protruding objects inside the water medium.
  - Shock due to pre-existing heart disease.
  - *Exhaustion:* Due to prolonged swimming.

WHAT ARE THE POSTMORTEM FINDINGS IN A CASE OF DEATH DUE TO DROWNING? (FM2.23)

What are the Difficulties Encountered When the Body is Decomposed?

Postmortem Findings

Nonspecific signs: External

- The external signs in drowning are:
  - The clothes and the hair will be wet.
  - Sand, mud and weed particles will be found adherent over the skin surface and on the clothing.
  - **Washer women hand:** The skin surface over the palm and soles become wrinkled, soddened and bleached. This is not an antemortem sign of drowning. It indicates the period of immersion of the body in water. Prolonged period of exposure with water increases the intensity of "washer women hand" **(Fig. 10.15)**.

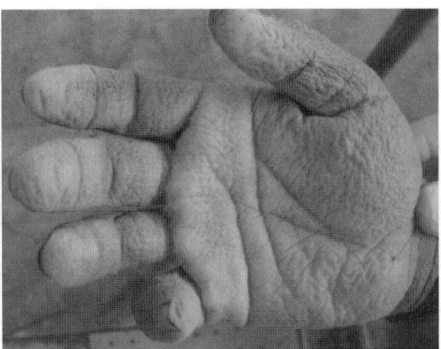

Fig. 10.15: Washerwoman's hand: A nonspecific external sign of death due to drowning *(For color version see Plate 7).*

- *Cutis anserina (goose skin):* It is due to contraction of the erector pylori muscle, which leads to puckered appearance of the hair follicle.
- Cyanosis, external injuries including broken nails and bleeding from ear can be seen. The injuries may be abrasions, lacerations or contusions and it has to be differentiated from the postmortem injuries caused by aquatic animals.
- In drowning the body floats over the water surface with face down position and hence postmortem hypostasis will be prominent over the face, front of chest and limbs.

Specific Signs

- The presence of fine, tenacious, white or blood tinged froth **(Fig. 10.16)** around the mouth and nostrils are an important finding in drowning. This froth reappears even if it is wiped off and if pressure is applied over the chest. This is an important antemortem sign of drowning and is called **"the sign of drowning"**.
- **Mechanism of formation of froth:** Water enters the lungs and damages the bronchial epithelium and the surfactant, there is residual air present in the

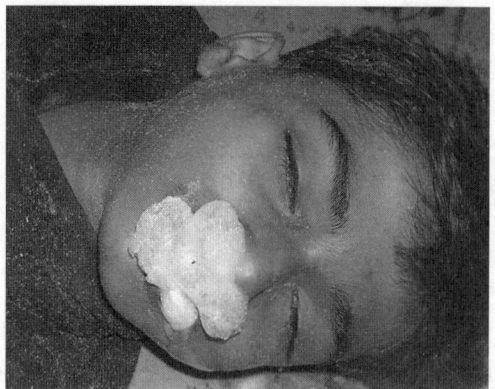

Fig. 10.16: Froth in the mouth and nostrils (the sign of drowning)—a case of sea water drowning *(For color version see Plate 7)*.

bronchioles with all these there are violent respiratory movements by the efforts of the victim for survival; all these results in chirring effect and results in the formation of the fine tenacious froth.

- **Cadaveric spasm:** While attempting to save oneself, the individual may tightly grasp the weeds and plants present in the drowning medium. During this process the individual develops sudden spasm due to development of instantaneous rigor. It indicates that the victim was alive when he entered into the water.

Nonspecific Internal Signs

- All the internal organs will be congested.
- Edema easily appreciable in lungs.
- The chambers of the heart may contain fluid blood.
- There will be multiple petechial hemorrhages (tardieu spots) over pleura and pericardium.
- Sand and mud particles can be seen in the nose, mouth or in oropharynx.
- Large quantity of water may be swallowed during the process of drowning, which will be detected in the stomach.

Specific Internal Signs

- **Emphysema aquosum:** Lungs are heavy and voluminous, water logged with prominent rib indentations on the surface. Multiple petechial hemorrhages on the sub-pleural surface and the intestinal spaces of the lung and are known as "paultaff's hemorrhages" cut section of the lungs will demonstrate frothy exudation. This lung picture of drowning is called emphysema aquosum.
- **Dissection of the bronchial tree:** It is always preferable to dissect the lung along the bronchial tree, which shows fine, leathery, tenacious white or blood stained froth in trachea and bronchi up to the terminal bronchiole. Sand, mud or sludge particles may be seen in the trachea, bronchi or primary and secondary bronchioles **(Fig. 10.17)**.

Floatation of the Body

- Floatation in water takes its own time and is mainly dependent on the temperature of the environment, as temperature directly influences the rate of decomposition.

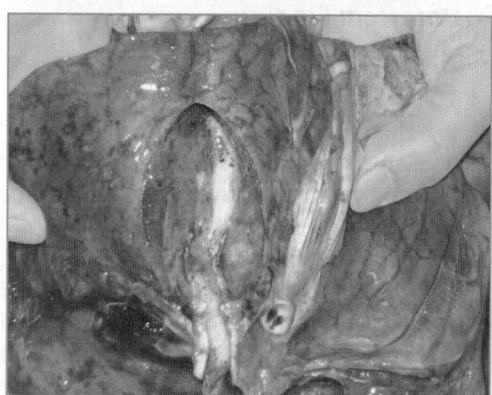

Fig. 10.17: Dissection of lung in case of death due to drowning—dissection along the bronchial tree, showing fine white, tenacious froth in the secondary bronchioles *(For color version see Plate 7)*.

- Once the body sinks under the water, it remains on the undersurface till enough gases accumulate inside the body, then the body comes back to the surface of water and float.
- Floatation of the body usually takes 18 to 24 hours in summer and 24–48 hours in winter.
- Rarely, drowned bodies may get entangled in the aquatic vegetations and may not come to the surface in a few days and may come out to surface after weeks in a bloated stage.
- Bodies drowned in deep lakes at hill stations, may not come up to the surface for a long period of time, as the extreme cold temperature markedly delays putrefaction shown in **Figure 10.18**.

Decomposition a Challenge to the Autopsy Surgeon

- When the body is fresh, the lung findings are easily appreciated in most cases and hence there exists no difficulty in finding out the cause of death in cases of drowning.
- But, it is unfortunate that many of the victim persons drown when nobody observes them and noticed only when the body comes to the surface of water after a reasonable period of time in a decomposed state.
- All the lung findings may disappear when the body is moderately decomposed. This is due to passive diffusion of water from the lungs into the body and decomposition of the lung parenchyma. Such cases are really a challenge to the forensic pathologist. However, a meticulous dissection of the bronchial tree for search of any minute foreign particles like mud, sand or any other materials which are present suspended in the drowning medium, will help to ascertain the cause of death.

WRITE SHORT NOTES ON DIATOMS? (FM2.23)

Laboratory Tests

- (i) Diatoms test; (ii) Getler's test; (iii) serum magnesium; (iv) serum strontium are available for testing antemortem drowning.
- In this Gelter's test and Diatoms tests are important.

Diatoms

- Diatoms are unicellular algae with their cell wall made of silica. It resists acid digestion.
- They are present in all types of water fresh, marine, river and lake water.
- There are more than 15 thousand species of diatoms; they are of different shapes and sizes.
- When an individual dies due to drowning; these diatoms enter the lung, carried into circulation to different parts of the body, including the bone marrow.

Isolation of Diatoms from Bones

- When decomposed bodies recovered from water are brought for autopsy, any of the

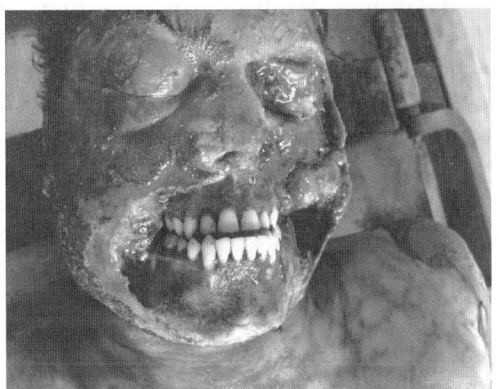

Fig. 10.18: A Case of drowning: Body recovered after 2 to 3 days—mutilation of the body by aquatic animals (For color version see Plate 7).

long bones or sternum is isolated and sent to the FSL.
- These bones are subjected to acid digestion and then centrifuged. The sediments are then examined under microscope for diatoms. Diatoms resist acid digestion, as they have a protective silica cell wall.

Medico-legal Importance of Diatoms

- Cause of death can be ascertained when decomposed or partially skeletonized bodies are recovered from water,
- *Place of drowning:* Comparison of diatoms present in the body with that of the diatoms present in the alleged drowning medium helps in concluding the place of drowning. Especially useful in cases of drowning in fast flowing water and in bodies recovered from ditches (diatoms help to find out antemortem drowning and place of drowning).
- While comparing the diatoms the number, size, shape and percentage of the diatoms are all taken into consideration.
- Diatoms test has got its own limitations of application and hence cannot be considered as a concrete proof of antemortem drowning. However, negative results may sometimes be helpful in ruling out the possibility of drowning.

WHAT IS GETTLER'S TEST? (FM2.23)

- This test is used to find out the chloride concentration from the right and left ventricular chambers of the heart.
- Normally concentration of chloride will be equal in both right and left side chambers of the heart.
- In case of fresh water drowning the chloride content will be low in the left ventricle due to hemodilution. In sea water drowning, the chloride concentration will increase by 40% due to hemoconcentration.
- This test is useful to differentiate sea water drowning from freshwater drowning. The significance of this test is highly doubtful and has less practical application.

WHAT ARE THE MEDICO-LEGAL ASPECTS ENCOUNTERED IN CASES OF DROWNING?

- Drowning is usually accidental, sometimes suicidal and rarely homicidal. It is difficult to distinguish the mode of drowning based on the postmortem findings. There could be signs of resistance in homicidal drowning and would be usually absent when the victim is pushed into water when he is unaware.
- Also it is not uncommon to kill the person by some other method and submerge the body in water, to simulate death due to suicidal drowning.

WHAT IS SHALLOW WATER DROWNING?

Shallow Water Drowning

- An intoxicated person may fall conscious by the side of a drainage channel and accidentally dip his head into water and death may result due to aspiration. At autopsy, the sewage material may be found in the respiratory tract indicating death due to drowning, this is also called as "shallow water drowning".
- It is always difficult to opine about the manner of death in drowning, as the postmortem findings may be similar in all the cases of accidental, suicidal or homicidal drowning. There may be some signs of resistance in case of homicidal drowning and these signs of struggle will be absent when the victim is unaware. Hence, opining about the manner of death in drowning is much of uncertainty.

MULTIPLE CHOICE QUESTIONS

1. **Surest sign of antemortem hanging is:**
   a. Oblique ligature mark
   b. Dried salivary stains at the angle of mouth
   c. Glove and stockings distribution of postmortem staining
   d. Pale, dry and parchmentized tissues underneath the ligature abrasion
2. **Hangman fracture is an usual phenomenon in:**
   a. Complete hanging
   b. Partial hanging
   c. Lynching
   d. Judicial hanging
3. **Adduction fracture of hyoid bone is most commonly seen in:**
   a. Hanging
   b. Bansdola
   c. Manual strangulation
   d. Ligature strangulation
4. **A person can successfully commit suicide by the following, *except*:**
   a. Throttling
   b. Strangulation
   c. Hanging
   d. Drowning
5. **Surest sign of antemortem drowning:**
   a. Froth in mouth and nostrils
   b. Cutis anserina
   c. Water in stomach
   d. Washer women skin
6. **Gettler's test is done to estimate:**
   a. Magnesium
   b. Potassium
   c. Strontium
   d. Chloride
7. **The term 'typical hanging' means:**
   a. Knot is at occiput
   b. Knot is at the side of neck
   c. Knot is under the chin
   d. None of the above
8. **Trachea is obstructed by a constriction force of:**
   a. 2 kg
   b. 5 kg
   c. 15 kg
   d. 20 kg
9. **What is wrong about diatoms?**
   a. It is an algae
   b. Seen on the surface layers of water
   c. Has an outer coat of magnesium
   d. Seen in both fresh water and salt water
10. **'La facie sympathique' is a condition seen in cases of:**
    a. Hanging
    b. Strangulation
    c. Myocardial insufficiency
    d. Railway accidents
11. **In each freshwater drowning the death occurs within 4–5 minutes of submersion due to ventricular fibrillation. Which of the following reasons is responsible for this?**
    a. Total asphyxia is produced due to fresh water
    b. Laryngeal spasm causing vagal inhibition
    c. Hemoconcentration of blood caused by the osmotic pressure effect
    d. Hemodilution, overloading of heart and hemolysis resulting in release of potassium
12. **Postmortem lividity is unlikely to develop in a case of:**
    a. Drowning in well
    b. Drowning in a fast-flowing river
    c. Postmortem submersion
    d. Drowning in chlorinated swimming pool
13. **Feature indicative of antemortem drowning is:**
    a. Cutis anserina
    b. Rigor mortis
    c. Washerwomen's feet
    d. Grass and weeds grasped in the hand
14. **Hyoid bone fracture is commonly seen in:**
    a. Hanging
    b. Strangulation
    c. Throttling
    d. Choking
15. **Paltauff's hemorrhages in drowning are seen in:**
    a. Interstitial tissues of the lung
    b. Sub-mucosa of trachea
    c. Bronchioles
    d. Alveoli
16. **Burking consists of:**
    a. Traumatic asphyxia
    b. Smothering and traumatic asphyxia
    c. Choking and strangulation
    d. Gagging
17. **In which type of drowning, death is due to vagal inhibition:**
    a. Wet drowning
    b. Dry drowning

c. Secondary drowning
d. Immersion syndrome

18. **The most reliable evidence of death due to drowning:**
    a. Edema of lungs
    b. Froth in mouth and nostrils
    c. Diatoms in lung tissue
    d. Mud and sand particles in the bronchioles

19. **The 'knot' in judicial hanging is placed at:**
    a. Behind the neck
    b. Side of the neck
    c. Below the chin
    d. Choice of hangman

20. **Characteristics of strangulation are all, *except*:**
    a. Fracture of thyroid cartilage
    b. Bleeding from nose
    c. Saliva running out of mouth
    d. Transverse ligature mark

21. **'Café—coronary' refers to death in intoxicated person during meals due to:**
    a. Suffocation
    b. Cardiac arrest
    c. Chocking
    d. Smothering

22. **Not true about freshwater drowning:**
    a. Hyperkalemia
    b. Hypovolemia
    c. Ventricular fibrillation
    d. Hemolysis

23. **In dry drowning:**
    a. Death occurs in few days of submersion episode
    b. Death occurs due to sudden immersion in cold water
    c. Water does not enter lungs because of laryngeal spasm
    d. Seen in alcoholics who drown in shallow water

24. **Sexual asphyxia is:**
    a. Suicidal death
    b. Homicidal death
    c. Natural death
    d. Accidental death

25. **Not a feature of ligature strangulation:**
    a. Horizontal ligature mark
    b. Incomplete ligature mark
    c. Marked congested face
    d. Sub-conjunctival hemorrhage

26. **On postmortem examination, contusion of neck muscles is seen along with fracture of hyoid bone. The most probable cause of death is:**
    a. Smothering
    b. Mugging
    c. Burking
    d. Throttling

27. **Spanish windlass is practiced in which form of strangulation:**
    a. Bansdola
    b. Throttling
    c. Garroting
    d. Mugging

28. **A 5-year-old boy while having dinner suddenly becomes aphonic and is brought to the casualty with the complaint of respiratory distress. Appropriate management should be:**
    a. Cricothyroidotomy
    b. Emergency tracheostomy
    c. Humidified oxygen
    d. Heimlich maneuver

29. **All may cause traumatic asphyxia, *except*:**
    a. Railway accident
    b. Road traffic accident
    c. Accidental strangulation
    d. Stampede

30. **Not true about freshwater drowning:**
    a. Hyperkalemia
    b. Hypovolemia
    c. Ventricular fibrillation
    d. Hemolysis

31. **In case of drowning in sea water:**
    a. Hb increases
    b. Hb decreases
    c. Either
    d. No change

32. **Not seen in saltwater drowning:**
    a. Hyperkalemia
    b. Progressive hypovolemia
    c. Circulatory collapse
    d. Acute pulmonary edema

33. **Death occurs faster in:**
    a. Freshwater drowning
    b. Saltwater drowning
    c. Near drowning
    d. Warm water drowning

34. **Gettler's test is used to diagnose death due to:**
    a. Hanging
    b. Strangulation
    c. Burns
    d. Drowning
35. **Death due to drowning is suggested by all, except:**
    a. Profuse fine froth which increase on pressure on chest
    b. Cadaveric spasm
    c. Absence of mud/weeds in stomach
    d. Diatoms in bone marrow
36. **The best site for taking sample for diatoms test is:**
    a. Lungs
    b. Bone marrow of ulna
    c. Bone marrow of femur
    d. Muscle
37. **Sexual asphyxia is which manner of death?**
    a. Natural
    b. Suicide
    c. Homicide
    d. Accident
38. **To develop cyanosis, percentage of reduced hemoglobin exceeds:**
    a. 2 gm%
    b. 5 gm%
    c. 6 gm%
    d. 10 gm%
39. **In hanging last to be occluded is**
    a. Jugular vein
    b. Carotid artery
    c. Vertebral artery
    d. Trachea
40. **Death caused due to regurgitation and inhalation of food into the respiratory tract is called:**
    a. Smothering
    b. Burking
    c. Choking
    d. Gagging
41. **Sexual asphyxia is associated with:**
    a. Masochism
    b. Sadism
    c. Voyeurism
    d. Tribadism
42. **Traumatic asphyxia results from:**
    a. Cut injury of the windpipe
    b. Crush injury of the chest and abdomen
    c. Fall from height
    d. All of the above
43. **Reflex cardiac arrest is due to:**
    a. Sudden flow of water into the nasopharynx
    b. Sudden thrust of water over the abdominal region
    c. In both (a) and (b)
    d. Does not occur in drowning
44. **Acid digestion technique is used for:**
    a. Detection of aquatic vegetations in stomach content
    b. Detection of diatom in drowning
    c. Detection of fibers in stomach contents
    d. Detection of metallic pieces in tissues

ANSWERS

1. b	2. d	3. c	4. a	5. a	6. d	7. a	8. c	9. c	10. a
11. d	12. b	13. d	14. c	15. a	16. b	17. d	18. d	19. c	20. c
21. c	22. b	23. c	24. d	25. b	26. d	27. c	28. d	29. c	30. b
31. a	32. a	33. a	34. d	35. c	36. c	37. d	38. b	39. c	40. c
41. a	42. b	43. c	44. b						

CHAPTER 11

Death due to Starvation

> **KEY WORDS**
> Starvation, emaciation, brown atrophy of heart, intercurrent infections, Article 21.

FM2.26 Describe and discuss clinical features, postmortem findings and medico-legal aspects of death due to starvation and neglect.

WHAT IS STARVATION?

- Starvation is a condition in which there is deprivation of supply of essential nutrients, either due to inadequate food supply or due to non-intake of food for a long duration.
- Regular and constant supply of food is necessary for the maintenance of nutritional balance of the body.
- Starvation may be *acute or chronic*. Acute starvation results due to sudden and abrupt stoppage of food and water. Chronic starvation or malnutrition is due to deficient intake of food either quantitatively or qualitatively for a long period of time.

WHAT IS NORMAL BODY REQUIREMENT OF A HUMAN BEING?

- An adult requires minimum of 1800 calories of food per day to meet the dietary requirement. There is danger to life when 40% of the body weight is lost.
- Total deprivation water and food causes death in about 10 days. Without intake of food, if water along is consumed then the individual may survive for 50 to 60 days.

SIGNS AND SYMPTOMS OF ACUTE STARVATION (FM2.26)

Signs and Symptoms

- Acute feeling of hunger in 2 days
- Loss of body fat and emaciation starts appearing from 5th day, with progressive loss of body weight. Breath turns offensive.
- Pulse feeble, blood pressure falls and cardiac atrophy occurs.
- First there is constipation and later diarrhea.
- Temperature is sub-normal; urine scanty and dark in color.

- Skin becomes dry, fissured, pigmented, thin and drawn tight over bony prominences.
- Cheeks sunken; lips dry and cracked; tongue dry and coated.
- Abdomen scaphoid in shape and prominence of ribs with indrawing of intercostal space.
- In *chronic starvation*, in addition to the above mentioned features there will be ascites, oedema of the limbs and evidence of intercurrent infections.
- Hair becomes dry, lusterless and brittle; nails become brittle and ridged.
- The mind is usually clear till the end; some people may develop delirium just before death.

POSTMORTEM FINDINGS IN DEATH DUE TO STARVATION (FM2.26) (FIG. 11.1)

Postmortem Findings

Emaciation and all the external signs of starvation are present.

Internal:
- Loss of body fat and atrophy of muscles.
- **Stomach and intestines:** Empty, contracted and thinned out.
- **Gallbladder:** Full and distended with thick, tenacious bile.

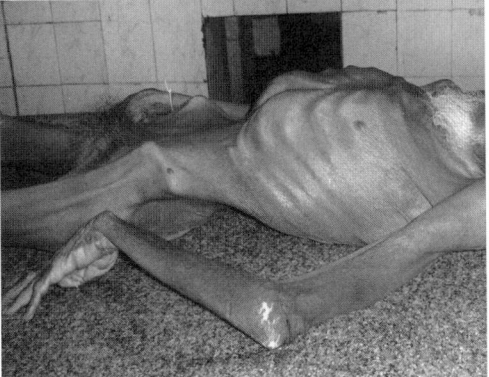

Fig. 11.1: Death due to starvation
(For color version see Plate 7).

- Loss of omental and mesenteric pad of fat.
- All internal organs except the brain are sunken and reduced in size; demineralization of bones and **'brown atrophy'** of heart muscles are evident.

FACTORS MODIFYING THE EFFECTS OF STARVATION

- **Age:** Old people withstand starvation better, due to lower food requirement.
- **Sex:** Females combat starvation better, since they have more body fat.
- **State of health:** Healthy people withstand better, due to higher muscle mass in the body.
- **Body fat:** Obese people withstand better.
- **Cold:** Extreme cold aggravates the effects of starvation, since cold accelerates the basal metabolic rate.

CAUSE OF DEATH IN STARVATION

- In acute starvation death is due to electrolytes imbalance, dehydration and circulatory failure.
- In partial or chronic starvation death results from loss of immunity and intercurrent infection.

MEDICO-LEGAL ASPECTS OF STARVATION (FM2.26)

- **Homicidal starvation:** Victims are usually infants and unwanted children. There is deliberate withholding of food by the parents or care givers.
- **Suicidal starvation:** It is rare but seen in mentally ill people and prisoners who go on hunger strike as protest. Political groups and other organizations venture on hunger strike to represent their views more strongly and as a mark of protest. However, in such situations they are not allowed to die of starvation. When they extend the starvation to such level

which threatens their life, treatment is done on compulsory basis without their consent.

- **The right for food** is not a basic right as per Article 21 of the constitution of India but guarantees **'right to life and liberty'** of all citizens.
- The Supreme Court has stated that the chief secretary of a state would be held responsible for all starvation deaths in the state, if reported and proved.

MULTIPLE CHOICE QUESTIONS

1. **Brown atrophy of heart is seen in:**
   a. Burns
   b. Cyanide poisoning
   c. Starvation
   d. Strangulation
2. **In death due to starvation, the gallbladder on autopsy shows:**
   a. Empty
   b. Full with bile
   c. Completely shrunken
   d. Partly filled with inspissated bile and gall stones

ANSWERS
1. c   2. b

SECTION 4

Forensic Traumatology

SECTION OUTLINE

Chapter 12: Mechanical Injuries
Chapter 13: Regional Injuries
Chapter 14: Medico-Legal Aspects of Injuries
Chapter 15: Thermal Injuries
Chapter 16: Forensic Ballistics
Chapter 17: Electrical and Lightening Injuries

CHAPTER 12

Mechanical Injuries

KEY WORDS

Injury, wound, abrasion, grazes, imprint abrasion, contusion, ectopic bruise, artificial bruise, laceration, cut laceration, fracture, dislocation, incised wound, tailing of wound, cut wound, chop wound, stab wound, Langer's line.

FM3.3 Mechanical injuries and wounds: Define, describe and classify different types of mechanical injuries, abrasion, bruise, laceration, stab wound, incised wound, chop wound, defense wound, self-inflicted/fabricated wounds and their medicolegal aspects.

INTRODUCTION

- **Medical definition of injury**
    - Injury or **wound** is the "Breach in the natural continuity of any tissue of the living body".
    - Medically all injuries are wounds; these words injury and wound are often used interchangeably.
- **Legal definition of injury**
    - **Section 44 IPC** defines injury as "any harm whatsoever illegally caused to any person in body, mind, reputation or property".
    - Only bodily injuries are wounds. Hence, all wounds are injuries but all the injuries are not wounds.

Mechanical Injury (FM3.3)

- Injuries caused by application of physical force are called mechanical injuries.
- Character of an injury produced on the body depends upon the following factors:
    - Nature and shape of the weapon
    - The amount of force transmitted.
    - The rate of application of force.
    - The nature of the tissues involved.
    - The surface area over which energy is delivered.

CLASSIFY MECHANICAL INJURIES? (FM3.3)

- Mechanical injuries are classified according to the nature of force involved in production of the injury.
    - **Injuries caused by blunt force**:
        - Abrasion
        - Contusion
        - Laceration
        - Fracture and/or dislocation

- **Injuries caused by sharp edged weapons:**
  - Injuries caused by single edged light cutting weapons: Incised wound.
  - Injuries caused by heavy cutting weapons: Cut/chop wounds.
- **Injuries caused by pointed weapons:** Stab wounds
- **Firearm wounds:** Shot gun and rifled firearm injuries.
  Firearm wounds can also be grouped under mechanical injuries, since the projectile which produces the injury on the body is a pointed weapon. Hence, these injuries are also a form of stab injuries.

WHAT IS AN ABRASION? WHAT ARE THE TYPES OF ABRASION? (FM3.3)

What is Brush Burn and Imprint Abrasion?

Abrasion (Gravel Rash) (Fig. 12.1)

- Destruction of the skin, which involves only the superficial layers of the epidermis; i.e., injuries limited to only the cutidermis and does not involve the whole thickness of the skin.
- They are caused by a lateral rubbing, by a blow or a fall on a rough surface.
- Some pressure and movement of the agent (weapon/force) on the surface of the skin is essential to produce an abrasion.
- The damaged layers of the epithelium are heaped up towards one end of the wound, indicating the direction of application of force.
- The exposed raw surface is covered by exudation of lymph and blood, which produces a protective covering called as *"scab"*.
- Abrasions are usually simple injuries, as they cause less pain, bleed slightly and heal rapidly without leaving a permanent *scar*. However, abrasions over a large surface area of the body can cause severe pain and bleeding.

Types of Abrasion

There are mainly four types of abrasions:

Scratch Abrasion

- These are linear abrasions caused by a protruding object such as a thorn or nails.
- There is movement of the body or the weapon which produces linear scratch.
- These abrasions have a good length but relatively small breath.
- During the movement of the weapon or the body, the torn up epithelium are carried away towards the end of the wound, indicating the direction of force.
- Linear abrasions can also be caused by sharp weapons, not sharp enough to incise or cut. For example, a running victim is assaulted with a long cutting weapon through the clothing, now there is not enough force transmitted on the body and hence will result in a linear abrasion or linear abraded contusions.

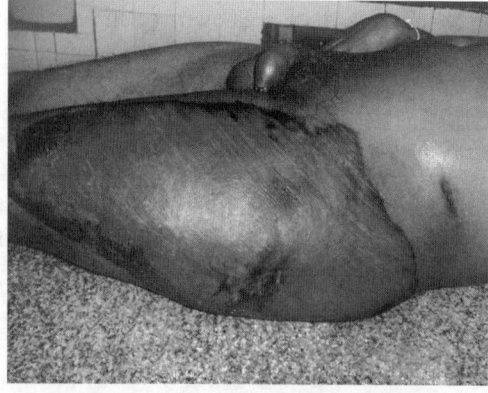

Fig. 12.1: Grazed abrasion caused in a road traffic accident *(For color version see Plate 8)*.

Grazed Abrasion

- Grazes are also called as brush burns or friction burns.
- Multiple linear abrasions over a larger area of the body are called as grazed abrasion.
- They are caused by rubbing of the body over a hard surface, usually seen in road traffic accidents; where the individual is dragged over the hard surface of the roads.
- Due to the uneven surface, the depth of the wound may not be uniform.
- Grazed abrasions are painful when it involves a large surface area and the depth is more, since the nerve endings are involved.
- During the rubbing process, there is production of heat between the body and the road, hence the ends of the wound may look like as if they are burnt; the wound is hard to touch and hence they are called as "**brush burns**" but they are not thermal injuries as they are not caused by heat and they are only mechanical injuries.

Pressure Abrasion

- They are also called as crushing or friction abrasions.
- These types of abrasions are caused by crushing of the epidermis by compressive blunt force. The skin is crushed by the pressure exerted by the offending object. These types of abrasions are usually associated with bruising of the surrounding areas.
- **Example:** Ligature abrasion of hanging and strangulation, bite marks, etc.

Impact Abrasion

- They are also called as "contact or **imprint** abrasions".
- These are abrasions caused by impact of a rough object perpendicular (at right angles) to the skin surface.
- The imprint of the weapon/offending object is left over on the skin.
- **Example:** Tyre mark in a run over accident, steering wheel impact in collision accidents, ligature mark produced by hard tough materials like that of plastic rope in cases of hanging and strangulation.
- Pressure abrasions and imprint abrasions are grouped under the category of "**patterned abrasions**" as the pattern of the weapon is seen on the skin surface, thus helps to corroborate the weapon responsible for causing the injury.

Atypical Abrasions

Some authors classify certain abrasions which does not fall into any of the four types such as crescentic abrasions caused by the finger nails, bite marks and tiger skin abrasion (thin linen clothing getting burnt due to heat generated by dragging and adherent on the surface, giving the appearance of tiger skin) as "Atypical abrasions" but abrasions caused by the nails are either pressure abrasions (applied at right angles as in throttling) or scratch abrasions (when applied tangentially producing linear scratches); bite marks are imprint or pressure abrasions; and tiger skin abrasion is brush burn (grazes).

HEALING OF AN ABRASION: MEDICOLEGAL IMPORTANCE OF ABRASIONS (FM3.3)

Healing of Abrasion (Table 12.1)

Age of an Abrasion

- Abrasion heals from the periphery with generation of new epithelial cells. The age of an abrasion can be assessed by examining the stage of healing of an abrasion.
- The time taken for healing mainly depends on the size, depth and area on the body.

TABLE 12.1: Healing of abrasion.

Time	Color
Fresh (<12 hours)	Bright red
12 to 24 hours	Bright red scab
2 to 3 days	Reddish brown scab
4 to 5 days	Dark brown scab
5 to 7 days	Black scab firmly adherent onto the base
7 to 10 days	Black scab loosely adherent onto the base; scab could have fallen off in the periphery
10 to 14 days	Scab completely fallen off, exposing the underlying pale dermis
With passage of time	Skin regains the original color, without any scar

- Abrasions are bright red in color when fresh, due to passage of time the color gradually changes to reddish brown and dark brown, finally becomes black in color in one week.
- From the color of an abrasion, the approximate time of infliction can be assessed.

Medicolegal Importance of Abrasions

- Abrasions are the most important medicolegal injury.
- Abrasions are produced at the site of impact and are useful to find out over which area of the body, force was applied.
- Indicates the direction of force: The torn layers of the epithelium are heaped up towards one end of the wound, indicating the direction of application of force/the direction of movement of the body, when hit or dragged over a fixed surface or object.
- It may be the only sign of a serious internal injury.
- Patterned abrasions helps to find out the object causing the injury.
  Example: Imprint of the tyre mark in a run over accident and pattern of the ligature material in case of hanging and strangulation.
- Age of the injury can be assessed which indicates the time of infliction of the injury.
- Relative position of the assailant and the victim can be assessed.
- Motive of the offence can be made out from site of injury for example, injuries over the breast, lips and genitals indicating sexual assault.
- Positive identification of the assailant can be made out; for example, from the pattern of bite marks (arrangement of teeth are unique to each individual) and tissue scrapings from the nail beds of the victim by DNA analysis.
- May give a clue to the place of incident by examination of the wound for dirt, dust, grease, sand or gravel.
- Manner of injury can be assessed (accidental, suicidal, homicidal or fabricated).
- Character and manner of abrasion gives a clue to the cause of death. For example, crescentic fingernail abrasions on the neck in throttling; pressure abrasion around the mouth and nose in smothering; abrasions on breast, genitals, inner aspect of thigh and around the anus in sexual offences like rape and sodomy.

CONDITIONS WHICH MIMICS AN ABRASION

Some of the skin lesions are frequently mistaken as abrasions; by careful examination these lesions could be easily differentiated.
- Erosions of the skin the body produced by ants after death.
- Excoriation of the skin by excreta; usually in babies when napkins are used and in old debilitated patients who do not have proper care takers to maintain hygiene when the patients are unable to take care of themselves.
- **Pressure sores (decubitus ulcer):** In old debilitated and bed ridden patients.

HOW TO DIFFERENTIATE ANTEMORTEM AND POSTMORTEM ABRASIONS? (TABLE 12.2)

- In routine circumstances, it is easy to differentiate antemortem and postmortem abrasions **(Figs. 12.2 and 12.3)** just by observation. Difficulties do arise in certain situations especially in decomposed bodies; sometimes it becomes difficult to differentiate abrasions produced just before or just after death even by microscopic examination.

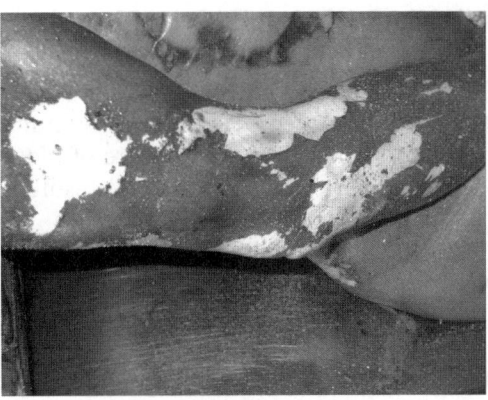

Fig. 12.2: Postmortem abrasion
(For color version see Plate 8).

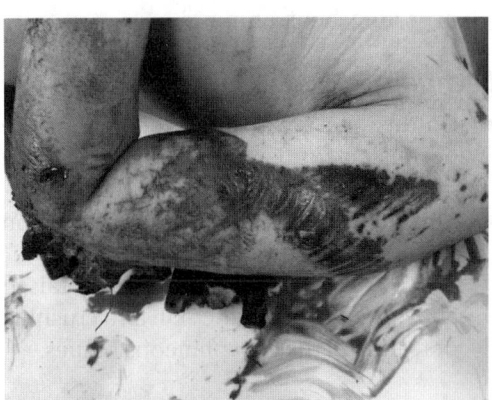

Fig. 12.3: Grazed abrasion (gravel rash)
(For color version see Plate 8).

TABLE 12.2: Differences between antemortem and postmortem abrasions.

Features	Antemortem abrasions	Postmortem abrasions
1. Site	Anywhere on the body	Over bony prominences
2. Oozing of lymph	Present	Absent
3. Scab formation	Present	Absent
4. Color changes	Present, if the victim survives some period of time	Absent, mostly yellowish without any change in color
5. Parchmentization	Absent	Present

WHAT ARE CONTUSION? (FM3.3)

Contusion/Bruise

- Contusions are caused by blunt trauma, due to which, there is rupture of blood vessels (arterioles or venules) resulting in extravasation of blood into the surrounding soft tissues.
- Contusions are caused by blunt force, such as fist, stone, stick, whip, bar, boot, or fall from height, etc.
- Contusions may develop not only under the skin and subcutaneous tissues, but also in the deeper layers of tissues in the body and also in the internal organs like liver, lung, brain or muscle.

Location

- Contusions are usually located in the dermis and subcutaneous tissues, often inside the fatty layers.
- Most of the time, there is no destruction of the skin.
- There is a painful swelling, slightly raised above the surface of the skin and crushing or tearing of the subcutaneous tissues.

Types of Contusion

- Superficial contusion or surface bruise **(Fig. 12.4)**
- Patterned bruise **(Fig. 12.5)**
- Deep bruise **(Fig. 12.6)**
- Bruise of internal organs **(Fig. 12.7)**
- Contre coup bruise
- Ectopic (gravity shifting) bruise
- Bruises may be seen in association with abrasion (abraded contusion) or lacerations (contused laceration) **(Fig. 12.8)**
- According to the size of the contusions, pinpoint contusions are called as **petechiae**; when the size is smaller than a few mm in diameter they are called as **ecchymosis** and when the size is more than a few cm in diameter they are called as **hematoma**.

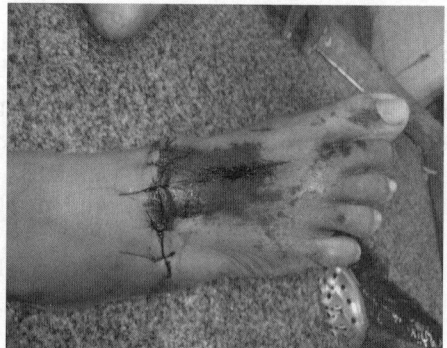

Fig. 12.4: Superficial contusion
(For color version see Plate 8).

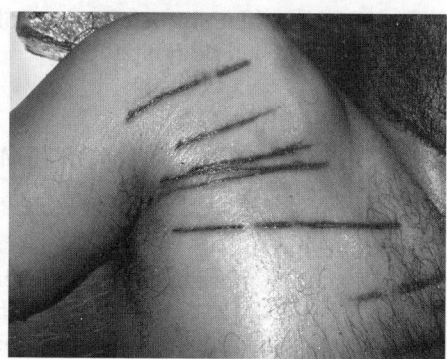

Fig. 12.5: Patterned contusion
(For color version see Plate 8).

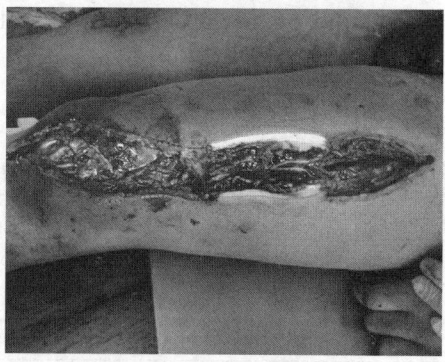

Fig. 12.6: Deep contusion
(For color version see Plate 8).

Color Changes of a Contusion: (Table 12.3)

Contusions are red in color when they develop after an impact. The contusions slowly resolve

CHAPTER 12: Mechanical Injuries

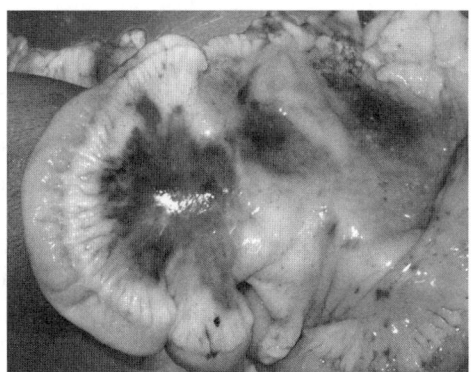

Fig. 12.7: Internal contusion
(For color version see Plate 9).

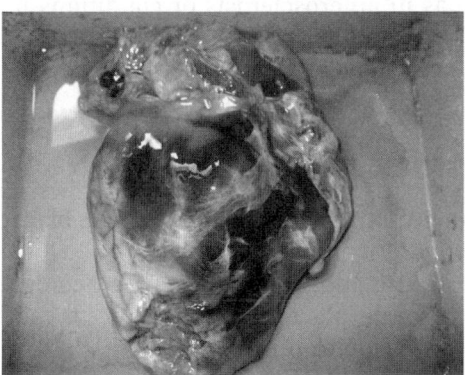

Fig. 12.8: Contusion of heart
(For color version see Plate 9).

in the process of healing; the color changes from time to time before the skin regains its original color; these color changes are used as indicators to assess the time of infliction of the injury.

Medico-legal Importance of Bruise

- It is a sign of violence.
- Bruise need not always be simple injuries.
- It is usually accidental or homicidal, and less commonly selfinflicted.
- Type of the object can sometimes be identified in cases of *patterned bruise*.
- Time of assault can be assessed by the color changes of the bruise.
- Motive of the offence can be identified from site of bruise.

CONDITIONS WHICH HAS TO BE DIFFERENTIATED CONTUSIONS?

How to Differentiate Contusion from Congestion and Livor Mortis?

Contusions has to be differentiated from:
- Postmortem staining
- Congestion
- Lesions produced by plant juices (artificial bruise)

Contusion and Postmortem Staining

- The difficulty with postmortem staining arises only in dead bodies, especially by 4 to 6 hours after death when the lividity is present in discrete patches before they coalesce with each other to form uniform postmortem staining by 6 to 8 hours.
- It is easy to differentiate by making an incision over the area, postmortem staining will show fluid blood, which oozes

TABLE 12.3: Healing of a contusion.

Time	Color	Pigment responsible
Fresh	Red	Due to extravasation of RBC
1 to 2 days	Reddish blue or blue	Due to deoxygenated blood
3 to 5 days	Reddish brown	Hemosiderin
5 to 7 days	Green	Biliverdin
7 to 10 days	Yellow	Bilirubin
10 to 14 days	Regains original skin color	Without leaving behind any scar

out and easily washed off under water. In contusion, there will be extravasation of blood into the layers of tissues and cannot be washed off under water.

Contusion and Congestion

The difficulty to differentiate with congestion arises both in living and the dead, especially in people with brown or fair complexion. Differences between bruise and congestion are described in **Table 12.4**.

WHAT IS A FALSE BRUISE? DIFFERENTIATE TRUE CONTUSION FROM FALSE CONTUSION? (TABLE 12.5)

False bruise or bruise like lesions (fabricated) may be produced, by application of irritant substances like chemicals, juices of marking nut or calotropis on the skin to bring a false charge of assault against somebody.

FACTORS WHICH DETERMINE THE APPEARANCE OF A BRUISE

- The production of a bruise is dependent upon a number of factors.
  - Vascularity of the tissues involved
  - **Site on the body:**
- Whether the tissues involved are loose or strongly supported; if the tissues are loosely arranged then the bruise appeared is marked, if the tissues are strongly supported then bruise is less pronounced.
  - *Age:* Children and old age people bruise easily.
  - *Sex:* Females bruise more readily, due to less muscle mass and more fat content.
  - *Complexion:* Bruises are more prominent in fair skinned individuals.
  - Pathological conditions
- When the blood vessels are diseased as in atherosclerosis or conditions like hemophilia, clotting factor deficiencies and blood discrasias, bruising occurs very easily and more marked.

ECTOPIC CONTUSION (FM3.3)

Gravity shifting contusion (Ectopic bruise) (Fig. 12.9)

- Bruise appears in a distant place other than the place of impact of force is called as "Ectopic bruise".
- It is due to the shifting of the blood from the ruptured site to the dependent part of the body due to gravity. Hence they are also called as "Gravity Shifting Bruise".

TABLE 12.4: Differences between bruise and congestion.

Factors	Bruise	Congestion
Causative agent	Mechanical force	Pathological condition like inflammation, capillary stasis due to hypoxia, etc.
Level of the tissue involved	Diffusion of blood at the SC or submucous level with rupture of capillaries	Intravascular phenomenon with engorgement of capillaries (stasis of blood inside the capillaries)
Color	Changes from red to blue, brown, green and yellow	It is all along dusky red without any change
Margins	Diffuse	Well defined
Dissection	Cut surface stained due to extravasation which is not washable	Bleeding which occurs from the engorged vessels during dissection is washable

CHAPTER 12: Mechanical Injuries

TABLE 12.5: Differences between bruises, and bruise like lesions produced by chemicals or plant juices.

Features	Bruise	False bruise
Shape	Regular	Irregular
Margins	Diffuse and ill-defined	Clear and sharply demarcated
Swelling	Slight	No swelling
Abrasion of the surrounding area	May be present	Not present
Small blisters	Not present	May be present
Itching	Absent	Present
Color changes	Occur as the age of the bruise progress	No color change
Similar lesions	May be present elsewhere in the body even if sustained accidentally or caused by someone (homicidal)	Usually present around the nail beds due to itching and many other parts of the body wherever he scratches after itching the affected area
Cause	Mechanical force	Contact with chemicals or plant juice
Extravasation of blood	Present in the subcutaneous tissue	Not present
Chemical test of skin scrapping	Detects nothing; extravasation can be demonstrated by HPE	Detects the chemical or the plant juice used

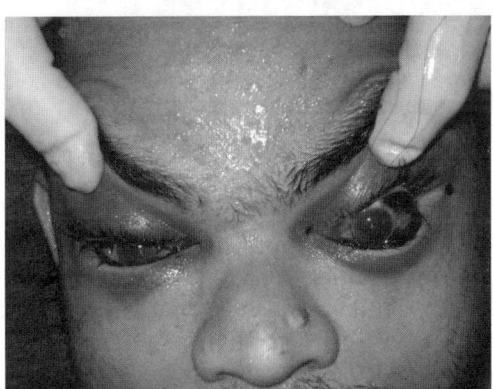

Fig. 12.9: Ectopic contusion *(For color version see Plate 9).*

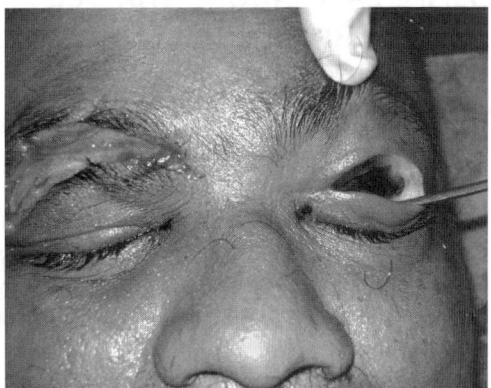

Fig. 12.10: Ectopic contusion–dissection of the eyelids to demonstrate the contusion; also there is laceration on the eyebrow of the opposite eye *(For color version see Plate 9).*

- **Examples:** (i) Injury to the forehead producing periorbital bruising (Raccoon eye or black eye) shown in **Figure 12.10;** (ii) Injury to the lower part of the thighs result in collection of blood around the knee joint; (iii) Injury to the legs, leading to collection of blood around the ankle joint.

DELAYED BRUISING

- A superficial bruise appears within a short span of time as a dark-red swelling. Whereas a deep bruise may take several hours or even 1 to 2 days to appear.

Sometimes, a deeper extravasation of blood may not become externally visible at all. Hence, in any case of suspected blunt force injury it is advisable to repeat the examination after 48 hours, to check for deep contusions.
- Also when the rupture of minute arterioles or venules takes place there is slow collection of blood and it may take time for appearance of a contusion.

DIFFERENTIATE ANTEMORTEM AND POSTMORTEM BRUISE?

- In antemortem bruise, there is swelling, extravasation, coagulation and infiltration of blood into the tissues; there will be visible color change if the individual has survived for reasonable period of time after the infliction of injury.
- In postmortem bruise all these signs are absent.

DEFINE LACERATION? WHAT ARE THE GENERAL FEATURES OF A LACERATION? (FM3.3)

- **Lacerations** are injuries in which the tissues are crushed/torn as result of application of blunt force. They involve all the layers of the skin and may also involve the deeper layers like muscles, vessels and nerves. Healing of laceration is by secondary intension with resultant scar formation.
- **General features of a laceration:**
    - The shape of laceration is always irregular; the edges of the wound are ragged, bruised and undermined **(Fig. 12.11)**.
    - Margins are irregular with abraded contusions surrounding the margins of the injured tissues **(Fig. 12.12)**.
    - The floor of the laceration shows tags of tissue over riding each other to a varying depth. This is called **bridging of tissues**—diagnostic of laceration.
    - The level of tissue damage is gross and severe in laceration.
    - Blood loss is usually minimal due to crushing of the lumen of blood vessels.
    - In lacerations involving scalp there is crushing of hair bulbs, which is useful to differentiate a laceration from incised wound of the scalp **(Fig. 12.13)**.
    - Foreign material like dust, gravel, sand, etc., may be present in a laceration.
    - Healing is by secondary intension with resultant scar formation.

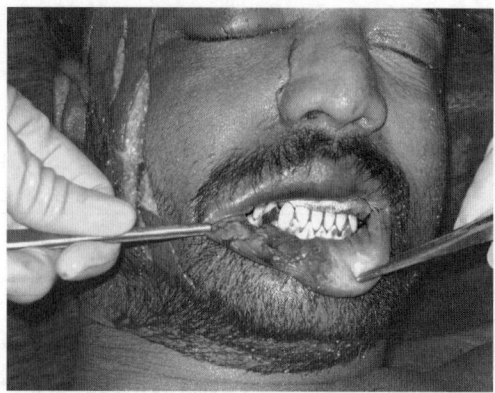

Fig. 12.11: Laceration of inner surface of lips caused by teeth *(For color version see Plate 9)*.

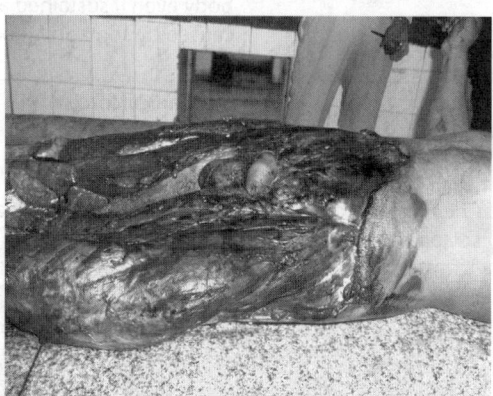

Fig. 12.12: Crush laceration of thigh caused in road traffic accident *(For color version see Plate 9)*.

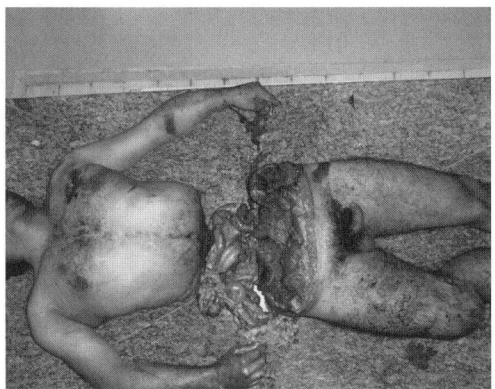

Fig. 12.13: Transaction of the body in a run-over train accident *(For color version see Plate 10)*.

WHAT ARE THE TYPES OF LACERATION?

- **Split laceration:** It also called as "**incised looking laceration**". These lacerations are present on the areas where there are lesser amount of subcutaneous soft tissues between the skin and the underlying bone. A blunt impact or trauma over such areas will result in splitting of the skin producing injuries which looks like an incised or cut wound. But these types of injuries can be easily identified as lacerations, by examination such injuries using a hand lens, which will show the irregular ragged and bruised margins.
- **Stretch laceration:** Results due to abnormal stretching of the skin as a result of localized pressure and pulling of the skin at site of impact. These lacerations result when the starching effect exceeds the elasticity of the skin.
- **Tear laceration:** These types of lacerations are as a result of stretching effect combined with compression of the tissues, under the hard object.
- **Avulsion:** Otherwise called shearing laceration, the shearing and grinding force of a heavy object or a vehicle producing separation of the skin from the underlying tissues (like lifting a flap of skin) over a larger area.
- **Internal laceration:** This may occur with or without any evidence of external injury.
- **Crush laceration:** A laceration involving a wider surface area of the body or a limb with extensive laceration of the skin, connective tissues, muscles, tendons, vessels and nerves with compound comminuted fracture of the underlying bones.

MEDICO-LEGAL SIGNIFICANCE OF LACERATION

- It is a sign of violence.
- The place of occurrence can be identified by the presence of foreign material such as mud, dust, gravel, etc.
- Laceration over the face is considered as a grievous injury, since it produces a permanent scar which amounts to disfiguration of face.
- Lacerations heal by secondary intension with the resultant of scar formation. Large laceration over a joint result in the formation of an extensive scar, which restricts the movement of a joint, resulting in permanent disability, thus amounts to grievous hurt.
- Scars so formed may sometimes be helpful in personal identity.
- Lacerations are usually accidental or homicidal and rarely suicidal.
- Age of the injury cannot be determined from lacerations due to extensive variation in the rate of healing of such injures.

DESCRIBE INJURIES CAUSED BY SHARP FORCE? (FM3.3)

What are the Features of an Incised Wound?

There are three main types of sharp force injuries:

i. Incised wound
ii. Cut wound and
iii. Chop wound.

Incised Wound (Cut, Slash)

- These are wounds produced as a result of slashing or cutting motion with a light cutting weapon such as a knife.
- The primary characteristic of an incised wound is the length of the wound is more than depth of the wound.
- It produces uniform and clear division of the skin and underlying soft tissues.

Features of Incised Wound

- The margins of the wound are clean cut, regular and well defined; usually there is no bruising along the margins of the wound.
- Predominantly incised wounds are linear with everted margins, but in areas where skin is loosely applied to the body such as scrotum or axilla, the margins might appear inverted and jagged (with multiple folds).
- The length is the greatest dimension and it does not have any relationship with length of the blade.
- The breath of the wound depends on the extent of gaping of the margins and the elasticity of the skin; the breath of the wound has a relationship with the thickness of the blade.
- The wound will be deeper at the site of commencement and it becomes progressively shallow as the weapon is drawn over the surface of the skin. This is known as "**tailing of the wound**" shown in **Figure 12.14**.
- Tailing of the wound indicates the direction of application of force and the relative position of the assailant and the victim.
- The **shape** of the injury will be fusiform or spindle due to comparatively more retraction of the edges in the center. When inflicted on the convex surface of the body

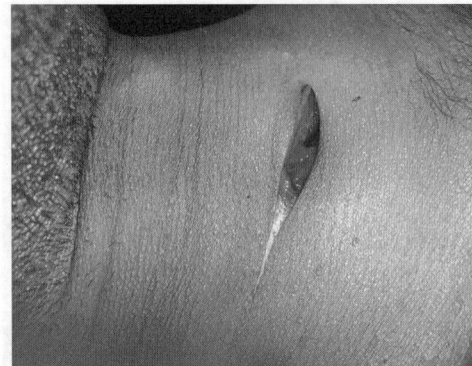

Fig. 12.14: Incised wound with tailing of wound
(For color version see Plate 10).

like the occipital region or buttocks, the wound may be crescentic or semilunar in appearance shown in **Figure 12.15**.
- Profuse bleeding is present, as the vessels are perpendicularly clean cut.
- In case of an oblique slash by a sharp edged weapon, beveling of the edges may be present indicating the angle at which the weapon was applied.
- Incised wounds will produce a skin flap when the weapon is struck nearly horizontal to the body.
- In the event of death, in such cases, the cause of death is predominantly due to shock and excessive bleeding.

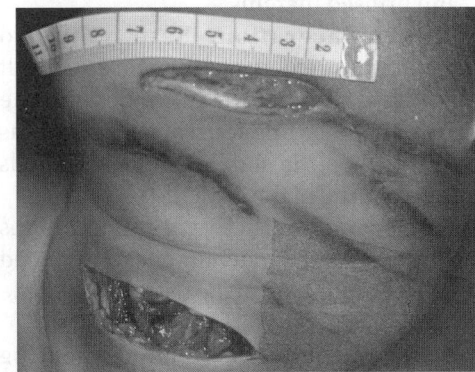

Fig. 12.15: Multiple incised wounds on the neck
(For color version see Plate 10).

CHAPTER 12: Mechanical Injuries

- In case of cut-throat injury, in addition to hemorrhagic shock, death may occur due to asphyxia as a result of aspiration of blood into the respiratory passage.
- In case of homicidal injuries, incised wounds or cut wounds seen on the palmar and dorsal aspects of hands or on the posteromedial aspect of the forearm is indicative of defense injuries.
- Multiple, parallel superficial incised wounds **(Fig. 12.16)** seen over the wrist or neck or elsewhere on accessible parts of the body are hesitation cuts indicative of suicidal tendencies.

Cut Wounds (Fig. 12.17)

- Cut wounds are produced by a perpendicular strike, using a heavy cutting weapon such as a chopper or long cutting weapon.
- The resultant injury depends on the weight of the weapon and the force used.
- The injuries are usually severe in nature; it may involve all the layers of tissues like skin, muscles, and also the bones. On the bone, there would be linear fissured fracture or a cut fracture dividing the bone into two; the margins of the cut ends are cleanly divided.

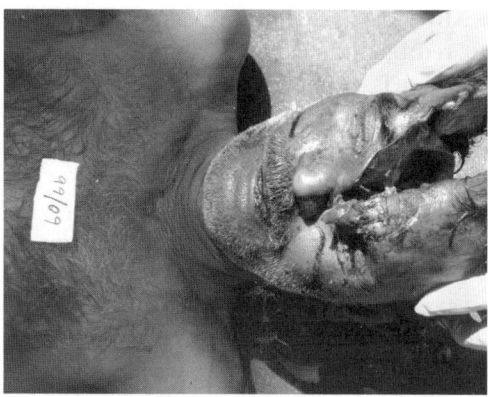

Fig. 12.17: Cut wound
(For color version see Plate 10).

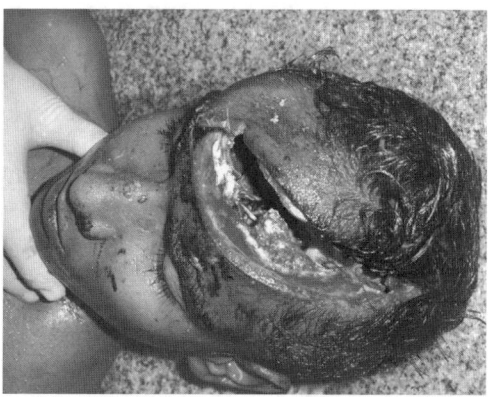

Fig. 12.18: Chop wound
(For color version see Plate 10).

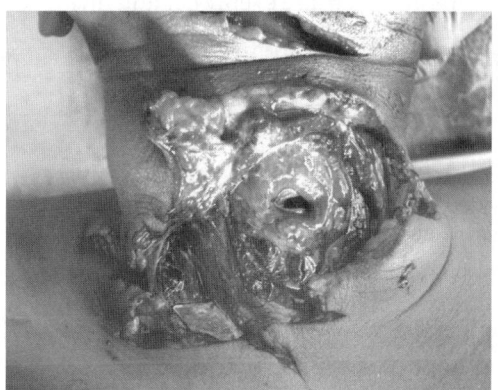

Fig. 12.16: Multiple overlapping incised wounds on the neck *(For color version see Plate 10).*

Chop Wounds (Fig. 12.18)

Injuries produced by heavy cutting weapon when the striking force is in a tangential manner. A flap may be lifted or the injured part may be severed from the body.

HOW DOES HEALING OF AN INCISED WOUND TAKES PLACE?

- **When fresh:** Bleeding may be still present or fresh soft clot is found loosely adherent onto the base; margins are red, slightly swollen and tender.

- **By 12 hours:** The margins are swollen and red; blood and lymph dry up; histologically, there is leucocytic infiltration.
- **By 24 hours:** There is proliferation of connective tissue cells and vascular endothelium.
- **By 36 hours:** There is capillary network formation and fibroblastic infiltration.
- **By 48 hours:** Capillary network is complete and fibroblasts run across the new vessels
- **By 3–5 days:** Blood vessels are thickened and many new vessels obliterate. Healing of the wound by scar formation starts and advances; and by the end of 6th day the scar formation is complete.
- The scab over the wound falls off or can be taken out easily, leaving a soft, tender, reddish scar, which in the course of weeks or months becomes whitish and firm.
- **Note:** Incised wound produced by **saw like** movement of the weapon over those parts of the body covered with loose tissue may appear irregular and ragged and give the impression of lacerated wound.

Postmortem Incised Wound

- Incised wounds may sometimes be produced on the dead body, which are though rare, may be related with sexual perversion. These incised wounds are made to mutilate the body particularly the private parts, after forceful sexual intercourse and killing of the victim by any means like injuries or strangulation.
- Sometimes after killing a person, the body is cut into multiple pieces for disposal.
- In cases of murder, the face of the victim is mutilated by multiple incisions to obliterate the feature of identification.
- These postmortem incised wounds are easily recognized as such by absence of wound gapping, less or no bleeding and absence of spurting of blood even if a major artery is cut.

DIFFERENTIATE INCISED WOUND FROM LACERATION? (TABLE 12.6)

- Laceration is a blunt force injury which is caused by shearing stress force which when exceeds the elasticity of the tissues results in tearing of the tissues irregularly and the architecture of the tissues is altered. The tags of torn tissues are usually present in a laceration.
- Incised wounds are caused by sharp light cutting weapons such as blade or hand knife in which there is clean cut division of the skin and underlying layers. All the tissue layers are evenly cut and divided.

TABLE 12.6: Incised wound vs laceration.		
Features	Incised wound	Laceration
Margins	Regular and clean cut	Irregular bruised and ragged margins
Bridging of tissues	All tissues are evenly divided and no bridging of tissues is seen	Bridging of tissues present
Blood vessels and bleeding	Blood vessels are clean cut and bleeding is more	Blood vessels are crushed and bleeding is relatively less
Hair pulp (mainly on scalp)	Hair pulps are intact and evenly divided	Hair pulps are crushed
Healing and timing of wound	Healing is by primary intension and timing of injury can be assessed	Healing is by secondary intension and assessing the time of injury is less probable

- As such it is not very difficult to distinguish a laceration from an incised wound but difficulties do raise in case of incised looking lacerations, in which the laceration on the parts of the body where the shin is not supported by subcutaneous tissues and lies over the bone. Even in those cases using a hand lens or taking a photograph and enlarging the picture we can easily differentiate a laceration from incised wound by the irregular, bruised and ragged margins.

DIFFERENTIATE SUICIDAL CUT THROAT FROM HOMICIDAL CUT THROAT INJURY? (TABLE 12.7)

- In cases of death by cut throat injury, it is very crucial to determine whether it is a case of suicide or murder. When proper reliable witness is not available for the investigation team, they may have to solely depend on the medical witness to find out whether it is a case of suicide or murder.
- Even though the medical witness may not be able to say 100% whether it is a case of suicide or homicide only based on the pattern of the wound on the neck. Many points will surely help the doctor to differentiate whether it is a case of suicidal or homicidal cut throat.

INJURIES CAUSED BY POINTED WEAPON; TYPES OF STAB WOUND; WHAT ARE THE FEATURES OF A STAB WOUND? (FM3.3)

- Stab wounds **(Fig. 12.19)** are injuries produced with a pointed weapon. The weapon need not always be sharp. It can be a sharp pointed weapon like a knife or only a pointed weapon like the end of an umbrella or a broken branch of tree.
- If weapon is sharp, then less force is needed to thrush the weapon into the body and marginal bruising is less or absent; but when the weapon is pointed and not sharp, then more force is necessary to stab the victim and there is a large abrasion around the wound **(Fig. 12.20)**.

Stab wounds are of two types: **(Fig. 12.21)**

(i) Penetrating Wounds

The wound enters the body through one cavity and ends at one point or organ, without producing any wound of exit.

(ii) Perforating Wounds

When the weapon enters the body through a cavity and exits out of the body, thus producing two surface wounds (entry wound and exit wound). Multiple stab wound depicted in **Figure 12.22**.

Features of a Stab Wound

- **Breath:** The breath of a stab wound usually does not correspond to the thickness of the blade, because of the gapping of the wound margins produced by skin elasticity. But when the edges are approximated, it corresponds to the thickness of the weapon.
- The depth of the wound which corresponds to the length of the track is a guide to the length of the blade inserted into the body.
- The length of the wound has some relationship with the breath of the blade.
- In a stab wound when the force is applied with a thrust, the resulting injury will have a depth which is more than the length of the weapon. This is commonly seen in abdominal wall injuries where the yielding nature of the abdominal wall makes the depth of the injury more than that of the length of the weapon causing it. For example, a 4 inch pocket knife when applied with thrust can produce a stab injury of 6 or 7 inches in depth.

TABLE 12.7: Differences between suicidal and homicidal cut throat injury.

Features	Suicidal cut throat	Homicidal cut throat
Site	Mostly on the left side and front of the neck, and partly on right side of neck, in case of right handed person	Mostly, in front and partly on either or both sides of the neck
Situation	High up on the neck	At a lower level
Direction	From left to right and above downward in a right handed person	Depends on the position of the assailant and the victim. If the assailant was on the right side of the victim, then direction of the wound would be from left to right
Tailing	Present at the right end of the wound in right handed person	May be present on either side depending on the position of the assailant
Hesitation cuts	Present	Absent
Severity of the wound	All the incisions are superficial except one or two wounds which is fatal	Usually, all injuries are of equal severity
Defense cuts	Absent	Present
Signs of struggle	Absent	Present
Secondary wounds	Self-inflicted incised wounds may be present on other accessible parts of the body	Other homicidal wounds, defense cuts, marks of resistance may present on other parts of the body
Weapon	Held in the hand in case of cadaveric spasm or present nearby	Usually absent. Sometimes after killing, the victim, the weapon is placed in the hand of the victim, to simulate suicide
Vessels	Carotid arteries are usually spared because before injuring himself the individual stretches his neck upward, when these arteries shift behind the sternomastoid muscles	The vessels remain vulnerable to injury due to lack of this maneuver
Bleeding	Suicidal injuries on the neck are produced in standing or erect position so, a good amount of blood trickles down in front of chest and abdomen	In most cases, the assailant cuts the neck of the victim in lying position, blood trickles down by the sides of the neck
Foreign materials like hair, etc.	Materials like foreign hair, shirt button, etc., will not be present in the hand of the victim	May be present in the hand of the victim, due to the grip in a state of cadaveric spasm
Corresponding cuts on clothes	Absent as the person cautiously removes the clothes to get a clear field to cut the neck	Cuts may be present on clothes as the assailant being in haste is unmindful about the clothes
Circumstance	Closed room bolted from inside or secluded place, which appears undisturbed; the body may be found in front of a mirror	Place of occurrence remains approachable to others which appears disturbed due to struggle with the assailant, latent fingerprint, belongings of assailant may be available in the scene of crime
Suicidal note	May be present	Absent

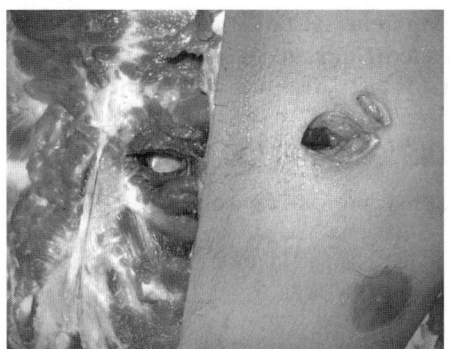

Fig. 12.19: Stab wound on the chest, the wound enters into the thoracic cavity through the intercostal space *(For color version see Plate 11).*

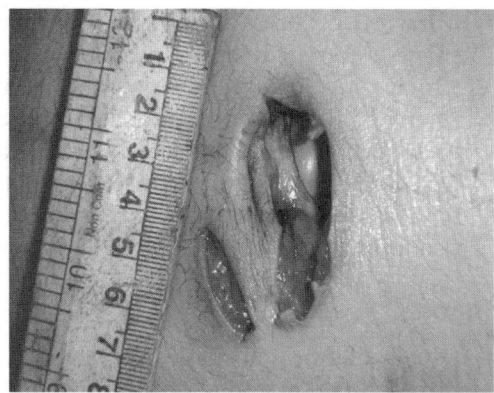

Fig. 12.22: Multiple stab wounds on the abdomen *(For color version see Plate 11).*

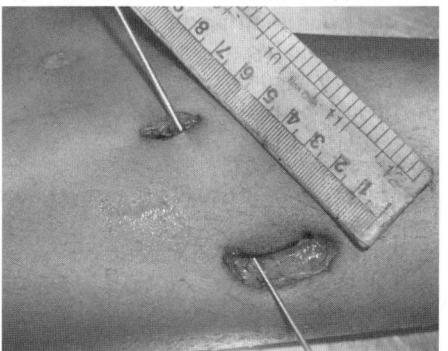

Fig. 12.20: Probing of stab wound on the thigh, to demonstrate the tract of the wound *(For color version see Plate 11).*

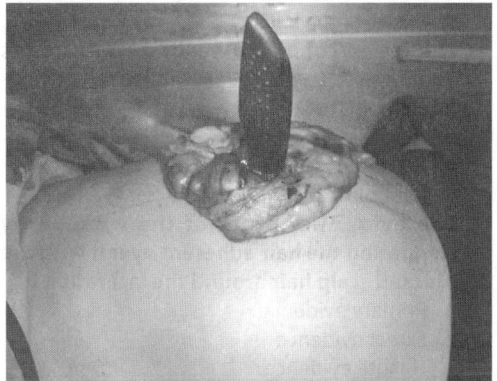

Fig. 12.21: Stab wound on the abdomen *(For color version see Plate 11).*

- The lung if punctured, may collapse and be drawn upwards and backwards when the impact is from the side of the chest, thus giving increased measurements at autopsy.
- The depth and direction of the stab wound depends on the relationship of intra-abdominal organs at the time of assault (whether the victim was standing erect, bent or lying).
- Track of the stab wound indicates direction of the wound.
- Probing is not advisable in living individuals, as it may dislodge some clot or creates false passage.
- Depth should be determined by dissecting the track of the wound in layers during operation or autopsy.

Margins

- Margins are inverted. Margins can be everted when the wound is situated over the fatty area such as abdomen or gluteal region; but the margins of exit wound are always everted.
- When a sharp cutting weapon has been thrust, the margins are clean cut without bruising.

- Abrasion or bruising of the margins suggests complete insertion of the blade which produces an imprint abrasion of the hilt or handle. The suspected weapon if available must be examined for compatibility of the shape of the hilt of the handle with that of the abrasion or contusion present on the body.

Shape

- Usually elliptical in shape, but may vary (like V, square, diamond, cruciate, satellite shapes, etc.)
- The size, shape and configuration of a stab wounds are influenced by a number of endogenous and exogenous factors.
- The elastic tissues of the dermis and the deeper layer of the skin have considerable bearing upon the shape of the wound.

LINES OF LANGER

- The dermal collagen and elastic fibers are arranged in definite pattern and are flowing along imaginary lines present all over the body.
- The pattern of fiber arrangement are the lines of cleavage of the skin and their linear representations on the skin are known as "Langer's line of cleavage".
- These cleavage lines correspond to the creases of the body surface and these are held in tension. When an injury cuts these lines perpendicularly (at right angle) there is wide gapping of the resultant wound.
- A stab wound with long axis at right angles to the cleavage lines of Langer, will gape open with edges pulled apart.
- A stab that is inflicted parallel to these lines will appear slit-like or wedge shaped (dimension of blade will fairly match with the injury).

Competency (CBME): Defense wound, Self-inflicted/Fabricated wounds and their Medico-legal aspects–**discussed in Chapter 14.**

MULTIPLE CHOICE QUESTIONS

1. **Brush burn is a type of:**
   a. Thermal injury
   b. Mechanical injury
   c. Chemical injury
   d. Electrical injury
2. **Medicolegally the most significant wound is:**
   a. Incised wound
   b. Lacerated wound
   c. Abrasion
   d. Stab wound
3. **The most significant difference between an incised wound and incised looking laceration over the scalp is:**
   a. Irregular margins
   b. Undermined edges
   c. Marginal abrasion
   d. Crushed hair bulb
4. **Split laceration is usually seen over all the regions, *except*:**
   a. Chin
   b. Forehead
   c. Shin
   d. Buttock
5. **Shape of a stab wound mostly depends upon:**
   a. Mode of withdrawal
   b. Amount of force
   c. Direction of force
   d. Shape of the knife
6. **The green color of a healing contusion is due to:**
   a. Hemoglobin
   b. Hemosiderin
   c. Biliverdin
   d. Bilirubin
7. **The evidential proof of the weapon by comparing the hair adherent over it with the plucked scalp hair around the laceration is:**
   a. Primary evidence
   b. Direct evidence
   c. Hirsute evidence
   d. Secondary evidence

8. Scab or crust of abrasion appears brown:
   a. Between 12–24 hours
   b. Between 2–3 days
   c. Between 4–5 days
   d. Between 5–7 days
9. Wound caused by a curved weapon such as sickle is:
   a. Stab wound
   b. Incised wound
   c. Stab and incised wound
   d. Laceration
10. Concealed puncture wounds are seen over the following regions, *except*:
    a. Naph of neck
    b. Inner canthus of eye
    c. Wrist
    d. Vagina
11. Which one of the following is true of antemortem abrasions?
    a. Bright red color
    b. Exudation of serum is more
    c. Vital reactions are seen
    d. All of the above
12. A person will bruise readily in all the following, *except*:
    a. Hemophilia
    b. Scurvy
    c. Vitamin K deficiency
    d. Anemia
13. Minor trauma results in major damage in all the following sites, *except*:
    a. Neck
    b. Abdomen
    c. Back of trunk
    d. Scrotum
14. Parallel bruise (double line with an intervening space) could be caused by:
    a. Whip
    b. Wrist
    c. Cycle chain
    d. Double edged weapon
15. All are true regarding a bruise, *except*:
    a. Turns blue in a day
    b. Green in 5 to 7 days
    c. Final color is yellow
    d. By the end of two weeks, only a scar is present
16. Bite marks is an example of:
    a. Pressure abrasion
    b. Grazed abrasion
    c. Scratch abrasion
    d. Patterned abrasion
17. No color change is seen in subconjunctival hemorrhage is due to:
    a. Continuous CO_2 supply
    b. Little amount of blood is present
    c. Continuous O_2 supply
    d. Color change do occurs but not visible to naked eye
18. The commonest type of abrasion seen in road traffic accidents is:
    a. Scratch abrasions
    b. Graze abrasions
    c. Contact abrasions
    d. Imprint abrasions
19. Graze abrasions mimics:
    a. Eczema
    b. Pressure sore
    c. Burns
    d. Scalds
20. Brush burn is injury due to:
    a. Friction
    b. Electrocution
    c. Hot liquid
    d. Burns
21. Ligature mark in hanging is an example for:
    a. Linear abrasion
    b. Pressure abrasion
    c. Superficial bruise
    d. Sliding abrasion
22. An auto rickshaw ran over a child's thigh, there is a mark of the tyre tracks, it is an example of:
    a. Patterned bruise
    b. Patterned abrasion
    c. Pressure abrasion
    d. Graze abrasion
23. Blue color of contusion is due to:
    a. Bilirubin
    b. Hemosiderin
    c. Hematoidin
    d. De-oxyhemoglobin
24. Prominent bruise with minimum force is seen in:
    a. Soles
    b. Scalp
    c. Face
    d. Palm

25. **Split lacerations are due to:**
    a. Blunt object
    b. Sharp object
    c. Pointed object
    d. Sharp heavy object
26. **Split laceration resembles:**
    a. Incised wound
    b. Gunshot wound
    c. Stab wound
    d. Contusion
27. **Sites notorious for incised looking wound are all,** *except:*
    a. Zygoma
    b. Chest
    c. Iliac crest
    d. Shin
28. **Flaying is seen in which type of lacerated wound:**
    a. Stretch
    b. Split
    c. Cut
    d. Avulsion
29. **Tissue bridges are seen in:**
    a. Abrasion
    b. Contusion
    c. Laceration
    d. Stab wound

ANSWERS

1. b	2. c	3. d	4. d	5. a	6. c	7. c	8. b	9. c	10. c
11. d	12. d	13. c	14. a	15. d	16. d	17. c	18. b	19. c	20. a
21. b	22. b	23. d	24. c	25. a	26. a	27. b	28. d	29. c	

CHAPTER 13

Regional Injuries

KEY WORDS

Head injury, intracranial hemorrhages, cerebral concussion, lucid interval, skull fracture, pond fracture, fracture ala signature, coup and contre coup injury, cardiac tamponade, whiplash injury, railway spine, primary impact, secondary impact, second impact.

FM3.11 Describe and discuss regional injuries to head (scalp wounds, fracture skull, intracranial hemorrhages, coup and contrecoup injuries), neck, chest, abdomen, limbs, genital organs, spinal cord and skeleton.

FM3.12 Describe and discuss injuries related to fall from height and vehicular injuries—primary and secondary impact, secondary injuries, crush syndrome, railway spine.

INTRODUCTION

Regional injuries: Regional injuries are produced in various parts of the body, either as a result of trauma or violence. Among the regional injuries the commonly occurring condition is head injury. However, injuries to other body parts like injury to the chest including rib fractures, heart and lung injuries, damage to the abdominal visceral organs, pelvic injury, injury to the spinal cord and injuries to the extremities are not uncommon.

DEFINE HEAD INJURY: MECHANISMS OF SKULL FRACTURES? (FM3.11) (FIG. 13.1)

- Head injury includes injury to the scalp, skull and to the brain. Any injury which produces structural and/or functional damage to head and brain are head injuries.
- Injury to the skull could be to the cranial vault or base of the skull.

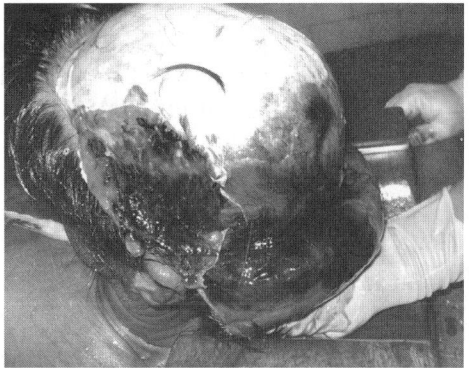

Fig. 13.1: Scalp contusion
(For color version see Plate 11).

Skull Fractures

There are two mechanisms by which skull fracture may be caused.
1. **Direct violence:** An object in motion striking the head or a moving head striking a stationary object. Compressions of head under the motor wheel, a stone thrown on the head or a hammer striking the head are examples of direct violence.
2. **Indirect violence:** Injury to the skull from a force transmitted from elsewhere. Examples: Injury to the skull occurring due to fall on the feet or buttock. Here the impact sustained by the feet or buttock is transmitted through the spinal column resulting in injury to the base of the skull (***ring fracture***).

Mechanism of Skull Fracture

There are two mechanisms by which skull fractures are produced.
1. **Fracture due to local deformation:** When the skull receives a focal impact, the area under the point of impact bends inwards and hence, compensatory bulging occurs at other areas. The contents of skull are virtually incompressible. When the distortion of the bone exceeds the limit of elasticity, then both these intruded and extruded areas may get fractured.
2. **Fracture due to general deformation:** When the skull is compressed in between two external objects, such as the ground on one side and the wheel of a vehicle on the other side, causing distortion and bulging of the part distal to the point of impact, which may result in fracture.

TYPES OF SKULL FRACTURES (FM3.11)

Fissured Fracture (Fig. 13.2)

- These are linear fractures produced by general deformation of the skull.

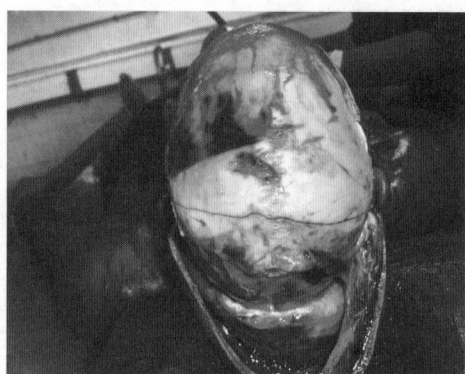

Fig. 13.2: Fissured fracture
(For color version see Plate 11).

- These are likely to be caused by forcible contact with a broad hard surface or blows with an agent having a relatively broad striking surface.
- The outer table is capable of rebounding to its normal shape whereas the more brittle inner table gets fractured.
- Fissured fractures do not tend to cross bony buttresses, such as glabella, frontal and parietal eminences, and occipital protuberances (this is called as "**Puppy's Rule**").

Depressed Fracture

- These fractures are produced by focal application of force. Localized depressed fractures are caused by blows from heavy weapon with a small striking surface. Example: Hammer
- It results in local deformation of the skull and the fractured fragment may sometimes be driven inwards into the skull cavity.
- When a hammer is used, the fracture is circular or an Arc of a circle, having the same diameter as the striking surface, thus giving a clue to the weapon used.
- Sometimes the fracture radiates in all direction from the center point of application of force. The part of the skull which is struck first shows maximum

depression. Then it is called "depressed comminuted fracture". This is also called as **"fracture ala signature"** as the pattern resembles like a signature.

Comminuted Fracture: (Comminuting–Fragmentation) (Fig. 13.3)

- It is often a complication of fissured and depressed fracture.
- In a comminuted fracture there are two or more intersecting lines of fracture, which divide the bone into three or more fragments.
- When there is no displacement of fragments, it resembles a **spider's web** or mosaic pattern **(Fig. 13.4)**. When the force is high, the fragments may get displaced and some of the fragments may enter the brain.
- Comminuted fractures are caused by a fall from a height on a hard surface or blows by weapons with large striking surface.

Pond or Indented Fracture

- This type of fracture usually occurs only in infants. There is a shallow depressed fracture forming a concave "pond" (dent) like appearance.

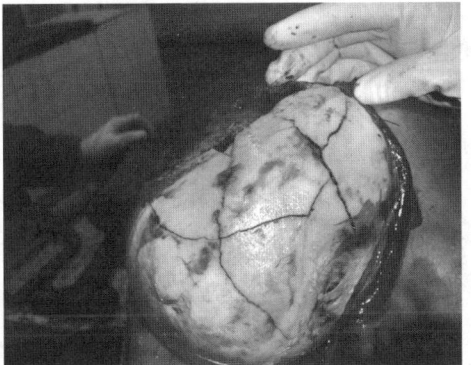

Fig. 13.3: Comminuted fracture
(For color version see Plate 12).

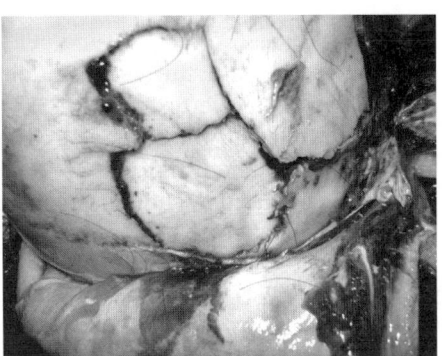

Fig. 13.4: Depressed fracture
(For color version see Plate 12).

- It is more common in the pliable bones of infants; these are caused by obstetric forceps, blow by a blunt object or impact against some hard protruding object.
- Sometimes there is no fracture of inner table, but a fissured fracture may occur in the outer table around the periphery of the dent.

Gutter Fracture

- In this type of fracture, the full thickness of the bone is not involved, it is only the outer table which is removed as a result of the tangential movement and the glancing effect of the moving object. When a part of bone is removed, it forms a gutter like shape as in a case of a bullet injury.
- Sometimes it is associated with irregular depressed fracture of inner table of skull.

Ring Fracture or Foramen Fracture

- It is a fissured fracture around the foramen magnum which encircles the base of the skull. It is always due to transmitted force from a distant site of impact.
- The fracture runs about 3 to 5 cm outside the foramen of magnum at the back and sides of skull, due to which the skull is separated from the spinal column.

Causes

- Fall from a height on the feet or buttock, a severe blow to the vertex.
- A forceful blow on the chin, as in a road traffic accident and fisting.
- May also be caused by sudden violent turn of the head on spine.

Perforating Fracture

- Caused by firearms and pointed sharp weapons like daggers, knives, and axe.
- The weapon passes through both the tables of the skull.
- The size and shape correspond to the cross section of the weapon.

Diastatic or Sutural Fracture (Figs. 13.5 and 13.6)

- Fracture on the sutural lines which results in separation of the sutures. When force is transmitted on the skull over a larger area and not hard enough to compress the skull to cause a comminuted fracture. Example: when the individual tries to pull the cement bags, vegetable, or rice bags and many of those bags fall on the person's head.
- It is commonly seen in young adult individuals, in whom the skull sutures are not fused completely. It may be associated with other type fractures.

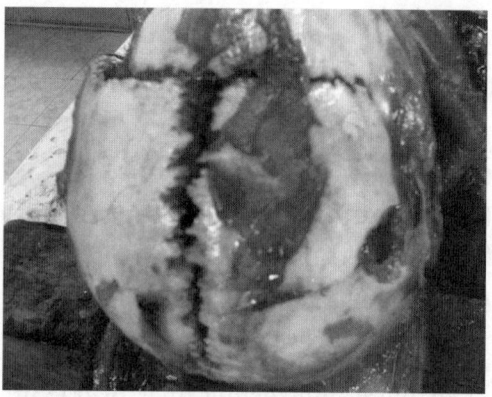

Fig. 13.6: Diastatic fracture *(For color version see Plate 12).*

Cut Fracture

Caused by heavy cutting weapon such as chopper. The scalp, skull and brain tissues are all cut along the plane of the injury. The severity and depth depend on the weight of the weapon and force involved.

Fractures of Base of the Skull (Fig. 13.7)

- The base of skull fracture may be produced by a force applied directly at the level of base, or due to general deformation of skull.
- It may also occur as an extension of force from the vault and by the force applied

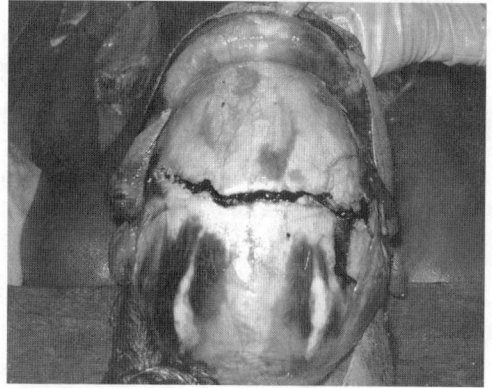

Fig. 13.5: Sutural fracture *(For color version see Plate 12).*

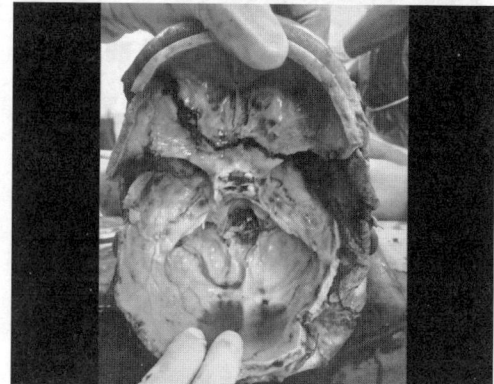

Fig. 13.7: Fracture base of skull on the anterior cranial fossa *(For color version see Plate 12).*

to the base through the spinal column or face.
- Fractures of the base of skull may be:
  - *Longitudinal:* As in case of front to back or back to front compression, e.g., run over.
  - Transverse fracture due to Side to side compression, and
  - Ring fracture.
- Fracture of anterior cranial fossa can be indicated by discharge of blood through mouth and nostrils.
- Fracture of the middle cranial fossa diagnosed by loss of blood from mouth and ears. Fracture of petrous temporal bone, allows blood and CSF to escape through the ears.
- Fracture of the posterior cranial fossa results in extravasations of blood is behind the mastoid process, or a large hematoma in the soft tissues of back of the neck.

COUP AND CONTRE COUP INJURIES (FM3.11)

- **Coup injury:** Means the injury which is caused at the point or beneath the area of impact and results directly from the impacting force.
- **Contre-coup injury:** Here the resultant injury or damage is produced at the diagonally opposite to the point of impact.
- A line drawn between the centers of coup and contre coup injury indicates the direction of the force of impact; contre coup injuries are common only on the brain.

Mechanism of Contre Coup Injury

- The injury depends upon the acceleration and deceleration force.
- Occur only when a moving head is struck or suddenly stopped by a stationary object.
- When the individual is in motion, the skull moves forward, the brain which lags behind is also in motion towards the same direction. When the moving head is suddenly stopped, the brain hits over the skull, bounces back and hit over the opposite side of the skull which results in injury at that point. This is called "contre coup" injury.
- Contre coup injuries will not occur when the head is well fixed at the time of impact or held immovable and cannot rotate. In other words, for a contre coup injury to occur the head should be in motion and/or free to rotate.
- Contre coup injuries are due to shearing strain of brain and meninges.

Impact area	Contre coup lesion
Occipital region	Under surface of frontal lobes and parts of temporal lobe
Parietal region	External surface of frontal and temporal lobe of opposite side

- When both coup and contre coup injuries are present, then the contre coup lesions are more severe than the coup one.
- Contre coup injuries are rare before the age of three years, as the skull is more flexible.

Medico-legal Importance

- The point of impact can be identified, especially when only contre coup injury is present.
- When both coup and contre coup injuries are present, it should not be mistaken for two different impacts.
- Indicates whether the head was fixed or mobile at the time of impact.

WHAT IS CONCUSSION OF BRAIN OR COMMOTIO CEREBRI? (CEREBRAL CONCUSSION)

- It is a state of temporary unconsciousness due to head injury which is seen

immediately after impact, and is always followed by amnesia. It tends to recover spontaneously.
- Concussion most often occurs with acceleration or deceleration injuries, when the head is moving or is freely movable. This is a popularly known as 'stunning of the brain'.

Symptoms and Signs

- The patient recovers completely after a brief period of unconsciousness with symptoms of "post-concussion syndrome".
- Recovery from concussion is often followed by complete loss of memory to recent events (**retrograde amnesia**).
- This retrograde amnesia is often due to injury to the frontal lobes.
- It has medico-legal significance as it may be associated with Post-traumatic automatism.
- In rare circumstances, the patient may die without regaining consciousness when the shock due to concussion is severe.

PM Findings

- May not be rewarding, but some cases may show Petechial hemorrhages over cerebral cortex at the junction of gray and white matter.
- Naked eye examination does not reveal any structural damage to the brain; however, on microscopy retraction bulbs may be demonstrated.

TYPES OF INTRACRANIAL HEMORRHAGES (FM3.11)

- Intracranial hemorrhages are mainly of four types.
  1. Extradural/epidural hemorrhage
  2. Subdural hemorrhage
  3. Subarachnoid hemorrhage
  4. Intracerebral hemorrhage

- Bleeding over a large area of brain surface, as a thin film is called as hemorrhage. If it is large, well circumscribed and space occupying, it is called as hematoma.
- According to their situation in relation to the membranes, intracranial hemorrhages are classified as extradural, subdural, subarachnoid and intracerebral hemorrhages.
- Intracerebral hemorrhage may be: cerebellar, cortical, thalamic, pontine, medullary.

DISCUSS THE FEATURES OF EDH? WHAT IS LUCID INTERVAL? (FM3.11)

Extra Dural/Epidural Hemorrhage (Fig. 13.8)

- Bleeding occurs in between inner table of the skull and the dura matter.
- Mostly traumatic in origin and occurs usually on the same side of impact (coup injury).

Causes

- Impact over the lateral convexity of the head may result in rupture of the middle meningeal artery or any its branches; less commonly, the posterior meningeal artery.

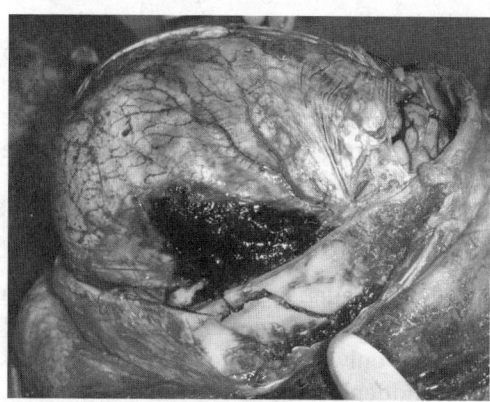

Fig. 13.8: Extra-dual hemorrhage
(For color version see Plate 12).

- EDH is seen in common association with fracture of squamous part of temporal bone.
- The middle meningeal artery is embedded deep in the groove within the skull and remain firmly attached to the dura. Fracture of the skull bones causes stretching of the vessel which leads to rupture of the artery.
- Rupture of anterior branch of middle meningeal artery, usually compresses motor area of the brain of the same side.
- In infants and old age EDH is not common, as the dura remains tightly adherent to skull.

Salient Features of EDH

The clot will press the brain inwards, producing signs and symptoms similar to that of space occupying lesions and increase in intracranial pressure. The clot produces a localized concavity or flattening of external surface of brain.

Clinical Features of EDH

- Following injury patient looses consciousness due to cerebral concussion.
- After some time he regains consciousness. Later on, due to continued bleeding cerebral compression occurs and the patient goes into permanent unconsciousness (coma).
- Death results from respiratory failure due to compression of brain stem.
- Nearly 25–50% of cases may end fatally.

Medico-legal Importance of EDH

- The period of consciousness between two bouts of unconsciousness is called "lucid interval". Early diagnosis by CT scan and surgical intervention by craniotomy and evacuation of the blood clot usually saves the patient. EDH is the only intracranial hemorrhage where the chance of survival by surgical intervention is more, and hence the doctor may be held liable for death of such patients.
- In all cases of head injury the patient must be kept under observation for a minimum period of 24 hours. A charge of negligence may be filed against the doctor if the he fails to keep the patient under observation. Repeat X-ray and CT scan are advisable to confirm no EDH is present before deciding the patient is fit for discharge.

SUBDURAL HEMORRHAGE (FIG. 13.9)

- Hemorrhage occurring inside the subdural space is subdural hemorrhage.
- Subdural space is the narrow space in between the dura and arachnoid mater; it contains a small amount of fluid, which permits the tough arachnoid to move towards the dura.
- This is the most common type of intracranial hemorrhage.
- It is invariably traumatic in origin following a blow or fall. SDH may occur even without any fracture of skull or injury to the scalp.
- Subdural hemorrhage is essentially venous or capillary bleeding and not arterial bleeding.

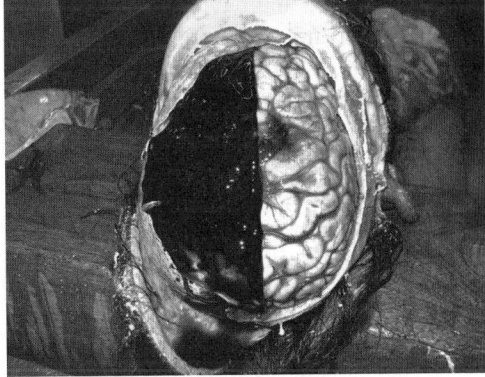

Fig. 13.9: Sub-dural hemorrhage
(For color version see Plate 12).

Causes of SDH

- SDH commonly occurs due to
  - Rupture of bridging veins or communicating veins when brain moves across the dura;
  - Rupture of inferior cerebral veins, entering the sinuses at the base of the skull;
  - Rupture of dural venous sinuses following a blow, or
  - Injury to the cortical veins.
- SDH also occurs due to lacerations or contusions of brain and dura, injury to the old adhesion between the brain and dura; and due to cerebral neoplasm, aneurysm, superior sagittal sinus thrombosis or bleeding disorder.
- The volume of blood varies from a few drops or a thin layered effusion to 150 mL or more. Death may occur if the hemorrhage exceeds 50 mL.
- SDH could be acute, sub-acute or chronic:
  - Acute subdural hemorrhage: (immediate)
    - *Clinical symptoms:* There may be slight confusion and forgetfulness, but no lucid interval.
  - *Sub-acute SDH:* (several days to 2–3 weeks)
    - In sub-acute type the brain may or may not be damaged.
  - *Chronic SDH:* (Pachymeningitis Hemorrhagica Interna)
    - It presents usually 3 to 6 weeks after the injury.
    - It is a frequent incidental finding at autopsy in old persons.
    - The blood collected in subdural space cannot be reabsorbed as dura and arachnoid has no mesothelial lining.
    - By 3–4 weeks the hematoma gets completely encapsulated.
    - Death is very common due to secondary pressure on brain stem.

SUBARACHNOID HEMORRHAGE (FIG. 13.10)

- The space between the arachnoid and the pia mater is the subarachnoid space.
- It is filled with CSF produced by the choroid plexuses of the lateral and fourth ventricles.
- In all cases of significant brain injury some degree of SAH is found.
- Subarachnoid hemorrhage usually spreads out, rarely forms a hematoma and removed by phagocytosis.

Causes of Subarachnoid Hemorrhage

Non Traumatic

- Common in young adults due to rupture of minute developmental aneurysms of the vessels of circle of Willis.
- In elderly subject's spontaneous rupture of anterior and posterior cerebral arteries.

Traumatic Causes

- Commonly associated with traumatic head injuries.
- Blow over the jaw or on the sides of upper part of the neck may cause rupture of vertebral artery with basal SAH.

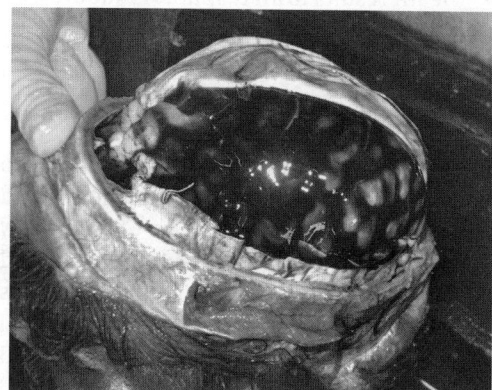

Fig. 13.10: Subarachnoid hemorrhage
(For color version see Plate 13).

Clinical Features

- **Diagnostic features of SAH:** Sudden onset of intense headache with stiffness of the neck and photophobia, followed by unconsciousness.
- The diagnosis is confirmed by lumbar puncture which reveals CSF intimately mixed with blood coming out under pressure.

INTRACEREBRAL HEMORRHAGE (FIG. 13.11)

What is Dementia Pugilistica?

- This may be found on the surface or in the substance of the brain.
- It occurs most frequently and spontaneously in the elderly and middle-aged hypertensives, due to rupture of lenticulostriate artery in the basal ganglia, pons, etc.
- Large areas of hemorrhage may occur at the junction of gray and white matter of the frontal and temporal lobes.
- Causes of ICH other than trauma are arterial thrombosis, fat embolism, cerebral aneurysm; patients under anticoagulant (warfarin) therapy; angioma, brain tumor or metastasis.
- When starts the hemorrhage may be small but will enlarge due to gradual oozing, leading to edema and softening of brain; ultimately rupture into the ventricle to cause death known as "**delayed traumatic apoplexy**".

Punch Drunk Syndrome (Dementia Pugilistica)

- Is a state that occurs in boxers due to the tiny hemorrhages in the brain?
- The patient suffers from post-traumatic psychosis, loss of memory, tremors, rigidity of the limbs and dysarthria.

RAILWAY SPINE (FM3.12)

- Railway spine is due to concussion of Spinal cord.
- Usually caused by forcible blow over the back or rarely by fall from a height.
- There could be injury to spinal column, and it can occur without any evidence of external injury to the spinal column.
- Commonly seen in railway accidents and motor car collisions, hence called as railway spine.

Signs and Symptoms

- Associated with paralysis of upper and lower limbs, with or without involvement of bladder and rectum.
- There may be inability to walk, irritability of temper, loss of sexual power. But, the patient may improve gradually with in 48 hours.

Medico Legal Importance

May involve compensation in civil suits.

WHIPLASH INJURY (FM3.12)

- Whiplash injury of spinal cord is due to sudden hyperflexion and hyperextension.
- Usually sustained by occupant of a car due to sudden stoppage of a high speed vehicle or sudden movement of a

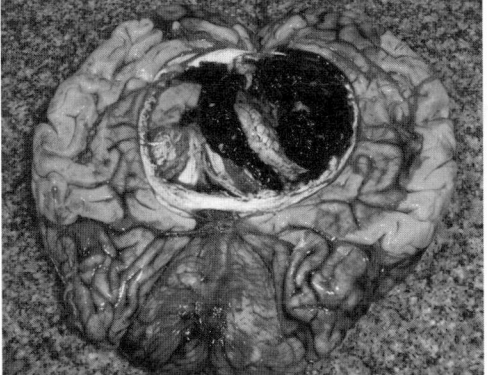

Fig. 13.11: Intracerebral hemorrhage
(For color version see Plate 13).

resting vehicle, which results in sudden hyperflexion followed by hyperextension (or hyperextension followed by hyper flexion) of the head.
- Resulting in fatal contusion or laceration of spinal cord without fracture of spine.

DISCUSS ABOUT CARDIAC TAMPONADE?

- It is the accumulation of blood in the pericardial sac.
- Accumulation of 400–500 mL of blood will be sufficient to cause death.
- **Mechanism:** Collection of blood in pericardial sac, which prevents ventricular dilatation in diastolic phase, thus compresses the right atrium and venous openings, resulting in progressive failure of circulation, leading to fall in arterial pressure and rise in venous pressure.

Causes

- Penetrating wounds of heart and great vessels.
- Contusion and laceration of pericardium and heart, by the fractured ends of ribs or sternum.
- Rupture of heart or aorta from indirect force and old myocardial infarction.
- Accidentally occurs during sternal puncture or intra cardiac injections in emergency.
- With intact parietal pericardium cardiac tamponade will be rapid. It will be slow when the parietal pericardium is punctured or lacerated since the blood can escape out.

WHAT ARE THE TYPES OF TRANSPORTATION INJURIES? (FM3.12)

Transportation injuries are caused by blunt force with powerful impact, which could result in three types of injuries:

1. Primary impact injuries
2. Secondary impact injuries
3. Secondary injuries

Primary Impact Injuries

- These are injuries caused when the vehicle hits the victim (pedestrian).
- It depends on the position of the victim and the part of the vehicle which comes into contact with the pedestrian.
- It bears the design of that part of the vehicle which struck, in the form of an imprint abrasion or a patterned bruise.

Secondary Impact Injuries

- These are injuries sustained by the victim after being knocked down by the vehicle. It is due to fall and friction or by the impact on the ground the individual.
- Injuries may be of any blunt impact injuries like abrasions, grazed abrasions, stretch lacerations, etc.

Secondary Injuries

- Injuries sustained as a result of impact between the body and the vehicle for the **second time**.
- The injuries may be run over injuries (crush injuries or internal lacerations and fractures) or avulsions (avulsed lacerations, stretch lacerations or brush burns, etc).

MULTIPLE CHOICE QUESTIONS

1. **The most common intracranial hemorrhage following blunt impact to the head is:**
   a. EDH
   b. SDH
   c. SAH
   d. Brain stem hemorrhage
2. **The commonest source of hemorrhage in extradural hemorrhage is:**
   a. Anterior meningeal artery
   b. Posterior meningeal artery

c. Middle meningeal artery
d. Middle meningeal vein

3. **Fracture of overlying skull bone is virtually always present with:**
   a. Epidural hemorrhage
   b. Subdural hemorrhage
   c. Subarachnoid hemorrhage
   d. Intracerebral hemorrhage

4. **The most common cause of spontaneous subarachnoid hemorrhage is due to rupture of:**
   a. Arteriosclerotic aneurysm
   b. Berry aneurysm
   c. Cirsoid aneurysm
   d. Mycotic aneurysm

5. **The following are the similarities of epidural and subdural hemorrhage, *except*:**
   a. Symptoms of cerebral compression
   b. Traumatic episode
   c. Swelling of temporalis muscle
   d. Existence of lucid interval

6. **The most common cause of death of a boxer during or soon after the fight is:**
   a. Epidural hemorrhage
   b. Subdural hemorrhage
   c. Subarachnoid hemorrhage
   d. Intracerebral hemorrhage

7. **One of the following skull fracture is caused by combined effects of local indentation and general deformation of skull:**
   a. Spider web fracture
   b. Depressed fracture
   c. Depressed comminuted fracture
   d. Fissured fracture

8. **One of the following lesion due to trauma is never be due to contre coup force:**
   a. Brain contusion
   b. Brain laceration
   c. Subdural hemorrhage
   d. Epidural hemorrhage

9. **The commonest site of contre coup fracture in an occipital fall is:**
   a. Parietal bone
   b. Temporal bone
   c. Orbital roof
   d. Ethmoidal bone

10. **Whiplash injury occurs in _____**
    a. Pedestrian hit from front
    b. Pedestrian hit from behind
    c. Occupant of a car
    d. Any of the above

11. **A sack of rice falls on the head of a 22-year-old male. The likely fracture is:**
    a. Comminuted
    b. Sutural
    c. Depressed
    d. Gutter

12. **Concussion is characterized by:**
    a. Contusion of brain
    b. Post-traumatic amnesia
    c. Irreversible brain damage
    d. None of the above

13. **Fracture ala signature is:**
    a. Gutter fracture
    b. Depressed fracture
    c. Ring fracture
    d. Sutural separation

14. **Pond's fracture is most common in:**
    a. Children
    b. Elderly
    c. Adolescent
    d. Middle aged women

15. **A depressed fracture of the skull is caused by:**
    a. A light blunt force
    b. A heavy blunt force
    c. Fall on a level road
    d. A heavy blunt object with a small striking surface

16. **Gutter fractures of the skull are most often seen with:**
    a. Axe injury
    b. Stick injury
    c. Stone injury
    d. Bullet injury

17. **Impact fracture are characteristically found in:**
    a. Pelvis
    b. Skull
    c. Vertebra
    d. Calcaneum

18. **The commonest site of rupture of heart due to blunt injury chest is:**
    a. Right ventricle
    b. Left ventricle
    c. Left auricle
    d. Right auricle

19. **Teardrop sign is seen in:**
    a. Fracture medial wall of orbit
    b. Fracture lateral wall of orbit
    c. Fracture floor of orbit
    d. Fracture roof of orbit

20. Characteristic of anterior cranial fossa fracture:
    a. Pupillary dilatation
    b. CSF otorrhea
    c. Black eye
    d. Hemotympanum
21. Best prognostic indicator for head injured patients:
    a. GCS score
    b. Age of the patient
    c. CT findings
    d. History
22. Primary impact injury to brain:
    a. Concussion
    b. Hypoxic injury
    c. Cerebral edema
    d. Intracerebral hematoma
23. Secondary brain injury is:
    a. Concussion
    b. Diffuse axonal surgery
    c. Depressed skull fracture
    d. Intracerebral hematoma
24. Antero-grade amnesia is seen in:
    a. Post-traumatic head injury
    b. Drug induced
    c. Electroconvulsive therapy
    d. Stroke
25. Shearing damage is seen in:
    a. Heart
    b. Brain
    c. Liver
    d. Spinal cord
26. Diffuse axonal injury is characterized by lesion at:
    a. Junction of gray and white matter
    b. White matter
    c. Basal ganglia
    d. Corpus callosum
27. Brain hemorrhage limited by sutures:
    a. SAH
    b. SDH
    c. EDH
    d. ICH
28. Most common manifestation of increased intracranial pressure a patient with head injury is:
    a. Change in the level of consciousness
    b. Ipsilateral pupillary dilatation
    c. Retching and vomiting
    d. Bradycardia
29. The following are the clinical features of raised intracranial tension, *except:*
    a. Headache
    b. Bradycardia
    c. Insomnia
    d. Papilledema
30. Subdural hemorrhage is due to rupture of:
    a. Middle meningeal artery
    b. Dural venous sinus
    c. Cortical bridging veins
    d. Rupture of intracranial aneurysms
31. A 14-year-old boy was hit on the side of the head with a baseball bat during practice. A laceration with palpable bone fragment was found in the wound. After 5 hours the boy died, the most likely cause of death is:
    a. Subarachnoid hemorrhage
    b. Epidural hemorrhage
    c. Subdural hemorrhage
    d. Intracranial hemorrhage
32. CT of subdural hematoma will show:
    a. Biconvex hyperdense opacity
    b. Biconcave hyperdense opacity
    c. Concavo-convex opacity
    d. Hyperdense diffuse lesion
33. Circle of Willis is not formed by:
    a. Anterior choroidal artery
    b. Anterior cerebral artery
    c. Posterior cerebral artery
    d. Anterior communicating artery
34. A female presented with severe headache of sudden onset. On CT scan, a diagnosis of subarachnoid hemorrhage is made. Most common cause is:
    a. Hypertension
    b. Berry aneurysm rupture
    c. Basilar artery rupture
    d. Subdural venous sinuses rupture
35. Investigation of choice in SAH:
    a. X-ray
    b. MRI scan
    c. CT scan
    d. Radionuclide scan
36. Cause of berry aneurysm:
    a. Degeneration of internal elastic lamina
    b. Degeneration of media/muscle cell layer
    c. Deposition of mucoid material in media
    d. Low grade inflammation of vessel wall
37. Traumatic bleeding may include all, *except:*
    a. Subarachnoid hemorrhage
    b. Epidural hemorrhage

c. Subdural hemorrhage
d. Intracerebral hemorrhage

38. **Most common location of hypertensive intracranial hemorrhage is:**
    a. Subarachnoid space
    b. Cerebellum
    c. Basal ganglia
    d. Brainstem

39. **A 45-year-old hypertensive male patient presented in the casualty with 2 hours history of sudden onset of severe headache associated with nausea and vomiting. On clinical examination, the patient had neck stiffness and right sided ptosis. The rest of the neurological examination was normal. Diagnosis is:**
    a. Hypertensive brain hemorrhage
    b. Migraine
    c. Aneurysmal subarachnoid hemorrhage
    d. Arteriovenous malformation rupture

40. **Hinge fracture is:**
    a. Depressed fracture
    b. Sutural fracture
    c. Orbital fracture
    d. Basilar fracture

41. **Concussion causes:**
    a. Small hemorrhages and swelling of brain tissues
    b. Momentary interruption of brain function with transient loss of consciousness
    c. Tearing or shearing of brain structures
    d. Bruising of the brain

42. **Primary impact injury (1°) most commonly seen in:**
    a. Head
    b. Thorax
    c. Legs
    d. Abdomen

43. **Bumper fracture is:**
    a. Primary impact injury
    b. Secondary impact injury
    c. Tertiary impact injury
    d. Secondary injury

44. **Whip-lash' injury is caused due to:**
    a. Fall from a height
    b. Acute hyperextension of the spine
    c. Blow on top to head
    d. Acute hyperflexion of the spine

45. **Most common organ injured in blunt trauma to the abdomen:**
    a. Liver
    b. Spleen
    c. Pancreas
    d. Intestine

ANSWERS

1. b	2. c	3. a	4. b	5. d	6. b	7. a	8. d	9. c	10. c
11. b	12. b	13. b	14. a	15. d	16. d	17. b	18. d	19. c	20. c
21. a	22. a	23. d	24. a	25. b	26. a	27. c	28. a	29. c	30. c
31. b	32. c	33. a	34. b	35. c	36. b	37. d	38. c	39. c	40. d
41. b	42. c	43. a	44. b	45. b					

CHAPTER 14

Medico-Legal Aspects of Injuries

KEY WORDS

Simple injuries, grievous hurt, dangerous injury, antemortem and postmortem injury, shock, primary neurogenic shock, hypovolemic shock, bomb blast injuries, primary, secondary and tertiary injuries, defense wound, fabricated wound, hesitation cuts, self-inflicted wounds.

FM3.4	Define injury, assault and hurt. Describe IPC pertaining to injuries.
FM3.5	Describe accidental, suicidal and homicidal injuries. Describe simple, grievous and dangerous injuries. Describe antemortem and postmortem injuries.

INTRODUCTION

Legal Definition of Injury (FM3.4)

- **Section 44 IPC** defines injury as "any harm what so ever illegally caused to any person in body, mind, reputation or property".
- Only bodily injuries are wounds. Hence, all wounds are injuries but all the injuries are not wounds.

Hurt (Section 319 IPC)

Any bodily pain, disease or infirmity caused to any person is called hurt.

Assault (Section 351 IPC)

Any offer of threat or attempt to apply force to the body of another in a hostile manner. Execution of such act amounts to '**battering**'.

HOW DO WE CLASSIFY INJURIES?

Injuries are classified in three ways:
1. Medical classification
2. Legal classification
3. Medico-legal classification

Medical Classification of Injuries

- **Mechanical injuries:** Injuries caused by application of physical force.
- **Chemical injury:** Corrosive acids and alkalis
- **Thermal injury:**
  - Due to cold: (i) Frost bite, (ii) Trench foot, (iii) Immersion foot.
  - Due to heat: (i) Burns-dry heat. (ii) Scalds-wet heat.
- **Miscellaneous:** (a) Electrical injury (b) Radiation injuries (c) Firearm injuries (d) Explosive injuries.

Legal Classification of Injuries

Legally, injuries are classified according to the severity of the injury:
- Simple injury
- Grievous hurt
- Dangerous injury—in living
- Fatal injury—in dead.

Medico-legal Classification of Injuries

For medico-legal interpretation, injuries are classified as:
- Accidental injuries.
- Suicidal injuries (self-inflicted injuries).
- Homicidal injuries.
- Defense injuries.
- Fabricated injuries.

WHAT ARE SIMPLE INJURIES; GRIEVOUS HURT AND DANGEROUS INJURIES? (FM3.5)

Simple Injuries

Injuries that are neither serious nor dangerous to life, not causing severe pain, heals easily without leading to any complications and usually heals without leaving any scar are called as simple injuries. Example: Abrasions, skin deep laceration on the limbs, etc.

Grievous Hurt

Section 320 IPC enumerates eight clauses of injuries which constitute grievous hurt. All other injuries which do not fit into any of the clauses of grievous hurt are simple injuries.

Grievous Hurt (FM3.5)

Section 320 IPC defines grievous hurt as:
- Emasculation
- Permanent privation of sight of either eye
- Permanent privation of hearing of either ear.
  - Permanent privation of any member or a joint.
- Permanent destruction of power of any member or a joint.
- Permanent disfiguration of head or face.
- Fracture or dislocation of a bone or tooth.
- Any hurt which endangers life, or
  - Any injury which causes the victim to be in severe bodily pain, or
  - Any injury which prevents the person from following his ordinary pursuits of life for a minimum period of twenty days.

Dangerous Injury (FM3.5)

Any injury which causes imminent threat to the life of the individual is a dangerous injury. An endangering injury is one for which if the individual is not admitted to the hospital for life saving treatment and surgical intervention had not been done, he could have died.

When the injury leads to death of an individual, then it is called as fatal injury.

Example: Incised wound on the wrist resulting in cut of the radial artery; if surgical intervention is done there is no threat to the life of the individual. This is an endangering injury. But, if not treated by surgical intervention, profuse bleeding would result in death of the victim in a few minutes to an hour; if death occurs, it becomes a fatal injury.

Dangerous Weapon

- Any weapon used for cutting, stabbing or shooting or any weapon used as a weapon for assault of an individual is like to cause endangering injuries or death is a called as dangerous weapon.
- Any routinely used objects can be used as a dangerous weapon. Like the iron chairs, wooden stools when used for assault are likely to cause death. Even the hand kerchief can be used to for choking and the "dupatta" (scarf) can be used to strangulate an individual.

- Hence, basically any weapon used for cutting stabbing or shooting is always dangerous weapons and carrying any such weapons, the individual is liable for carrying dangerous weapon.

SECTIONS OF IPC RELATED TO INJURIES (FM3.4)

Homicide

Homicide is killing of a human being by another.

Justifiable Homicide

The homicide is justified under the particular circumstance. Example:
- In administration of justice such as execution of capital punishment.
- In the maintenance of justice as like suppression of riots or while executing an arrest of criminals.
- A woman who kills a person who attempts to rape her.

Excusable Homicide

This is homicide caused unintentionally:
- Killing in self defense
- Death by accident or misadventure
- Death following lawful operation, done in good faith, not intended or known to cause death.
- Homicide by an insane person.

Culpable Homicide (Section 299 IPC)

Culpable homicide is causing death of a person by an act done:
- With the intension of causing death.
- With the intension of causing such bodily injuries which are likely to cause death.
- With the knowledge that such act is likely to cause death.

Murder (Section 300 IPC)

Culpable homicide is murder if:
- The act was done with the intension of causing death.
- If done with the intension of causing such bodily injuries which are likely to cause death.
- With the knowledge that such bodily injuries would cause death in ordinary course of nature'.

Exceptions

- Culpable homicide does not amounts to murder, if such act was done under:
  - Grave provocation
  - Done in private defense
  - Without premedication
  - For public justice
  - When the person above 18 years takes the risk of death with his own consent, as like death occurring in complicated life saving surgical treatments.

Section 302 IPC

- Punishment for murder. Death or life imprisonment, and also fine.
- Life imprisonment implies imprisonment till the end of life and/or imprisonment not <14 years.

Section 304 IPC

Punishment for culpable homicide not amounting to murder. Imprisonment up to 10 years and also fine.

Section 304 (A) IPC

Causing death by rash and negligent act not amounting to culpable homicide. Imprisonment for 2 years, with or without fine.

Section 304 (B) IPC (Dowry Death)

Causing death of a female by any bodily injuries or burns or which occurs otherwise than the normal circumstances within 7 years of marriage. Whoever commits dowry death shall be punished with imprisonment of not <10 years, which may extend to life.

Sections of IPC Relating to Hurt

- **Section 44 IPC:** Defines injury as "any harm whatsoever illegally caused to any person in body, mind, reputation or property".
- **Section 319 IPC:** Defines hurt as "any bodily pain, disease or infirmity caused to any person".
- **Section 320 IPC:** Definition of grievous hurt.
- **Section 321 IPC:** Voluntarily causing hurt.
- **Section 322 IPC:** Voluntarily causing grievous hurt.
- **Section 323 IPC:** Punishment for voluntarily causing hurt. Imprisonment upto one year, or fine up to ₹ 1000 or both.
- **Section 324 IPC:** Voluntarily causing hurt with dangerous weapon. Imprisonment up to 3 years.
- **Section 325 IPC:** Punishment for voluntarily causing grievous hurt. Imprisonment up to 7 years, and also fine.
- **Section 326 IPC:** Voluntarily causing grievous hurt by dangerous weapon. Imprisonment up to 10 years, and also fine.
- **Section 326 (A) IPC:** Voluntarily causing grievous hurt by throwing acid. Imprisonment not <10 years, but may extend to life and with fine.
- **Section 326 (B) IPC:** Voluntarily throwing or attempt to throw acid on a person. Imprisonment not <5 years and with fine.

DIFFERENTIATE ANTEMORTEM FROM POSTMORTEM INJURIES? (FM3.5)

There is not much difficulty in finding out the nature of the injury as antemortem or postmortem in nature. A trained medical expert can easily find it out by just seeing the wound. But difficulties are encountered while examining injuries caused just before death and injuries caused just immediately after death **(Table 14.1)**.

CAUSES OF DEATH FROM WOUNDS

The causes of death from wounds could be (i) Immediate causes and (ii) Remote or delayed causes.

Immediate Causes

Shock

Shock is circulatory disturbance resulting in hypo-perfusion of tissues due to either reduction in the cardiac output or reduction in the volume of blood in the circulation.

- **Primary shock or neurogenic shock:**
  - Vaso-vagal shock or reflux cardiac arrest results from sudden reduction in the venous return to heart resulting from pooling of blood in the peripheral vessels by neurogenic vasodilatation caused by sudden reflex vagal inhibition.
- **Hypovolemic shock (hemorrhage)**
  - Hemorrhage is escape of blood from the cardiovascular system. The source of hemorrhage could be capillary, venous, arterial or direct trauma to the heart. The resultant hemorrhage could be external hemorrhage (due to injuries on the body surface) or internal hemorrhage (bleeding within the body, where blood escapes from the circulation but gets collected in

TABLE 14.1: Antemortem wounds vs postmortem wounds.

Features	Antemortem wounds	Postmortem wounds
Hemorrhage	Usually copious, showing signs of arterial spurting	Comparatively very less, may even be absent
Wound edges	Swollen, everted and retracted except; wound gapping present due to elasticity of the skin	Not swollen or retracted wound gapping is absent because the skin looses elasticity immediately after death
Extravasation of blood	There is extensive infiltration of blood in and around the injured areas, which cannot be washed off	No extravasation and infiltration of blood into the tissues, even if the surrounding tissues show staining it is easily washed off
Blood clot	Coagulated blood is noticed in and around the injured tissues. The clot is laminated and firmly adherent to the lining endothelium. The clot cannot be easily separated and when detached the fibrin network imprint in present of the tissues where the clot was adherent	Blood is usually not clotted. The clot, if found, is nonlaminated and weakly adherent to the lining endothelium
Consistency of the blood clot	Clot is rubbery and firm. On being pulled out from the vessel, it will come out like a horse tail because of fibrin and platelet aggregation	The clots are soft and friable. On being pulled, will invariably break due to absence of platelet aggregation
Lines of Zahn	The surface shows apparent lines of Zahn. These lines are formed by alternate areas of light stained (aggregated platelets admixed with fibrin meshwork) and dark stained layers (red cells)	The surface is yellow (chicken fat) in appearance. There is separation of plasma and leucocytes covering the dark red cell constituents (currant jelly) due to sedimentation of blood after death
Microscopy of the blood clot	Microscopically: composed of fibrin, platelets and RBCs	Mainly composed of fibrin and RBCs
Vital reaction	Signs of inflammation and repair are demonstrable depending upon the age of the wound/injury	No signs of inflammation and repair
Microscopy	Leucocytic emigration appreciable in the surrounding tissue as to the age (neutrophils dominating for the first 6–24 hours)	Vessels distended with postmortem clot without showing any cells outside the vessel wall
Enzyme histochemistry	➢ Adenosine triphosphatase +ve (as early as 1 hour) ➢ Aminopeptidase +ve (at about 2 hours) ➢ Acid phosphatase +ve (at about 4 hours) ➢ Alkaline phosphatase +ve (at about 8 hours)	No enzyme activity
Wound biochemistry	➢ Serotonin peak (within about 10 minutes) ➢ Free histamine peak (within about 20–30 minutes)	Nil Nil

the body cavities, as in penetrating stab wounds, gunshot wounds or internal lacerations of major organ like liver, lung or spleen, etc.) either of them results is reduced cardiac output and reduction in the circulating blood volume.
- Anyway, could be the source of hemorrhage reduction in one third of circulating blood volume causes death by irreversible hypovolemic shock.
- **Secondary shock (delayed shock):**
  - This condition is more serious and many a times fatal. There is progressive circulatory failure and resultant tissue damage. Due to diminished perfusion of the tissues intracellular metabolism is disturbed with anaerobic glucose metabolism and increased production of lactic acid which causes disruption of lysosomes. There is a decrease in production of ATP, metabolic acidosis, electrolyte disturbance and renal insufficiency.
- **Septic shock:**
  - Most of the cases of septic shock are caused by endotoxin producing gram-negative bacilli such as *E. coli*, *Klebsiella*, *Proteus*, *Pseudomonas*, *Pneumococci* and *Streptococci*.

Remote Causes

- **Infection:**
  - Infection is the most important complication. The skin protects us from access of infection but when an injury is sustained, depending on the size of body surface involved and the severity of injury the bacteria gain easy access into the body and both local and systemic infections are the most common complication of injuries.
- **Embolism:**
  - Pulmonary air embolism (entry or air through ruptured veins) and fat embolism (from fractured long bones) are expected in extensive injuries of limbs, usually lower limb.
- **Gangrene and necrosis:**
  - When there occurs severe crush injury, the blood vessels are ruptured and the distal part usually limbs undergo gangrenous change, necrosis and putrefaction of the dead tissues.
- DIC and renal failure are also expected complications of injuries.

EFFECTS OF BOMB EXPLOSIVE INJURIES

Identification of Mutilated Bodies

- The effects of all explosive bomb injuries are accompanied by complex waves. There are two components of such complex waves:
  i. Blast wave (dynamic overpressure) with positive and negative phase.
  ii. Blast wind (Mass movement of air).
- The resultant injuries are mainly due to the initial shock waves followed later and aggravated by the sub atmospheric phase.
- When body is impacted by a blast pressure wave, it sets up series of stress waves injuring organs at air fluid inter-phases (ears, lungs, heart and GIT).
- Blast injuries are divided into four categories: Primary, secondary, tertiary and quaternary injuries.

Primary Injuries

- These injuries are unique to high explosives and are presented as over-pressurization blast waves with body surface and usually there is absence of external injuries.
- These primary injuries most commonly involve air-filled organs and air-fluid interfaces, mainly middle ear, lungs and gastrointestinal tract.

Types of injuries produced are:

Blast lung

Shock wave transit through the lungs can tear the alveolar septa and give rise to alveolar hemorrhage. Other findings in the lungs may include sub-pleural patchy hemorrhages (often in the line of ribs) and intrapulmonary hemorrhages. The air passages may be filled with bloody froth causing airway obstruction and hypoxia in addition to the primary damage. Later, neutrophilic reaction may develop around the hemorrhagic areas and those can progress onto bronchopneumonia. The pulmonary injury is a specific injury of the air blast and is sometimes called as **'blast lung'**.

- **Other major injuries produced are:**
    - Tympanic membrane (TM) rupture (acoustic barotrauma).
    - Abdominal hemorrhage and perforation (colon, stomach, small intestine, caecum).
    - Traumatic brain injury (TBI) without physical signs of head injury.

Secondary Injuries

- These secondary injuries are due to flying debris and bomb fragments which affects part of the body which results in penetrating ballistic or blunt injuries.
- These are the leading causes of death in military and civilian terrorist attacks except in cases of major building collapse.
- Wounds may be grossly contaminated.
- Thoracic trauma (lacerations over heart and great vessel) is a common cause of death.

Tertiary Injuries

- Tertiary injuries are due to the persons being thrown onto fixed solid objects by the blast wind of explosions and are also due to structural collapse and fragmentation of building, and vehicles. This may cause extensive blunts and penetrating trauma and these injuries would show features of peppering effect with a triad of abrasion, contusion and puncture lacerations.
- Bone fractures and countercoup injuries are also seen.
- Children are at high risk due to their lesser body weight.

Quaternary Injuries

- Quaternary injuries are also called as miscellaneous injuries and they include:
    - Injuries not included in the first three categories. Example: Flash burns, crush injuries, fall resulting from the explosion and respiratory injuries (toxic dust, gas) or radiation exposure.
    - Post-traumatic psychiatric effects are most common which could be due to neurological damage caused during the blast.
    - Post-traumatic stress disorder may affect people who were otherwise uninjured.
    - The sequelae of these traumatic injuries would also result in crush syndrome, acute renal failure and compartment syndrome.

Identification of the Dead in Bomb Blast Injuries

- Full body X-ray for findings like pacemaker or some old fracture/bony changes that the alleged victim was known to have.
- Many a times, the body could be fragmented into many pieces and thrown at some distance and are also frequently intermixed with fragmented body parts of different victims. In such cases first aligning the body parts is done using the knowledge of anatomy. Complexion, size of the body parts are all considered for

segregating and aligning the body parts to fix a complete body.
- Some of the body parts may not be traceable or disintegrated and may not be recovered at all in such circumstances the following data are useful in fixing the identity of the individual:
  - Dentition (dental pattern) and artificial dentures may help in identification.
  - Fingerprints are sometimes helpful if previous records are available.
  - Blood grouping and DNA profile may also be useful in some cases for identification.
  - Anthropometry may also be useful in some cases.

DESCRIBE BLAST LUNG

Shock wave transit through the lungs can tear the alveolar septa and give rise to alveolar hemorrhage. Other findings in the lungs may include sub-pleural patchy hemorrhages (often in the line of ribs) and intrapulmonary hemorrhages. The air passages may be filled with bloody froth causing airway obstruction and hypoxia in addition to the primary damage. Later, neutrophilic reaction may develop around the hemorrhagic areas and those can progress onto bronchopneumonia. The pulmonary injury is a specific injury of the air blast and is sometimes called as **'blast lung'**.

DEFENCE WOUNDS (FM3.3) (FIGS. 14.1 AND 14.2)

- They are the result of immediate and instinctive reactions of the victim to save himself, either by raising the arm to prevent the attack or by grasping the weapon.
- If the weapon is blunt, abrasions and bruises are produced on the back of forearms, wrist or back of the hands.

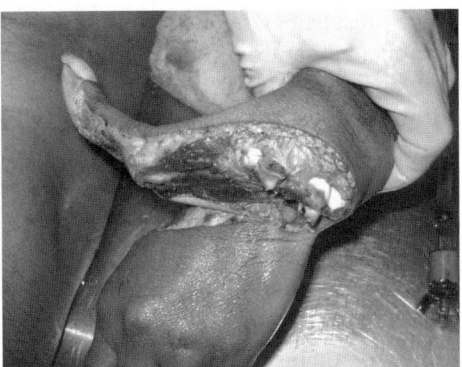

Fig. 14.1: Defense wound
(For color version see Plate 13).

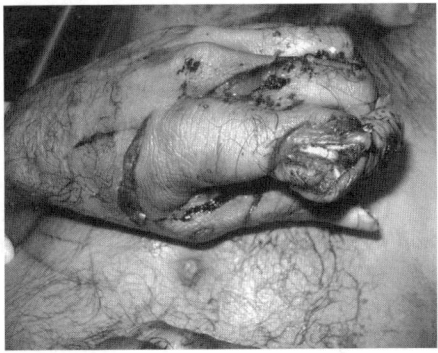

Fig. 14.2: Multiple cut wounds—defense wounds
(For color version see Plate 13).

- The size and shape depends upon the type and shape of the weapon.
- When sharp weapons were used, the injuries produced will depend upon the mode of application of force.
- In stabbing with a single edged weapon, if the weapon is grasped, a single cut is produced on the palm of the hands or on the creases of the fingers and/or thumb.
- If the weapon is double edged, then cut injuries are produced both on the palmar aspect and the fingers. The cuts may be irregular and ragged, because of the gripping movement of the hand.
- A typical defense wound is seen in the web between the base of the thumb and index finger, when the blade is grasped.

- The presence of defense wounds indicate homicidal nature of the injuries and may be absent if the victim is incapacitated, unconscious, intoxicated or attacked by surprise.

SELF INFLICTED WOUNDS/ FABRICATED WOUND? (FM3.3)

- Self-inflicted wounds are those inflicted by a person on his own body.
- Fabricated wounds (**fictitious, forged or invented wounds**) are inflicted by a person on his own body or by another person with his consent.
- These types of wounds are inflicted:
    - To charge an enemy with assault or attempt murder.
    - By the policemen and watchmen acting in collision with robbers to show that they were defending the property.
    - By the prisoners to bring a false charge of torture against the officers.
    - By the recruits of uniformed services to escape hard work.
    - By women to bring a false charge of sexual assault or cruelty against them.
- The commonest injuries fabricated are incised wounds; many a times false contusions and sometimes stab wounds and burns. Lacerated wounds and true contusions are least fabricated.
- Self-inflicted incised wounds are usually multiple, superficial, shallow and parallel to each other, present on the accessible parts of the body and does not involve any vital parts like face.
- The direction is from behind forwards on the top of the head; from above downwards on the outer side of upper arm; from below upwards on the front of forearms; variable on lower extremities, chest and abdomen.
- Burns are superficial and usually on the left upper arm.
- Clothes are not cut, and if cut are not compatible with the nature of the wounds.
- The history of the assault is usually not compatible with the injuries present on the body.
- Fabricated bruises are also produced using plant juices of semecarpus anacardium and calotropis; which can be easily made out by an expert by examination of the margins for the presence of vital reactions, color changes, blister formation and itching.

WHAT ARE HESITATION CUTS?

- Hesitation cuts are also called *tentative cuts* or *feeler strokes*.
- These are multiple, superficial, horizontal and linear injuries almost parallel to each other. These injuries are never deep.
- The tentative cuts are always superficial because it is the basic instinct of a human to preserve his life, that he cannot inflict painful deep injuries to himself.
- The presence of hesitation cuts indicates the suicidal nature of the injury.
- Commonly present in cut-throat injuries on the neck around the main wound, which indicates the half-heartedness and the divided state of mind.
- They are present only on the accessible parts of the body, commonly present on the front of forearm, wrist or elsewhere on the body.
- These types of injuries are also inflicted to annoy or threaten the people close to them.

DISCUSS ABOUT ANESTHETIC AND SURGERY RELATED DEATHS AND ITS LEGAL IMPLICATION?

These deaths could be categorized as:
- Deaths occurring during administration of anesthesia

- These could be related to:
  - The serious disease or injury for which surgery was preferred has caused death and anesthesia could have precipitated death.
  - The patient could have been suffering from undiagnosed disease which could have caused death and anesthesia could have precipitated death.
- Deaths directly related to administration of anesthesia:
  - These could be due to:
    - Inexperience of the doctor who administer anesthesia like failure to adopt adequate precautions and faulty techniques due to inexperience.
    - Technical mishaps like equipment failure, reduced oxygen supply, acute neurogenic cardiovascular arrest, etc.
- Deaths due to hypovolemia:
  - This may occur during the surgical procedure which are directly related to failure to recognize or replace blood/fluid volume as necessary by calculating the amount of blood loss.
- Deaths and complications related to administration of anesthesia:
  - A large number of unexpected complications of anesthesia vary from minor to fatal events.
- Malignant hyperthermia:
  - Even though fatal complication is rare due to drugs using in general anesthesia like halothane and succinylcholine.
- Postmortem examination and investigation of such deaths:
  - Chemical analysis to detect the anesthetic drug administered and incidence of over dosage if any.
  - Brain should be fixed and sent for histopathological examination.
- All deaths/complications may not be due to errors, most of the time it is the disease process in the patient and/or the response of the individual to the anesthetic drug administered.
- To fix the liability and find out where the sequence went wrong and how death has resulted is a difficult task for the autopsy surgeon. He should consider the following aspects when conducting autopsy on such death:
  - Complete history of the patient's disease condition before surgery.
  - Details of anesthesia administration: The expected adverse effects of the drugs administered.
  - Details of surgical procedure and the level of risk involved in that particular surgical procedure should be considered.
  - Preanesthetic drugs used.
  - Details of blood transfusion before, during and after surgery.
  - Details of resuscitation attempted
  - Equipments used and whether the correct qualified person handled it.

Medico-legal issues relating to operational deaths:

- Whether the surgery is a life saving surgery or an optional surgery:
  - If it is a life saving surgery that is, if the patient dies directly due to the effects of the disease problem or condition for which surgery was done, then there lies no liability on the part of the surgical team because even if surgery is not opted then also the patient would have died directly due to disease or the condition, he was suffering from. Example: Cardiac surgeries like valvular replacement, coronary artery bypass, severe traumatic injury, etc.
  - If it is an optional surgery then there lies more liability on the part of the

surgical team because if surgery is not done he could have been very well living as the disease, problem he was suffering from was not dangerous enough to cause death. Example: Surgeries done for deviated nasal septum, squint, cosmetic surgeries, etc.

- Even in an important surgery like cardiac or brain surgery, if death is due to any gross negligent act on the part of the anesthetist or surgeon or anyone of the team then they are liable for compensation.

MULTIPLE CHOICE QUESTIONS

1. **The similarity between legal and medical definition of injury is:**
   a. Injury to the body
   b. Injury to the mind
   c. Damage to property
   d. Damage of reputation

2. **A 25-year-old person sustained injury in right eye. He developed right corneal opacity following the injury. Left eye was already having poor vision. Corneoplasty of right eye was done and vision was restored medico-legally such injury is labeled as:**
   a. Grievous
   b. Simple
   c. Dangerous
   d. Serious

3. **Killing in self defense comes under:**
   a. Murder
   b. Justifiable homicide
   c. Excusable homicide
   d. Culpable homicide

4. **A person has been brought in casualty with history of road accident. He had lost consciousness transiently and then gained consciousness but again became unconscious. Most likely, he is having brain hemorrhage of:**
   a. Intracerebral
   b. Subarachnoid
   c. Subdural
   d. Extradural

5. **Self-inflicted artificial bruises are characterized by all of the following, *except*:**
   a. Small in number
   b. Not extensive
   c. Only on accessible parts
   d. Typical color changes

6. **Causing death under the following conditions does not amount to murder, *except*:**
   a. Premedication
   b. Provocation
   c. Private defense
   d. Public justice

7. **The following are medico-legal significance of defense wounds, *except*:**
   a. Sign of instinctive reaction of the victim
   b. Mandatory in all homicides
   c. Nature of weapon can be identified
   d. Relative position of the victim and assailant can be presumed

8. **The following grievous wounds can be certified without consultation of an expert, *except*:**
   a. Simple fracture of tibia
   b. Erectile dysfunction
   c. Partially broken central incisor
   d. Nasal bone fracture

9. **Tentative cut is a feature of:**
   a. Fall from the height
   b. Homicidal assault
   c. Accidental injury
   d. Suicidal attempt

10. **Punishment for culpable homicide not amounting to murder is dealt under:**
    a. Section 299 IPC
    b. Section 300 IPC
    c. Section 302 IPC
    d. Section 304 IPC

11. **IPC section dealing with dowry death:**
    a. 307 IPC
    b. 304 IPC
    c. 304-A IPC
    d. 304-B IPC

12. **As per the Dowry Prohibition Act 1961, penalty awarded in case of death is imprisonment for:**
    a. More than 5 years
    b. Up to 7 years
    c. 7 years to life imprisonment
    d. Up to 10 years

13. **If a woman is assaulted by her husband, then he is charged under:**
    a. Section 498-A IPC
    b. Section 304-A IPC
    c. Section 304-B IPC
    d. Section 504 IPC
14. **Which one of the following is not a grievous hurt:**
    a. Loss of left little finger
    b. Loss of hearing in one ear
    c. Loss of vision of one eye
    d. A large abrasion on the face
15. **Neurogenic shock is characterized by:**
    a. Cool and moist skin
    b. Increased cardiac output
    c. Decreased peripheral vascular resistance
    d. Bradycardia and hypotension
16. **Not a manifestation of anaphylactic shock:**
    a. Hypotension
    b. Vasoconstriction
    c. Bronchospasm
    d. Laryngeal edema
17. **Risk of thromboembolism is highest with:**
    a. Deep femoral vein thrombus
    b. Anterior tibial vein thrombus
    c. Posterior tibial vein thrombus
    d. Popliteal vein thrombus
18. **Fat embolism commonly occurs in:**
    a. Scurvy
    b. Fracture of long bones (femur)
    c. Paget's disease
    d. Psoriasis

ANSWERS

1. a	2. a	3. c	4. d	5. d	6. a	7. b	8. b	9. d	10. d
11. d	12. c	13. a	14. d	15. c	16. b	17. a	18. b		

CHAPTER 15

Thermal Injuries

 KEY WORDS

Burns, scalds, thermoregulation, hypothermia, heat cramps, sun stroke, frost bite, trench foot, epidermal burns, rule of nine, pugilistic attitude, soot particles, COHb.

FM2.24	Thermal deaths: Describe the clinical features, postmortem finding and medico-legal aspects of injuries due to physical agents like heat (heat-hyperpyrexia, heat stroke, sun stroke, heat exhaustion/prostration, heat cramps (miner's cramp) or cold (systemic and localized hypothermia, frostbite, trench foot, immersion foot).
FM2.25	Describe types of injuries, clinical features, pathophysiology, postmortem findings and medico-legal aspects in cases of burns, scalds, lightening, electrocution and radiations.

INTRODUCTION

Thermal injuries are injuries due to heat and cold:
- Thermal injuries are as a result of the systemic and/or localized effects to excessive heat or cold.
- The factors determining the effects of heat are:
  - Temperature (the intensity of heat)
  - The duration of contact of heat on the body.
- According to Mortiz and Henriques: The lowest temperature that would produce burns was 44°C and the time required was 5 hours, whereas at 60°C only 3 seconds is required to cause localized burns.

DISCUSS THE MECHANISM OF THERMOREGULATION?

- There is always a delicate balance between heat production and heat loss.
- **Internal body factors:** The amount of heat generated by oxidation of metabolic products (internal factor).
- Environmental heat from the Sun (external factor) is influenced by:
  - Moisture content of the air
  - Wavelength of the light
  - Spectral distribution
  - Absorption by ozone layer
- Heat load results from combination of both internal and environmental factors.
- Whenever, heat load exceeds heat loss, the temperature of the body rises. The

dispersion of heat takes place, mainly by sweating and vaporization from the respiratory passages.
- When the body is exposed to high temperature, there is vasodilatation of blood vessels of the skin due to inhibition of sympathetic centers in the posterior hypothalamus. When the environmental temperature increases to a point beyond lose of temperature by convection and radiation, results in sweating.
- Temperature varies in different parts of the body. The inner body temperature always remains constant, except when the individual develops fever.
- The skin temperature rises and falls with the temperature of the surroundings.
- The average body temperature is 98° to 98.6°F when measured orally. It is higher by 1° when measured rectally and lower by 1° when measured under the axilla.

CLASSIFY THERMAL INJURIES? (FM2.4)

Thermal injuries are either effects of heat or effects of cold **(Flowchart 15.1)**.

Effects of Heat

- **Generalized effects:** Heat stroke, heat cramps and heat exhaustion.
- **Localized effects:** Burns (due to dry heat) and scalds (due to wet heat).

Effects of Cold

- **Generalized effects:** Hypothermia.
- **Localized effects:** Frostbite, trench foot and immersion foot.

DISCUSS THE SYSTEMIC EFFECTS OF HEAT? (FM2.24)

Heat Cramps

Painful spasm of voluntary muscles, especially extremities and abdominal wall. This is due to loss of water content, sodium and chloride ions from the body as in severe dehydration.

Heat Exhaustion

- This is due to inadequate replacement of water and salts lost in perspiration, due to thermal stress.
- Usually occurs after several days of exposure to high temperature. In this condition body temperature does not exceed 102°F.
- The symptoms are: Tiredness, increased thirst, headache, irritability, subjective feeling of exhaustion and incapacity to work, sweating, fainting and peripheral vascular collapse.

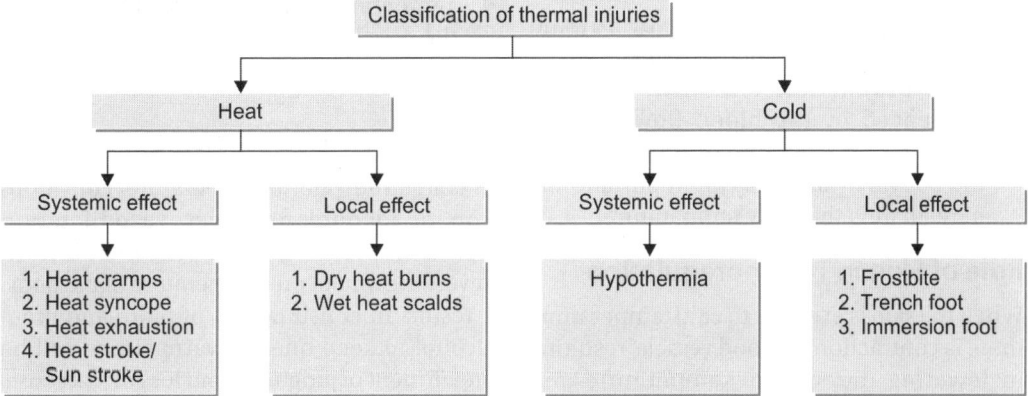

Flowchart 15.1: Classification of thermal injuries.

Heat Syncope (Heat Collapse)

It is due to loss of vasomotor tone resulting in peripheral pooling of blood usually in the lower limbs due to dilatation of blood vessels. This results in reduction of blood flow to the heart. There is hypotension and reduced blood supply to the brain. Commonly seen in soldiers standing for a long time in parades under hot sun; recovery is usual.

Heat Stroke (Sun Stroke)

- It results in absence of sweating, increase in body temperature to 106°F or more.
- Onset is acute or sometimes insidious. The skin is flushed, hot and dry.
- The pulse will be rapid, threading and BP may be normal or reduced.
- The individuals may suffer neuromuscular paralysis.
- Death is commonly due to low BP or disseminated intravascular coagulation (DIC).

DISCUSS ABOUT HYPOTHERMIA? (FM2.24)

Pathophysiology of Hypothermia

- Temperature of peripheral parts of the body varies from time to time depending on the atmospheric temperature. But the inner core temperature of the body is always maintained constant by thermoregulation and controlled by thyroid hormone, and muscular activity.
- Heat production and heat loss are influenced by the blood flow through the skin and sweating. Clothes covering the body may also play an important role in regulating the body temperature.

Role of Skin in Thermoregulation

When the skin is exposed to cold temperature, there is contraction of blood vessels, resulting in lowering the surface temperature and conservation of body heat. This produces a feeling of chill. Continued exposure results in injury to the superficial surface as well as loss of body heat.

Thermoregulation by Lungs

- Lungs are one of the major sources of heat exchange.
- During the process of respiration, equilibrium is maintained between the body temperature and the external environment.
- Therefore, continued breathing of cold air results in a massive loss of body heat, which leads to lowering of the inner body core temperature.

Phases of Hypothermia

- **First phase:** No clinical significance; rectal temperature is between 90° to 98.4°F. Feeling of cold and shivering is present. Responds well to simple resuscitation measures.
- **Second phase:** Rectal temperature is between 75° to 90°F. The subject is depressed; there is progressive fall in pulse, BP and respiration. Sense of shivering ceases below 85°F.
- **Third phase:** Rectal temperature is below 75°F, temperature regulatory center ceases to function and there occurs progressive cooling; survival is rare at this phase.
- Temperature difference of 10°C between the core body temperature and the atmosphere is enough to cause hypothermia.

Alcohol and Hypothermia

In cold atmospheric temperature, consumption of alcohol produces vasodilatation resulting in heat generation which in turn lowers the inner core temperature of the body. It results in consumption of more and more alcohol to keep oneself warm. There will be impairment of judgment and loss of risk sense.

Mechanism of Death in Hypothermia

- As the body core temperature falls, there is progressive decrease in the dissociation of oxyhemoglobin, which leads to reduced oxygen supply to the tissues.
- This in turn, depresses the oxidative process in the tissues and results in stagnation of blood, leading to tissue hypoxia (stagnant anoxia).
- Death is due to circulatory collapse.

Autopsy findings: Depends on the intensity of cold and the duration of exposure.

External findings:
- Body surface is usually pale, with irregular dusky red patches of frost erythema, particularly on the exposed parts, large joints and extensor surfaces of the body.
- Postmortem staining is usually pink in color; the extremities are cyanosed.

FROSTBITE AND TRENCH FOOD (FM2.24)

Frostbite

Frostbite is localized effect of cold due to impaired local circulation as a result of exposure to freezing temperature (-2° to -8°C). Signs of vital reaction like erythema, swelling and indurations can be seen around the involved surface. Exposure to extreme cold temperature results in sudden vasospasm, ischemia and localized necrosis beyond the line of inflammatory demarcation of the tissues. Occurs in the exposed parts of the body such as ears, nose and extremities like toes and fingers, etc.

Trench Foot

Prolonged exposure of the extremities to cold (nonfreezing temperature 5° to 8°C) for many hours, leads to trench foot or Immersion foot. Blister formation and localized dry gangrene formation occurs, typically seen in soldiers in winter warfare especially in trenches and in persons exposed to prolonged immersion and exposure to cold sea water.

Internal Findings

- Internal findings are predominantly due to avascular necrosis. Subcutaneous tissues are relatively avascular and blood, if present is often bright red in color.
- **GIT:** Multiple patches of acute sub-mucosal hemorrhages may be seen in the stomach and duodenum (appears dark red due to presence of altered blood). If the individual survives, the mucosa over the hemorrhages may slough out leaving shallow ulcers.
- **Brain:** Shows perivascular hemorrhage in the 3rd ventricle with chromatolysis of ganglion cells.
- **Pancreas:** There is variable degree of fat necrosis in the pancreas, ranging from small patches to extensive nonhemorrhagic pancreatitis. This leads to high serum amylase levels, often with fatty necrosis of the adjacent mesentery.
- Multiple visceral infarcts caused by ischemia and evidence of venous thrombosis may be found.

WHAT IS BURNS? CLASSIFY BURNS? (FM2.25)

- It is a condition due to the local effect of dry heat, either due to direct contact with flame or any heated object like wire, hot metals or heated glass.
- In household accidents burns develop as result of explosion of cooking stoves or gas cylinders resulting in ignition of the clothes worn by the victim. Depending on the intensity of spread either part or whole of the garments catches fire.
- Upon contact with the skin surface the flame produces burns involving the epidermis, dermis and the deeper structures. Depending on the duration of contact and the extent of involvement burn

injuries are classified into three degrees. First degree burns (involving only the epidermis), second degree burns (involving up to the dermis) and third degree burns (involvement of deeper layers of tissues).

Classification of Burns

Epidermal Burns

- This type of burns involves only the epidermis and are superficial in nature. It results in reddening (erythema and blistering without involvement of the dermis) of the skin.
- Followed by capillary dilatation and transudation of fluid into the tissues resulting in swelling.
- The blisters contain fluid rich in albumin and are covered by white avascular epidermis surrounded by a zone of hyperemia.
- These blisters may resorb and the layers of dermis are peeled off exposing dark red dermis, replaced by growth from the periphery.
- Blisters are painful because of involvement of nerve endings and usually heal without leaving a permanent scar.

Dermo-epidermal Burns

- Burns involves the whole thickness of the skin including hair follicles, sweat glands and sebaceous glands.
- Extremely painful as they affect the sensory nerve endings
- Heals with resultant scar formation.

Deep Burns

- Destruction of deeper tissues, varying from damage to the subcutaneous soft tissues, muscles, bones, etc.
- The burnt areas may be completely charred.
- They are relatively painless, as the nerve endings are completely destroyed.
- **Prognosis:** Depends upon the extent of body surface involved, rather than the degree of burns. First degree burns involving a larger area of body surface is more fatal than a third degree burns with focal involvement.

WHAT IS RULE OF NINE? (TABLE 15.1)

- This is a method used to calculate the extent of body surface involved in burns. It is useful in assessing the prognosis of the patient. The body surface is divided into 11 parts and each part is given a score of 9%.
- Burns involving 50% or above is invariably fatal and 30% is sufficient to cause death.

Rule of Palm

In cases where the distribution of burns is scattered, the percentage is calculated with the presumption that the surface area of a person's palm, is taken as 1% of the total body surface.

CAUSES OF DEATH IN BURNS (FM2.25)

Causes of Death in Burns

- **Immediate causes of death:**
    - *Suffocation:* Due to inhalation of smoke, CO and other irrespirable gases.

TABLE 15.1: Rule of nine.

Part of the body	Percentage
Head and face	9%
Right upper limb	9%
Left upper limb	9%
Front of chest	9%
Front of abdomen	9%
Back of chest	9%
Back of abdomen	9%
Front of right lower limb	9%
Front of left lower limb	9%
Back of right lower limb	9%
Back of left lower limb	9%
Genitalia	1%
Total	**100%**

- **Primary neurogenic shock:** Death within a few hours.
- Secondary shock due to hypovolemia within 24 to 48 hours. It is usually associated with renal failure due to hypoperfusion resulting in acute tubular necrosis.
- Death due to accidental injuries.
- **Delayed causes of death:**
  - *Toxemia:* It is due to absorption of toxic products from the surface of the body, generated during the process of burning.
  - *Infections:* Prolonged exposure of the burnt skin surface to micro organisms may favor the development of infections; these infections affect other vital systems and leads to meningitis, bronchopneumonia, pericarditis, etc., and death due to septicemia.
  - Few individuals may develop complications like curling's ulcer (duodenal ulcer) due to prolonged bed rest.

AGE OF BURNS INJURY

Age of the burns can be accessed from the external appearance like:
- **Erythema (redness):** Which occurs immediately.
- **Vesication:** 2 to 3 hours
- **Exudates begins to dry:** By 24 to 48 hours (dry brown crest).
- **If infected:** Pus is formed in 2 to 3 days; superficial slough separates out by 4–6 days; deeper slough separates out within 2 weeks. Then granulation tissue begins to cover the raw areas; scar is formed after several weeks or months.

WHAT ARE THE POSTMORTEM FINDINGS IN DEATH DUE TO BURNS?

What is Pugilistic Attitude? (FM2.25)

- **Examinations of clothes:** For evidence of burns and for the presence of any characteristic smell, like that of kerosene, petrol or any other combustible substances should be looked for. Clothes which are in close contact with the body gets damaged completely. Synthetic materials like terylene, nylon may be found closely adherent onto the skin surface.
- Skin surface covered by tight clothing like undergarments are usually spared from damage, if exposure to fire is for a short duration.

External Findings

- If the body is fully burnt all the surface of the skin might have been damage **(Fig. 15.1)**. If some unburnt skin is present adjacent to the damaged areas, vital reactions in the form of reddish borders adjoining the burnt areas can be seen. The epidermis may be burnt completely, exposing the underlying dermis which is usually pink in color depicted in **Figure 15.2**, indicating the antemortem nature of the burns.
- Scalp hair and body hair are found burnt and singed.
- Blood tinged froth may be seen around the mouth and nostril, due to development of pulmonary edema. This is due to the irritation produced by inhalation of hot air.

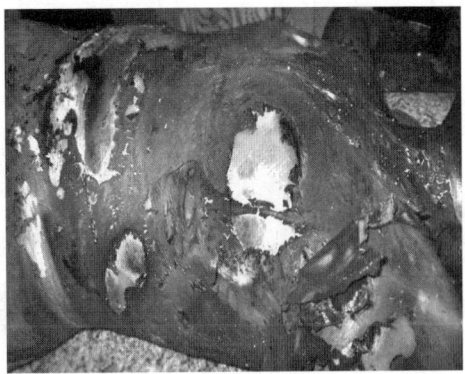

Fig. 15.1: Extensive superficial burns with charring *(For color version see Plate 13).*

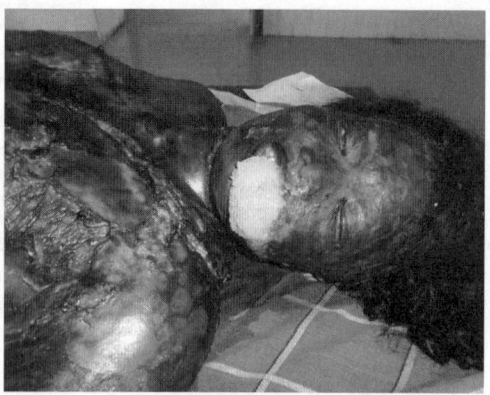

Fig. 15.2: Dermo-epidermal burns exposing underlying pink dermis—antemortem burns *(For color version see Plate 13).*

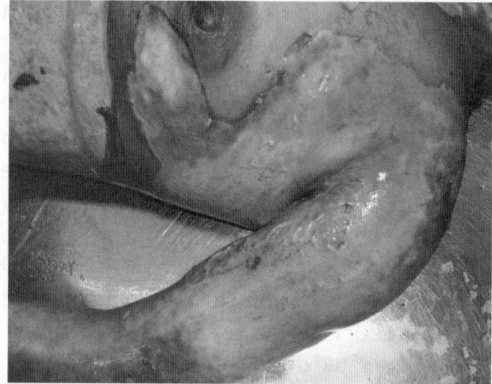

Fig. 15.4: Infected burns—death due to septicemia *(For color version see Plate 14).*

Pugilistic Attitude (Universal Flexion/Boxers Attitude)

- When the body is exposed to prolonged and sustained heat, it results of contraction of the muscle fibers due to coagulation of muscle proteins. This produces flexion of all the joints which simulates the position of boxer. This is called as "pugilistic attitude". This is not antemortem sign of burns; a dead body thrown into fire will show this change **(Fig. 15.3)**.
- Infected burns—death due to septicemia, shown in **Figure 15.4**.

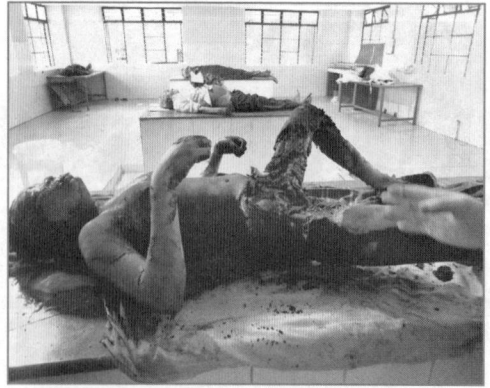

Fig. 15.3: Burns with heat stiffening—pugilistic attitude *(For color version see Plate 14).*

Heat Ruptures

This is seen in fleshy areas like calf muscles, thighs, etc., when there is sustained exposure of the body to fire. This can be differentiated from laceration or incised wounds by the absence of blood clots, intact blood vessels and absence of inflammatory infiltrations, as heat ruptures are postmortem in nature.

Internal Findings

- Blood is usually cherry red if death has occurred due to inhalation of carbon monoxide.
- Mucosa of the stomach and duodenum are frequently hyperemic and may show ulcers.

Heat Hematomas

These are areas of collection of blood clots inside the cranial cavity. It is usually seen over the frontal and occipital regions. The size of the hematoma corresponds to the external damage and charring effect to the skull.

Respiratory Passage

Soot particles: These are the deposition of burnt carbon particles which are found adherent to the edematous mucosal surface of the respiratory passage. Demonstration of soot particles over the mucosal surface of the respiratory passage up to the secondary bronchioles are diagnostic of antemortem burns.

WHAT ARE THE MEDICO-LEGAL ISSUES IN DEATH DUE TO BURNS?

What are the Signs of Antemortem Burns? (FM2.25)

- **Identity of the deceased:** Identity of the deceased in cases of burns throws a big challenge to the investigators. Remnants of clothing, other articles, X-ray of the entire body and dental pattern may help in establishing the identity.
- **Whether burns are antemortem or postmortem:** The points in favor of antemortem burns are the following.
- **Cutaneous reaction to heat or flame:**
  - Presence of vital reactions (red flare/red line) on the intact skin adjacent the burnt area.
  - *Blister formation:* These blisters contain a serous fluid of albumin and chlorides; base is inflamed and red with erythematous borders. Postmortem blisters contain traces of albumin and chlorides and more of gas; the base is dry, hard and yellow.
- Presence of smoke and soot particles in the respiratory passage.
  - Evidence of injury to the respiratory tract by fumes and hot gases: Inhalation of hot fumes causes acute laryngeal oedema resulting in sudden asphyxiation.
- **Elevated levels of carboxy hemoglobin:** Incomplete combustion of any organic matter leads to production of carbon monoxide. CO has got high affinity to Hb resulting in increased levels COHb.
- More than 10% of Hb saturation with CO, usually indicates that the victim has inhaled CO; however, in chain smokers the normal level itself is 8–10%.
- Presence of elevated levels of other toxic gases in the blood like HCN, ammonia, NO, CO_2 and H_2S are also indicative of antemortem burns.
- **Histological evidence:** Histochemical reaction shows presence of nonspecific esterase (within 45 minutes), leucine aminopeptidase (within 2 hours), increase in reaction of alkaline phosphatase (within 3 hours) and leucocytic infiltration and staining for DNA and RNA (within 6 hours) is indicative of antemortem burns.

HOW TO ASSESS THE MANNER OF DEATH IN BURNS?

Suicidal

- Not uncommon.
- Suicide by burning in domestic environment is much more common among females.
- Usually, some inflammable material like kerosene is used.
- At times, superficial burns may be inflicted over the accessible parts of the body to make a false accusation against the enemy.

Accidental

- Majority of cases occur when the victim is trapped inside the burning buildings or vehicle.
- Some accidents do occur in the kitchen, while cooking.
- Children, epileptics, old people and grossly intoxicated individuals are the usual victims.

Homicidal

- Though not common, incidences of homicidal burns are reported worldwide.
- Killing the victim by some other means and then burn the body to simulate

accidental/suicidal burns are also regular phenomenon. Postmortem nature of burns injury and finding out the real cause of death like throttling will help solve such cases easily.
- When death is due to burns and there is a suspicion/allegation of homicidal burns, the medical expert should examine the pattern of burns on the body and assess how the fuel could have been poured. Whether from head to toe (suicidal) of splashed by the assailant in which case there will be burns on one side of the body and the opposite sideburns would be absent. Also, more and deep burns on the front of chest and abdomen as the fuel could have been splashed on the victim. Examine the palm as a mechanism of instinctive self-defense, the victim could have attempted to blocked the fuel by hands and the palm could be exposed to more fuel and hence palm would show extensive and deep burns.

WHAT IS SCALDS? FEATURES OF SCALDS INJURY (FM2.25)

Scalds

- These are injuries caused by moist heat. Hot liquids of temperature above 60°C cause scalds (**Fig. 15.5**).

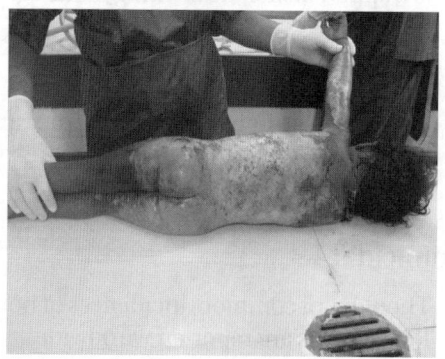

Fig. 15.5: Infected scalds
(For color version see Plate 14).

- The protection offered by the skin and the short duration of contact of the hot liquids prevents inward conduction of heat into the deeper layers, and hence generally only the superficial layers of the skin are involved in scalds.
- However, the extent of scalds greatly depends on the latent heat (heat retention capacity) of any liquid. Scalds produced by sticky viscous liquids are very high due to the high degree of penetration of heat; example; hot tar, syrups, oil, etc. Injuries caused by these liquids are comparatively deeper than the one caused by hot water.

General Features of Scald Injury

- The liquid responsible for scalding may be seen on the clothing and the body; smell of the liquid may be present. Scalding usually occur through the intact clothing and the degree of scalds depend upon the permeability of the liquid.
- Injury is usually limited to the areas of contact and more severe at the point of initial contact. Scalding is severe at the point of initial contact and at places where the liquid has come into contact with the body for a longer duration. As the liquid runs down, the degree of scalding progressively diminishes.
- Redness appears at once and blistering (vesication) takes place within a few minutes.
- Vesicles are abundant along the course of the running liquid; there is usually a demarcated edge, corresponding to the limit of contact of the liquid.
- The blisters have a hyperemic zone surrounding them.
- Reddening and swelling over the surface can be made out in the floor of the blisters.
- If the skin over the blisters is removed, the floor appears reddish with serosanguinous discharge.

CHAPTER 15: Thermal Injuries

- Postmortem blisters contain gas with scanty fluid, which has a less proteins and chloride content. All the antemortem reactions like redness and swelling are absent.
- Features of injuries caused by dry heat, like burning of clothes, singeing of hair, deposition of carbon particles on the burnt skin surface and respiratory passage, and charring of tissues are absent in scalds.

HOW WILL YOU DIFFERENTIATE BURNS FROM SCALDS? (FM2.25)

Table 15.2 is depicted the differentiate between burns and scalds.

CIRCUMSTANCES OF SCALDS INJURIES

- Usually, accidental due to splashing of fluid.
- Children may upset the vessels containing hot liquids or may accidentally fall into the vessels containing hot liquids. They may sometimes sucks the spouts of the kettles containing hot milk or water, resulting in severe scalds of the mouth and throat.
- Boiling water may be thrown with the intention to injure or annoy any individual.
- Deliberate scalds using hot fluid are common in child abuse.
- Suicidal scalding is rare because they are extremely painful and moreover, does not guarantee death.

WHAT IS RESPIRATORY BURNS?

Respiratory Burns

- This condition is produced by exposure of the respiratory passage to super heated steam or vapors.
- Steam or hot air may be inhaled, causing thermal injury to the respiratory tract. During this there is excessive production of thick tenacious mucus plugs and edema of the mucus membranes, resulting in obstruction of the airway. This produces death by asphyxia.
- Exposure of skin over the face to super heated steam can produce soddening of the skin, which becomes dirty white in color.

WHAT IS PARADOXICAL UNDRESSING?

Paradoxical undressing refers to cold exposed hypothermic condition in which the person taking of his clothes and undresses himself just before death.

TABLE 15.2: Burns vs scalds.

Features	Burns	Scalds
Source	Dry heat	Wet heat
Clothing	Burnt	Not affected
Singing of hair	Present	Absent
Charring and blackening of tissues	Present	Absent
Nature of injury	At and above the level of contact	At and below the level of contact, gradually reducing
Soot particles in respiratory tract	Present	Absent
Carboxy hemoglobin	May be present in blood	Absent
Fatality	Usually fatal	Less fatal

Mechanism

Hypoglycemia leads to reduced parasympathetic activity, which in turn paralyses the thermal regulatory mechanism leading to dilatation of cutaneous blood vessels. This dilatation increases the skin temperature and the individual gets a spurious feeling of warmth. He experiences burning sensation of skin due to the hypothermic condition, he is already exposed, to get rid of the warmth, he undresses himself.

This happens in the terminal stage of hypothermia just before death and is usually associated with mental confusion, delirium and hallucinations.

Hide and Die Syndrome

This may be seen sometimes in association with undressing. The person may hide himself in corners of rooms, cupboards or under the furnitures. He may be in a naked or semi-naked condition. There will be great disturbance in the scene giving the suspension of some crime.

Medico-legal Importance

Condition of the body and disturbance in the scene of crime gives a suspension of some serious crime as like sexual offences.

Visit to the scene of crime by an experienced forensic pathologist and corroboration of autopsy findings will help to reconstruct the sequence of events

MULTIPLE CHOICE QUESTIONS

1. All of the following are systemic effects of heat exposure, *except:*
    a. Internal organ burn
    b. Heat syncope
    c. Heat exhaustion
    d. Heat rigor
2. The following are signs of antemortem burns, *except:*
    a. Soot in the stomach
    b. Soot in the bronchi
    c. Pugilistic attitude
    d. Carboxy hemoglobin
3. Flame burns differs from scalding in the following aspects, *except:*
    a. Soot deposition
    b. Blistering
    c. Charring
    d. Singeing
4. The following are the findings of heat hematoma in antemortem burns, *except:*
    a. Charring of the overlying bone
    b. Spongy in texture
    c. Chocolate brown in color
    d. Absence of carboxy hemoglobin
5. What is wrong about heat hematoma?
    a. It is antemortem
    b. Friable
    c. Seen in charred body
    d. Frontal area
6. A 25-year female was found in a room with 100% burns on her body. The tongue was protruding out; body was in pugilistic attitude with heat ruptures, peeling of skin, and heat hematoma and heat fractures of skull. Carboxy-hemoglobin was 25% and soot particles were present in trachea. Which of the combinations of two findings will establish that the burns were antemortem in nature?
    a. Heat hematoma and heat ruptures
    b. Heat fracture of skull and peeling of skin
    c. Heat hematoma and pugilistic attitude
    d. Carboxy-hemoglobin (25%) and soot particles in trachea
7. Paradoxical undressing is seen in:
    a. Hyperthermia
    b. Hypothermia
    c. Transvestism
    d. Immersion syndrome
8. A person working in hot environment who consumes more water without salt is likely to develop a condition called:
    a. Heat stroke
    b. Heat exhaustion
    c. Heat cramps
    d. Heat hyperpyrexia
9. Not seen in heat stroke:
    a. Hypovolemic shock
    b. Pancreatitis
    c. Rhabdomyolysis
    d. Cerebral edema

10. **Characteristic features of superficial burns are all, *except*:**
    a. Damage no deeper than papillary dermis
    b. Blisters absent
    c. Loss of epidermis
    d. Pinprick is not painful
11. **Blister formation in burn is classified as:**
    a. First degree
    b. Second degree superficial
    c. Second degree deep
    d. Third degree
12. **Most important aspect of management of burn injury in the first 24 hour:**
    a. Dressing
    b. Escharotomy
    c. Fluid resuscitation
    d. Antibiotics
13. **Best fluid for resuscitation in burns:**
    a. Dextran
    b. Albumin
    c. Hartmann's solution
    d. Ringer lactate
14. **Sweating is absent in:**
    a. Heat syncope
    b. Heat exhaustion
    c. Heat stroke
    d. Heat cramps
15. **A 65-year male weighing 50 kg was admitted with 80% burn and RL was transfused with Parkland method. How much fluid should be infused in first 8 hours:**
    a. 200 mL/hr
    b. 500 mL/hr
    c. 1000 mL/hr
    d. 8000 mL/hr
16. **Most common cause of death in thermal burns is:**
    a. Convulsion
    b. Hypovolemic shock
    c. Aspiration pneumonia
    d. Arrhythmias
17. **Not an indication for admission in burns ward:**
    a. Acid burns
    b. Inhalational injury
    c. 5% surface area superficial burns in an unmarried female
    d. 10% deep burns in a male
18. **Cause of late death in burn patients is:**
    a. Neurogenic shock
    b. Cardiogenic shock
    c. Hypovolemic shock
    d. Sepsis
19. **Pugilistic attitude is due to:**
    a. Lipolysis
    b. Protein coagulation
    c. Carbohydrate coagulation
    d. Lipogenesis
20. **True about pugilistic attitude:**
    a. Indicate antemortem burns
    b. Indicate postmortem burns
    c. Cannot differentiate between ante- or postmortem
    d. Indicate defense by victim
21. **Appearance of burn hematoma:**
    a. Honeycomb like
    b. Disc shaped
    c. Stellate shaped
    d. Smooth and rubbery
22. **Bone pearl's or wax drippings is pathognomonic of:**
    a. Burns
    b. Lightening
    c. Scalds
    d. Electrocution
23. **Muir and Barclay formula is for:**
    a. Colloid resuscitation in burns
    b. Polytrauma fluid resuscitation
    c. Crystalloid in trauma
    d. Dextran in burns
24. **Parkland formula for burns is for:**
    a. Ringer lactate
    b. Glucose saline
    c. Normal saline
    d. 25% dextrose
25. **All are features of deep burn, *except*:**
    a. Leathery skin
    b. No blister/vesicles
    c. Painful
    d. Involvement of fat
26. **In adults, circulatory collapse occurs after a minimum of what percentage burns of total body surface area:**
    a. 10%
    b. 15%
    c. 30%
    d. 50%
27. **Head and neck burns in infant constitute of burns:**
    a. 9% of burns
    b. 18% of burns

c. 24% of burns
d. 36% of burns
28. **Feature of ruptured skin caused by excessive heat:**
    a. Clear regular margin
    b. Contused margin
    c. Abraded margin
    d. Irregular margin
29. **In hypothermia, cause of death is:**
    a. Stroke
    b. Cardiac arrest
    c. Pulmonary embolism
    d. Asphyxia
30. **Color of postmortem lividity in hypothermic deaths:**
    a. Purple
    b. Deep red
    c. Cherry red
    d. Bright pink

ANSWERS

1. a	2. c	3. b	4. d	5. a	6. d	7. b	8. c	9. b	10. d
11. b	12. c	13. d	14. c	15. c	16. b	17. c	18. d	19. b	20. c
21. a	22. d	23. a	24. a	25. c	26. b	27. b	28. d	29. b	30. d

16 CHAPTER

Forensic Ballistics

KEY WORDS

Ballistics, shot gun, rifled firearm, choking, bore, caliber, cartridge, entry wound, exit wound, scorching, smudging, singeing, stippling, abrasion collar, dirt collar, grease collar, range, contact range, close range, near range, distant range, smokeless gunpowder, nitrocellulose, dum dum bullet, souvenir bullet, gunshot residues, dermal nitrate test, neutron activation analysis, atomic absorption spectrometry.

FM3.9 Describe different types of firearms including structure and components. Along with description of ammunition propellant charge and mechanism of firearms, different types of cartridges and bullets and various terminology in relation of firearm—caliber, range, choking.

FM3.10 Describe and discuss wound ballistics—different types of firearm injuries, blast injuries and their interpretation, preservation and dispatch of trace evidences in cases of firearm and blast injuries, various tests related to confirmation of use of firearms.

INTRODUCTION

- **Ballistics** is the science which deals with the study of firearms and ammunition.
- The experts who deal with this branch of science are called as "ballistic experts".
- **Proximal ballistics:** It is the study of firearm and projectiles.
- **Intermediate ballistics:** Study of motion of the projectile, after being ejected from the firearm till the time it hits the target.
- **Terminal ballistics:** Study of the damages (effects) caused by the projectile on the human body, and hence called "**wound ballistics**". Doctors are the experts in this area of ballistics.

DEFINE A FIREARM? WHAT IS AMMUNITION? (FM3.9)

Firearm

Firearm is a mechanical device equipped to create an explosion, which in turn forces out a projectile at high velocity in order to hit the target at a distance.

Ammunition

Ammunition refers to materials used for causing the explosion, along with the projectile. One complete round of ammunition is called the cartridge.

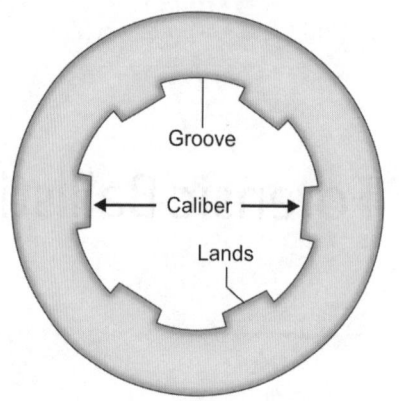

Fig. 16.1: Cross-section of barrel in rifled firearm.

General Makeup of a Firearm/Mechanism

- Any firearm consists of a barrel, a chamber and a triggering mechanism.
- The barrel consists **(Fig. 16.1):** A hollow metal cylinder of varying length, which is closed at the back (breech end) and open at the front (muzzle end).
- The chamber consists of a cabin which can accommodate the cartridge situated at the breech end.
- Trigger and the firing pin initiate the process of firing.

Cartridge (Fig. 16.2)

- Consists of an outer case in which the explosives or chemicals required to ignite the gun powder and the projectile are packed.
- The igniting chemical is the detonator (primer).
- The projectile is either bullets (rifled firearms) and pellets or shots (shot guns).

CLASSIFY FIREARMS: WHAT IS SHOT GUN AND RIFLED FIREARM? (FM3.9)

Firearms are classified as:
- Shot guns
- Rifled firearms
- Air guns or gas operated firearms
- Country made firearms

Shot Gun

These are smooth bored firearm; the inner surface of the barrel is smooth without any rifling. Shot gun could be:
- **Single barreled or double barreled:** There could be one barrel or in some guns there could be two barrels and each firing two cartridges would be fired out.
- **Breach loader or muzzle loader:** Whether the firing materials are loaded into the gun through the breach end muzzle end? When it is breach loader, cartridges are used for ammunition. When it is muzzle loader all the components of firing are loaded through the muzzle end using thin iron rod, keeping the firing pin under lock. There is always a chance of sudden misfortunate firing in cases of muzzle loader guns. However, these types of muzzle loader guns are not in much use now a days as illegal cartridges are available even for country made firearms.
- **Cylindrical or choked (Figs 16.3 and 16.4):** The diameter of the barrel is uniform from the breach end to the muzzle end. There is dispersion of pellets immediately as the leave the muzzle end of the barrel. Choking of a shotgun depicted in **Figure 16.5** and effects of choking depicted in **Figure 16.6**.

Rifled Firearms (Fig. 16.7)

- On the inner surface of the barrel of the gun there are twisted spiral grooves internally. This is called as **rifling of a firearm.** The projecting ridges between the grooves are called as lands. The diameter of the bullet is equal to the distance between two diagonally opposite lands.
- Rifling gives the bullet a spinning motion, thus increases the power of penetration and prevents wobbling of the bullet when it is traveling in the air.

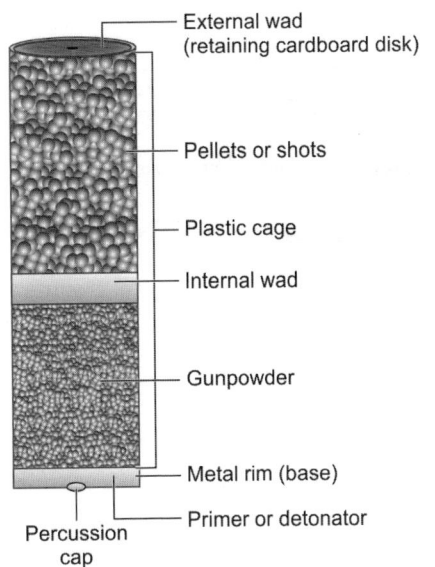

Fig. 16.2: Shotgun cartridge.

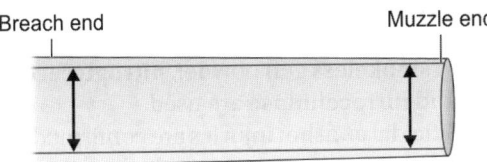

Fig. 16.3: Barrel of shotgun (smooth bored) cylindrical gun.

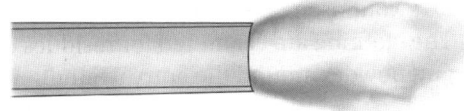

Fig. 16.4: Dispersion of pellets in cylindrical gun.

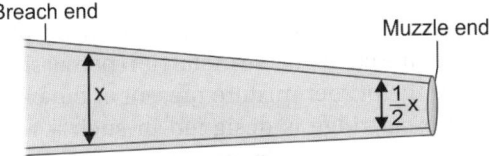

Fig. 16.5: Choking of a shotgun.

- Rifled firearms could be:
  - *High velocity guns:* Shoulder arms (machine guns, stun guns, AK 47)

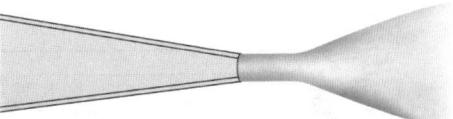

Fig. 16.6: Effects of choking—prevents early dispersion of pellets.

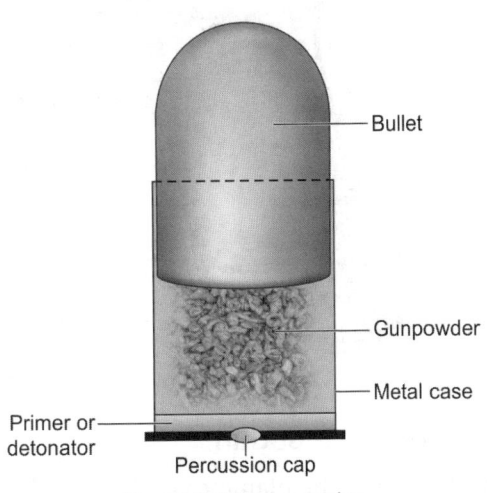

Fig. 16.7: Rifled cartridge.

They can hit the target exactly even if fired from a very long distance. It may be manual, semi-automatic or fully automatic in their makeup.
- *Low velocity guns (Fig. 16.8):* Hand guns (revolver and pistol).

WHAT IS CHOKING? DESCRIBE CALIBER OF SHOT GUN? (FM3.9)

Choking of a Firearm

It is done only in case of shot guns. In these shot guns, the terminal portion of the barrel is constricted. Depending upon the degree of choking it may quarter choke, half choke or full choke. Choking is done to prevent the early dispersion of the pellets after the pellets are discharged from the forearm through the breach end.

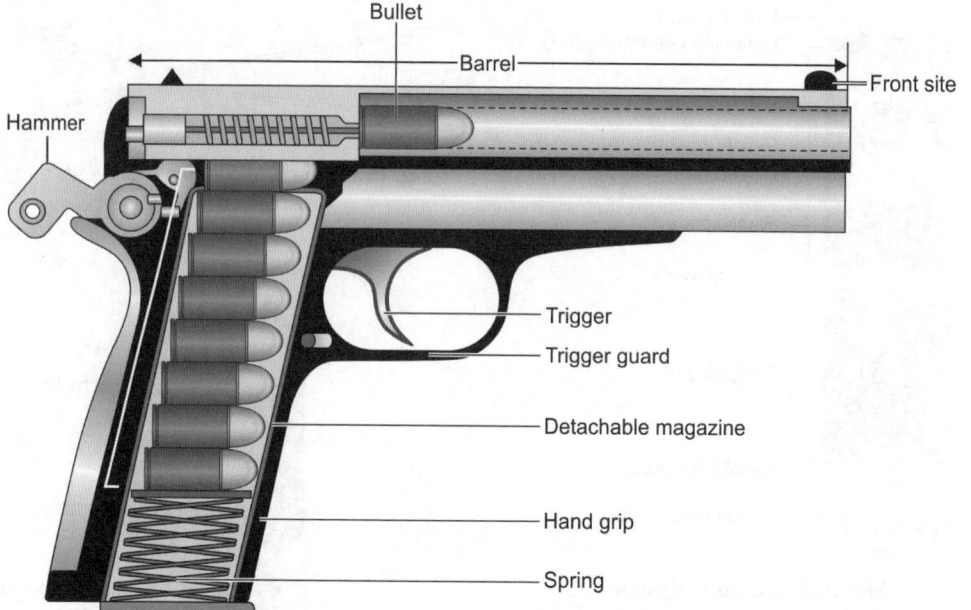

Fig. 16.8: Pistol (handgun—low velocity firearm).

Caliber of a Shot Gun

- Caliber is the diameter of the barrel in sooth bored firearms.
- It is the number of lead balls of equal size and shape made from and out of one pound of pure lead. When one such ball exactly fits into the inner barrel of the gun, then the number of balls made out of one pound of lead is called the bore of the gun. For example, if 12 balls are made from one pound of lead and one ball exactly fits into the size of the barrel, then it is designated as twelve bore gun.

WHAT IS GUN POWDER; COMPOSITION OF GUN POWER?

- This is the principle requirement of the propellant; explodes rapidly and is capable of generating enormous amount of gas, which in turn pushes the projectile at high velocity.
- Usually, **black gun powder** is used and is composed of **potassium nitrate, charcoal and sulfur.**
- In **smokeless** gun powder, **nitroglycerine and nitrocellulose** are used.
- Suicidal gunshot injuries are confirmed by residues of gun powder in the hands.
- Preautopsy X-ray of whole body is a must in all cases of gunshot injuries both shot guns and rifled firearms, even if corresponding exit wounds are present.
- The clothing are examined for residues of gun powder around the entry wound.

WHAT IS THE MECHANISM OF FIRING OF A FIREARM? (FM3.9)

When the trigger is pressed the firing pin strikes the center of the metal rim (percussion cup). The primer mixture present at the base of the cartridge is designed in such a way that it gets ignited by minimum amount of heat. The primer is the **brain** of the cartridge. The minimum amount of heat generated by the striking of the firing pin ignites the primer. Once the primer is ignited it ignites the gun powder. The gun power is designed in such a way that, once ignited it produces enormous amount of gas under pressure. This pressurized gas pushes the projectile (pellets in shot gun and bullet in case of rifled firearm) out through the barrel. The projectile travels in air and ultimately hits the target. All these takes place in fraction of a second.

DISCUSS THE FEATURES OF ENTRY WOUND OF A RIFLED FIREARM? (FM3.10)

Short notes on: Abrasion collar; Contusion collar, Grease collar; Scorching; Smudging; Stippling; Lead ring.

General Features of an Entry Wound

- **When the bullet pierces through the skin:** Due to the spinning motion of the bullet, the edges of the wound may be abraded and is called as "**Abrasion collar**". Usually, it extends up to 0.3 cm around the entry wound.
- In some cases, there may be a contusion in addition to the abrasion. This is called **Contusion collar.**
- The diameter of the entry wound together with the abrasion collar gives the approximate diameter of the bullet.
- **Grease collar or dirt collar (0.7 cm):** The barrel of the firearm is cleaned using lubricant (grease). When a bullet is fired, the projectile will carry a coating of the grease and while it enters the target, it is whipped off around the entry wound. This is called as "grease collar". It will be absent if firing has taken place through the clothing.
- **Burning (scorching or singeing):** It is due to the effect of the flame or fire which travels along with the projectile, up to a certain distance. When the target is within the range of the distance travelled by the flame, then evidence of burning like scorching of skin, singeing of hair follicles can be appreciated around the entry wound. Evidence of such findings can be made out in the clothes when firing has taken place through the clothing.
- **Blackening or smudging:** Results from superficial deposit of smoke on the skin surface. Smudging may not be visible to naked eyes when smokeless gunpowder is used. In such cases, infrared or ultraviolet photography will help to visualize the smudging.
- **Tattooing (peppering or stippling):** Results from the grains of gunpowder (partially burnt and unburnt) being driven into the skin, each grain acting as a minute missile. The extent of tattooing depends upon the caliber of the weapon, the type of gunpowder used and the range of firing. Tattooing may be absent if firing has taken place through the clothing.
- **Lead ring:** It is a line of deposition of the metallic particle around the circumference of the entry wound which can be detected by neutron activation analysis.
- Firearm wounds are generally easily recognized as such, but sometimes wounds caused by red hot pokers or a burning pointed stick may simulate a firearm entry wound.
- Conversely, glancing injuries caused by rifled firearms may be confused with incised wounds or lacerated wounds.
- The shape of the entry wound depends upon the angle of entry of the bullet.

DEFINE RANGE OF A FIREARM INJURY? (FM3.10)

Range

- The distance travelled by the bullet from the muzzle end of the firearm to the target is the range of a firearm. The range of a firearm injury is exactly determined only by ballistics experts using test firing methods.
- Determination of accurate range in meters is not necessary in all cases and it is enough if we could find out the approximate range of firing.

- By examination of the characteristics of the entry wound as a medical expert we can easily group the injury into any of the four ranges.
    1. *Contact range:* The muzzle end is in contact with the body.
    2. *Close range:* Within the distance travelled by flame.
    3. *Near range:* Within the distance travelled by smoke, unburnt and partially burnt gun powder particles.
    4. *Distant range:* Beyond the distance travelled by flame, smoke and gunpowder.

DESCRIBE DIFFERENT RANGES OF A RIFLED FIREARM INJURY? (FM3.10)

Contact Range

- Contact shot over a dense area such as the cranial vault is usually large and cruciate in shape, due to the explosive effect of the gases liberated.
- The imprint of the muzzle of the weapon may be found stamped on the skin.
- Burning, smudging and tattooing are usually absent and in some cases slightly appreciable.
- Contact wounds over thin bones, chest or abdomen are usually circular in shape and are surrounded by abrasion collar and/or contusion collar.
- Hair follicles surrounding the contact wound are singed.
- Muscles and soft tissues along the track of the wound may be cherry red in color due to carbon monoxide.
- Contact shots have a varying size and shape and it will be larger than the size of the bullet due to the explosive effect.
- All the contents of the cartridge, bullet, burnt and partially burnt gunpowder, smoke and fire and are all pushed into body through the entry wound. The exit wound is larger than the size of the entry wound due to the exploding effect of the gases.

Close Range

- Close shot is the distance travelled by the flame from the muzzle end. Usually, flame travels approximately up to 7.5 cm in case of a revolver or pistol and 15 cm in case of a rifle (shoulder arms—high velocity firearms).
- Wounds are circular; margins are inverted and are surrounded by scorching, smudging and singeing of hair. They are absent if firing has taken place through the clothing but evidence of such findings will be noticed on the clothing.
- Abrasion collar and contusion collar are present; grease collar and tattooing may or may not be present, but will be present on the clothing if firing has taken place through the clothing.

Near Range

- The distance travelled by smoke, unburnt and partially burnt gunpowder particles; usually unburnt gunpowder travel up to 60 cm in revolver and 75 cm in case of a rifle.
- Entry wound is circular or oval in shape, with inverted margins.
- Singeing of hair and scorching are absent.
- Tattooing is seen up to a maximum of 90 cm.
- Abrasion collar and grease collar are present around the entry wound.

Distant Range

- Beyond the distance travelled by flame, smoke and gunpowder.
- Entry wound is circular with inverted margins.
- Scorching, smudging and tattooing are all absent.
- Distant shot suggests a range beyond self-infliction.

FEATURES OF EXIT WOUND OF RIFLED FIREARM INJURY

- Exit wounds vary greatly in size, shape and configuration.
- They are usually larger than their corresponding entry wounds and edges may be everted.
- All the findings of the entry wound, such as abrasion collar, grease collar, scorching, smudging and tattooing are absent.
- Evidence of exploding effect can be noticed in the exit wound except when it is supported by hard surface.

WHAT ARE THE DIFFERENCES BETWEEN ENTRY WOUND AND EXIT WOUND?

See **Table 16.1**.

DISCUSS THE FEATURES OF A SHOT GUN ENTRY WOUND?

Generally, when the shot gun is fired:
- Fire may travel up to 30 cm and produces burning and singeing on the skin.
- Smoke will spread up to 45 cm and produce smudging.
- Unburnt and partially burnt gunpowder will move up to 60 cm and cause tattooing
- Wad may travel up to 2 to 5 meters
- Pellets move out as single mass up to 2 meters and starts dispersion after that.

DISCUSS THE RANGE OF SHOT GUN FIREARM INJURY?

Contact Shot

- Contact shot with a shot gun causes explosion and gross destruction of the tissues. If the injury is on the head, the skull and brain may shatter with explosive destruction of skull bones and brain tissues. Extensive mutilation may occur because the gases have limited space to expand.
- The contact shot on chest and abdomen are round or oval in shape, massive destruction usually not present as like head because these cavities can accommodate large amount of expelled gas.
- There would be burning inside the wound, smoke and unburnt gunpowder particles will be present inside the wound. The wound will be cherry red in color due to carbon monoxide. The torn parts of the clothing are driven into the wound.
- Exit wound of contact shot may not be present on the head. In other parts of the body, the exit wound will have everted margins and extrusion of tissues. Not all the pellets may come out through the exit wound, many of the pellets may get

TABLE 16.1: Differences between entry wound and exit wound.

Character	Entry wound	Exit wound
Size	Smaller than the diameter of the bullet	Larger
Edges	Inverted	Everted
Abrasion collar and grease collar	Present	Absent
Scorching, smudging and tattooing	May be present	Absent
Bleeding	Less	More
Fat extrusion	Absent	May be present
Atomic absorption spectrometry	Positive	Negative
Cherry red color	May be present	Absent

embedded into the body tissues, especially those pellets which strike on the bones.

Close Shot

- Close shot is for a distance up to 30 cm (up to the range of flame).
- Entry wound is large circular (when fired perpendicularly) or oval (when fired at an angle) in shape surrounded by burning, smudging and tattooing are present. Tattooing is for a few cm in diameter around the entry wound and the pallets enters into the body as a single mass.

Near Shot

- Near shot is for a distance of more than 1 meter and less than 4 meters.
- For a distance of less than 2 meters, the pellets may enter as a single mass producing a round hole (**Rat hole**) with irregular margins.
- After 2 meters the pellets starts dispersion. For a distance of 2 meters, there would be large central hole with a few small individual pellet holes surrounding it.
- As the distance increases, the size of the central hole will decrease more individual pellet holes dispersed around the central entry wound.
- Over 2 meters there is complete dispersion of pellets and no central hole will be present. Burning, smudging and tattooing would be absent. The wad can travel up to 4 meters and may make an abrasion on the skin.

Distant Shot

- Any distance beyond 4 meters is distant shot.
- The dispersion of pellets is complete and each pellet enters the body by making individual holes. The entrance wound is distributed and there is no central hole. The more the distance the more the dispersion of pellets.

- The spread of pellets will be more if the pellets colloid each other while they travel through the air and the shot pattern would simulate longer range. This phenomenon is called "Billiard ball ricochet effect".
- As the distance increase, the velocity of the pellets is reduced and none of the pellet exit out from the body and would be embedded into the body tissues. The more the distance the pellets may be seen just embedded beneath the skin with wide dispersion.

DUM DUM BULLET

It is a type of bullet in which the jacket does not cover the whole of the base; hence there is a tendency for the core to explode leaving the jacket inside the barrel which hinders the loading of the next round.

RICOCHET BULLET

Ricochet effect of bullet:
- When a bullet is fired from the weapon, it gets deflected from its course by striking an intervening object in its way, before striking the target. This is called "Ricochet bullet".
- **Medicolegal importance:** Culpable homicide not amounting to murder if it is proved that the injury is due to ricochet effect of the bullet. Since, the intension is not to kill the affected victim.

TANDEM BULLET

- Tandem bullet is due to "**Piggy back bullet/phenomenon**".
- Due to faulty ammunition like deposition of rust or due to prolonged non-usage of the firearm, the fired bullet may get struck inside the barrel and when the next round is fired, two bullets come out and enter the target through the same entry wound or two different entry wounds as a result back to back firing of the bullet.

SOUVENIR BULLET

- Encapsulation of the bullet inside the body of a victim for a long period.
- The foreign body may get covered within the soft tissues producing slow absorption of the heavy metals, resulting in chronic poisoning.
- This is a rare occurrence.
- The original entrance wound may be seen as a tiny scar in such cases.

FRANGIBLE BULLET

They are bullets designed to fragment upon striking the target, often to the point of total disintegration. They are mostly made up of lead or iron. Chronic heavy metal poisoning in such individuals is common. The object of designing a frangible bullet is to make the recovery and matching with a test bullet difficult. If a bone is penetrated, they are recovered in a deformed state. These bullets do not ricochet inside the body.

WHAT IS KENNEDY PHENOMENON?

- Surgical alteration by suturing and extending the entry/exit wound will create problems in interpretation and evaluation at autopsy.
- This is called as "Kennedy Phenomenon". In this condition, it is difficult to differentiate entry and exit wound of a firearm.

WHAT ARE THE PRIMARY AND SECONDARY MARKINGS ON BULLETS?

When a **Crime bullet** (exhibit bullet) is recovered, it has to be found out which kind of weapon fired the bullet and also the exact weapon from which the bullet was fired. This objective is achieved by checking for primary and secondary markings on the bullet.

- **Primary markings:**
  - These are class characteristics (primary markings) made on the bullet by the manufacturer; which would be in the diameter, numbering and codes imprinted on the metal case of the bullet. Such types of primary markings are also present on the gun, which are the primary principles of identification like:
    - Caliber of the gun
    - Number and width of the rifling groves
    - Direction of rifling groves (left or right twist), etc.
  - These class characteristics of the gun are the specifications of the manufacturer, design and dimensions.
- **Secondary markings on the bullet:**
  - In all rifled firearm, the diameter of the bullet is slightly larger than diameter of the barrel; hence, when the bullet is fired, as it travels through the barrel of the gun, the inner grooves of the barrel leaves its signature on the bullet and are called the secondary markings on the bullet.
  - Identification of the bullet is by the caliber, direction of twists of rifling, rate (number) of groves and width of the groves produced on the bullet by the firing gun.

TESTS FOR GUNSHOT RESIDUES: DERMAL NITRATE TEST; NAA AND AAS (FM3.10)

- **Harrison and Gilroy Test (Dermal nitrate test):** The principle behind this test is that when a weapon is fired some traces of the gunpowder residues gets deposited over the dorsum of the hand close to the index and the thumb fingers. Evidence of presence of gunpowder residues in an individual confirms usage of firearm by him. Dermal nitrate test is performed to find out the presence of antimony, barium and lead.

Neutron Activation Analysis (NAA)

- It's a chemical method to detect even minute traces of elements present in hair, nails, soil, glass pieces, paints, drugs and gunshot residues.
- This test is useful when a comparative sample is available; residues from the suspect's hands are removed by paraffin casting or swabs dipped in 5% nitric acid.
- The atoms of an element present in the specimen are bombarded with neutrons in a nuclear reactor; some of the nuclei of those atoms capture neutrons and they become radioactive. The radioactivity is measured using an analyzer.
- Residues of the primer, antimony and copper are detected by this method.

Atomic Absorption Spectrometry (AAS)

- Used for measurement of antimony, barium and copper in gunshot residues. This test uses high temperature to vaporize the metallic elements of the primer residues to detect and to measure the quantity.
- NAA and AAS are used to:
    - Identify the holes in the clothing, tissues or wood, as whether they were caused by a bullet or not.
    - To find out the range of firearm (concentration of antimony and lead around the bullet entry wound).
    - Determine the common origin of bullet fragments from different places (in shot gun pellets: By the concentration of antimony, arsenic, copper and silver).
    - Find out gunshot residues on the hands, whether the person has fired the gun (presence of lead, antimony and barium in the hands).

MULTIPLE CHOICE QUESTIONS

1. Black gunpowder is composed of all the following, *except:*
    a. Sulfur
    b. Potassium nitrate
    c. Nitrocellulose
    d. Charcoal
2. The following are features of gunshot exit wound, *except:*
    a. Bigger than the entry wound
    b. Everted edges
    c. Protrusion of soft tissues
    d. Singeing and smudging
3. The purpose of choking of a firearm is to:
    a. Prevent the early dispersion of pellets
    b. Minimize sound
    c. Minimize smoke emission
    d. Cause maximum destruction
4. Death by suicidal gunshot wound usually can be confirmed by:
    a. Fingerprint on the gun
    b. Blood on the gun
    c. Gun in hand
    d. Gunshot residues in the hand
5. Punched out inner table and craterlike outer table in the skull means_____
    a. Chop wound
    b. Pond fracture
    c. Entrance wound
    d. Exit wound
6. Presence of wad inside the entrance wound suggests all the following, *except:*
    a. Contact shot
    b. Close shot
    c. Smoothbore firearm
    d. Cannot be homicidal
7. Tandem bullet is:
    a. Where nose is cut off
    b. Back to back fired bullet
    c. Is seen in case of defective weapon
    d. Present in body for long time
8. What is paradox gun?
    a. A shot gun with smooth barrel
    b. A shot gun whose muzzle end is rifled
    c. A shot gun whose muzzle wider
    d. A rifle that fires a single ball

9. Gunshot residue on hands can be detected by:
   a. Phenolphthalein test
   b. Dermal nitrate test
   c. Benzidine test
   d. Hydrogen activation analysis
10. In which of the following weapons empty cartridge case is ejected after firing?
    a. Short gun
    b. Revolver
    c. Pistol
    d. Rifle
11. In firearm injury, entry wound blackening is due to:
    a. Flame
    b. Hot gases
    c. Smoke
    d. Unburnt powder
12. Blackening and tattooing of skin and clothing can be best demonstrated by:
    a. Luminol spray
    b. Infrared photography
    c. Ultraviolet light
    d. Magnifying lens
13. A stellate wound is produced when the projectile is discharged at a distance of:
    a. Contact range
    b. Close range (up to 1 meter)
    c. Near range (up to 4 meters)
    d. Long range (above 4 meters)
14. Caliber of a rifled firearm is calculated by:
    a. Distance between a land and a groove
    b. Distance between two diagonally opposite lands
    c. Distance between two diagonally opposite grooves
    d. The number of lead balls that could be made from one pound of lead
15. Bullet that fragments on impact is called:
    a. Duplex bullet
    b. Dum-dum bullet
    c. Frangible bullet
    d. Soft point bullet
16. In a firearm injury, there is burning, blackening, tattooing around the wound and is circular in shape is a:
    a. Close shot
    b. Close contact shot
    c. Contact shot
    d. Distant shot
17. Brain of the cartridge is:
    a. Gunpowder
    b. Projectile
    c. Primer
    d. Wad
18. All are tests for detection of metals around entry wound is done by all, *except*:
    a. Harrison and Glory test
    b. Atomic absorption spectrometry
    c. Neutron activation analysis
    d. Paraffin test
19. In blast injuries, the most common internal organ to be affected is:
    a. Eardrum
    b. Stomach
    c. Lungs
    d. Liver
20. Terminal ballistics refers to:
    a. Study of behavior of the missile once it penetrates the target
    b. Study of the effects of missile on the living tissue
    c. Study of ammunition
    d. Study of muzzle end of a barrel
21. Not a part of firearm:
    a. Breech
    b. Piston
    c. Barrel
    d. Muzzle
22. Not a constituent of a cartridge:
    a. Primer
    b. Propellant
    c. Projectile
    d. Lubricant
23. Function of wad in the shotgun cartridge is:
    a. Sealing effect
    b. To prevent dissipation of gases
    c. To keep gunpowder and shots in place
    d. All of the above
24. Ratio of semi-smokeless gunpowder is:
    a. 50% Black powder: 50% smokeless powder
    b. 75% Black powder: 25% smokeless powder
    c. 80% Black powder: 20% smokeless powder
    d. 70% Black powder: 30% smokeless powder
25. Priming mixture constitutes all, *except*:
    a. Barium nitrate
    b. Lead styphnate
    c. Antimony sulfide
    d. Charcoal

SECTION 4: Forensic Traumatology

26. Surgical alteration or suturing of gunshot wounds create problems in interpretation of gunshot wounds. This is called as:
    a. Formication phenomenon
    b. Gordon phenomenon
    c. Cookie cutter phenomenon
    d. Kennedy phenomenon
27. A case of homicide with gunshot was reported and bullet was recovered from the body. Primary and secondary markings on the bullet can be used for:
    a. Identification of weapon
    b. Range of firing
    c. Severity of tissue damage
    d. Time of crime
28. In a firearm injury, singeing seen around the entry wound is due to:
    a. Flame
    b. Smoke
    c. Unburnt powder
    d. Hot gases
29. In a firearm injury, blackening seen around the entry wound is due to:
    a. Flame
    b. Smoke
    c. Unburnt powder
    d. Hot gases
30. Tattooing in entry wound of a firearm injury is due to:
    a. Burns
    b. Smoke
    c. Gunpowder
    d. Wads
31. A man was found with suicidal gunshot on right temple with the gun in his right hand. The skull was burst open. There was charring and cherry red coloration in the track inside. Range of the shot is:
    a. Contact shot
    b. Close shot at a distance of 1 feet
    c. Shot within range of 2 feet
    d. Shot within range of 3 feet
32. Tattooing around the entry wound is seen in:
    a. Contact shot
    b. Near shot
    c. Distant shot
    d. All of the above

ANSWERS

1. c	2. d	3. a	4. d	5. d	6. d	7. b	8. b	9. b	10. c
11. c	12. b	13. a	14. b	15. c	16. a	17. c	18. d	19. a	20. a
21. b	22. d	23. d	24. c	25. d	26. d	27. a	28. a	29. d	30. c
31. a	32. b								

17
CHAPTER

Electrical and Lightening Injuries

KEY WORDS

Electrocution, joule burns, ventricular fibrillation, lightening, filigree burns, entry wound, exit wound, flash burns, spark burns.

FM2.5 Describe types of injuries, clinical features, pathophysiology, postmortem findings and medico-legal aspects in cases of burns, scalds, lightening, electrocution and radiations.

INTRODUCTION

Electrocution (Pathophysiology) (FM2.5)

- Deaths due to electrocution are relatively common in domestic and industrial settings. It is mainly due to carelessness or improper knowledge about electrical appliances and electricity. Death due to electrocution is most commonly accidental.
- Injuries produced on the body depends upon:
  - *Kind of electric current:* Both direct current (DC) and alternate current (AC) can produce deleterious effects. Alternate current is 5 to 6 times more dangerous than direct current of the same voltage, since AC results in titanic stimulation which induces muscle spasm and does not allow the patient to release contact of current.
  - *The amount of current:* Electrocution is rare below 100 volts. Domestic supply is between 220 to 240 volts in the form of alternating current at 50 cycles per second.
  - *Path of the current inside the body:* When current flows through the heart or brain, death is imminent. Severity is directly proportional to the duration of flow. Current takes the easiest path inside the body and not the shortest path.
- **Mode of electrocution:** For electric shock to occur there must be contact of the body with both positive and negative pole or alternatively, the earth; when earthing of the body is poor (when the individual stands on a wooden platform) fatal electrocution is uncommon, he may

experience only a shock and he can get himself released from the contact source.
- The effects of electricity depend upon the resistance offered by the body.

Electric Burns Injury ("Joule Burn") (FM2.5)

- The injury produced on the body is due to resistance offered by the body tissues. Electrical burns injuries are usually present at the point of entry and also at the point of exit shown in **Figures 17.1 and 17.2** respectively. They are absent when the hands and feet were wet. Since wetness allows the current to flow easily into the body, as the resistance offered by the body tissues is greatly reduced by wetness.

Joule Burn

- Round or oval shallow craters of 1 to 3 cm in diameter. The floor looks pale, depressed and sometimes burnt, hard to touch, usually extending into the underlying deep tissues to some extent; surrounded by an elevated hyperemic margins which are visible after thorough washing and viewed with hand lens in good light. The extent of tissue involvement can be made out easily by dissection. If hairs are present at the point of contact it appears burnt and singed. When the period of contact is prolonged charring and blackening are also seen.
- This characteristic appearance will not be seen in any other types of injury. The exit wound is almost similar to the entry wound in appearance but less hard; blackening and singing of hair are usually absent at the point of exit.
- When a larger area of the body comes in contact with a broad bare wire, then long and linear injuries are produced. In such cases, the clothing also catches fire and whole body may catch fire and get burnt in a short span of time. These cases may be presented as case of death due to burns.
- Difficulty arises only when the entry and exit wound are absent.

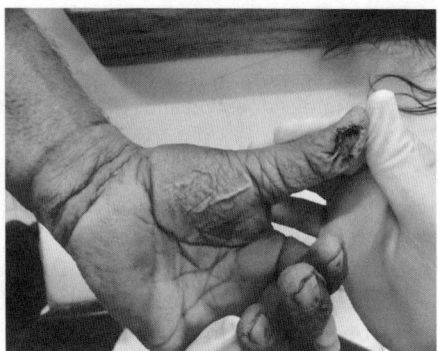

Fig. 17.1: Electrical entry wound on the hands *(For color version see Plate 14).*

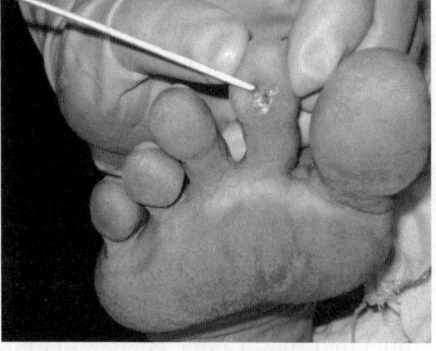

Fig. 17.2: Electrical exit wound on the sole of foot *(For color version see Plate 14).*

What is the Mechanism of Death in Electrocution? (FM2.5)

- When current enters the body through the point of contact, it travels along the body to the contact point of exit. When it passes through the heart, it produces conduction defects, leading to increase in the heart rate. This leads to ventricular tachycardia and death may ensure in a short span of time due to ventricular fibrillation. When

the passage of current is through the brain, death may result due to paralysis of respiratory center.
- Passage of current for a short duration may not result in death of the individuals, however, the patient may develop a stage of suspended animation which simulates death. Strict caution is required in declaring death in such situation to avoid any premature certification of death. Timely resuscitation measures will help in reviving this condition.

WHAT IS FLASH BURN/SPARK BURN?

It occurs in high voltage electricity. Direct contact is not required in such instances. When there is a gap between the source of electricity and the body, the intense heat results in flash-over and produce thermal burns. Usually there will be deposition of trace metallic particles over the burnt surface, which is transferred from the metallic wire.

POSTMORTEM FINDINGS IN ELECTROCUTION (FM2.5)

External Autopsy Findings

Entry wound in the form of **joule burn** and exit wound are usually present, except when the contact surface is wet.

Internal Autopsy Findings

- *Heart:* Multiple sub-epicardial and sub-endocardial petechial hemorrhages in the heart more on the left ventricle and also on the root of aorta is seen. In doubtful circumstances bits from left ventricle can be subjected for Histopathological examination. This reveals elongation of the myocardial fibers, with movement of nucleus towards the periphery of the cell, as current flows through the heart and compensatory vacuolization on the opposite end of the cell due to sudden movement of the nucleus towards the direction of current flow. Peticho-ecchymotic hemorrhage on the surface of left ventricle of heart—a case of death due to electrocution shown in **Figure 17.3**.
- *Lungs:* Multiple sub-pleural petechial hemorrhages on the surface of both lungs, more concentrated on the inter-lobar surface (pleura offers some resistance when current travels from one lobe to another). Intraventricular hemorrhage in electrocution depicted in **Figure 17.4**.
- All the internal organs will be congested.

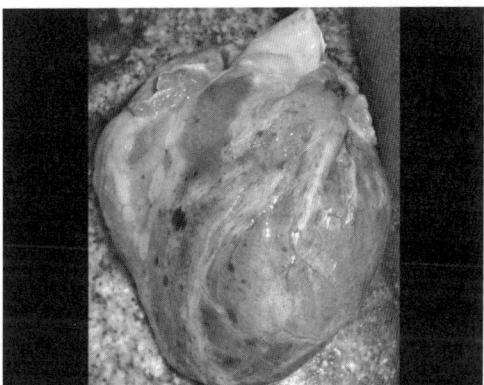

Fig. 17.3: Peticho-ecchymotic hemorrhage on the surface of left ventricle of heart—a case of death due to electrocution *(For color version see Plate 14).*

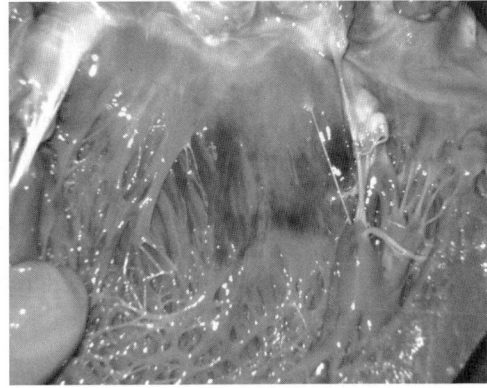

Fig. 17.4: Intraventricular hemorrhage in electrocution *(For color version see Plate 15).*

- **Note:** When entry and exit wounds are present on the body, cause of death can be opined without any ambiguity. In the absence of visible external findings, opinion about death due to electrocution can be construed, based on the internal findings of the heart, lungs and histopathological observations. An attempt to visit the scene of occurrence will also help in forming a clear opinion about the cause of death in such cases.

INTRODUCTION OF LIGHTENING

- Lightening is a phenomenon which occurs due to generation of very high voltage current from the clouds which is transmitted to the earth through a medium like trees, or high raised buildings or tall metallic poles. The transmission of electricity from the clouds to the earth is called as lightening stroke.
- Lightening chooses the easiest but not the shortest route and hence it sometimes takes a wandering, zigzag path.
- The lightening stroke has a potential of 1000 million volts, and when it passes through the body, results in lethal electrocution.
- Lightening differs from electrocution only in degree of electric current. Skin and dry clothes are relatively bad conductors than wet skin and wet clothes. The effects of lightning are similar to that of electrocution but the severity is high. The body and clothing may be completely burnt. Linear burns of 3 to 30 cm length and 0.6 to 2.5 cm in breath can be seen, usually in moist areas of the body.
- The external appearance in case of death due to lightening is the presence of filigree burns (arborescent burns).

Filigree Burns (Lichtenberg Figures) (FM2.5)

- It is otherwise called as arborescent burns.
- It is a superficial, thin, irregular, tortuous marking on the skin. They resemble the branching pattern of a tree or fern leaf.
- This is usually mistaken for the marbling appearance found on decomposed bodies. Filigree burns are brownish black in color as compared to the bluish green discolouration in marbling. Difficulty may arise in differentiating marbling appearance from filigree burns especially when the body is recovered after a few days.

What are Surface Burns?

These are burns produced due to heating up of metallic objects worn or carried by the individual; when lightening strikes the body, these metallic objects generate enormous heat and produce surface burns on the body. Sometimes, the object becomes magnetized which can be ascertained by pocket compass.

Associated Findings of Lightening

- Clothes may be torn and burnt.
- Shoes may burst open.
- Rupture of tympanic membrane often present.
- Burns injuries may extend deep into subcutaneous tissues, muscles or bones.
- Petechial hemorrhages may be seen in spinal cord and brain. On HPE, chromatolysis and fragmentation of axons can be made out.

MULTIPLE CHOICE QUESTIONS

1. **Which one of the following causes "joule burns":**
   a. Lightening
   b. Electrocution
   c. Radiation injury
   d. Thermal injury
2. **Arborescent burns is caused by:**
   a. Physical force
   b. Hot flame
   c. Radiation
   d. Electricity
3. **A dead body is found to have marks like branching of a tree on front of chest. The most likely cause of death could be due to:**
   a. Firearm
   b. Lightening injury
   c. Injuries due to bomb blast
   d. Road traffic accident
4. **Filigree burns are:**
   a. Lightening burns
   b. Thermal burns
   c. Chemical burns
   d. Radiation burns
5. **Electrocution is rare below:**
   a. 100 volts
   b. 150 volts
   c. 200 volts
   d. 240 volts

ANSWERS

1. b   2. d   3. b   4. a   5. a

SECTION 5

Sexual Jurisprudence

SECTION OUTLINE

Chapter 18: Virginity
Chapter 19: Impotence, Sterility and Artificial Insemination
Chapter 20: Pregnancy and Delivery
Chapter 21: Abortion and MTP Act 1971
Chapter 22: Infant Deaths
Chapter 23: Sexual Offences and Paraphilias

18

CHAPTER

Virginity

 KEY WORDS

Virginity, labia majora, labia minora, fourchette, rugosity, virgin, false virgin, defloration, carunculae hymenalis, carunculae myrtiformis.

FM3.18 Describe anatomy of male and female genitalia, hymen and its types. Discuss the medico-legal importance of hymen. Define virginity, defloration, legitimacy and its medico-legal importance.

INTRODUCTION

For proper medico-legal examination and certification in cases relating to virginity, pregnancy, delivery, abortion and sexual offences good knowledge of anatomy of the female genital organs is mandatory and hence, anatomy of the female genital organs are discussed in brief.

DESCRIBE THE ANATOMY OF FEMALE GENITAL ORGANS? (FM3.18)

- The labia majora are two elongated folds of skin projecting downwards and backwards from the mons veneris; they meet together in the front in the anterior commissure and on the back in the posterior commissure (in front of the anus).
- In a virgin, the labia majora are thick, firm, elastic and rounded, and lie in close apposition with each other and thus completely close the vaginal orifice.
- The labia minora are two thin folds of skin, just within the labia majora, not usually visualized externally in a virgin; the lower portion of the labia minora fuse in midline and forms the fourchette; the depression between the fourchette and the vaginal orifice is called the fossa navicularis.
- The labia minora are soft, pink in color and sensitive to touch.
- The vaginal canal is a pocket like structure, triangular in shape about 7.5 cm long; shorter in its anterior wall (6 cm) and longer in its posterior wall (9 cm). The mucosa of the vaginal canal is reddish in color, with multiple folds of rugosity and the walls are well approximated.
- Frequent sexual intercourse makes the vaginal canal more elongated, up to the posterior fornix, with loss of rugosity; a

single intercourse does not alter the parts much except for rupture of the hymen and elongation of the posterior vaginal wall.
- In the women who have undergone full term pregnancy and delivery, the labia majora will be separated, exposing the labia minora and the vaginal canal.

WHAT IS VIRGINITY? (FM3.18)

- Virginity is a state of a female who has not experienced sexual intercourse even once.
- Virginity is otherwise called as "**chastity**" or "**virgo intacta**".
- Defloration means loss of virginity, which means the female has experienced sexual intercourse at least once.
- The question of virginity may arise in situations like rape, nullity of marriage and divorce.

WHAT IS HYMEN? WHAT ARE THE TYPES OF HYMEN? (FM3.18)

- Hymen is a thin fold of mucus membrane about 1 mm in thickness and situated at the vaginal outlet; adult hymen consists of folds of membrane having crescentic or annular shape.
- In children, the hymen appears as a tight membrane and lies relatively at a higher level in the vaginal canal. It descends to the lower level (normal level) with the formation of series of folds, when the woman attains menarche.
- The hymen has a central orifice, which usually does not admit more than the tip of the little finger in a virgin and this opening is for the menstrual flow.
- Depending on the size and shape, the hymen is classified into the following types.

Types of Hymen

- **Semilunar or crescentic:** Semilunar in shape and the opening is placed anteriorly.
- **Annular:** The opening is oval or circular and is situated near the center.
- **Infantile:** A small linear opening in the middle.
- **Cribriform:** Consists of several opening.
- **Vertical:** Opening is vertical.
- **Septate:** Two lateral openings side by side, separated by a thin strip of tissue.
- **Imperforate hymen:** In this type the hymenal orifice is absent. At the time of attainment of menarche, there will be gradual accumulation of menstrual blood, which makes the hymen bulging with severe lower abdominal pain. In such situations, a small incision is made to create hymenal opening, through which the accumulated menstrual blood is let out.
- **Fimbriated or notched:** The edges of the hymenal orifice show multiple small projections in its circumference.

WHAT ARE THE PRINCIPAL SIGNS OF VIRGINITY? (FM3.18)

- Breasts are hemispherical, firm and rounded. Nipples are small with pinkish areola.
- Labia majora appears thick, firm and rounded; fleshy and elastic. Lies in close opposition to each other and hence the labia minora and the vaginal orifice are not visible externally.
- Labia minora is soft and small in size; pink in color and sensitive to touch and not visible externally, since it is completely covered by labia majora.
- The vagina is narrow and tight; triangular in cross section. Rugosity is more prominent, its walls can be approximated, the vaginal canal is not roomy and the vaginal orifice remains closed. The orifice admits only the tip of the little finger and is painful. The hymen, posterior commissure, fossa navicularis and fourchette will be intact in virgins.

CHAPTER 18: Virginity

VIRGINITY VS DEFLORATION

Table 18.1 is depicted the differences between virgin and deflorated woman.

WHAT ARE THE CAUSES OF RUPTURE OF HYMEN?

- Hymen may be ruptured due to:
    - Sexual intercourse

TABLE 18.1: Difference between virgin and deflorated woman.

Virgin woman	Deflorated woman
Breast: Hemispherical Firm and rounded Nipples are small and pinkish *Areola:* Pink in color	Enlarged Loses firmness and slightly pendulous Nipples are large and raised *Areola:* Dark brown or black
Labia majora: ➢ Thick and firm ➢ Fleshy, elastic and rounded ➢ Lie in opposition to each other and hence labia minora is not visible externally ➢ Completely closes the vaginal orifice	➢ Lax ➢ Not rounded and dark in color ➢ Not in opposition with each other and labia minora is exposed outside ➢ Gap is present in between the two sides, and the vaginal orifice may be visible externally
Labia minora: ➢ Soft and small in size ➢ Pink, sensitive to touch and completely covered by labia majora ➢ Depression is present in between the fourchette and the vaginal orifice ➢ Vaginal orifice remains closed	➢ Enlarged ➢ Dark or blackened in color and may also show pigmentation ➢ Project much outside the labia majora, the depression and folds are lost ➢ Vaginal orifice is visible externally
Vagina: ➢ Narrow and tight ➢ The canal is triangular in cross section ➢ Rugosity is present and sensitive to touch ➢ Its walls are approximated, ➢ Not capacious	➢ Widened and loose ➢ The canal is oval or rounded in cross section ➢ Rugosity is decreased/lost and sensitiveness is reduced ➢ Walls are not approximated and are separated ➢ Roomy and spacious
Vestibule: Admits tip of little finger and painful	Admits more than two fingers without pain
Posterior commissure: Intact in virgins	Loose or not prominent due to repeated sexual intercourse in deflorated woman
Fossa navicularis: Closed/intact in virgins	Disappear in deflorated woman
Fourchette: Intact in virgins	Ruptured and old healed tear/scaring may be present
Hymen is intact	Hymen ruptured and only remnants of tags of the hymen may be present along the margins after multiple acts of coitus

- *Accidental:* Heavy exercise like cycling, gymnastics, etc.
- *Masturbation:* Using fingers or foreign body insertion.
- *Ulceration:* From diphtheria, repeated fungal infection.
- Rarely by uncleanliness, poor personal hygiene and sanitary tampons.
- Surgical and gynecological operations.
- There are a number of reasons for rupture of hymen other than sexual intercourse. Ruptured hymen cannot be said as a sign of defloration. The same way, an intact hymen is not a proof of virginity, as the hymen may be elastic and the female is as a false virgin.

WHO IS A FALSE VIRGIN?

False virgin is a female who has experienced sexual intercourse, but retains an intact hymen. In few females, the hymen may remain intact even after multiple acts of coitus; this is due to elastic, thick, tough, fleshy or loose hymen.

MEDICO-LEGAL IMPORTANCE OF HYMEN/VIRGINITY (FM3.18)

- The presence of an intact hymen at the time of marriage is considered to be proof of virginity by the society and the law.
- Presence of an intact hymen is presumed to be a sign of virginity, but is not an absolute proof (false virgin). Similarly, a ruptured hymen may not necessarily be due to an act of coitus.

Medico-legal Importance of Virginity

- **Nullity of marriage:** (S-12 Hindu Marriage Act)
  - If the woman was pregnant at the time of marriage or the male was already married/impotent, then the marriage is said to be null.
- **Divorce:** (S-13 Hindu Marriage Act)
  - If either of the couple is proved to have a committed the offence of adultery, then it is a ground for divorce.

CARUNCLUNAE HYMENALIS AND CARUNCLUNAE MYRTIFORMIS

Carunclunae Hymenalis

Multiple ruptures of hymen with presence of tags of the hymenal tissue on the margins. It is seen in woman habituated to sexual intercourse.

Carunclunae Myrtiformis

In this condition, hymen is almost abolished, with remnants of hymenal tissues attached to the margins, as a thick rim of residual tissue. This is seen after pregnancy and delivery.

MULTIPLE CHOICE QUESTIONS

1. **'Carunculae myrtiformes' on hymen is:**
   a. Seen after pregnancy
   b. Seen after rape
   c. Sign of virginity
   d. Seen after vaginoplasty
2. **False virgin is one who:**
   a. Has never taken part in sexual intercourse
   b. Retains an intact hymen even after multiple sexual intercourse
   c. Congenital absence of hymen
   d. Is a virgin but hymen is torn
3. **Medico-legal importance of fimbriated hymen:**
   a. Hymen lies at a lower level for easy examination
   b. There is no central opening for menstrual blood to be let out
   c. Implies the female is used to masturbation
   d. Is a virgin but looks like a deflorated woman

ANSWERS

1. a   2. b   3. d

CHAPTER 19

Impotence, Sterility and Artificial Insemination

 KEY WORDS

Impotence, sterility, frigidity, quad, vaginismus, sterilization, artificial insemination, posthumous child, test tube baby, atavism, paternity, legitimacy, surrogate motherhood.

FM3.22 Define and discuss impotence, sterility, frigidity, sexual dysfunction, premature ejaculation. Discuss the causes of impotence and sterility in male and female.

FM3.23 Discuss sterilization of male and female, artificial insemination, test tube baby, surrogate mother, hormonal replacement therapy with respect to appropriate national and state laws.

DEFINE IMPOTENCE? (FM3.22)

- Impotence is the inability to perform or take part in sexual intercourse by a male.
- In the act of sexual intercourse male is the active partner, who has to develop and maintain penile erection sufficient enough to accomplish the act.

WHAT IS STERILITY? (FM3.22)

- Sterility is the inability to procreate by a male or conceive children in a female.
- An impotent person may be fertile and capable of procreating; similarly, a potent individual capable of performing intercourse may not be able fertilize, due to defective production of sperms.

WHAT IS PREMATURE EJACULATION? (FM3.22)

It is a condition in which ejaculation of semen occurs before the complete act of coitus, either immediately before or immediately after penetration.

WHAT IS SEXUAL DYSFUNCTION? (FM3.22)

- Any defect either structurally or functionally, which makes the person unable to achieve sexual gratification, is termed as "sexual dysfunction".
- A person is said to physiologically impotent at the extremes of age. Same way, after several years of marriage a male

may be impotent towards his wife, but potent towards many other females; this is also a form of physiological impotence.

DESCRIBE THE CAUSES OF IMPOTENCE IN MALE? (FM3.22)

Organic Causes (Congenital)

- Klinefelter's syndrome and primary testicular failure, mainly cryptorchidism.
- Phimosis, paraphimosis, epispadias, hypospadias, accessory penis and bent nail syndrome.

Acquired Causes

- Partial or complete amputation of penis.
- Prepubertal castration.
- **Local diseases:** Large hydrocele, scrotal filariasis, gonorrhea and carcinoma of the penis.
- **General diseases:** Diabetes, PT and endocrine disorders.

Neurological Causes

- Paralysis of the motor nerves supplying the genitalia, autonomic neuropathy, tumors of cauda equina, lesions in the CNS or spinal cord.
- **Hemiparesis or paraplegia:** Either due to trauma or cerebrovascular accident (CVA), general paralysis of insane (GPI in tertiary syphilis) and drugs.

WHAT ARE THE FUNCTIONAL CAUSES OF IMPOTENCE? (FM3.22)

Functional Causes

- They are predominantly psychogenic in nature.
  - First night impotence or bridegroom impotence:
    - Fear, timidity and anxiety are responsible.
- *Impotentia quad persona:* In this condition a man is impotent towards a particular woman. He is potent with others.
- *Sexual aversion disorder:* Persistent or recurrent aversion, thus avoid genital sexual contact with a woman.
- Excessive passion and overindulgence.

WHAT IS FRIGIDITY? WHAT ARE THE CAUSES OF FRIGIDITY IN A FEMALE? (FM3.22)

Frigidity

- Sexual unresponsiveness in females is called frigidity: it is similar to that of impotence in males.
- In frigidity, there is inability to initiate or maintain sexual arousal pattern.
- It may be considered as absence of desire for sexual intercourse.
- The true meaning of frigidity means abnormal aversion towards sexual intercourse.

Causes of Frigidity

- Sedatives or depressant drugs.
- Local diseases
- Systemic diseases: Hypothyroidism.
- Physiological causes: Prepuberty and menopause state.
- Psychological causes: Vaginismus.
  - Frigidity may be temporary or permanent. Temporary frigidity always manifest as female sexual aversion disorder. It may be due to vaginismus.

Vaginismus

Hyperesthesia leading to painful spasm of sphincter muscles and levator ani with simultaneous contraction of adductor muscles of the thigh and erector spinae making penetration impossible.

Dyspareunia

- There is severe pain in the lower abdomen and perineum at the time of coitus.
- Permanent frigidity is invariably psychogenic in nature, which results due to sexual abuse during childhood or traumatic sexual assault in adulthood.

DEFINE INFERTILITY: WHAT ARE THE CAUSES OF ABSOLUTE INFERTILITY? (FM3.22)

Infertility means incapability of fertilization or reproduction.

Absolute Infertility

- Inability to conceive due to structural or functional defects in the genital organs; which is complete and irreversible.
- **Relative infertility:** Diminished capacity to produce offspring, which can be rectified.

Causes of absolute infertility in females are:
- Congenital defects (defect in uterus, cervix or fallopian tubes).
- Acquired causes (infection and surgery on uterus).
- Hormonal dysfunction.
- Chromosomal defects (Turner's syndrome).
- Local conditions like recto-vaginal fistula.
- Chronic poisoning (like arsenic and lead).

DEFINE STERILIZATION; MEDICO-LEGAL ISSUES OF STERILIZATION?

What is "Wrongful Conception"? (FM3.23)

- Sterilization is a procedure which makes a person sterile, without affecting his/her potency or sexual function.
- Medico-legal importance of sterilization:
  - Failure of sterilization in a male may result in the wife becoming pregnant this leads to suspecting the fidelity of the wife, which in turn leads to situations like divorce, legitimacy of the child and disputed paternity.
  - Failure of sterilization in is the most common basis for the birth related actions called "**wrongful conception**" or "wrongful pregnancy" which may bring conflicts in the life between the husband and wife as suspicion of adultery (if husband is sterilized) and if the female has been sterilized then doctor who performed the surgery may have to bear the expenditure cost of the child growth as it is an unwanted child in their family.
  - Doctor may be implicated if he/she perform sterilization without proper indication.
  - Healthy unmarried individuals and married individuals, who don't have any siblings, should not be permanently sterilized even if they volunteer for the same.

DESCRIBE ARTIFICIAL INSEMINATION; WHAT ARE THE INDICATIONS OF AI? WHAT ARE THE ETHICAL AND LEGAL ISSUES OF AI? (FM3.23)

- It is a method of assisted reproductive technique, by which healthy semen is deposited into the vagina, cervix or uterus by instruments to bring about pregnancy. There are three types:
  1. Artificial insemination homologues (AIH)
  2. Artificial insemination donor (AID)
  3. Artificial insemination homologues donor (AIHD): ***Pooled semen***

Indications

- When the husband is impotent but fertile (AIH, AIHD).
- When the husband is sterile (AID, AIHD).
- Rh incompatibility (AID).
- When the husband is suffering from hereditary diseases (AID).

Guiding Principles (Ethical Issues)

- Informed consent of both spouses has to be obtained after explaining the procedure, its legal implications, etc.
- The identity of the donor and recipient must not be revealed to each other nor do the donors know the result of insemination.
- Donor must be below 40 years, preferably married, not related to either spouse and should have children of their own.
- The donor must be in good health, both physically and mentally.
- There must be similarity of race, religion and morphological appearance (as much as possible) between the donor and the husband of the recipient.
- It is better and advisable the physician who performs artificial insemination, avoid delivery of the child.

Legal Issues of Artificial Insemination

- Informed written consent of both the spouses donor and recipient. Improper consent would make the doctor face charges.
- **Legitimacy:** In cases of AID the husband is not the actual father of the child and therefore the child is illegitimate and the child has to be legally adopted.
- **Inheritance of property:** The child born of artificial insemination has to be legally adopted to inherit the property.
- **Natural birth:** If parents do not declare AI, child remains to be natural child for practical purposes.
- Unmarried woman/widow can procure child through AI but the status remains illegitimate.
- Litigation relating to nullity of marriage, divorce may rarely arise.

WHAT IS LEGITIMACY? (FM3.23)

- It is a legal status of a child or a person, born out of lawful wedlock. It includes children born to biological parents only. Persons born during the tenure of legal marriage or within 280 days of dissolution of marriage of the legally wedded couple.
- Legal Issues in relation to legitimacy are inheritance of property and use of title (of the husband of the mother) by the child.

Who is an Illegitimate Child? (FM3.23)

- Any child which is not born out of lawful wedlock is considered as illegitimate. A child is said to be illegitimate, if it is born out of extramarital relationship or through AID.
- Issues of legitimacy arise when the wife delivers a child when husband is sterile; or born when wife had no access to her husband during the probable period of conception.

What is Atavism?

- It is a condition in which the biological offspring does not resemble its parents, but resembles their grandparents. This is due to the presence of genes (recessive genes) which failed to express in the father but present in the child (Mendel's law of mutation).
- Paternal disputes are sorted out by HLA typing (up to 95% accuracy).
- Due to recent advances in DNA analysis they are concluded with 100% certainty.

Who is a Posthumous Child?

Any child born to a mother, within the period of gestation after the death of the husband, that means, if a child born within 280 days after the death of the biological father is a posthumous child. Legal issues arising out of posthumous child are inheritance of property, legitimacy and compensation.

WHAT IS TEST TUBE BABY? (FM3.23)

- **In-vitro fertilization** is test tube baby.
- It is a method of facilitating fertilization of the ovum and spermatozoa, outside the womb. It is adopted when the uterus is not conducive for the process of fertilization, to occur on its own.
- This is a process by which the ovum are surgically removed from the women, fertilized with the available sperms in a petri dish and the resultant embryo is implanted into the womb of the woman, who completes the pregnancy to its full term.

DISCUSS SURROGATE MOTHERHOOD (FM3.23)

It is a condition in which a woman agrees to bear the child for someone else on contractual basis.

Methods

- By way of artificial insemination.
- By fertilization of a mature healthy ovum of the wife with husband's sperm and implanting the embryo into the hired woman's (surrogate's) womb.

Types of Surrogacy

- **Full surrogacy:** Situation where the embryo is provided by the commissioning couple.
- **Partial surrogacy:** When the carrying woman has her own egg fertilized outside and later implanted into the uterus.

Indications for Surrogate Motherhood

- Inability of the wife to conceive or carry the child to term.
- Genetic defects or inherited diseases.
- Wife does not wish to take time to carry the fetus through.
- Wife may suffer from anxiety or labor phobia.

Medico-legal Aspects

- **Consent:** Written informed consent of the deserving couple and the surrogate mother.
- Custody of child is to legal parents.
- For the entire period, surrogate mother has to be given expenses for diet and medicines.
- **Adoption of the child:** After delivery by the surrogate mother, the child has to be legally adopted by the couple to make the child legitimate.

MULTIPLE CHOICE QUESTIONS

1. **"Quod" is a term which denotes an individual who is:**
   a. Absolutely impotent
   b. Relatively impotent
   c. Selectively impotent
   d. Impotent and sterile
2. **Posthumous child means child born within ____ days of death of biological father:**
   a. 120 days
   b. 280 days
   c. 310 days
   d. 1 year
3. **Atavism is useful in disputes of determination of:**
   a. Race
   b. Age
   c. Sex
   d. Paternity

SECTION 5: Sexual Jurisprudence

4. **The cause of sterility in the male includes:**
   a. Caude equina syndrome
   b. Excessive tranquilization
   c. Loss of both testicles
   d. Tabes dorsalis
5. **Body fluid not responsible for the transmission of HIV:**
   a. Semen
   b. CSF
   c. Tears
   d. Breast milk
6. **Which of the following has more HIV load?**
   a. Urine
   b. Sweat
   c. Breast milk
   d. Saliva
7. **The first test tube baby in India was:**
   a. Durga (Kanupriya Agarwal)
   b. Bhavani (Sumungala Agarwal)
   c. Karthiyani (Shakthi Agarwal)
   d. Shwetambari (Kaamya Agarwal)
8. **Infertility can be defined as inability to conceive after:**
   a. 3 years of marriage
   b. 2 years of unprotected sexual intercourse
   c. 1 year of unprotected sexual intercourse
   d. 1 year of marriage
9. **Surrogacy in which baby's biological mother is the surrogate is called:**
   a. Altruistic surrogacy
   b. Commercial surrogacy
   c. Traditional surrogacy
   d. Gestational surrogacy
10. **All are steps of GIFT, *except*:**
    a. Ovulation stimulation
    b. Fertilization of oocyte in lab
    c. Oocyte retrieval
    d. Transfer of unfertilized eggs into the fallopian tube
11. **Quoad hoc means:**
    a. Medically impotent
    b. Legally impotent
    c. Impotent towards all women
    d. Impotent towards a particular woman
12. **Frigidity is:**
    a. Inability to initiate sexual arousal in female
    b. Inability to initiate sexual arousal in male
    c. Ejaculation occurring immediately after penetration
    d. Inability to conceive with particular male
13. **Test to differentiate between psychological and organic erectile dysfunction:**
    a. Pharmacologically induced penile erection therapy
    b. Nocturnal penile tumescence
    c. Sildenafil induced erection
    d. Squeeze technique
14. **Homologous sperm in IVF is:**
    a. Between donor and wife
    b. Between husband and wife
    c. Between husband and surrogate
    d. Between donor and surrogate

ANSWERS

1. c   2. b   3. d   4. c   5. c   6. c   7. a   8. c   9. c   10. b
11. d   12. a   13. b   14. b

CHAPTER 20

Pengancy and Delivery

 KEY WORDS

Pregnancy, delivery, pseudocyesis, fetus compressus, superfetation, superfecundation, lochia, suppositious child, nulliparous and multiparous uterus, concealment of birth.

FM3.19	Discuss the medico-legal aspects of pregnancy and delivery, signs of pregnancy, precipitate labor, superfetation, superfecundation and signs of recent and remote delivery in living and dead.
FM3.20	Discuss disputed paternity and maternity.

INTRODUCTION

Pregnancy

- Pregnancy is a physiological state, which occurs in a woman due to fertilization of the ovum by a spermatozoa and subsequent embedding of the fertilized ovum into the uterine cavity; it occurs during the reproductive age period of the female.
- Fertilization occurs in the isthmus of fallopian tubes and later on the products of conception get impregnated into the uterus.
- Fertilized ovum is called as zygote; after impregnation into the uterus it is called the embryo; from 9th week till term it is called as fetus.
- Pregnancy continues normally for 10 lunar months/40 weeks (9 calendar months + 7 days from the day of last menstruation).

WHAT ARE THE MEDICO-LEGAL ASPECTS OF PREGNANCY? (FM3.19)

Criminal Cases

- Pregnancy is considered as a valid ground for reducing capital punishment, when convicted of capital crime (Section: 416 IPC).
- A woman can plead for postponement of trial if she is pregnant.
- When pregnancy is claimed to be the result of rape, kidnapping and seduction, then this pregnancy is helpful to prove the crime and such pregnancies can be legally terminated under MTP Act 1971.
- Pregnancy in an unmarried girl of 16 years or less, and in a married woman of 15 years or less point towards commission of rape.
- Charge of breach of trust is filed if the female becomes pregnant and the man refuses to marry her.

- **Blackmailing:** A pregnant woman may force a man to marry her or pay compensation as she is pregnant and alleges that the pregnancy is due to sexual intercourse with that man.
- **Adultery:** When pregnancy has resulted due to sexual intercourse with a third person.
- Abortion or concealment of birth cases can be brought against a woman who was said to be pregnant.

Civil Cases

Pregnancy plays an important role in cases pertaining to nullity of marriage, divorce, inheritance of property, compensation cases, illegitimate child and additional leave facilities.

HOW DO WE DIAGNOSE PREGNANCY? (FM3.19)

Diagnosis of pregnancy can be made by the following:
- Presumptive signs
- Probable signs
- Positive signs

Presumptive Signs of Pregnancy

Amenorrhea, morning sickness (hyperemesis gravidarum), enlargement of breast and appearance of Montgomery follicles, pigmentation of skin and Chadwick's sign are some of the presumptive signs of pregnancy.

Probable Signs of Pregnancy

"Quickening" (coming to life)
- The movement of the fetus is felt by the mother for the first time and is evident by 14 to 20 weeks.
- Enlargement of the abdomen, Hegar's sign, Goodeell's sign (softening of cervix), Braxton Hick's sign (intermittent uterine contractions), ballottement, palpation of fetal parts, uterine soufflé and urinary HCG are probable signs of pregnancy.

Positive Signs of Pregnancy

- **Fetal heart sounds:**
  - It can be heard from 18 to 20 weeks of pregnancy.
  - By 5th month fetal heart rate is 160/min, and by 9th month it is 190/min.
  - It is not synchronous with mother's pulse.
  - Heart sounds are not heard in dead fetus, excessive liquor, fatty abdomen, and in fetus less than 18 weeks.
  - *Funic soufflé:* It is a hissing sound, which is synchronous with fetal pulse.
- **X-Ray diagnosis:**
  - Detection of fetal parts can be made from 16th week of gestation by X-ray examination.
    - Annular shadow for skull,
    - Small dots with linear arrangement for vertebral column,
    - Series of parallel lines for ribs,
    - Linear shadow for limbs.
  - Radiological examination will be useful in the diagnosis of twin pregnancy, fetal abnormalities, intrauterine death and hydatidiform mole.
- **Ultrasonography:** More reliable.
  - By 5 to 6 weeks: Gestational sac and cardiac activity are made out.
  - By 8 weeks: Echo from Gestational ring/blighted ovum.
  - By 12 weeks: Fetal heart beat and heart rate can be recorded.
  - By 14 weeks: Fetal head and thorax can be identified.
- **Fetal ECG:** Will show evidence of the cardiac activity of the fetus and is more accurate above 17 weeks of gestation.

HOW TO DIAGNOSIS OF PREGNANCY IN THE DEAD? (FM3.19)

During autopsy pregnancy can be confirmed by the presence of enlarged uterus, presence of embryo/fetus/placental tissue and corpus luteum in an ovary in its progressive or regressive phase. Fetus of three months gestation present inside the uterus in the amniotic fluid sac depicted in **Figure 20.1**.

WHAT IS PSEUDOCYESIS?

- Pseudocyesis is also called as spurious pregnancy or false pregnancy or phantom pregnancy.
- It is usually seen in young woman who have an intense desire to bear a child.
- Also common in woman nearing menopause; it is associated with psychic or hormonal disorder.
- Patients with this condition may present with all the subjective symptoms of pregnancy. If not diagnosed in time, the patient may go through full term of pregnancy and may even have false labor pains of delivery.

WHAT IS FETUS COMPRESSUS?

- Fetus compressus is also called as fetus papyraceous.
- It is a rare form of twin pregnancy, in which the 1st fetus may grow and develop more at the cost of the other. The latter may eventually die, get compressed and gradually gets flattened.

WHAT IS SUPERFETATION? (FM3.19)

- It is a type of twin pregnancy in which there is fertilization of 2nd ovum in an already pregnant woman.
- Two fetuses are born either at the same period showing different stages of development. Or, first a fully developed fetus is born; then after a period of one to three months another fetus is born.

WHAT IS SUPERFECUNDATION? (FM3.19)

- It is a type of twin pregnancy in which there is fertilization of two ova in the same ovulation cycle by two separate acts of coitus committed at short intervals. The incidence is 1.5% of all twin pregnancies.
- The two fertilized ova grow simultaneously; one may grow larger at the cost of the other.

Medico-legal Aspects of Superfetation and Superfecundation

Adultery, infidelity and disputed paternity, if the biological father of one child is different from that of the other.

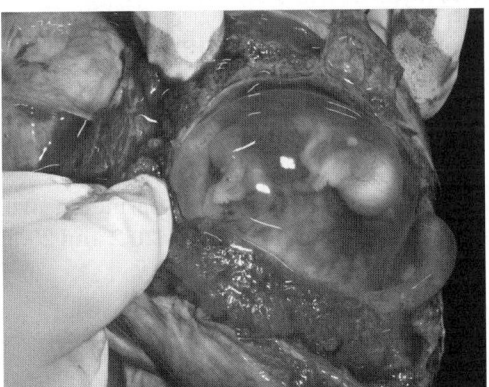

Fig. 20.1: Fetus of 3 months gestation present inside the uterus in the amniotic fluid sac *(For color version see Plate 15)*.

DELIVERY AND MEDICO-LEGAL ISSUES RELATED TO DELIVERY (FM3.19)

Delivery is defined as a process by which there is expulsion or extraction of the child from the uterus, with or without external help. It may be spontaneous or induced.

Medico-legal Aspects of Delivery

The question of delivery arises in situations like:
- Abortion
- Infanticide
- Concealment of Birth (Infanticide Section 318 IPC)
- Divorce and nullity of marriage
- Delivery is considered as a valid ground for delayed execution of judicial death sentence up to 6 months.

SIGNS OF RECENT DELIVERY IN LIVING; WHAT IS LOCHIA? (FM3.19)

General Appearance of Indisposition

- The woman looks pale and sick, with shrunken eyes for the first 2 to 3 days.
- Presence of dark colored pigmentation over the lower eyelids.
- Pulse and body temperature are slightly raised.

Changes in the Breast

- Breasts are full and prominent, having a knotty or nodular feeling and tender.
- **Nipples:** Enlarged, surrounded by darkened areola and Montgomery's tubercles.
- Nipples on squeezing yield milk or colostrums.

Abdominal Changes

- Abdomen is lax, flabby and the skin over the abdomen appears wrinkled.
- Striae gravidarum, linea albicantes and linea nigra are seen due to over stretching of the skin over the abdomen during pregnancy.
- Intermittent painful uterine contractions are felt by the patient for 4 to 5 days.
- The uterus gradually diminishes in size at the rate of 1.5 cm/day.
- On 6th day, the height of the uterus is midway between umbilicus and the Pubis; on 14th day, fundus is at the level of pubic symphysis. The uterus comes back to normal position by 9 weeks.

Labia Majora and Labia Minora

Swollen, tender, bruising and laceration of the labia may be present.

Fossa Navicularis and Posterior Commissure

Shows tears which may extend up to perineum in primigravida.

Changes in the Vagina

- Vagina is spacious with loss of rugosity and the walls are relaxed.
- May show recent tears which heal by 7th day and the rugae reappear in about 3 weeks.

Bruising and tear in the perineum with vaginal wall shows in **Figures 20.2 and 20.3**.

Changes in the Cervix

- Cervix is soft and patulous.
- Internal Os closes by 24 hours and the external Os appears soft and admits two fingers.
- After 1 week, the external Os admits one finger with difficulty and it closes by 2nd week.

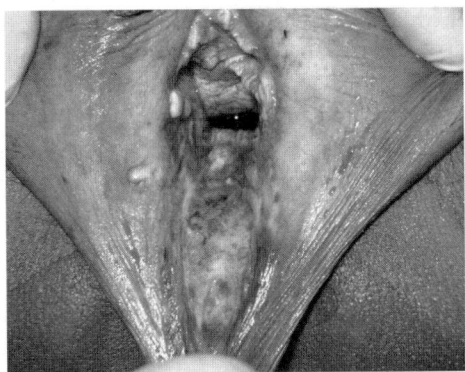

Fig. 20.2: Bruising and tear in the perineum *(For color version see Plate 15).*

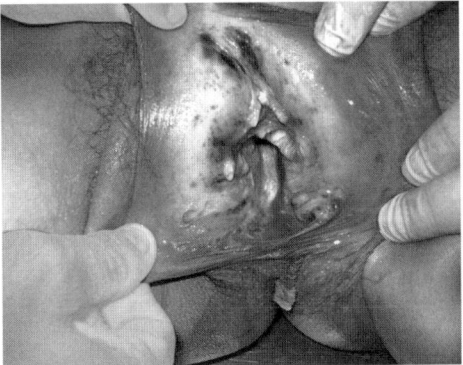

Fig. 20.3: Bruising of the vaginal wall with tear in the perineum *(For color version see Plate 15).*

Lochia

- It is a discharge from the vagina, which is present for a period of 2 to 3 weeks after delivery. It has peculiar disagreeable odor; it gradually changes in color and consistency. Lochia is of three types depending on its color.
- **Lochia rubra:** It is bright red containing blood clots; it is thick in consistency and is present for the first 4 to 5 days after delivery.
- **Lochia serosa:** During the next 4 to 5 days, the lochia changes in color and appears serous. The consistency becomes gradually thin and pale.
- **Lochia alba:** From the 9th day onwards, the color is yellowish gray which becomes white and turbid and finally disappears in two weeks.
- **Laboratory findings:** Urine shows presence of HCG even after delivery. It can be detected in traces up to two weeks after delivery.

SIGNS OF RECENT DELIVERY IN THE DEAD (FM3.19)

- All external signs and local signs seen in living persons can be made out. In addition to that, on internal examination, the uterine wall appears 4 to 5 cm thickness.
- Uterine cavity is obliterated by apposition of anterior and posterior walls.
- After 6 weeks thickness of the uterus is about 1 to 2 cm.

On Dissection of the Uterine Cavity

- The area of the placental attachment **(Fig. 20.4)** shows irregular, nodular, and elevated raw surface **(Fig. 20.5)** of about 15 cm in diameter. It gradually diminishes in size when the uterus contracts. By end of 2nd week, its 3 to 4 cm in diameter and by 6th week, it is 1 to 2 cm in diameter.

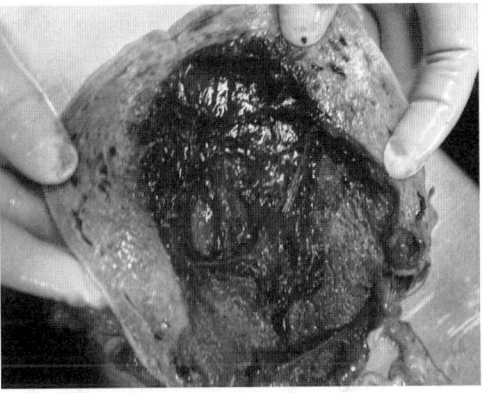

Fig. 20.4: Inner surface of uterus showing retained placenta *(For color version see Plate 15).*

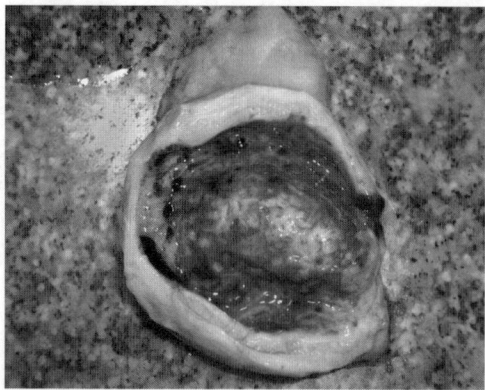

Fig. 20.5: Inner surface of uterus showing irregular nodular areas of placental attachment *(For color version see Plate 15).*

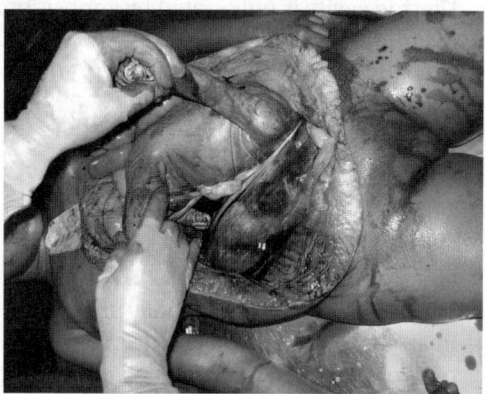

Fig. 20.6: Prolonged obstructed labor resulted in rupture of the uterus and the dead fetus is present in the abdominal cavity with bruising of the peritoneum *(For color version see Plate 16).*

- Peritoneum covering the lower part of uterus is arranged in folds. Prolonged obstructed labor resulted in rupture of the uterus and the dead fetus is present in the abdominal cavity with bruising of the peritoneum shown in **Figure 20.6.**
- Bladder is hyperemic and submucosal hemorrhages may be present.
- The changes in the labia and vagina are similar to that of in the living.
- Perineum shows old tears and healed scars.

DIFFERENCE BETWEEN NULLIPAROUS AND MULTIPAROUS UTERUS?

Features	Nulliparous uterus	Multiparous uterus
Size	Small and thin; about 7 cm long	Large and thick; about 9 cm long
Weight	Lighter about 40–60 g	Heavier about 80–120 g
Proportion with cervix	Body of the uterus and cervix are of equal length	Body of uterus is twice the length of the cervix
Fundus	Less convex and at the level of broad ligament	More convex and at a higher level than broad ligament
Cavity	Triangular and the walls are convex	Rounded and walls are concave
Cervix	Surface is smooth, regular without any scars	Surface is rough, irregular and edges shows scars of delivery

WHAT ARE THE SIGNS OF REMOTE DELIVERY IN LIVING AND THE DEAD?

- Externally abdomen lax and flabby.
- Linea albicantes present in all the cases and striae gravidarum may be seen in some cases.

Breast

- Breast will be soft and pendulous. Nipples are larger, darker and appear raised.
- Areola is dark with Montgomery's tubercles.
- On palpation the breasts are nodular in consistency and in some multipara, striae may be present on the surface of the breasts.

External Genitalia

- Labia majora is dark and are not in close apposition with each other.

- Labia minora is pigmented, dark and protrude out through the gap in between the two sides of labia majora.
- Fourchette and posterior commissure may show lacerations.
- **Vagina:** Looks capacious, dilated and the walls appear relaxed.
- **Hymen:** Absent and represented by carunculae myrtiformis.

WHAT IS PATERNITY? (FM3.20)

- Paternity is the legal status of a child said to be born to a particular father and mother.
- It is decided by paternal likeliness, atavism, blood groups and DNA finger printing.

Disputed paternity: Issues of disputed paternity arises in
- In hospital birth (interchange of newborn by mistake or intentionally).
- In alleged suppositious child.

WHO IS A SUPPOSITIOUS CHILD?

- A woman presents a child, as she is said to have delivered the child; but the fact is that she has not delivered any such child.
- Examination of the female for signs of recent delivery and DNA analysis will be helpful to sort out the issue.
- **Legal issues:**
  - Inheritance of property.
  - Blackmailing a male.
  - When a widow claims higher compensation from her husband's employer.
  - Bringing a charge of breach of promise of marriage against a man, who is alleged to be the father of that child.

WHAT IS ABANDONING AN INFANT?

Section 317 IPC: Abandoning a child of <12 years by the father, mother or caretaker, shall be punished with imprisonment up to 7 years.

WHAT IS CONCEALMENT OF BIRTH?

Section 318 IPC: Whoever intentionally conceals the birth of a child; either dead born or still born and buries or disposes by other means, shall be punished with imprisonment up to 2 years.

MULTIPLE CHOICE QUESTIONS

1. Umbilical cord usually falls off by:
   a. 3–4 days
   b. 5–7 days
   c. 0–12 days
   d. 2 weeks
2. In India, the maximum punishment for the mother, if she is proved to have done infanticide is:
   a. 7 years
   b. 10 years
   c. Life imprisonment
   d. 5 years
3. First symptom of pregnancy is:
   a. Tingling in the breasts
   b. Amenorrhea
   c. Morning sickness
   d. Quickening
4. Quickening felt by mother at about:
   a. 6 weeks
   b. 8–10 weeks
   c. 16–20 weeks
   d. 20–24 weeks
5. Bluish discoloration of the vagina seen in pregnancy is known as:
   a. Chadwick's sign
   b. Goodell's sign
   c. Hegar's sign
   d. Palmer's sign
6. True about Braxton-Hick's contraction are all, *except*:
   a. Felt at 4th month
   b. Painful
   c. Contraction last for 1 minute
   d. Present even when fetus is dead
7. External ballottement can be done after how many weeks of gestation:
   a. 6 weeks
   b. 16 weeks
   c. 20 weeks
   d. 24 weeks

8. In a normal pregnancy, maternal HCG level is maximum at gestational age of:
   a. 8 to 10 weeks
   b. 12 to 14 weeks
   c. 16 to 18 weeks
   d. After 20 weeks
9. Definite diagnosis of pregnancy include all, except:
   a. Fetal heart sound
   b. Palpation of fetal parts
   c. Fetal skeleton on X-ray
   d. HCG in blood
10. Fetal parts are palpable at the earliest by:
    a. 16 weeks
    b. 18 weeks
    c. 20 weeks
    d. 28 weeks
11. Gestational sac can be seen using ultrasonography at the earliest by:
    a. 3rd week
    b. 4th week
    c. 5th week
    d. 8th week
12. Most accurate method of diagnosis of pregnancy at 6 weeks:
    a. Hegar's sign
    b. X-ray examination
    c. Palpation of fetal parts
    d. Fetal heart sound by USG
13. Twin pregnancy, but due to two different men is called:
    a. Superfetation
    b. Superfecundation
    c. Both of the above
    d. Not a realistic situation
14. Definitive finding in deflorate woman:
    a. Pigmented labia minora
    b. Roomy vagina
    c. Large clitoris
    d. Forn hymen
15. True about suppositious child:
    a. Child who is born after father dies
    b. Child born through artificial insemination
    c. Woman claim the child as her own
    d. Child born out of wedlock
16. Immediately after delivery, uterus is at the level of:
    a. Midway between the umbilicus and symphysis pubis
    b. Just at the level of umbilicus
    c. Midway between xiphisternum and umbilicus
    d. Descends into true pelvis
17. Rate of involution uterus following delivery:
    a. 1 cm/day
    b. 1.25 cm/day
    c. 2.25 cm/day
    d. 2.5 cm/day
18. Following delivery, uterus becomes a pelvic organ after:
    a. 2 weeks
    b. 4 weeks
    c. 6 weeks
    d. 8 weeks
19. Order in lochia:
    a. Serosa, rubra, alba
    b. Rubra, serosa, alba
    c. Alba, rubra, serosa
    d. Rubra, alba, serosa
20. Shape of nulliparous cervix is:
    a. Conical
    b. Circular
    c. Longitudinal
    d. Cylindrical
21. Divorce can be given if there is:
    a. Impotence
    b. Sterility
    c. Pre-existing mental illness
    d. Premature ejaculation
22. Fecundation ab extra means:
    a. Child having the characteristic of grandparents
    b. Birth of a child after the death of father
    c. Insemination without penetration of vagina by penis
    d. Sexual intercourse with blood relations
23. According to Hindu Marriage Act, 1955 following ground is considered as marriage is null and void:
    a. Bigamy
    b. Sterility
    c. Unemployment
    d. Chronic illness

ANSWERS

1. a	2. c	3. b	4. c	5. a	6. b	7. c	8. a	9. d	10. c
11. c	12. d	13. b	14. d	15. c	16. a	17. a	18. a	19. b	20. A
21. a	22. c	23. a							

CHAPTER 21

Abortion and MTP Act 1971

KEY WORDS

Abortion, premature labor, artificial abortion, criminal abortion, cupping, syringing, abortion stick, MTP act 1971, placenta.

FM3.27 Define, classify and discuss abortion, methods of procuring MTP and criminal abortion and complication of abortion. MTP Act 1971.

FM3.28 Describe evidences of abortion—living and dead, duties of doctor in cases of abortion, investigations of death due to criminal abortion.

WHAT IS ABORTION? WHAT IS PREMATURE LABOR? (FM3.27)

Abortion is a process by which the products of conception are expelled either spontaneously or by induction, before the viability of the child (28 weeks of gestation).

Legal Definition of Abortion
It is the expulsion of products of conception at any time prior to full term normal delivery.

Premature Labor
- Delivery of fetus after 28 weeks of pregnancy up to 40th week.
- Depending on the time of termination of pregnancy it is called as abortion in 1st trimester, miscarriage in 2nd trimester and premature labor in 3rd trimester.

CLASSIFY ABORTION? (FM3.27)

Abortion is classified into natural and artificial abortion.

Artificial Abortion
- Legal, justifiable or therapeutic abortion.
- Criminal abortion.

Natural Abortion
Natural abortion could be spontaneous or accidental.

Natural abortion usually by 2nd or 3rd months of pregnancy and the incidence is about 10% of all pregnancies; the causes may be maternal, placental or fetal.

Causes of Natural Abortion
- **Maternal causes:** Acute and chronic infections of genital tract; Rh incompatibility,

congenital defects of the uterus; poisons like phosphorus, lead, quinine and mercury; accidental injuries and metabolic disorders like diabetes and thyrotoxicosis.
- **Placental causes:** Acute hydramnios, hydatidiform degeneration of the placenta, placenta previa and other diseases involving decidua or placenta.
- **Fetal causes:** Developmental defects of the fetus, and intrauterine death of the fetus due to various reasons and effects of radiation.

WHAT IS CRIMINAL ABORTION? METHODS OF CRIMINAL ABORTION; WHAT IS ABORTION STICK? (FM3.27)

- Unlawful destruction or expulsion of the fetus or products of conception from the mother's womb, when there is no therapeutic indication to do so.
- **Usually undertaken by:**
  - Unmarried girls
  - Widows for remarriage
  - Married woman when they don't want children at that time
  - Female infanticide

Types of Abortionists

- Expert/medically qualified professionals.
- **Semiskilled abortionists:** Midwives, nurses, and chemists.
- **Unskilled abortionists:** Quacks, untrained dais.

Methods Adopted

- **Mechanical violence:** General or local
- Abortifacient drugs
- Instrumentation

Mechanical Violence

- **General violence:**
  - Acts indirectly on the uterus by promoting contraction of pelvic organs and thus causing hemorrhage between the uterus and placental membrane.
  - Application of severe pressure over the abdomen, violent exercise, cupping and application of very hot and cold water baths; application of leaches to pudenda, perineum and inner aspect of thighs.
- **Local violence:** Correction of retroverted uterus bimanually may lead to abortion.

Abortifacient Drugs

- **Ecbolics:** Act directly on the uterus and increase the uterine contractions. Example: Ergot, Quinine, Kmno4 tablets, lead pills and strychnine.
- **Emmenogogues:** Increases the menstrual blood flow. Act as abortifacient in large doses. Example: Savin, borax, prostaglandins and estrogens.
- Drugs which irritate the genitourinary tract and in turn provide reflex uterine contraction. Example: Oil of turpentine, cantharides, $KMNO_4$ (through vaginal route).
- Drugs which primarily irritate the gastrointestinal tract and reflexly stimulate the uterine contractions: It causes excitation of uterus to contract "in sympathy" with the violent contraction of the stomach, intestines and the colon. Example: Emetics (tartaric acid), purgatives (castor oil), croton oil, phenolphthalein and magnesium sulphate ($MgSO_4$).
- **Drugs which are primarily toxic to other systems:** Inorganic metallic irritants (lead, copper, antimony, mercury and arsenic) and organic irritants (bark of plumbago rosea, juice of calotropis, unripe fruit of papaya and pineapple).

Instruments

- **Those causing rupture of the membranes:** Uterine sound, catheter,

pencil, hairpin, knitting needle, stick and fingers.
- **Those causing dilatation of the cervix:** Bark of slippery elm; it is hygroscopic which absorbs the cervical and vaginal secretions to swell resulting in dilation of the cervix.

Instrumentation by Unskilled Abortionists

- Soft pieces of wood of different sizes with 3 mm thickness are passed into the cervical canal and are left in situ. It absorbs moisture and vaginal secretions, and swells up and thus dilates the cervical canal.
- **Disadvantages:** Unhygienic method and thus increase the chances of infection; it may also get lodged in bladder as a foreign body if improperly inserted and chances of perforation of the cervix or uterus is high.

Abortion Stick

- Thin bamboo stick or stem of calotropis plant, 12 to 18 cm long; one end wrapped with cotton wool or rag, whose greater part is soaked with juice of marking nut, calotropis or a paste made of arsenic oxide, sulfide or red lead, and is inserted into the uterus. This irritates the uterus and results in detachment of placenta from the uterus.
- **Air insufflations:** Air is instilled into the vagina by means of syringes or pumps, which results in separation of the placenta from its attachments. Air embolism is a commonest complication.
- **Electricity:** Positive pole is applied over the cervix and the negative pole over sacrum or lumbar vessels. Then current is passed, which leads to uterine contraction and thus brings about abortion.
- **Pastes:** Paste containing iodine, thymol or mercury is injected from a collapsible tube with uterine applicator into the uterus.
- **Cupping:** It is a method in which a cup is placed over the lower abdomen and vacuum is created inside, which in turn produces detachment of the placenta leading to abortion.
- **Syringing:** Enema syringe with a hard bulb is used to inject fluid into the uterus. Higginson's syringe is usually used; the suction valve is placed in a bowl of fluid and pressure is applied on the bulb. A mixture of air and fluid is forced into uterine cavity at high pressure; the fluid detaches parts of amniotic sac and placenta from the uterine walls. The uterus contracts causing hemorrhage and thus leads to abortion. Can be administered by patient herself or by an abortionist.

MEDICAL TERMINATION OF PREGNANCY: MTP ACT 1971 (FM3.27)

- Medical termination of pregnancy is guided by MTP act 34 of 1971.
- It came into force from 1st April 1972 in India except J&K.
- The Act imposes certain restrictions and aims at liberalizing the termination of pregnancy, in order to avoid illegal abortion by untrained abortionists.
- It lays down conditions under which pregnancies can be terminated.

Conditions under which pregnancy can be terminated:

- **Therapeutic:** Where continuation of pregnancy has a threat to the life of the mother.
- **Eugenic:** Where continuation of pregnancy may lead to the birth of congenitally defective children
- **Social grounds:** Where pregnancy is terminated to limit the size of the family in socially and economically underprivileged family.
- **Humanitarian:** When pregnancy is due to rape.

- **Persons authorized to perform MTP:**
  - Registered medical practitioner who has conducted or assisted minimum 25 abortions in authorized centers.
  - RMP with diploma or master degree in obstetrics and gynecology.

When can termination be done:
- MTP can be done only up to 12 weeks (3 months) of gestation.
- If any female goes to a doctor and tells that she doesn't want the child and if the gestation period is less than 3 months, then the doctor can very well go on with the induction of abortion (abortion on demand).
- If the period of pregnancy is more than 12 weeks (3 months) and less than 20 weeks (5 months) then opinion of two doctors is necessary for termination of such pregnancies (it's because sex determination becomes possible after 12 to 16 weeks USG, and hence there is always a chance of sex selection in abortion after 3 months and hence the opinion of two doctors is taken to do MTP between 3–5 months).
- After 5 months of gestation MTP should not be done and any doctor who indulges in such practice is said to have committed criminal abortion and is liable for the act.
- But during any period of gestation, if continuation of pregnancy has got an imminent threat to the life of the mother, then MTP can be done to save the life of the mother, even by the opinion of a single doctor alone.

Where termination should be performed:
Government, semi-government or private hospitals approved for this purpose.

Consent for MTP

- Written informed consent is necessary and consent of the guardian is required when age of the female is less than 18 years of age.
- Consent of the husband is not necessary, even if the female is married.

Maintain Records

- Records containing all the details of the patient on whom MTP was conducted.
- All forms filled for the procedure of conduction of MTP must be kept confidential and are not to be kept open.
- The consent form filled up by the patient together with the certified opinion of the doctor along with the intimation of termination of pregnancy should be kept in a sealed envelope and marked "SECRET" and then sent to chief medical officer of the state or head of the hospital and kept safe in the medical records department.

CAUSES OF DEATH IN CRIMINAL ABORTION

- **Immediate/rapid death:** Hemorrhage, perforation, vasovagal shock and fat/air embolism.
- **Delayed death:** Generalized peritonitis, complication of local infection, tetanus, septicemia and toxemia.
- **Remote causes of death:** Jaundice and renal suppression, bacterial endocarditis, pneumonia, pulmonary embolism, emphysema and meningitis; sometimes death is also due to the poisonous effect of the drugs used to procure abortion.

COMPLICATIONS OF CRIMINAL ABORTION (FM3.27)

- Endotoxemia, septic shock and death.
- Fatal hemorrhages.
- Necrosis of cervical canal.
- Delayed air embolism.

SIGNS OF RECENT ABORTION (FM3.28)

Local Examination

- Undergarments show some staining with blood and occasionally with liquid abortifacient agent which is used.

- Labia majora and minora appear congested and may show some injuries.
- Posterior commissure, fourchette and vaginal wall are congested with reduced rugosity.
- Vagina shows presence of blood clots.
- **Cervix:** Congested and Os shows abrasion and tears; cervix remains dilated for a few days after abortion.
- The woman remains indisposed for 1 to 2 days with slight increase in body temperature.
- Serum and urine of the woman remains positive for HCG tests up to about 7 to 10 days.
- Evidence about the method used to procure abortion may be present.
- Discharge of milk or colostrums on squeezing the breast.

POSTMORTEM FINDINGS IN A CASE OF DEATH DUE TO ABORTION (FM3.28)

Postmortem Findings

External Findings

- Undergarments may be blood stained or show clots and stains.
- Body may look extremely pale and PMS not prominent due to loss of blood before death.
- Pigmentation of breast and abdomen may be present.
- **Breasts:** Enlarged with dark areola, montgomery's tubercles and large raised nipples.
- Abdominal wall is lax with linea nigra and occasionally striae gravidarum.
- If cupping is done to induce abortion, then a circular mark may be noticed on the wall of lower abdomen.
- Labia majora appears laxed; labia minora is pigmented, injured and may be stained with blood. Injuries on fourchette and posterior commissure are commonly seen.

Internal Examination

- Uterus, ovary and vagina are dissected enmass for detailed examination.
- Injury to the intra-abdominal organs may be present.
- **Vagina:** Vaginal wall may show perforations near the fornix; the walls may be stained according to the chemical used with excoriation of epithelium.
- **Uterus:** Enlarged, soft and congested with prominent surface vessels; on cut section the walls will be thickened; cavity may contain the products of conception in full or some remnants of products of consumption. There may be presence of blood clot, hairpin, nail or root of a plant inside the uterine cavity.
- Both the internal and external Os are congested and distorted with injuries.
- **Ovaries:** Either of the ovaries will show presence of an active corpus luteum.
- **Lungs:** Evidence of air/fat embolism may be seen, with marked congestion.

If general anesthetic agents like ether were used, smell of ether will be present.

In cases of death due to hemorrhage the lungs will appear pale.

MEDICO-LEGAL IMPORTANCE OF PLACENTA

- From the size and weight the period of gestation can be made out.
- Its mere presence (even in pieces) along with blood clots, confirms abortion or delivery.
- Chemical examination of placenta can detects the type of systemic abortifacient used.

WHAT IS AMNIOTIC FLUID EMBOLISM? (FM3.28)

- Mostly occur during the phase of active labor and rarely in 1st or 2nd trimester

abortions following trauma and amniocentesis.
- The amniotic fluid enters the maternal venous circulation and results in pulmonary microvascular obstruction and results in severe vasospasm of pulmonary vasculature and hypoxia; usually death occurs in the 1st hour.
- If death is not immediate, then disseminated intravascular coagulation and fibrin deposition occurs in most internal organs.
- Diagnosis is by demonstration of fetal squamous cells, meconium, lanugo hair, fat globules, chorionic and amniotic cells in the lung by HPE.

SECTIONS OF IPC RELATED TO ABORTION

Section 312 IPC

Voluntarily causing criminal abortion with the consent of the woman. Both the woman and the abortionist are liable for imprisonment up to 3 years, with or without fine. If the woman is quick with the child, the imprisonment may extend up to 7 years.

Section 313 IPC

When abortion is caused without the consent of the woman, the punishment extends up to 10 years.

Section 314 IPC

If a pregnant woman dies, from an act intended to cause miscarriage, the punishment shall not be less than 10 years and fine up to 2 lakhs.

Section 315 IPC

A person doing an act intended to prevent the child from being born alive or to cause of the child, is liable for imprisonment up to 10 years.

Section 316 IPC

Causing death of a quick unborn child by any act, amounts to culpable homicide. The punishment may extend up to 10 years.

Section 317 IPC (Abandoning an Infant)

Abandoning a child of less than twelve years by the father, mother or caretaker, shall be punished with imprisonment upto up to 7 years.

Section 318 IPC (Concealment of Birth)

Whoever intentionally conceals the birth of a child; either dead born or still born and buries or disposes by other means, shall be punished with imprisonment up to two years.

MULTIPLE CHOICE QUESTIONS

1. **All the following are duties of a doctor in criminal abortion cases, *except*:**
   a. Should maintain professional secrecy
   b. Treat the patient
   c. Arrange for dying declaration
   d. Should issue death certificate if the woman dies
2. **An abortifacient which causes partial deafness includes:**
   a. Nerium
   b. Digitalis
   c. Aconite
   d. Quinine
3. **The maximum period of pregnancy, up to which MTP can be done:**
   a. 10 weeks
   b. 15 weeks
   c. 20 weeks
   d. 28 weeks
4. **Abortion in a 30 kg wt woman (unmarried) is to be considered on _____ grounds.**
   a. Medical
   b. Eugenic
   c. Social
   d. Humanitarian

5. All statements are true regarding MTP act, except:
   a. MTP act was passed in 1971
   b. MTP act has brought down the incidence of illegal abortion
   c. In an emergency pregnancy can be terminated by a single doctor even after 20 weeks without consulting a second doctor
   d. MTP can be done after 20 weeks of gestation, if the two doctors agree together
6. Indications for medical termination of pregnancy as per MTP ACT 1971 are all, except:
   a. Social
   b. Altruistic
   c. Therapeutic
   d. Eugenic
7. Complications of illegal/criminal abortion are all, except:
   a. Cerebral hemorrhage
   b. DIC
   c. Septicemia
   d. Acute renal failure
8. Most common cause for 1st trimester abortion is:
   a. Chromosomal defect
   b. Endocrine disturbance
   c. Infection
   d. Anatomical abnormalities in the uterus
9. Mechanism of action of abortion stick used in criminal abortion:
   a. Necrosis of endometrium causing infection
   b. Uterine contraction
   c. Stimulation of nerve
   d. Uterine relaxation
10. MTP can be done by one doctor if the gestation period is up to:
    a. 12 weeks
    b. 20 weeks
    c. 34 weeks
    d. 28 weeks
11. Lendrum's stain is useful to detect:
    a. Amniotic fluid embolism deaths
    b. Air embolism death
    c. Septicemia
    d. Fat embolism
12. Emmenagogues—MAO is:
    a. Increased menstrual flow
    b. Increased uterine contraction
    c. Reflex uterine contraction
    d. Irritation of uterus
13. In 1970, the world medical association (WMA) adopted a resolution on therapeutic abortion, known as:
    a. Declaration of Berlin
    b. Declaration of Oslo
    c. Declaration of Tokyo
    d. Declaration of Denmark
14. Up to how many years from the last entry, should the admission registers of abortion cases be maintained:
    a. 2 years
    b. 6 years
    c. 1 year
    d. 5 years

ANSWERS

| 1. d | 2. d | 3. c | 4. d | 5. d | 6. b | 7. a | 8. a | 9. b | 10. a |
| 11. a | 12. a | 13. b | 14. d | | | | | | |

22 CHAPTER

Infant Deaths

 KEY WORDS

Infanticide, dead born, still born, live born, viability, rule of hasse, hydrostatic test, maceration, Spalding's sign, SIDS, battered baby.

FM2.27	Define and discuss infanticide, feticide and stillbirth.
FM2.28	Describe and discuss signs of intrauterine death, signs of live birth, viability of fetus, age determination of fetus, DOAP session of ossification centers, hydrostatic test, sudden infants death syndrome and Munchausen's syndrome by proxy.
FM3.29	Describe and discuss child abuse and battered baby syndrome.

INTRODUCTION (FM2.27)

- **Infanticide** is defined as killing a child under the age of one year.
- Only the mother of the child can be charged of the offence of infanticide, as she has the bound duty of protecting and taking care of the child, once she has delivered a child.
- In India there is no distinction between infanticide and murder of any individual.
- Other terms commonly used in medical science are:
    - *Feticide:* The killing of the fetus at any time prior to birth.
    - *Filicide:* The killing of a child by its parents.
    - *Neonaticide:* The killing of a child within 24 hours of birth.

Legal questions to be answered in infanticide:
- Whether the fetus have attained maturity/viability or not?
- Whether the child was dead born/still born/live born?
- If live born, then how long did the child survive and what was the cause of death?

WHAT IS DEAD BORN? WHAT ARE THE SIGNS OF MACERATION? (FM2.28)

- Dead born is a child which had already died inside the uterus and shows the following signs.
  Signs of maceration and rigor mortis at birth (rigor mortis only in viable fetus, as the myofibrils are developed only after 7 months of intra uterine life).

Maceration

- This is aseptic autolysis and occurs when the child remains in the uterus for about 3 to 4 days immersed in liquor amnii after death, but should be devoid of air.
- The earliest sign of maceration is skin slippage and seen in 12 hours after death inside the uterus.
- Maceration can be demonstrated by purple skin, air blebs, flexible bones and abnormal mobility of joints, soft viscera, and rarely mummification.
- Loss of alignment and overriding of skull bones of the cranial vault due to shrinkage of the brain after death. This is called **Spalding sign** and it is seen 48 hours after death of the fetus inside the uterus, which is due to loss of intracranial tension.
- **Robert's sign:** There is appearance of gas shadow in the chambers of the heart and aorta, which is evident by 12 hours of death of the fetus inside the uterus.

DEFINE STILL BORN; CAUSES OF STILL BIRTH? (FM2.28)

- A stillborn child is one, which is born after 28th week of pregnancy but did not show any signs of life, after it has been completely expelled from the vaginal canal.
- The child was alive inside uterus but did not come to life at all and is considered to be due to defects in the birth process.
- The incidence is about 5% and is seen more frequently in immature male children.
- Prolonged labor, which is shown by presence of caput succedaneum and severe molding of head, and negative hydrostatic test are indicative of still birth.
- In these cases, the body is sterile and decomposition occurs only by aseptic autolysis.

Common Causes of Stillbirth

- Prematurity.
- Anoxia and birth trauma.
- Placental abnormalities and toxemia of pregnancy.
- Erythroblastosis fetalis and congenital defects of the fetus.

WHAT IS VIABILITY? (FM2.28)

- Viability is the physical ability of a fetus to lead a separate existence of its own, outside the womb of the mother, by virtue of a certain degree of development.
- A child is said to be viable after 210 days of intrauterine life. However, the minimum period of viability is 180 days (6 months).

DIFFERENCE BETWEEN DEAD BORN AND STILL BIRTH (FM2.28)

Table 22.1 is depicted the differences between dead born and still born.

DISCUSS THE SIGNS OF LIVE BIRTH?

Short Notes: Hydrostatic Test; Rule of Hasse (FM2.28)

- **Live born** child is one which is born alive and showed signs of life after it has been completely delivered out of the mother. Causing death of such a child is regarded as infanticide (homicide).
- The law presumes that every newborn child found dead was born dead, till the contrary is proved.
- In civil cases, any sign of life such as hearing of a cry, movement of limbs or even feeble respiration, after complete birth of the child is accepted as proof of live birth.
- Whereas, in criminal cases live birth has to be demonstrated by postmortem examination.

Signs of Live Birth

Postmortem Examination

- Assessment of intrauterine age of the fetus by **Rule of Hasse**. Crown heal length

TABLE 22.1: Dead born vs still born.

Features	Dead born	Still born
Definition	Fetus died inside the uterus and shows signs of maceration	Viable fetus which was alive inside the uterus but did not show any signs of life after it being completely delivered from the vaginal canal
Inside the uterus	Died inside the uterus and either spontaneously expelled or the doctors induces labor and delivers it after confirming the baby died already	Alive inside the uterus but dies during the process of delivery
Findings at postmortem	Rigor mortis, signs of maceration, Spalding's sign, Robert's sign, mummification	Signs of prolonged labor such as caput succedaneum, cephalhematoma, etc.
Predominance	No such predominance	Preterm male and primigavida
Causes	Congenital anomaly, ABO or Rh incompatibility	Anemia, toxemia, birth trauma, prematurity

of the fetus is measured and if the length is less than 25 cm, then the square root of the length will give the approximate age of the fetus in months. If the length is more than 25 cm, then it is divided by 5, which will give the gestational age of the fetus. Example: If the length is 16 cm, then the age of the fetus is 4 months and if the length is 35 cm, the age of the fetus is 7 months.

- **Shape of chest:** Before respiration, the chest is flat and its circumference is 1 to 2 cm less than the abdomen at the level of umbilicus; after respiration, the chest becomes arched, and the circumference of chest is 1 to 2 cm more than that of abdomen.
- Abdominal cavity is opened first to check the level of diaphragm.

Position of Diaphragm

Diaphragm is found at the level of 4th or 5th rib before respiration; after respiration, the diaphragm is pushed downwards to the level of 6th or 7th ribs (decomposition alters the finding).

Lungs

- **Volume:** Fully respired lungs fill the whole of the thoracic cavity and the margins of the lungs overlapping on the pericardium of the heart; whereas unrespired lung appears collapsed towards the hilum.
- **Margins:** Margins are usually sharp before respiration, but becomes rounded after the first respiration, even if feeble respiration has taken place; presence of bullae suggests some form of obstruction and evidence of respiration.
- **Consistency:** Lungs are dense, firm and non crepitant like liver before respiration. It becomes soft, spongy, elastic and crepitant if respiration takes place.
- **Weight:**
  - *Fodere's test:* The average weight of the lungs before respiration is 30 to 40 g and it becomes 60 to 70 g after respiration due to increase in blood flow.
  - *Ploquet's test:* After respiration, due to increased blood flow in the lung, their weight gets doubled from 1/70 of body weight to 1/35 of body weight.

Hydrostatic Test

- Hydrostatic test is done to find out whether the lung has respired or not.
- **Principle:** Before respiration the lungs are of same consistency as that of liver and do not float in water. After respiration, the specific gravity of lung is decreased which makes the lungs to float in water.
- **Procedure:** A ligature is applied to dissect the entire lung and is placed on water. If the entire lung floats, then each lung is cut into 12 to 20 pieces and then placed on water; a small piece of liver is kept as control (if liver floats, it indicates decomposition has set in and the test is invalid). Whole lung is put in water with liver as control shown in **Figure 22.1**.
- If the lung pieces still float, then they are squeezed under water to see if any bubbles escape. Then, the lung bits are wrapped in piece of cloth and squeezed to remove the residual air. The squeezed lung pieces are again put in water. If the pieces still float, it indicates that active respiration has taken place shown in **Figure 22.2**. If they sink, it indicates that respiration has not taken place.
- If some pieces sinks and some floats, then it indicates feeble respiration has taken place.
- **Respired lung may sink:** False negative results may occur in pneumonia, atelectasis and obstruction by alveolar duct membrane.
- **Unrespired lung may float:** False positive results may occur in decomposition and artificial respiration.

Medico-legal Aspects of Live Birth

- Autopsy carries crucial values.
- Death could be due to an act of omission e.g., failure to give feeds, not protecting the baby with proper coverings, etc., or by an act of commission like throttling, strangulation **(Fig. 22.3)**, foreign body in the larynx and trachea, poisoning or even injuries (usually concealed puncture wounds)
- A detailed postmortem examination will demonstrate the exact cause of death **(Fig. 22.4)** it also helps to assess the exact intrauterine age of the fetus by demonstration of the various ossification centers like sternum, lower end of femur, calcaneum and talus.

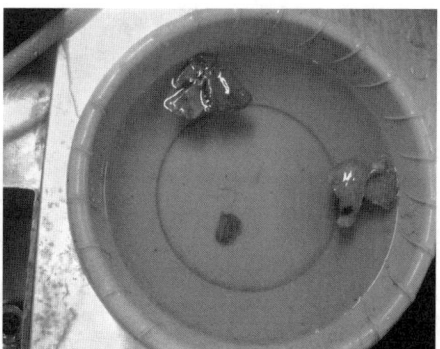

Fig. 22.1: Whole lung is put in water with liver as control *(For color version see Plate 16)*.

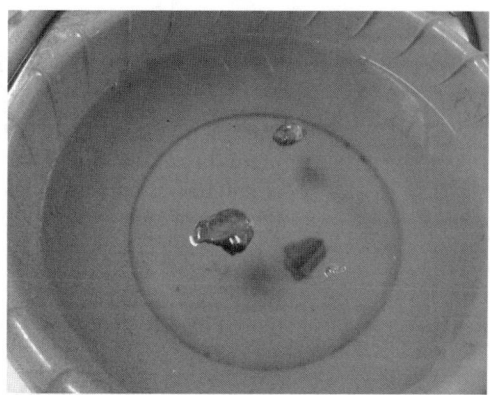

Fig. 22.2: Pieces of lung after squeezing are put into water with liver as control. Pieces of lung floats and liver sinks–positive hydrostatic test, indicating live birth *(For color version see Plate 16)*.

DIFFERENCE BETWEEN STILL BORN AND LIVE BORN? (FM2.28)

See **Table 22.2.**

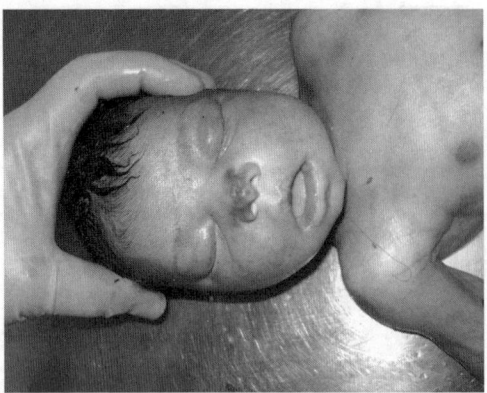 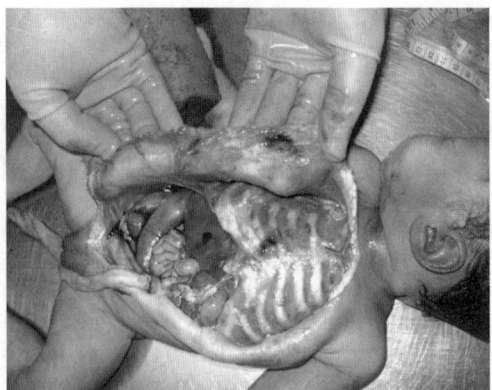

Fig. 22.3: A case of smothering showing bruising of nostrils *(For color version see Plate 16).*

Fig. 22.4: Punctured wound on the right side of abdomen entering into the liver *(For color version see Plate 16).*

TABLE 22.2: Still born vs live born.

Features	Still born	Live born
Definition	Viable fetus which was alive inside the uterus but did not show any signs of life after it being completely delivered from the vaginal canal	The baby was born alive, showed signs of life like cry and respiration and later on died due to some causes
Causes	Anemia, toxemia, birth trauma, prematurity	The death of the baby could be by act of omission or commission
Signs	Signs of prolonged labor such as caput succedaneum, cephalhematoma, etc.	No such signs
Level of diaphragm	At the level of 4th or 5th rib	At the level of 6th or 7th rib
Lungs	Small condensed towards the hilum, not occupying the whole of thoracic cavity and not covering the heart. Lungs are dark red or brown in color	Lungs fully expanded, occupying whole of the thoracic cavity, overlapping the pericardium. Lungs are pink in color
Margins	Sharp	Rounded
Weight	1/70 of body weight. Weighs around 30 to 40 g	1/35 of body weight; weighs 60 to 70 g
Consistency	Firm, noncrepitant and liver like	Soft, spongy and crepitant
Hydrostatic test	Negative	Positive
Medico-legal importance	No crime against anybody; allegation of medical negligence may be raised against the doctor who conducted delivery	Charge of infanticide against the mother

MUNCHAUSEN'S SYNDROME BY PROXY (FM2.28)

- This is a type of child abuse, involving the mother.
- It consists of repeated pretentions of illness or repeated infliction of minor injuries.
- The child is brought to the hospital for induced signs and symptoms with fictitious injuries.

- The child is frequently admitted into the hospital for medical evaluation of any nonexistent conditions.

Example of Few Cases of Munchausen's Syndrome

- The mother may prick her fingers and add the blood drop to the urine of the child and take the sample to the doctor with complains of hematuria by the child.
- The child is repeatedly smothered to unconsciousness, then resuscitated and taken to the hospital.

SUDDEN INFANT DEATH SYNDROME (SIDS, CRIB DEATHS, COT DEATHS) (FM2.28)

- It is sudden death of an infant which cannot be explained and the cause of death in such cases remains a mystery, even after a complete autopsy and analysis of clinical history and death scene investigation.
- The incidence is 2 to 3 per 1000 live births; with male preponderance.
- Most common age is 2 weeks to 2 years; maximum in between 3 to 7 months.
- Twins are at greater risk.
- Commonly occurs at night and usually there is a history of running nose or coryza.

Autopsy Findings

- Blood stained froth in the mouth, evidence of laryngitis, trachea-bronchitis or congenital heart disease.
- Multiple petechial hemorrhages are often found on the heart, lungs and thymus.
- **Aetiology:** The hypothesis of SIDS include:
    - Prone sleeping position
    - Prolonged sleep apnea
    - Hypotonic babies, whose neck position reduces airway lumen due to obliteration of the air passages.
    - Dust, mite and cow's milk allergy and anaphylaxis of unknown origin.
    - Calcium and selenium deficiency.
    - Viraemia.

BATTERED BABY SYNDROME (FM3.29)

- The other synonyms for this condition are: **Caffey's syndrome**, child abuse or maltreatment syndrome.
- Battered child is one who receives repetitive nonaccidental physical injuries, usually inflicted by the parents or guardian.
- In addition to these injuries, there may be deprivation of nutrition, care and affection.
- The classical features are obvious discrepancy between the nature of injuries and the explanation offered by the parents. There will be unexplained delay between the time of sustaining such injuries and seeking medical attention.
- There is constant repetition of injuries, often progressive from minor to major injuries.
- Children of low socio-economic group, broken families, illegitimate and unwanted children are the usual victims.
- There is often a history of financial and emotional problems in the parents.
- Many of the fathers have criminal records and mothers have social and psychiatric deviations.

Manifestations

- Relatively more in male children and the age group is 2 to 5 years.
- Child may reflect fear and despair.
- Bruises around the wrist, forearm, thighs and ankles, which are due to rough handling and violent swinging of the child.
- Buttocks may show burns often with cigars and whip marks.
- Face and lips bruised, and frenulum of tongue may be torn.

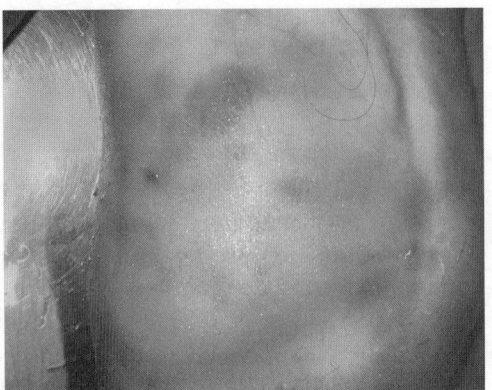

Fig. 22.5: The multiple bruises on chest and abdomen caused by poking with the fingers (six penny bruises) *(For color version see Plate 16).*

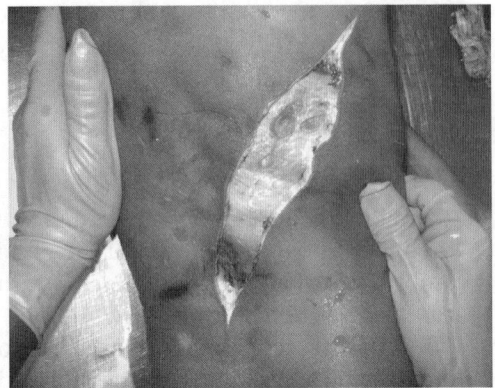

Fig. 22.7: Demonstration of the bruises of the underlying subcutaneous tissues and muscles by dissection *(For color version see Plate 17).*

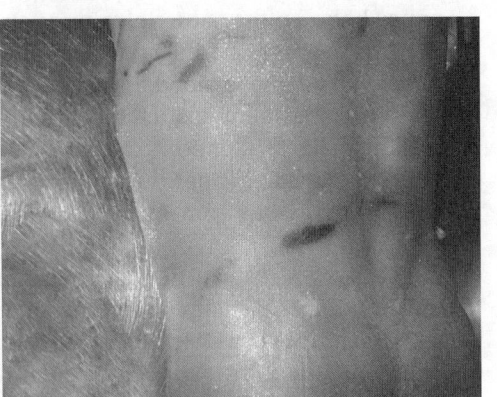

Fig. 22.6: Linear bruise caused by whipping with blunt weapon like a stick *(For color version see Plate 17).*

- Circular bruises of 1 to 2 cm in diameter, due to pocking of adult fingers on the chest, abdomen and thighs. These are called as **six penny bruises**, shown in **Figure 22.5**.
- Multiple rib fractures may be seen; limb fractures (fresh and old unhealed) mostly in regions of epiphysis of growing bones with periosteal separations.
- Crack fractures of skull associated with intracranial hemorrhages.
- Evidence of multiple external injuries of varying degrees under different stages of healing can be noticed depicted in **Figures 22.6 and 22.7.**
- Rarely these children may die of these injuries and brought for autopsy with fabricated history of sustaining these injuries accidentally. The autopsy surgeon must be aware of the probability of these conditions and help the investigation team as well as the court appropriately so that the culprits do not escape from the law.

SHAKEN BABY SYNDROME (FM3.29)

- Is a variant of battered baby syndrome and is serious form of child abuse.
- It results from extreme rotational movements, cranial acceleration and deceleration injuries produced by violent shaking.

Clinical Features

- They are popularly known as 'whiplash shaken baby syndrome'. It is characterized by retinal hemorrhage, SDH and/or SAH. There may be little or no evidence of external injuries.
- Shaking itself may cause serious and fatal injuries; there may also be other forms of head trauma, including impact injuries by throwing the child on the walls "Shaken slam syndrome" or "Shaken impact syndrome".

- The victims need not be babies alone, the age of the affected individuals may vary extensively.
- Intractable crying of the baby may lead to tension and frustration for the parents or guardians resulting in aversion towards the victim.
- The caretakers are of abusive behavior and have unrealistic expectation of their children. Many of them may expect their needs to be met with by the children.

Investigations

- CT scan is the choice and may reveal SDH, mass effects and diffuse axonal injuries.
- The mortality rate is 15 to 30%
- **Autopsy findings:** External examination may show injuries which corresponds to violent shaking of the child. Internally, SDH, SAH, cerebral edema, intracranial or retinal hemorrhages, and multiple fractures of skull, long bones and ribs are seen.

Cinderella Syndrome

Sometimes in a family, a single child is chosen to receive the battering (commonly the youngest or the eldest) and repeatedly thrashed, while the other children are spared.

MULTIPLE CHOICE QUESTIONS

1. **The most reliable evidence for respiration in new born child is derived from:**
   a. Hydrostatic test
   b. Breslan's test
   c. Microscopic test
   d. Fodere's test (static test)
2. **Spalding's sign is evident in:**
   a. 2 days
   b. 14 days
   c. 5 days
   d. 7 days
3. **How many ossification centers will be seen in the sternum of a full-term fetus?**
   a. 3
   b. 4
   c. 5
   d. 6
4. **Aseptic autolysis' occurs in:**
   a. Decomposition
   b. Maceration
   c. Mummification
   d. Still birth
5. **The test performed to compare weight of the lung with the weight of the body is:**
   a. Getler's test
   b. Raygat's test
   c. Ploucquet's test
   d. Foedere's test
6. **Hydrostatic test is done in:**
   a. Dry drowning
   b. Wet drowning
   c. Near drowning
   d. Infant deaths
7. **In a 3-month fetus, characteristic feature seen is:**
   a. Nails are visible
   b. Limbs well formed
   c. Anus is seen as dark spot
   d. Meconium is found in duodenum
8. **Lanugo hair first appears in a fetus at:**
   a. 2nd month
   b. 3rd month
   c. 4th month
   d. 5th month
9. **The center of ossification used as medico-legal evidence for fetal viability:**
   a. Head of femur
   b. Distal end of femur
   c. Talus
   d. Calcaneum
10. **Testes completely descend in the scrotum by the:**
    a. End of 7th month
    b. End of 8th month
    c. End of 9th month
    d. After birth
11. **Center of ossification of lower end of femur appears at:**
    a. 36 weeks
    b. 38 weeks
    c. 40 weeks
    d. 28 weeks
12. **Rule of Hasse is used to determine:**
    a. Age of fetus
    b. Height of an adult
    c. Race of a person
    d. Identification
13. **At what age, does the birth length doubles:**
    a. 1 year
    b. 2 years

c. 3 years
   d. 4 years
14. **Not true about cephalhematoma:**
   a. Not limited by sutures
   b. Swelling develops in 12–24 hours after birth
   c. Swelling subsides in 2–3 months
   d. Caused by periosteal injury of skull
15. **Caput succedaneum in a newborn is:**
   a. Collection of blood under the pericranium
   b. Collection of sero-sanguineous fluid in the scalp
   c. Edema of the scalp due to grip of the forceps
   d. Varicose veins in the scalp
16. **Birth weight triples at:**
   a. 9 months of age
   b. 1 year of age
   c. 2 years of age
   d. 2.5 years of age
17. **The following are the characteristics of caput succedaneum, *except*:**
   a. It is present at birth
   b. It does not cause jaundice in newborn
   c. It is limited to individual bone
   d. It disappears within a few hours of birth
18. **All tests are used to detect live birth, *except*:**
   a. Ploucquet's test
   b. Fodere's test
   c. Gettler's test
   d. Raygat's test
19. **Raygat's/Hydrostatic test is based on:**
   a. Weight of lung
   b. Specific gravity of lung
   c. Consistency of lung
   d. Volume of lungs
20. **False negative hydrostatic test in live born:**
   a. Atelectasis
   b. Meconium aspiration
   c. Emphysema
   d. Congenital heart disease
21. **Dead-born fetus does not show:**
   a. Rigor mortis at birth
   b. Adipocere formation
   c. Maceration
   d. Mummification
22. **Spalding sign usually seen in:**
   a. Abortion
   b. Stillbirth
   c. Intrauterine death
   d. Infanticide
23. **Presence of gas shadow in the heart and great vessels suggestive of intrauterine death. This is called:**
   a. Chadwick's sign
   b. Osiander's sign
   c. Robert's sign
   d. Spalding sign
24. **All are true about stillbirth, *except*:**
   a. Fetus was alive in utero
   b. Birth weight <1000 g
   c. Diaphragm at 4–5th rib level
   d. Hydrostatic test is negative
25. **An infant is brought to casualty with reports of violent shaking by parents. Most characteristic injury is:**
   a. Long bone fracture
   b. Ruptured spleen
   c. Subdural hematoma
   d. Skull bone fracture
26. **Munchausen by proxy includes all, *except*:**
   a. Acceptance of abuse by parents
   b. Illness does not suggest particular disease
   c. Child becomes ill in presence of the caregiver
   d. Laboratory and X-ray findings are negative
27. **Concealment of birth is punishable under:**
   a. Section 320 IPC
   b. Section 312 IPC
   c. Section 317 IPC
   d. Section 318 IPC

ANSWERS

1. a	2. a	3. c	4. b	5. c	6. d	7. b	8. c	9. c	10. c
11. a	12. a	13. d	14. a	15. b	16. b	17. c	18. c	19. b	20. a
21. b	22. c	23. c	24. b	25. c	26. a	27. d			

23 CHAPTER

Sexual Offences and Paraphilias

 KEY WORDS

Sexual offence, section 375, 376, 377 IPC, unnatural offence, perversions, rape, adultery, incest, sodomy, habitual passive agent, lesbianism, buccal coitus, bestiality, necrophilia, necrophagia, pederasty, indecent assault, fetishism, transvestism, sadism, masochism, voyeurism, peeping tom, froturism, troilism, exhibitionism.

FM3.13	Describe different types of sexual offences. Describe various sections of IPC regarding rape including definition of rape (Section 375 IPC), punishment for rape (Section 376 IPC) and recent amendments notified till date.
FM3.14	Describe and discuss the examination of the victim of an alleged case of rape, and the preparation of report, framing the opinion and preservation and dispatch of trace evidences in such cases.
FM3.15	Describe and discuss examination of accused and victim of sodomy, preparation of report, framing of opinion, preservation and dispatch of trace evidences in such cases.
FM3.16	Describe and discuss adultery and unnatural sexual offences sodomy, incest, lesbianism, buccal coitus, bestiality, indecent assault and preparation of report, framing the pinion and preservation and dispatch of trace evidences in such cases.
FM3.17	Describe and discuss the sexual perversions fetishism, transvestism, voyeurism, sadism, necrophagia, masochism, exhibitionism, frotteurism, necrophilia.

INTRODUCTION

Sexual Offences

- Both law and customs permits only heterosexual intercourse (penile–vaginal) between a man and his wife.
- Sexual offence is defined as "any form of sexual intercourse/abuse which deviates from the normal heterosexual penile-vaginal intercourse of a man with his own wife". Any act which deviates from this form of sexual intercourse is consequently contrary to law.

CLASSIFY SEXUAL OFFENCES? (FM3.13)

Sexual offences are broadly classified as:

Natural Sexual Offences

Rape, adultery and incest.

Unnatural Sexual Offences

Sodomy, lesbianism, buccal coitus and bestiality.

Sexual Perversions/Deviation/Paraphilias

- Fetishism and transvestism
- Sadism and masochism
- Exhibitionism and voyeurism
- Pedophilia and froturism
- Necrophilia and necrophagia
- Nymphomania and satyriasis, etc.

DEFINE RAPE? (FM3.13)

Section 375 IPC defines rape as: A man is said to have committed 'rape' if he:
- Penetrates his penis, to any extent, into the vagina, mouth, urethra or anus of a woman or makes her to do so with him or any other person; or
- Inserts, to any extent, any object or a part of body not being the penis, into the vagina, mouth, urethra or anus of a woman or makes her to do so with him or any other person; or
- Manipulates any part of the body of a woman so as to cause penetration into the vagina, mouth, urethra or anus of such woman or makes her to do so with him or any other person; or
- Applies his mouth to the vagina, anus or urethra of a woman or makes her to do so with him or any other person, under circumstances falling under any of the following seven descriptions:
    1. Against her will
    2. Without her consent
    3. With her consent, when her consent is obtained by putting her or any person in whom she is interested, in fear of death or bodily hurt.
    4. With her consent, when the man knows that he is not her husband, and that her consent has been given because she believes that he is the man to whom she is or believes herself to be lawfully married.
    5. With her consent when, at the time of giving such a consent, by reason of unsoundness of mind, or intoxication or the administration by him personally or through another of any stupefying or unwholesome substance, she is unable to understand the nature and consequences of that to which she gives consent.
    6. With or without her consent, when she is under 18 years of age.
    7. When she is unable to communicate consent.

WHAT IS THE PUNISHMENT FOR RAPE? (FM3.13)

Section 376 IPC: Prescribes punishment for rape:
- **Subsection 1:** Imprisonment for a term of at least 7 years which may extend to 10 years, with or without fine; unless the victim is his own wife and is not <12 years of age, in which case the maximum sentence is 2 years of imprisonment.
- **Subsection 2:** Punishment is extended up to 10 years when the offence committed is of:
    - Custodial rape
    - Institutional rape
    - Rape on a pregnant woman
    - Rape on a woman <12 years of age
    - Victim of gang rape.

Section 376A: A husband who has sexual intercourse with his own wife, who is living separately while divorce proceedings are pending in the court, can be punished with a maximum of 2 years imprisonment, with or without fine.

Section 376B, C, and D: A public servant, superintendent or member of the management or staff of any of the institutions, who has sexual intercourse with any inmates of such an institution even with consent, such sexual intercourse not amounting to rape, can be punished with imprisonment for a maximum period of 5 years, with or without fine.

DISCUSS THE RECENT AMENDMENTS IN RELATION TO SEXUAL OFFENCES? (FM3.13)

Recent Changes in Medical Examination of Sexual Violence

- Sexual violence is a significant cause of physical, psychological harm and suffering for women and children. Although sexual violence mostly affects women and girls, boys are also subject to child sexual abuse.
- The World Health Organization (WHO) defines sexual violence as "any sexual act, an attempt to obtain a sexual act, unwanted sexual comments/advances and acts to traffic, or otherwise directed against a person's sexuality, using coercion, threats of harm, or physical force, by any person regardless of relationship to the victim in any setting".
- The Criminal Law Amendment Act (CLAA) 2013 (after Delhi gang rape, Nirbhaya case) has expanded the definition of rape to include all forms of sexual violence—penetrative (oral, anal, vaginal) including by objects/weapons/fingers and nonpenetrative (touching, fondling, stalking, etc.).
- The consenting age for sexual act is 18 years (<18 years-statutory rape).
- Doctor can examine victims of sexual violence without police requisition, as per Section 357C CrPC (CLA). All these legal changes ensures the right of victim of sexual offence to voluntary report to the hospital instead of to the Police/Court after sexual violence and also that the medical examination of sexual violence victim is a medico-legal emergency.
- When such case comes to the hospital, the doctor/hospital must mandatorily inform the police. The problem with mandatory reporting is that, as per the MTP Act 1971 recognizes the right of the woman to MTP when her pregnancy is as a result of sexual violence. It also guarantees privacy and confidentiality of her information.
- Section 357C CrPC (CLAA) now mandates all hospitals irrespective of being government, public sector or private sector the responsibility of immediately providing first aid or medical treatment free of cost and medical examination of the victim, thus removing the major barrier which existed earlier of insisting government hospitals only.
- The examination need not be necessarily done by female doctor, any doctor with whom the female victim consented can carry out this examination in presence of female attendant. But, if the victim is a child, POCSO Act insists a female doctor only to examine a girl child (<18 years).
- During the examination, there should be a parent or any person whom she trust to be present throughout the examination. If such persons are not available then it is the duty of the hospital to provide one.

Importance of Presence of Injuries in Cases of Sexual Violence

- The WHO evidence states that in only 33% of cases of sexual violence there are injuries; that means out of three cases of sexual violence you do not find injuries in two cases.
- This absence of injuries could be due to various reasons—the victim being unconscious either due to trauma or being drugged/intoxicated, overpowered, silenced with fear.
- CLAA states that if someone does not resist the sexual violence that alone cannot be

construed as offering consent to the act. The Court wants at the time of incident, if the victim has said 'NO' then the law also does not question the woman for offering resistance.
- POCSO and CLAA specify that treatment should include care for injuries, HIV and other STD, pregnancy testing, emergency contraception, psychological counseling. The treatment should be free of cost and noncompliance of such treatment can drag the doctor to one year imprisonment and/or fine.
- CLAA also mandates every doctor/hospital should provide comprehensive care which also includes rehabilitation and follow up care.
- Past sexual practices still documented in sexual violence examination only in cases of chronic sexual abuse.
- Age estimation is required only when the documents or certificates are found to be fabricated or manipulated, then, the courts, the Juvenile Justice Board or the committee need to go for medical report for age determination.
- If the victim denies to give consent for examination: Law/court can't question the victim, but it can counsel the victim regarding consequences of not undergoing the examination.
- Doctor can treat the victim and informed refusal should be recorded.

Examination of Accused for Potency

Contrary to the earlier law we now have penetration by fingering or by objects and also nonpenetrative acts under the definition of rape/sexual assault. Thus doing a potency examination of the accused is not acceptable and it is irrelevant.

Provisional Opinion

- The doctor can provide provisional opinion about presence of injuries/spermatozoa if any, bodily injuries if any, and then age of injuries. Multiple contusions on the breast produced by biting and scratches by finger nails of the assailant indicates of rape **(Fig. 23.1)**. In a similar manner presence of injuries on the glans penis and ulcer on the skin coving the glans penis **(Fig. 23.2)** also indicates sexual offense.
- But as a defensive practice the doctor only opines—'reserved pending for want of FSL/laboratory reports', thus fixing the investigating officer in a spot of bother to proceed further in the case and worst the

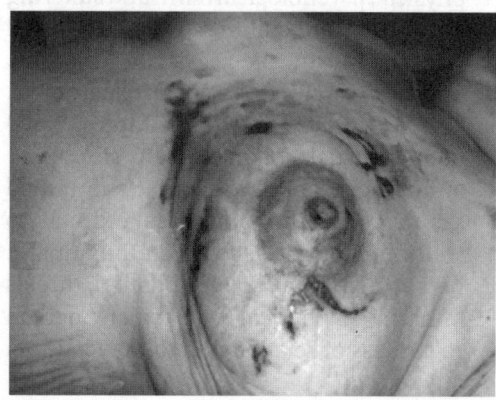

Fig. 23.1: Multiple contusions on the breast produced by biting and scratches by finger nails of the assailant *(For color version see Plate 17).*

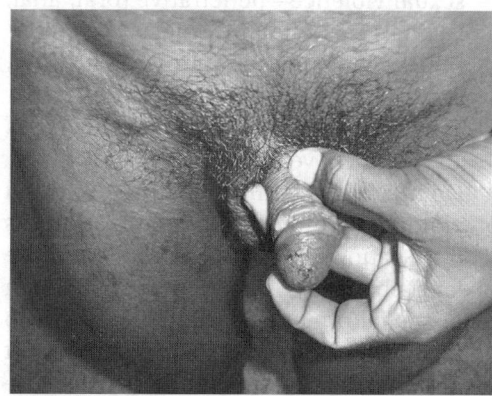

Fig. 23.2: Presence of injuries on the glans penis and ulcer on the skin coving the glans penis *(For color version see Plate 17).*

accused gets the benefit and may even get a bail as an outcome of defensive practices of doctors.
- Earlier courts were giving lot of credit to the medical evidence for proving a charge of rape/sexual assault when the law of rape was looking for penetrative penile-vaginal sexual intercourse. The law of rape/sexual assault is changed from recognizing even nonpenetrative acts and also penetrative acts into anus/oral/urethra/vagina by either penis or objects or body parts, there could be several situations of rape/sexual assault with no medical evidence at all.

Final Opinion

Law insists the doctor to provide a reasoned opinion and detailed report. Thus, the negative evidence, for example, absence of semen whether it's due to use of condom or due to washing of genitals/bathing or due to delay in medical examination etc., has to be explained.

Relevance of DNA in Cases of Sexual Violence

- DNA is crucial comparable evidence in sexual violence cases if collected and profiled properly. Courts are insisting for collection of DNA evidence in all cases of sexual violence, but our forensic science laboratories (FSL) are understaffed.
- Other problem with India is that we don't have DNA database of population or at least criminals; nor do we have more government forensic science laboratories neither private laboratories to test DNA.

Standard Uniform Guidelines

- The Ministry of Health and Family Welfare, Government of India Guidelines and Protocols—medico legal care for survivors/victims of sexual violence has been formulated.
- These guidelines includes medical examination, psychosocial care, treatment, issues in relation to dealing with children, disabled, transgender, intersex persons, persons with alternate sexual orientation, sex workers, people facing caste, class or religion based discrimination.
- They also have removed the insensitive practices in medical examination like two finger tests, over emphasis on hymen, built of the woman, past contraceptive practices, past consensual sexual acts, past abortions, etc.

CLA Legal Obligations of the Doctor in Cases of Sexual Violence

- Examination of a case of rape shall be conducted by a registered medical practitioner (RMP) employed in a hospital run by the government or a local authority and in the absence of such a practitioner, by any other RMP.
- Examination to be conducted without delay and a reasoned report to be prepared by the RMP.
- Informed consent should be obtained specifically for sexual assault examination, evidence collection and informing the police.
- Exact time of start and close of examination to be recorded.
- RMP to forward report without delay to investigating officer (IO), and in turn IO to magistrate.
- Providing necessary medical support to the survivor of sexual violence.
- Establishing a uniform method of examination and evidence collection by following the protocols [in the sexual assault forensic evidence (SAFE) kit].
- First contact psychological support and validation.

- Maintaining a clear and full-proof chain of custody of medical evidence collected.
- Referring to appropriate agencies for further assistance (e.g., legal support services, shelter services, etc.).
- Today with a lot of changes in the medical examination of sexual violence victims/survivors, adequate dissemination of this information to all stakeholders of healthcare sector along with proper training is required.

DISCUSS POCSO ACT (FM3.13)

The Protection of Children from Sexual Offences Act, 2012. Long title: An act to protect children from offences of sexual assault, sexual harassment and pornography and provide for establishment of special courts for trial of such offences and for matters connected therewith or incidental thereto.

Salient Features of the POCSO Act

- "Children" according to the act are individuals aged below 18 years. The act is gender-neutral.
- Different forms of sexual abuse including but not limited to sexual harassment, pornography, penetrative and nonpenetrative assault are defined in the act.
- Sexual assault is deemed to be "aggravated" under certain circumstances such as when the child is mentally ill. Also when the abuse is committed by the person in a position of trust such as a doctor, teacher, policeman, family member.
- Adequate provisions are made to avoid re-victimization of the child at the hands of the judicial system. The act assigns a policeman in the role of child protector during the investigation process.
- The act stipulates that such steps must be taken which makes the investigation process as child-friendly as possible and the case is disposed of within one year from the date of reporting of the offence.
- The act provides for the establishment of special courts for the trial of such offences and matters related to it.
- Under Section 45 of the act, the power to make rules lies with the central government.
- To monitor the implementation of the act, the National Commission for the Protection of Child Rights (NCPCR) and State Commissions for the Protection of Child Rights (SCPCRs) have been made the designated authority. Both being statutory bodies.
- Section 42A of the act provides that in case of inconsistency with provisions of any other law, the POCSO act shall override such provisions.
- The act calls for mandatory reporting of sexual offences. A false complaint with intent to defame a person is punishable under the Act.

POCSO Act: General principles: The Protection of Children from Sexual Offences Act, 2012 mentions 12 key principles which are to be followed by anyone, including the State Governments, the Child Welfare Committee, the Police, the Special Courts, NGOs or any other professional present during the trial and assisting the child during the trial. These include:

- **Right to life and survival:** A child must be shielded from any kind of physical, psychological, mental and emotional abuse and neglect.
- **Best interests of the child:** The primary consideration must be the harmonious development of the child.
- **Right to be treated with dignity and compassion:** Child victims should be treated in a caring and sensitive manner throughout the justice process.
- **Right to be protected from discrimination:** The justice process must be

transparent and just; irrespective of the child's cultural, religious, linguistic or social orientation.
- **Right to special preventive measures:** It suggests, that victimized children are more likely to get abused again, thus, preventive measures and training must be given to them for self-protection.
- **Right to be informed:** The child victim or witness must be well informed of the legal proceedings.
- **Right to be heard and to express views and concerns:** Every child has the right to be heard in respect of matters affecting him/her.
- **Right to effective assistance:** Financial, legal, counselling, health, social and educational services, physical and psychological recovery services and other services necessary for the child's healing must be provided.
- **Right to privacy:** The child's privacy and identity must be protected at all stages of the pretrial and trial process.
- **Right to be protected from hardship during the justice process:** Secondary victimization or hardships for a child during the justice procedure must be minimized.
- **Right to safety:** A child victim must be protected before, during and after the justice process.
- **Right to compensation:** The child victim may be awarded compensation for his/her relief and rehabilitation.

Complaint Mechanism of POCSO Act

An online complaint management system, POCSO e-box was launched in New Delhi by the Union Ministry of Women and Child Development in order to facilitate easy and direct reporting of sexual offences against children and timely disposal of the cases under POCSO Act 2012.

WRITE THE SCHEME OF EXAMINATION OF AN ALLEGED VICTIM OF RAPE? (FM3.14)

- There are two main responsibilities for a Doctor in the examination of an alleged victim of rape.
  1. *Medical responsibility:* To treat the patient for the complications arising due to the alleged offence, giving appropriate counseling and rehabilitation measures.
  2. *Legal responsibilities:* Thorough and complete examination along with collection of trace evidences to establish the offence of rape and facilitate proper delivery of justice to the victim.
- **Note:** The scheme of examination and certification of both the victim and the accused are discussed under the practical heading.

Evidence of Rape

- Marks of violence on victim and the accused.
- Marks of violence about the genitals.
- Presence of stains of blood and/or semen on the clothes and body of the victim.
- Presence of seminal matter in the vagina.
- Pregnancy or existence of STD in both the parties.

WHAT IS ADULTERY? (FM3.16)

Consented extra-marital sexual relationship is considered as adultery. Section 497 and 498 IPC deals with adultery.

Section 497 IPC

Whoever has sexual intercourse with a person whom he knows or has reasons to believe to be the wife of another man; such sexual intercourse not amounting to rape, is guilty of the offence of adultery and liable for punishment of imprisonment for 2 years.

Section 498 IPC

- Enticing or detaining a married woman, with criminal intension.
- Charge of adultery can be filed only against the adulterous man; and he should know or have reasons to believe that she is lawfully wedded to another man.
- If proved, then it's a ground for divorce for the husband of the adulterous woman.

WHAT IS INCEST? (FM3.16)

- Consented natural sexual intercourse between a man and a woman, who are prevented by the society to get married.
- Incest is not an offence in India, since marriage between close blood relatives is an accepted practice in India.
- Sexual contact within the same nuclear family is not accepted by any religious customs.

UNNATURAL SEXUAL OFFENCES: SECTION 377 IPC (FM3.15)

Unnatural Sexual Offences

- Sodomy
- Lesbianism
- Buccal coitus
- Bestiality

Section 377 IPC

Whoever voluntarily has carnal intercourse against the order of nature with any man, woman or animal shall be punished with imprisonment for life, or with imprisonment of either description for a term which may extend to 10 years, and shall also be liable for fine.

SHORT NOTES ON SODOMY (FM3.15)

Sodomy

- **Sodomy** denotes male homosexuality and involves penile-anal intercourse.
- Anal intercourse with a female is called **buggery**.
- The offender is the active agent; the other partner is the passive agent.
- If the passive agent is a child, the practice is known as **pederasty**.
- Habitual passive agents are called **catamites** (fairies, gays or queens).
- In India, **Hijras** (castrated males) and **Zenanas** (male transvestites) are the habitual passive agents of sodomy.

Local examination: The findings of examination are totally different on an individual who is not used to an act of sodomy and a habitual passive agent.

Victim not Used to Sodomy

- Pain and tenderness are always present.
- Lubricant used and loose pubic hair in and around the anus.
- Perianal abrasions and bruising are always present; sometimes with anal laceration.
- Fresh/dried stains of semen and blood may be recoverable.
- Digital examination is painful and does not allow more than two fingers.

Habitual Passive Agent

- Blood stains are usually not present.
- Lubricant and loose foreign pubic hair may or may not be present.
- Perianal hair is shaved and local hygiene scrupulously maintained.
- Thickening and keratinization of the perianal skin due to constant friction.
- No pain or tenderness during examination.
- Lateral buttock traction test is positive (funnel shaped depression of the anus).

- **Anus:** Dilated, patulous and loss of rugosity of mucus membrane. Fresh and old fissures and/or sinuses (tunneling) is a common finding.
- **Rectum:** Prolapsed mucosa, with thickening and disappearance of radial folds.
- Evidence of STD (condylomata, chancre and gonorrheal discharge) may be evident.
- **Digital examination:** Allows three to four fingers easily and pain is highly improbable.

WHAT IS LESBIANISM? (FM3.16)

- Lesbianism denotes female homosexuality; it is also called as **tribadism or sapphism**.
- Typically, it involves mutual masturbation and occasionally an active-passive relationship, by bilateral/digital/lingual, vaginal stimulation, or the use of vibrators or artificial phalluses (**Dildoes**).
- Active lesbian is known as **butch** or **dyke**, the usual passive agent is called **femme**.
- Habitually active lesbians have a strong aversion to normal sexual behavior.
- Whereas the passive agent is not so, and in fact frequently bisexual.

Medico-legal Aspects

- Lesbianism is extremely difficult to prove: Traces of fresh and dried saliva and/or mucosal cells can be detected on/around the external genitalia, or
- Injuries are present if there has been forcible introduction of a grossly disproportionate artificial phallus.

WHAT IS SIN OF GOMORRAH? (FM3.16)

Buccal Coitus

- Buccal-penile intercourse is called **fellatio**; the partner who performs the act is called the **fellator;** and on whom it is performed is the **fellate**.
- Buccal-vaginal stimulation is referred to as **cunnilingus.**

Medico-legal Aspects

The only material evidence of commission of the offence would be:
- Spermatozoa of the fellate in the buccal cavity of the fellator, or
- Fresh or dried saliva and/or mucosal cells on the penis of the fellate, or vulva of the subject of cunnilingus.

WRITE SHORT NOTES ON BESTIALITY (FM3.16)

- Sexual intercourse with a lower animal is called as bestiality and it is a crime throughout the world.
- The animal usually selected are cows, bitches, female sheep/goat/donkey and large birds in males and bulls, horses, dogs, male sheep/goat/donkeys by the females.

Medico-legal Aspects

- Difficult to prove unless the accused is caught during the act.
- Young adult male, usually mentally challenged are the affected people.
- Injuries inflicted by the animal, hair/feathers and/or blood stains of the animal on the clothing or on the individual may be present.

WHAT IS AN INDECENT ASSAULT? (FM3.16)

- Indecent assault generally means sex-linked misbehavior towards a person of opposite sex or the same sex.
- Any offence committed towards a female with the intention or knowledge to outrage the modesty of the female.
- **Section 509 IPC:** Whoever, intending to insult the modesty of a woman, utters

any word, makes any sound or gesture, or exhibits any object shall be punished with imprisonment which may extend to one year.

DISCUSS ABOUT SEXUAL PARAPHILIAS? (FM3.17)

- Achievement of sexual gratification by means other than sexual intercourse; they are called as sexual deviations, perversions or paraphilias.
- These form a group of psychosexual disorders, which involves involuntary, repetitive, unusual acts, on which sexual arousal and orgasm are dependent.

Fetishism (Fetishism)

- Sexual focus is on relatively indestructible objects intimately associated with human body.
- Male are the affected; attraction is mainly on the clothes and articles which were in close intimation with the female body. Example: Panties, petticoat, handkerchief, etc.
- Orgasm is obtained usually by masturbation.

Transvestism

Cross dressing or eonism; dressing in the opposite sex, for the purpose of arousal and as an adjunct in sexual intercourse or masturbation.

Sadism

Male are the affected; sexual arousal and orgasm linked to active infliction of injuries or torture of the sexual partner.

Masochism

- Female are the usually affected; sexual excitement linked with passive experience of physical or emotional humiliation or torture.

- There arises no problem when a sadistic male and a masochist female go hand in hand.

Lust Murder

Lust murder is an extreme form of sadism, where the sadistic male may pass a ligature around the neck of the female and strangle her (may also be a part of masochistic activity) during the act of sexual intercourse; at the moment of attainment of orgasm, he may tighten the ligature and hold it tight for some reasonable period of time and the woman may die due to ligature strangulation, this is called as lust murder. There is no intension to kill, but death is due to accidental strangulation.

Exhibitionism

Exhibitionism involves repeated acts of exposing one's genitals to a female, who may even be a stranger or unsuspected person.

Voyeurism/Scoptophilia

Perversion with desire to observe the genitals or other private parts of the female, while they are bathing, or go still perverted and like to watch them urinating or defecating and orgasm is obtained by masturbation.

Peeping Tom

Watching people engaged in sexual activity without their knowledge.

Troilism

Extreme form of peeping tom, where the pervert gets sexual gratification by inducing his wife to sexual intercourse with another person and like to witness the same.

Frotteurism

Practiced by a male pervert in a crowded place to drive sexual gratification by rubbing his private parts against a female's body.

Necrophilia

- Sexual arousal and orgasm can be attained by intercourse with a corpse.
- Mortuary workers are the usual sufferers, as they have the access; people addicted to alcohol and who are impotent may involve in these types of activities.

Necrophagia

- Necrophagia is an extreme form of necrophilia where in sexual gratification is attained by tearing out the genitals or other part of body of a corpse and eating them.
- Necrophilia and necrophagia are punishable under section 297 IPC.

Section 297 IPC

Whoever with the intention of offering any indignity to any human corpse, shall be punished with imprisonment of either description for a term which may extend to one year, or with fine, or both.

Pedophilia

Preferential sexual activity with children. Indulging the children in sexual activity by touching their private parts, kissing, hugging and make the children touch and fondle on their private parts; they make the children indulge in buccal coitus also.

Satyriasis

Excessive sexual desire among males. These subjects are liable to commit sexual offences.

Nymphomania

Excessive sexual desire among woman; they make indulge in sex with multiple sex partners and when the access to sex is restricted, they make indulge in lesbianism.

AUTO-EROTIC ASPHYXIAS/SEXUAL ASPHYXIA

Discussed in asphyxial death.

MULTIPLE CHOICE QUESTIONS

1. **The sign of recent rape:**
   a. Fourchette congestion
   b. Bleeding hymeneal tear
   c. Motile spermatozoa
   d. Patulous vagina
2. **One of the following sections of IPC prescribes punishment for sodomy:**
   a. 375
   b. 376
   c. 377
   d. 366A
3. **The following is a proof of penetration after 48 hours:**
   a. Nonmotile spermatozoa
   b. Fragmented spermatozoa
   c. Acid phosphatase
   d. Alkaline phosphatase
4. **The tear in one of the following site of hymen is an absolute proof of penetration:**
   a. 12 O'clock position
   b. 2 O'clock position
   c. 9 O'clock position
   d. 7 O'clock position
5. **Impotence is pleaded as a defence in the following,** *except:*
   a. Divorce
   b. Rape
   c. Sadism
   d. Adultery
6. **Statutory rape is** _____
   a. Sex with a girl aged above 16 years
   b. Sex with a girl aged below 16 years
   c. Sex with a girl aged below 18 years
   d. Sex with a wife aged below 16 years
7. **All are wrong statement,** *except:*
   a. If a case of criminal abortion comes to the hospital, the attending doctor is not bound to inform the police
   b. Attempt to commit suicide is not an offence in India

c. There is no punishment for incest in India
d. Maximum punishment for rape is life imprisonment

8. Normal amount of acid phosphatase in human semen is:
   a. 250 bodansky units
   b. 350
   c. 450
   d. 2500 BU

9. Best method to detect blood from an old stain is:
   a. Spectroscopy
   b. Absorption elution
   c. Hemochromogen
   d. None

10. Lust murder is an extreme form of:
    a. Sadism
    b. Masochism
    c. Frotteurism
    d. Fetichism

11. Which of the following tests is used to detect semen?
    a. Phenolphthalein test
    b. Reine's test
    c. Barberio's test
    d. Paraffin test

12. Kastle-Meyer test is known as:
    a. Precipitin test
    b. Phenolphthalein test
    c. Benzidine test
    d. Hemochromogen test

13. Which one of the following is the best test for seminal stains?
    a. Teichmann test
    b. Alkaline phosphate test
    c. Acid phosphatase test
    d. Precipitin test

14. Locard's principle is classically observed in:
    a. Drowning
    b. Putrefaction
    c. Sexual offences
    d. Planned homicide

15. Sexual pleasure is obtained by wearing clothes of opposite sex is:
    a. Transvestism
    b. Fetichism
    c. Masochism
    d. Tribadism

16. Exhibitionism and voyeurism are punishable under:
    a. Section 377 IPC
    b. Section 354 IPC
    c. Section 294 IPC
    d. Section 376 IPC

17. In sodomy if the passive agent is a child, then he is called as:
    a. Catamite
    b. Pedophile
    c. Pederast
    d. Femme

18. Sexual gratification by urinating on the partner is:
    a. Urolagnia
    b. Uranism
    c. Necrophagia
    d. Scopophilia

19. Gerontophilia is:
    a. Preferential sexual activity with children
    b. Preferential sexual activity with cadavers
    c. Preferential sexual activity with elderly
    d. Preferential sexual activity with animals

20. Rape is defined under:
    a. Section 320 IPC
    b. Section 375 IPC
    c. Section 376 IPC
    d. Section 351 IPC

21. It is considered rape even after consent if:
    a. Age <16 years
    b. Age <18 years
    c. Age <21 years
    d. Age <25 years

22. A 24-year-old man gets married with 14-year-old female. Having sex with her will be considered rape because:
    a. No consent taken from wife
    b. Wife age <18 years
    c. Wife age <15 years
    d. Wife age <17 year

23. 2-year-old girl with sexual abuse presented with bleeding from genitals and fracture pelvis. Appropriate sequence of management is:
    a. Internal iliac artery ligation, blood transfusion, inform police, medico-legal report
    b. Blood transfusion, internal iliac artery ligation, medico-legal report, inform police

c. Blood transfusion, medico-legal report, internal iliac artery ligation, inform police
d. Inform police, medico-legal report, blood transfusion, internal iliac artery ligation

24. **Punishment for rape under Section 376(1) IPC:**
   a. 3 years imprisonment + fine
   b. 5 years imprisonment + fine
   c. 7 years imprisonment + fine
   d. Death sentence + fine

25. **Husband had intercourse with wife during separation without consent. Section which deals with it:**
   a. 376-A IPC
   b. 376-B IPC
   c. 376-C IPC
   d. 376-D IPC

26. **Most common position of hymen rupture in a virgin is:**
   a. Anterior
   b. Anterio-lateral
   c. Posterior-lateral
   d. Posterior

27. **Motile spermatozoa found in wet mount of vaginal secretions are indicative of intercourse within the past:**
   a. 6 hours
   b. 12 hours
   c. 24 hours
   d. 48 hours

28. **In sexual assault of a child, the hymen is usually not ruptured due to:**
   a. Deep seated
   b. Underdeveloped
   c. Too tough to rupture
   d. Distensible

29. **Test for vaginal cells collected for investigation for rape:**
   a. Lugol's iodine test
   b. Acro-reaction test
   c. Precipitin test
   d. Barberio's test

ANSWERS

1. c	2. c	3. c	4. d	5. c	6. c	7. c	8. b	9. b	10. a
11. c	12. b	13. c	14. c	15. a	16. c	17. b	18. a	19. c	20. b
21. b	22. c	23. b	24. c	25. b	26. c	27. b	28. a	29. a	

SECTION
6

Forensic Psychiatry

SECTION OUTLINE

Chapter 24: Symptoms of Psychiatry and Mental Health Act 1987

CHAPTER 24

Symptoms of Psychiatry and Mental Health Act 1987

KEY WORDS

Psychiatry, mental illness, insanity defense, delirium, delusion, illusion, hallucination, impulse, obsession, fugue, phobia, psychosis, sociopath, neurosis, somnambulism, somnalentia, hypnosis, mental retardation, epileptic psychosis, lactational psychosis, GPI, delirium tremens, feigned insanity, restraint of an insane, testamentary capacity, criminal responsibility, Mc Naughton's rule, Curren's rule, Durham's rule, irresistible impulse test.

FM5.1	Classify common mental illnesses including post-traumatic stress disorder (PTSD).
FM5.2	Define, classify, and describe delusions, hallucinations, illusion, lucid interval and obsessions with exemplification.
FM5.3	Describe civil and criminal responsibilities of a mentally ill person.
FM5.4	Differentiate between true insanity from feigned insanity.
FM5.5	Describe and discuss Delirium tremens.
FM 5.6	Describe the Indian Mental Health Act, 1987 with special reference to admission, care and discharge of a mentally ill person.

INTRODUCTION

Forensic Psychiatry

Psychiatry is a branch of medical science which deals with diagnosis, treatment, and rehabilitation measure of the mentally ill people.

Forensic Psychiatry

- Forensic psychiatry is a subspecialty of psychiatry which deals with the application of knowledge of psychiatry in legal issues.
- In general it represents interference between law and psychiatry.
- The term "insanity" is loosely used to refer any mental disorder or mental illness.
- However, it is commonly used in legal context such as "insanity defense".
- The IPC employs the term: "unsoundness of mind" while referring to insanity.

DEFINE MENTAL ILLNESS?

Mental illness is a sociological concept accordingly a "**mentally ill person**" may be designated as that member of the community who is unable to look after himself or manage his own affairs or is dangerous to himself or to others.

WHAT IS LEGAL INSANITY?

The mental illness may be of such gravity that it becomes advisable in the interest of the patient or the community to segregate such an individual and deprive him of his liberty and rights as a citizen.

WHAT IS RECEPTION ORDER?

It is an order issued by the court for admission and detention of a mentally ill person in a psychiatric hospital or nursing home.

WHAT IS DELIRIUM?

Delirium is a disorders of consciousness.
- There is disturbance of consciousness and orientation is impaired.
- Thought content is irrelevant or inconsistent.
- In the early stage the patient is restless, uneasy, and sleepless.
- Later, he loses self-control, becomes excited and talks furiously.
- Delusions and hallucinations may be present at this stage; and he becomes impulsive and may commit any crime, for which he is not liable.
- Usually occurs in **physical disease.**
- Example: Continuous high fever, mental stress, or drug intoxication.

DESCRIBE DELUSION AND DIFFERENT TYPES OF DELUSIONS? (FM5.2)

Delusion is a disorder of thought. False belief in something which is not a fact; and continues to persist even after the falsity is clearly demonstrated.

Types of Delusions

- **Delusion of grandeur or exaltation:** This is a pleasant delusion. The individual is actually very poor but thinks that he is very rich and spends money so much lavishly.
- **Delusion of persecution:** This is an unpleasant delusion and usually co-exists with delusion of grandeur. The individual thinks that because he is rich and got lot of money, people closely associated with him (wife, children, relatives, or friends) are trying steal his money and also believes that they are even trying to kill him or poison him to take away his imaginary property and money.
- **Delusion of reference:** He feels that whatever he hears or comes across, he is being referred to.
- **Delusion of influence:** He believes that all his actions are influenced by some external agency; he receives imaginary commands and obeys them (like telepathy).
- **Delusion of infidelity:** The male are the sufferers; he suspects the fidelity of his wife; even though she is not like that in reality and is gem of a female; they are usually addicted to alcohol and may also be impotent.
- **Delusion of self-reproach:** He accuses himself for all the bad and mishaps in his life.
- **Nihilistic delusion:** He does not believe in the worldly existence at all.
- **Hypochondriacal delusion:** The individual is relatively healthy, but thinks that he suffers from a number of diseases, goes from doctor to doctor with cluster of imaginary complaints. Once the doctor says he is completely normal after necessary investigations, he changes over to a new doctor with new imaginary complaints.
- **Erotomaniacal delusion:** Females are the usual sufferers; usually people at a lower level develop some imaginary intimate affection towards one of a higher level and starts believing that they are also reciprocating.

WHAT IS HALLUCINATION? WHAT ARE THE TYPES OF HALLUCINATIONS? (FM5.2)

Hallucination is a disorder of perception in which there is false sense perception without any external object or stimuli to produce it. This is purely imaginary and may affect any or all of the special senses. Depending on the various special senses it may be:
- **Visual hallucination:** He sees something when actually nothing is present there.
- **Auditory hallucination:** He hears some imaginary sounds, which do not exist.
- **Olfactory hallucination:** He perceives some smell, when no such odor is present.
- **Gustatory hallucination:** He feels some taste when nothing is there in the mouth.
- **Tactile hallucination:** He feels some insects are crawling over his body, which are actually not there. This type of hallucination is also called "***Magnan's symptom***" or "***Formication***". It commonly occurs as withdrawal symptom of chronic cocaine poisoning and are referred to as "***Cocaine Bugs***".
- **Psychomotor hallucination:** He feels that some part of the body, usually the limbs are getting elongated, goes away from his body, performs some activity and come back.

WHAT IS AN ILLUSION? (FM5.2)

- Illusion is also a disorder of perception. There is misinterpretation of a real existing stimulus or object.
- **Example:** Seeing a rope, he may mistake it as a snake; the weight of the blanket may be mistaken as that of the weight of a collapsed building, etc.
- Under certain circumstances even sane people will have illusion, but when the reality is exposed, the sane person is able to understand his misinterpretation but an insane will continue to perceive the same even after clearly proving the misinterpretation.

WHAT IS AN IMPULSE? WHAT ARE THE TYPES OF IMPULSES? (FM5.2)

- Impulse is defined as sudden irresistible desire/force compelling a person to the conscious performance of some act for which there is no motive or forethought.
- Every individual may have impulsive behavior at any one time due to emotional imbalance. But, a sane person is capable of controlling his impulse but an insane person cannot control the impulses.
- **Types of impulse:**
    - *Kleptomania:* Irresistible desire to steal articles of little value.
    - *Pyromania:* Irresistible desire to set fire.
    - *Mutilomania:* Irresistible desire to mutilate lower animals (pet animals)
    - *Dipsomania:* Irresistible desire to drink alcohol in excess amount
    - *Sexual impulse:* Irresistible desire to engage in some form of sexual activity.
    - Suicidal impulse: Irresistible desire to commit suicide.
    - *Homicidal impulse:* Irresistible desire to kill someone.

WHAT IS AN OBSESSION? (FM5.2)

- Obsession is a disorder of the content of thought.
- A single idea, thought or emotion is constantly entertained by a person which he himself recognizes as irrational but persists in spite of all efforts to drive it from his mind.
- Any attempt to resist makes them appear more insistent, and yielding is the inevitable outcome.
- It is a ***borderline*** between sanity and insanity.

- Usually occurs in neurotic people, who are very well able to discharge their ordinary responsibilities of life.

WHAT IS FUGUE STATE? (FM5.2)

- It is a state of altered awareness during which an individual forgets part or whole of his past life, leaves home and wanders away; he has a state of complete amnesia for the period.
- He regains his memory once he comes back to the same situation after a lapse of time but will forget the events which happened in between the period.
- It is more of self-induced to escape from the unpleasant situations of life, like heavy financial debuts, family problems, etc.
- Occurs commonly in Hysteria and also in depressive illness and schizophrenia.

WHAT IS PHOBIA? WHAT ARE THE TYPES? (FM5.2)

Fear is an inbuilt attitude of any human being. Some persons may have fear of particular issues. But excessive or irrational fear of a particular object or situation is called "phobia". Depending on the type of fear an individual has, it could be:
- **Claustrophobia:** Fear of staying in a closed place
- **Nyctophobia:** Fear of darkness
- **Agoraphobia:** Fear of open space
- **Acrophobia:** Fear of height
- **Mysophobia:** Fear of dirt
- **Hydrophobia:** Fear of water.

WHO IS A PSYCHOPATH? (FM5.1)

- Psychopath is also known as sociopath.
- A person who is neither insane nor mentally defective but fails to conform to normal standards of behavior.
- Psychopaths have abnormal personality and persistently behave in an antisocial or disruptive manner.
- There is failure of maturation of the personality and the individual retains a childlike selfishness.
- There is no abnormality of thought, mood or intelligence.
- It's not a ground for insanity defense but may provide a plea of diminished responsibility.

WHAT IS A PSYCHOPATHIC DISORDER? (FM5.1)

It's a persistent disorder or disability of mind, which results in abnormally aggressive or seriously irresponsible conduct on the part of the person.

WHAT IS PSYCHOSIS? (FM5.1)

- Psychosis is characterized by a withdrawal from reality and living in a world of fantasy.
- Mental illness supervenes upon a normally developed mental faculty.
- There is disorientation in the personality and progressive loss of contact with reality.
- He totally loses touch with reality and lives in his own imaginary world.

WHAT IS NEUROSIS? (FM5.1)

- The patient suffers from emotional and intellectual disorders but does not lose touch with reality. Hence, he is capable of living a normal life in the society.
- Neurosis is commonly seen in anxiety, depression, or hysteria.
- The effect may be mild or may cause considerable disturbance.

WHAT IS AFFECTIVE DISORDER? (FM5.1)

- Affect means Emotion, Feeling or Mood
- Affective disorder:
- Psychiatric disorder in which the chief feature is a relatively prolonged affective change of an abnormal degree; it consists of two phases namely, Mania (elevation) and Melancholia (depression) hence also called as "bipolar disorders".

WHAT IS LUCID INTERVAL OF INSANITY? (FM5.2)

- The period of sanity in between two bouts of insanity is called "lucid interval".
- All the symptoms of insanity disappear, and the person is completely normal.
- He can make a valid will during this period and is legally responsible for all his acts if it is proved that he was under lucid interval when he committed that act.
- Difference between lucid interval of insanity and lucid interval of head injury tabulated in **Table 24.1**.

TABLE 24.1: Difference between lucid interval of insanity and lucid interval of head injury.

Insanity	Head injury
History of insanity is present	History of head injury is present and usually occurs in extra-dural hemorrhage
Predisposing symptoms of insanity present	Predisposing symptoms of cerebral concussion is present
Following symptoms of insanity present	Symptoms of cerebral irritation and brain compression are present
Occurrence is frequent	Occurs only once, and then the person undergoes permanent unconsciousness and death follows

WHAT ARE THE CAUSES OF INSANITY? (FM5.1)

- **Hereditary:** Huntington's chorea, family idiocy, etc.
- **Environmental:** Faulty parental attitude and lack of mental hygiene.
- **Psychogenic:** Unsuccessfully repressed mental conflict.
- **Precipitating:** Financial worries, frustrations and disappointment in sexual affairs, death of close relative, etc.
- **Organic causes:** Head injury, atherosclerosis, senile degeneration, myxedema, pernicious anemia, etc.
  - International classification of diseases-ICD 10th edition. 1992, classifies psychiatric diseases for the purpose of treatment and Chapter F deals with psychiatric disorders.

CLASSIFICATION OF INSANITY (WHO 1965) (FM5.1)

- ICD classification is an elaborate one and is followed all over the world and more useful for clinician who treats the psychiatric problems.
- For legal purposes WHO classification holds good for all purposes.
- WHO classification of psychiatric diseases is simple and also widely accepted even today, especially for legal issues.

Psychoses

- **Organic psychoses:** Senile and presenile dementia, associated with disease, tumors, and endocrine, metabolic, and nutritional disorders.
- **Functional:** Schizophrenia and affective disorders.

Neuroses

- Anxiety neurosis
- Hystcrical neurosis

- Phobic neurosis
- Obsessive compulsive neurosis
- Depressive neurosis
  - Personality disorders (psychopath)
  - Sexual deviations
  - Drug dependence (drug induced)
  - Mental sub-normality (amentia)
- In mental sub-normality (**mental retardation**) there is defective development of mental maturity and intelligent quotient of an individual is taken into consideration.
  - *Idiocy:* IQ 0 to 20 and mental is 3 years.
  - *Imbecility:* IQ 20 to 50 and mental age is 7 years.
  - *Moron or feeble mindedness:* IQ 50 to 75 and mental age is 12 years.

WHAT IS THE RELATIONSHIP OF ALCOHOLISM AND PSYCHOSIS? WHAT IS DELIRIUM TREMENS? (FM5.5)

- Alcohol is a CNS depressant and prolonged consumption of large quantities leads to psychiatric problems. Some of the important conditions related to alcohol are:
  - *Alcoholic blackouts:* These are episodes of amnesia which occur after a sudden heavy alcoholic drink and the individual has a complete amnesia of the sequence of events which occur during this phase.

Delirium Tremens

- Delirium tremens is a withdrawal symptom of chronic alcoholism; occurs 2 to 3 days after the last drink and may persist for 3 weeks; it is a consequence of sudden abstinence in a chronic drunkard.
- Injuries, infection, and shock may be precipitating factors.
- The patient becomes sleepless, restless, and irritable; then develops disorders of perception and coarse muscular tremors of the peripheries, mainly face, tongue and hand.
- He is prone to commit some offences during this phase, especially assault, sexual offences, suicide, or murder.
- He is totally exempted from the law for any of the offences committed during this period, since delirium tremens is a psychotic condition.

Alcoholic Hallucinosis

The patient may suffer from different types of hallucinations and may also develop illusions due to chronic alcoholism.

Korsakov's Psychosis

Characterized by loss of memory for recent events, both retrograde and anterograde amnesia; the individual remains responsive and alert despite the severe memory loss and learning impairment.

Wernicke's Encephalopathy

- The physical components of Korsakov's psychosis consist of ophthalmoplegia, ataxia and peripheral neuritis and is known as Wernicke's encephalopathy.
- Delusions of infidelity and delusions of jealousy may develop due to the effects of chronic alcoholism.

WHAT IS GPI? (GENERAL PARALYSIS OF INSANE)

- Usually associated with meningovascular syphilis and tabes dorsalis.
- Chronic psychoorganic syndrome characterized by temperamental and personality changes, leading to paralysis and dementia.
- Memory is impaired and retarded thoughts are present.

EFFECTS OF EPILEPSY ON PSYCHOSIS

Epilepsy is usually not associated with psychiatric symptoms; but 10% of patients suffering from epilepsy may have associated psychiatric problems; and may occur at any of the three phases:
1. **Postepileptic confusional state:** A state of confusion and irritability occurring just prior to the epileptic fits.
2. **Postepileptic automatism:** Occurs immediately after the epileptic fits and the individual may commit any offence like assault or theft after the epileptic phase and usually same type of act is done repeatedly, after every attack of fits.
3. **Epileptic equilent or masked epilepsy:** The epileptic fits phase may be completely replaced by some criminal act; the individual may even commit murder. This is also called psychomotor epilepsy or psychic epilepsy.

WHAT ARE THE EFFECTS OF PREGNANCY AND CHILDBIRTH TO PSYCHOSIS?

- Psychosis may occur any time from the beginning of pregnancy to the end of lactation: delusions are common and dislike or hatred towards the husband may occur, and the patient may develop suicidal tendencies.
- Postpartum psychosis may take a great variety of forms:
- The commonest being mania and the women may commit infanticide.

WHAT IS LACTATIONAL PSYCHOSIS?

May occur after six weeks of confinement.
- Characterized by mental confusion, hallucinations, and depression.
- Delusion of persecution may develop, which may lead to suicide and infanticide.

HOW TO DIAGNOSE INSANITY? (FM5.1)

- Insanity is usually a slowly developing disease and the people close to the patient who are present around the individual can very well make out the difference if observed carefully. It may take two to ten years for the development of full-blown psychosis.
- But in a less percentage of cases it may be sudden in onset; especially in emotionally instable individuals who have some traumatic episode of events in their life, like sudden loss of someone who were very close and on whom they were much dependent in life.
- In typical cases the diagnosis is easy, but in early stages and in borderline cases, the correct diagnosis becomes very difficult.
- The objectives of clinical examination are to form an opinion about the patient's mind and the degree of responsibility.

Preliminary Particulars

- **Family history:** Psychosis, chorea, epilepsy, etc.
- **Personal history:** Previous mental illness and treatment, environmental factors, emotional conflict and anxiety, drugs, frustrations in life, love, etc.

Physical Examination

- Manner of dress and walk.
- Examine for deformities and organic diseases which may lead to psychosis.
- Pulse and temperature (may be increased).
- **Tongue:** Furred and coated.
- **Skin:** Dry and Wrinkled.

Mental Condition

- **Talk:** Mutism, distraction, and irrelevant talk.

- **Speech:** Incoherent, slurred and stammering of speech.
- **Writing:** Flight of ideas, insulting language, meaningless and unintelligible.
- **Behavior:** Lazy, impulsive, stereotypy and echopraxia.
- **Mood:** Highly variable mood; emotion, euphoria, joy, anger, apathy, irritable, etc.
- **Memory:** Impaired and amnesia usually present.
- **Sleep:** Insomnia, hyposomnia, somnambulism, somnolentia.
- **Walk and gait:** Staggering gait.
- **Sex behavior:** Abstinence or perverted.
- **Attention:** Focusing the attention to a particular object or incident is very difficult and concentration power is very much lowered or even absent.
- Thought process and thought content are irrelevant and inconsistent.
- **Investigations:** Blood, Urine, CSF, X-ray, EEG.
- But the results of the investigations may not show any diagnostic feature of abnormality.

WHAT ARE THE METHODS OF OBSERVATION AND CERTIFICATION OF INSANITY? (FM5.4)

- No certificate of mental illness is to be issued by a single examination; minimum three examinations on different day and different times, before a certification of insanity is issued.
- The patient is admitted and kept under observation for 10 days in the first slot, if no clear opinion could be arrived in ten days, then it can be extended to another 10 days to a maximum of 30 days.
- The patient is observed when he is unaware that he is being observed; now a days hidden cameras are used for continuous secret observation.
- No single feature is diagnostic, but many of the following findings are useful to arrive at a conclusion of insanity.

HOW TO DIFFERENTIATE TRUE INSANITY FROM FEIGNED INSANITY? (FM5.4)

Table 24.2 is depicted the differences between true insanity and feigned insanity.

WRITE SHORT NOTES ON THE MENTAL HEALTH ACT 1987 (FM5.6)

The Mental Health Act 1987

- **Replaced Indian Lunacy Act 1912:** The basic of the Lunacy Act was to prevent ourselves from the mentally ill people. Due to the advancements in the field of psychiatry, the basic aim of the Mental Health Act is preserve the rights of the mentally ill people.
- **MHA is divided into 10 chapters consisting of 98 sections:** Chapter 1 deals with definitions.

Psychiatric Hospital or Nursing Home Means

- It is a hospital for the mentally ill maintained by the government or private authority with facilities of outpatient treatment and registered with appropriate licensing authority.
- Admitting a mentally ill person to a general nursing home is an offence.

Psychiatrist Means

A RMP with postgraduate or diploma degree in psychiatry recognized by the MCI (MD in psychiatry or DPM).

Mentally Ill Person

- A person who is in need of treatment for any mental disorder other than mental retardation.
- MHA 1987 lays down stringent guidelines for admission, treatment and discharge of psychiatric patients in registered psychiatric hospitals. If a psychiatric

TABLE 24.2: Difference between true insanity and feigned insanity.

True insanity	Feigned insanity
Onset: Gradual	Usually sudden, after committing an offence
Motive: 100% no motive	Obvious motive (diagnostic)
Predisposing factors of insanity are present	No predisposing factors—absent
Signs and symptoms: Uniform irrespective of whether he is being observed or not	Signs and symptoms: Present only when observed by someone
The symptoms are uniform and fall into any one of diagnosable psychiatric illness	The symptoms are varying and will not fall into any diagnosable psychiatric illness
Physical signs of insanity are present: Face will have the classical feature called—vacant look (without any expression)	Physical signs of insanity are absent: Changing facial expressions
Filthy behavior and worst hygiene	Hygiene and filthy behaviors are not to that extent as these cannot be mimicked
Can withstand hunger, insomnia and exertion for a very long period of time	Cannot withstand hunger, insomnia and exertion and hence becomes exhausted soon
Does not mind frequent examinations	Resists frequent examinations, for fear of being detected

patient is not properly received, for such improper reception of psychiatric patients in psychiatric hospitals, the punishment is imprisonment up to 2 years and fine of ₹ 1000 or both.
- As per the MHA 1987, there are specified methods for restraint of an insane under different circumstances.

WHAT ARE THE VARIOUS METHODS OF RESTRAINT OF THE INSANE? (FM5.6)? WHAT ARE THE METHODS OF ADMISSION INTO A PSYCHIATRIC HOSPITAL?

Immediate Restraint

- Anyone who is present nearby can restrain a mentally ill person if:
  - He is dangerous to himself or to others
  - He is likely to injure himself or others
  - He wastefully spends his money
  - Persons suffering from delirium due to disease, and
  - Delirium tremens.

METHODS OF ADMISSION OF A PATIENT IN PSYCHIATRIC HOSPITAL

Admission on Voluntary Basis

- The patient himself or his relatives approaches the hospital for admission; such application has to be supported by medical certificates from two doctors (psychiatrists) and one of them should preferably be a government doctor.
- If the hospital has enough facilities, even without such medical certificate admission can be made after examining by two psychiatrists from their hospital itself.
- When he is admitted on voluntary basis, if request for discharge is made, then he has to be discharged within 24 hours of such request, even if he is not fully cured of the problem.
- For a patient to get admitted into the hospital on voluntary basis, there has to be "insight".
- **Insight** is the ability of the individual to recognize that he is having some mental problem and because of that he is unable

to adapt to the required standards of life; thus seeks the help of someone (usually psychiatrist) to get cured of his illness.

Admission Under Special Circumstances

- **Reception order on application:**
  - The relatives can make an application to the magistrate along with two medical certificates and get a reception order for admission; when such individual applies for discharge, then he will be discharged only after information to the magistrate, and he has to wait for the period of time for completion of the process to get discharged.
- **Reception order on production of mentally ill person before the magistrate:**
  - A wandering psychiatric patient can be produced in front of the magistrate by the police of that jurisdiction and obtain a reception order for detention and admission of such patients. When some relative of such an individual comes forward after a period and requests for discharge, he cannot be discharged if he is not fully cured.
- **Admission after judicial inquisition:**
  - When a person accused of a crime, takes a defend on the grounds of insanity, then the magistrate issues a reception order for detention, observation, and certification of mental illness.
- **Admission of mentally ill prisoner:**
  - When a person convicted of a crime is found/proved to be insane, then he cannot be imprisoned; he has to be admitted and treated in a psychiatric hospital under the reception order of the magistrate; when such an individual is cured of his mental illness, then the doctor informs the magistrate and he may be discharged or imprisoned under the orders of the court.
- **Admission of an escaped mentally ill person:**
  - When a mentally ill person escapes from the hospital, on production of the individual in the court, he can be admitted again on obtaining a reception order.

WHAT ARE ALL THE CIVIL RESPONSIBILITIES OF AN INSANE (FM5.7)? WHAT IS TESTAMENTARY CAPACITY?

- **Management of property and affairs:**
  - The insanity is of such a degree as to make him incapable of managing his property and affairs; then the court may appoint a manager (when he is unable manage the property) or a guardian (when he is unable manage the property and as well as his own affairs) depending on the condition of the patient, on opinion of two psychiatrists.
- **Consent:** Consent given by an insane person is not a valid consent.
- **Contract:** An insane person cannot sign a contract and is invalid; if any of the partner was proved to be insane at the time of signing a contract, then the contract goes invalid, but if he has signed in the period of lucid interval, then it becomes a valid contract.
- **Marriage:** If anyone of the parties was proved to be insane at the time of marriage, the marriage is declared as null or void (invalid marriage). But anyone of the parties became insane after marriage then it can be a ground for divorce by the other party, provided he/she has made enough efforts to treat the mental illness for a reasonable period of time.
- **Competency as witness:** An insane person is not competent to be a witness in the court of law unless he is in the period of lucid interval.

- **Testamentary capacity:** It is the mental ability of a person to make a valid will.
- **The requirements are:**
  - A written, properly signed and witnessed document.
  - The testator must be a major and of sound disposing mind (Compos mentis) and it should be certified by a doctor.
  - Force, undue influence, or dishonest representation of facts, should not have been applied by others.
  - None of the witnesses should be beneficiaries of such a will.
  - Bed ridden and aphasic individuals are not prevented from making a will; provided they understand what the property they've got, to whom they are giving and why they are giving to them.
- **Holograph will:** (2 Marks)
  - It is a will which is written by the testator in his/her own handwriting.
  - Many a time's doctors are called upon to witness the execution of the will of a sick, and the doctor should check whether the individual is in compos mentis (sound disposing mind).

WHAT IS SOMNAMBULISM? (FM5.3)

- Sleep walking
- During sleep, the individual may leave the bed and walk out of the house; he is not asleep but in a state of dissociated consciousness, in a hallucinatory state.
- His mental faculties are partially active and are so concentrated towards one particular idea (that he may solve a difficult problem, which he was unable to do after working for hours on it to solve the issue)
- He may commit any crime or suicide, or meet with an accident, but rarely injures himself.
- There is no recollection of the events, but in some cases the events of one episode are remembered and consequently repeated in the next time.
- Such people are usually well adjusted in life, socially well behaved and are not aggressive.
- They are not criminally liable for any offence committed during this phase.

WHAT IS SOMNOLENTIA? (FM5.3)

- **Semi-somnolence:** (sleep drunkenness) It's midway between sleep and awake.
- When a person is in the phase of deep sleep and suddenly aroused, especially when he is in a dream at that time (deep sleep pattern), he has a confused state of mind and may commit any crime during this period.
- They are not criminally liable for their acts during this phase, as they are in a confused state of mind.

WHAT ARE THE EFFECTS OF HYPNOTISM AND MESMERISM IN PSYCHIATRY? (FM5.3)

- Hypnotism is asleep like condition induced by artificial means.
- The individual during the hypnotic trance may perform some act suggested by the hypnotist, but does not remember them afterwards.
- Medical hypnosis is safe and is used for treatment of many psychiatric conditions.
- Usually, the hypnotized individual cannot be made to do some immoral activities.
- An individual doing a crime under this phase is criminally liable, since even though he is under hypnotism, he will be able to regulate his conduct to the needs of the law and can prevent himself from doing such crimes.
- It's said that the brain of a hypnotized person is under the control of the hypnotist and hence *doctrine of diminished responsibility* may be applied if such a

person commits any grave crime under the influence of hypnotism.

WHAT IS THE CRIMINAL RESPONSIBILITY OF AN INSANE? (FM5.3)? WHAT IS MC NAUGHTEN'S RULE?

- The law presumes that every individual is sane and is responsible for his actions.
- The law also presumes that for every criminal act there must be criminal intend.
- Every crime has two components, a criminal mind, and the physical component execution of the crime. Criminal mind (MENS REA) and ACTUS REUS (the actual physical act doing the crime).

Mc Naughten's Rule: The Right or Wrong Test

- An accused person is not legally responsible, if it is **clearly proved** that:
  - At the time of committing the crime,
  - He was suffering from such a defect of reason
  - Due to disease of the mind that
  - He did not know the nature and quality of his act he has done,
  - or that what he was doing was wrong and contrary to the law.

Section 84 IPC

Nothing is an offence which is done by a person, who at the time of doing it, by reason of unsoundness of mind, is incapable of knowing the nature of the act, or that what he is doing is either wrong or contrary to law.

NAME SOME ADVANCEMENTS IN PSYCHIATRY TAKEN PLACE IN ADVANCED COUNTRIES?

- **Durham's rule**
  - An accused person is not criminally responsible, if his unlawful act is the product of mental disease (mental disorder) and mental defect (mental retardation).
- **Curren's rule**
  - An accused person is not criminally responsible if at the time of committing the act, he did not have the capacity to regulate his conduct to the requirements of the law, as a result of mental disease or mental defect.
- **The irresistible impulse test:** (The New Hampshire Doctrine)
  - An accused person is not criminally responsible even if he knows the nature and quality of his act and knows that it is wrong' if he is incapable of restraining himself from committing the act, because the free agency of his will has been destroyed by mental disease.
  - In this test whether the impulse was strong (and irresistible) or the offender is weak (not resisting the impulse voluntarily) is the question for which the psychiatrist or the law does not have any proper answer, and hence this test is never used alone and is always used along with the 'right or wrong test'.
- **The American Law Institute Test:**
  - A person is not criminally liable, if at the time of such conduct, he lacks adequate capacity either to appreciate the criminality of the conduct or to

adjust his conduct to the requirements of the law, as a result of mental disease of defect.

- **The Federal Rule (USA):**
  - An accused person is not criminally responsible, if at the time of commission of the act which constitutes an offence, as result of severe mental disease or defect the defendant was unable to appreciate the nature, quality or wrongfulness of his act.

MULTIPLE CHOICE QUESTIONS

1. Dementia pugilistica is a condition seen in:
   a. Sun stroke
   b. Head injury
   c. Chronic alcoholism
   d. Tertiary syphilis
2. A person in a state of Delirium tremens committing a crime, is not held responsible for his act, since he is:
   a. In a state of impulse
   b. In a state of unsoundness of mind
   c. In a state of intoxication
   d. Consumed alcohol under threat
3. Kleptomania is a type of:
   a. Delusion
   b. Hallucination
   c. Illusion
   d. Impulse
4. The most important characteristic of feigned insanity is:
   a. Sudden onset
   b. Obvious motive
   c. Changing facial expressions
   d. Exhibits symptoms only when watched by others
5. Criminal responsibility of an insane is defined under section ____ of IPC.
   a. 82
   b. 83
   c. 84
   d. 44
6. Magnan's symptom is a type of:
   a. Visual hallucination
   b. Olfactory hallucination
   c. Tactile hallucination
   d. Gustatory hallucination
7. A person is not held responsible for committing crime the following conditions, *except*:
   a. Hypnotism
   b. Post-traumatic automatism
   c. Delirium
   d. Somnambulism
8. A 20-years-old boy presents with fever along with hearing of voices, aggressive behavior muttering to self since 2 days, the diagnosis is:
   a. Dementia
   b. Acute psychosis
   c. Delirium
   d. Delusional disorder
9. One of the following delusion is known as "Othello syndrome":
   a. Delusion of persecution
   b. Erotomaniac delusion
   c. Delusion of infidelity
   d. Hypochondriacal delusion
10. The condition in which the weight of the blanket is mistaken for weight of the collapsed building is:
    a. Illusion
    b. Hallucination
    c. Obsession
    d. Delusion
11. The maximum period of observation to establish the diagnosis of feigned insanity is:
    a. 10 days
    b. 20 days
    c. 30 days
    d. 40 days
12. Will of the following is not valid, *except*:
    a. Persons under the influence of alcohol
    b. Out of a fixed delusion
    c. A mentally retarded person
    d. Senile dementia
13. Magnan's symptom is a/an:
    a. Illusion
    b. Formication
    c. Delusion
    d. Obsession
14. Mood disorder is:
    a. Psychosis
    b. Disorder of affect
    c. Anxiety
    d. Neurosis
15. Mental health act was enacted in:
    a. 1910
    b. 1921

c. 1985
d. 1987
16. **Curren's rule relates to:**
    a. Civil responsibility of insane person
    b. Hypnotism
    c. Criminal responsibility of insane
    d. None of the above
17. **Delirium is a disorder of:**
    a. Thought
    b. Perception
    c. Insight
    d. Cognition
18. **All are true about obsession, *except*:**
    a. Recurrent foolish thought
    b. Associated with dim light
    c. Attempts to resist intrusive ideas
    d. Associated depression
19. **The tests for determining criminal responsibility include:**
    a. Mc Naughten's rule
    b. Durham test
    c. Curren's rule
    d. All of the above
20. **Crime committed by which of the following is not criminally responsible:**
    a. Idiots
    b. Imbeciles
    c. In persons in whom cognitive functions are impaired
    d. All of the above
21. **Compos mentis denotes:**
    a. Coma
    b. Decomposed body
    c. Sound mind
    d. Unsound mind
22. **Dissociative fugue state:**
    a. Sudden onset of paralysis
    b. Fearful of a specified object
    c. Person has multiple identities
    d. Flees from an immediate life situation
23. **A 25-years-old university student had a fight with his neighbor. The next day he started feeling 2 policemen were watching his movements and would arrest him. His symptoms represent:**
    a. Delusion of persecution
    b. Nihilistic delusion
    c. Erotomania
    d. Thought insertion
24. **False perception without any external stimulus is:**
    a. Illusion
    b. Hallucination
    c. Delusion
    d. Delirium
25. **Obsession is a disorder of:**
    a. Perception
    b. Memory
    c. Thought
    d. Judgment
26. **Psychosis is not associated with:**
    a. Delusion
    b. Depression
    c. Phobia
    d. Mania
27. **Fear of open space:**
    a. Agoraphobia
    b. Acrophobia
    c. Claustrophobia
    d. Hydrophobia
28. **False but firm belief about something which is not a fact:**
    a. Illusion
    b. Hallucination
    c. Delusion
    d. Obsession
29. **Delusion is a disorder of:**
    a. Thought
    b. Perception
    c. Insight
    d. Cognition
30. **Delusion of grandiosity is commonly seen in:**
    a. Schizophrenia
    b. Depression
    c. Mania
    d. Dementia
31. **Depressive delusions that the world and everything related to it cease to exist is called:**
    a. Persecutory delusion
    b. Delusion of infidelity
    c. Nihilistic delusion
    d. Delusion of reference
32. **A 30-year-old unmarried woman of average socioeconomic background believes that her boss is secretly in love with her. She holds this belief, despite contradiction from her family members and his denial. She is most likely to be suffering from:**
    a. Depression
    b. Schizophrenia

c. Delusional disorder
d. No psychiatric ailment

33. **False perception without any external stimulus is:**
    a. Illusion
    b. Hallucination
    c. Delirium
    d. Delusion

34. **Olfactory hallucinations are seen in:**
    a. Temporal lobe epilepsy
    b. Schizophrenia
    c. Mania
    d. OCD

35. **All are true regarding hallucinations, *except*:**
    a. Represents a state of inner mind's spatial orientation
    b. Independent of the observer
    c. Under voluntary control
    d. Perception which occurs in the absence of stimulus

36. **Illusion is:**
    a. Misinterpretation of real objects
    b. False firm belief
    c. Absence of sensory stimulus
    d. Hearing of voices

37. **Kleptomania means:**
    a. Irresistible desire to steal things of low value
    b. Irresistible desire to drink
    c. Irresistible desire to dress like opposite sex
    d. Irresistible desire to set fire things

38. **Pyromania is a:**
    a. Conduct disorder
    b. Impulse disorder
    c. Personality disorder
    d. Conversion disorder

39. **Obsession is a disorder of:**
    a. Perception
    b. Thinking
    c. Memory
    d. Judgment

40. **Abreaction is:**
    a. Test for detecting injury due to electric shock
    b. Test for detecting injury due to lightning
    c. Test for detecting injury due to laser beam
    d. Reviving and bringing into consciousness, forgotten traumatic experiences from unconscious level by catharsis.

41. **Not a feature of dementia:**
    a. Loss of sensorium
    b. Wearing of dirty clothes

c. Forgetfulness
d. Loss of neurons in brain matter

42. **Mohan, 40 years, has recently started writing books. But the matter in this book could not be understood by anybody, since it contained words which are not there in dictionary and the theme was very disjoint. Likely diagnosis is:**
    a. Mania
    b. Schizophrenia/split personality
    c. Genius writer
    d. Delusional disorder

43. **Schizophrenia is characterized by:**
    a. Delusion and hallucination
    b. Tremor and delusion
    c. Obsession and delusion
    d. Autonomic disturbance

44. **Delusion of grandeur, persecution and reference is seen in:**
    a. Catatonic schizophrenia
    b. Paranoid schizophrenia
    c. Simple schizophrenia
    d. Disorganized schizophrenia

45. **Prognosis of schizophrenia is best, if:**
    a. Acute onset
    b. Insidious onset
    c. Family history is positive
    d. Negative symptoms

46. **Mood disorder is:**
    a. Psychosis
    b. Disturbance in affect
    c. Anxiety
    d. Neurosis

47. **Bipolar disorder is a:**
    a. Mood disorder
    b. Neurotic disorder
    c. Behavior disorder
    d. Personality disorder

48. **Repetitive hand washing is a symptom of:**
    a. Post-traumatic stress disorder
    b. Depression
    c. Anorexia nervosa
    d. Obsessive compulsive disorder

49. **A patient is always preoccupied with feeling of illness. Diagnosis is:**
    a. Hypochondriasis
    b. Somatization disorder
    c. Conversion disorder
    d. Obsession

SECTION 6: Forensic Psychiatry

50. **Classic tetrad of narcolepsy includes all, except:**
    a. Hypnagogic hallucination
    b. Sleep attacks
    c. Sleep paralysis
    d. Catalepsy

51. **A patient presents with a history of continuous headache for the past 8 years. Repeated examinations had failed to reveal any lesion. The patient is falsely convinced that he has a tumor in his brain. The diagnosis is:**
    a. Hypochondriasis
    b. Somatization
    c. Somatoform pain disorder
    d. Obsessive compulsive disorder

52. **Testamentary capacity refers to:**
    a. Criminal liability
    b. Right to vote
    c. Ability to give evidence
    d. Ability to make a valid will

53. **To plead for insanity in a court of law, the IPC is:**
    a. Section 84
    b. Section 85
    c. Section 88
    d. Section 90

ANSWERS

1. b	2. b	3. d	4. b	5. c	6. c	7. a	8. c	9. b	10. a
11. c	12. b	13. b	14. b	15. d	16. c	17. b	18. b	19. d	20. d
21. c	22. d	23. a	24. b	25. c	26. c	27. a	28. c	29. a	30. c
31. c	32. c	33. b	34. a	35. c	36. a	37. a	38. b	39. b	40. d
41. a	42. b	43. a	44. b	45. a	46. b	47. a	48. d	49. a	50. d
51. a	52. d	53. a							

SECTION 7

Medical Toxicology

SECTION OUTLINE

- **Chapter 25:** General Considerations of Poisoning
- **Chapter 26:** Agricultural Poisons
- **Chapter 27:** Corrosive Poisons
- **Chapter 28:** Metallic and Inorganic Irritants Poisons
- **Chapter 29:** Organic Irritant Poisons
- **Chapter 30:** Neurotoxic Poisons
- **Chapter 31:** Cardiac Poisons
- **Chapter 32:** Asphyxiants
- **Chapter 33:** Miscellaneous Poisons

CHAPTER 25

General Considerations of Poisoning

KEY WORDS

Toxicology, poison, toxinology, poison information centre, fulminant poisoning, acute poisoning, chronic poisoning, Section 85, 86 and 328 IPC, fulminant poisoning, acute poisoning, chronic poisoning, classification of poisons, stabilization, evaluation, poison elimination, emesis, gastric lavage, activated charcoal, antidotes, chelating agents, duties of doctor in poisoning, autopsy on poisoning cases, entomo-toxicology, thin layer chromatography, gas chromatography, liquid chromatography and atomic absorption spectroscopy.

FM8.1	Describe the history of toxicology.
FM8.2	Define the terms toxicology, forensic toxicology, clinical toxicology and poison.
FM8.3	Describe the various types of poisons, toxicokinetics, and toxicodynamics and diagnosis of poisoning in living and dead.
FM8.4	Describe the laws in relations to poisons including NDPS Act, medico-legal aspects of poisons.
FM8.5	Describe medico-legal autopsy in cases of poisoning including preservation and dispatch of viscera for chemical analysis.
FM8.6	Describe the general symptoms, principles of diagnosis and management of common poisons encountered in India.
FM8.7	Describe simple bedside clinic tests to detect poison/drug in a patient's body fluids.
FM8.8	Describe basic methodologies in treatment of poisoning: decontamination, supportive therapy, antidote therapy, procedures of enhanced elimination.
FM8.9	Describe the various types of poisons, toxicokinetics, and toxicodynamics and diagnosis of poisoning in living and dead.
FM8.10	Describe the general principles of analytical toxicology and give a brief description of analytical methods available for toxicological analysis: chromatography—thin layer chromatography, gas chromatography, liquid chromatography and atomic absorption spectroscopy.

HISTORY OF TOXICOLOGY (FM8.1)

- Mateu Joseph Bonaventura Orfila i Rotger was a 19th century Spanish chemist. He is considered the founder of modern toxicology due to his indisputable contributions to the field, which is rapidly evolving in modern times.
- Toxicology has been defined as the study of the adverse effects of xenobiotics and thus is a borrowing science that has evolved from ancient poisons. Modern toxicology goes beyond the study of the adverse effects of exogenous agents to the study of molecular biology, using toxicants as tools.
- The origin of toxicology in India can be traced to the Vedic period. The earliest mention of poisons is found in the Atharva Veda. Remedies for many ailments, including poisoning were discussed in this text. Another major work in this field was the Agnivesa Charaka Samhita.
- In 1832 police arrested John Bodle for lacing his grandfather's coffee with poison. Chemist James Marsh tested the drink in his laboratory, and confirmed the presence of arsenic by producing a yellow precipitate of arsenic sulfide.

Types of Toxicology

- **Analytical toxicology:** This includes the detection and evaluation of toxic chemicals.
- **Applied toxicology:** Applied toxicology is concerned with the application of modern technology in the early detection of toxicants.

INTRODUCTION: DEFINITIONS (FM8.2)

- **Toxicology** is the science which deals with properties, action, toxicity, fatal dose, detection, estimation and treatment of Poisons.
- **Forensic toxicology** deals with the medico-legal aspects of harmful effects of any poison on the human body.
- **Poison** is any substance (solid, liquid or gas) which if introduced into the human body or brought into contact with, will produce ill effect or death by its constitutional or local effect or both.
- **Clinical toxicology** deals with diseases caused by, or associated with abnormal exposure to chemical substances.
- **Toxinology** refers to toxins produced by living organisms which are dangerous to man. Example: Poisonous plants, venoms of snakes, spiders, bees, etc.

WRITE SHORT NOTES ON POISON INFORMATION CENTERS?

- The 1st PIC was established in Netherlands in 1949.
- A telephone answering service was introduced in Leeds, London in 1961.
- In 1963, a National Poison Information centre was established at Guys's Hospital, London. In the same year PIC was opened in Chicago, USA.
- Today more than 75 certified centers are there in USA alone. An intricate computerized information resource system (POISINDEX) is used, which covers more than 80,000 poisonous products.
- In India the National Poison Information Centre was established at AIIMS, New Delhi, in December 1994. Now, National Institute for Occupational Health, Ahmedabad, MMC Chennai, Industrial Toxicity Research Centre at Lucknow and Amrita Institute of Medical Sciences, Cochin has got well established WHO approved Poison Information Centers.
- The WHO has released its software (INTOX) which is used in India.

WHAT IS THE INDIAN STATUS ON DRUGS AND POISONS? (FM8.4)

There are various Acts in force with regard to poisons and drugs; the most important of these are:
- The Poisons Act 1919
- The Drugs and Cosmetics Act 1940
- The Drugs and Cosmetics Rules 1945.

The drug and cosmetics Act 1945 divides (groups) the drugs into various schedules:
- **Schedule C:** Biological Products, Sera, Vaccines, etc.
- **Schedule E:** Poisonous substances under ayurveda, siddha, and unani systems.
- **Schedule G:** Hormonal preparations, antihistamines and anticancer drugs.
- **Schedule H:** Barbiturates, amphetamines, reserpine, ergot and some sulfonamides.
- **Schedule L:** List of prescription drugs.

The other Acts in relation to the poisons and drugs are:
- The Pharmacy Act 1948. The Drugs Control Act 1950.
- The Drugs and Magic Remedies (Objectionable Advertisement) Act 1954.
- The Narcotic Drugs and Psychotropic Substances Act 1985.

Section 328 IPC: Whoever administers to any person any poison, or any stupefying, intoxicating or unwholesome drugs with the intent to cause hurt to such persons, shall be punished with imprisonment up to 10 years, and shall also be liable for fine.

Section 85 IPC: Criminal act done under involuntary intoxication.

When a person is intoxicated without his knowledge or against his will and he becomes incapable of judgment and commits a crime, he is not responsible for the crime.

Section 86 IPC: Criminal act done under voluntary intoxication.

When a person voluntarily consumes an intoxication drug, loses control and commits a crime, he is said to be responsible for the crime committed by him, even though he may have lost orientation. Since he has consumed the drug voluntarily it is presumed that he knew what he is doing, even though his intension to do so cannot be presumed.

WHAT ARE THE CHARACTERISTICS OF AN IDEAL HOMICIDAL POISON?

- An ideal homicidal poison should be:
  - Cheap
  - Easily available
  - Colorless, odorless and tasteless
  - Capable of being administered easily with food, drink or medicine, without producing any obvious (color) change to arise suspicion
  - Highly toxic
  - Signs and symptoms should mimic some natural disease
  - Effects must be delayed for sufficient long time for the accused to escape suspicion
  - Should not produce any specific postmortem change
  - Should not be detected by chemical analysis or tests.
- Organic compound of Fluorine (used as rodenticide) and thallium satisfy several of the above criteria. Arsenic and aconite are commonly used as homicidal poisons.

WHAT ARE THE CHARACTERISTICS OF AN IDEAL SUICIDAL POISON?

- An ideal suicidal poison should be:
  - Cheap
  - Easily available
  - Highly toxic
  - Tasteless or of pleasant taste
  - Capable of being easily taken with food or drink
  - Capable of producing painless death.
- Opium and barbiturates satisfy several of the above criteria.

- Organophosphorus compounds and endrin are commonly used suicidal poisons.

HOW DO WE CLASSIFY POISONS?

CINCAM

- **Corrosives:** Acids and alkalis
- **Irritants:** Organic and inorganic irritants; plants, animals and mechanical irritants.
- **Nervous poisons:**
  - *Cerebral (central:* Inebriants, depressants and deliriant poisons)
  - *Spinal poisons:* Strychnine
  - *Peripheral nerve poison:* Gelsemium
- **Cardiac poisons:** Aconite, digitalis, nicotine
- **Asphyxiants:** Carbon monoxide, cyanides
- **Miscellaneous:** Food poisoning—botulism.
- **Pesticides:** A separate group of compounds useful for agricultural purpose and are used as common suicidal poisons in India, due to the easy accessibility.

WHAT ARE MODES OF ACTIONS OF POISONING? WHAT ARE THE TYPES/STAGES OF POISONING? (FM8.3)

Action of Poison

Local Effects

- Local direct effect of the poison coming into contact with the body.
- **Example:** Corrosion caused by acids, inflammation caused by irritants, etc.

Remote Actions

- After the absorption of the poison from the gastrointestinal tract, the poison gets concentrated in the specific target organs and produce the ill effects.
- **Example:** Alcohol and morphine acts on the brain, Aconite on heart, phenol on kidney, etc.

Combined Effects

Local irritant and corrosive action combined with ill effects on the remote target organs.
Example: Carbolic acid, oxalic acid, etc.

Types of Poisoning

Fulminant Poisoning

Produced when a massive dose is taken on empty stomach, before complete absorption, death occurs rapidly sometimes without any preceding symptoms of poisoning.

Acute Poisoning

- Caused by excessive single dose or several small doses within a short interval of time.
- **Example:** Agricultural poisons, barbiturates, carbon monoxide, etc.

Chronic Poisoning

- Caused by small doses over a long period of time, due to cumulative accumulation of the poison in the target organs, symptoms of poisoning occurs slowly with gradual worsening of the patient symptoms.
- **Example:** Arsenic, lead, mercury, etc.,

Sub-acute Poisoning

Shows symptoms of both acute and chronic poisoning.

WHAT ARE THE GENERAL LINES OF MANAGEMENT OF A CASE OF POISONING?

Short Notes on: Activated Charcoal; Coma Cocktail (FM8.8)

The general line of management of any poisoning case are:
- Stabilization
- Evaluation
- Decontamination
- Poison elimination
- Antidote administration
- Nursing and psychiatric care.

Stabilization and Evaluation

When, the retention of CO_2 ($PaCO_2$ > 45 mm Hg) or hypoxia (PaO_2 < 70 mm Hg) are indications for assisted ventilation.

Coma Cocktail

- When a patient is on coma and the nature of the poison is unknown, then "coma cocktail" is used, which consists of:
  - Dextrose—100 mL of 50% solution IV
  - Thiamine—100 mg IV
  - Naloxone—2 mg IV
- Because, hypoglycemia and morphine are said to be the commonest causes of coma.

Decontamination

- There are various methods of decontamination: (i) Emesis; (ii) Gastric lavage; (iii) Catharsis; (iv) Activated charcoal; (v) Whole bowel irrigation.
- Decontamination can be done in any of these methods; forced emesis, gastric lavage and activated charcoal are commonly being used.

Emesis

- Forced emesis can be done and useful, when the poison was ingested within two hours.
- Concentrated solutions of sodium chloride, soapy water or lime water are generally used.
- Emesis can also be induced mechanically, by inserting the finger into the pharynx.
- Syrup of Ipecacuanha (ipecac) is much preferred; 30 mL for adults and 15 mL for children, followed by 250 mL to 500 mL of water.
- Patient must be in sitting position; if vomiting does not occur within 30 minutes then repeat the same dose once again.

Indications for Emesis by Using Ipecac:
- Conscious and alert patients who have ingested poison not more than 4 to 6 hours earlier.

Contraindication:
- **Relative contraindications:** Very young children, pregnancy, heart disease, bleeding disorders and cardiac poisons.
- **Absolute contraindications:** Convulsion, impaired gag reflex, coma, foreign body ingestion and corrosive poisons.

Gastric Lavage

- Indicated for ingested poisons, useful and effective within 2 to 4 hours (max 6–8 hours):
  Contraindications:
  - *Relative:* Comatose patients, convulsions, pregnancy and children.
  - *Absolute:* Corrosive poisons, convulsant, petroleum products and sharp objects.
- Boas tube (stomach wash tube) or ryles tube (for children) are used.

Activated Charcoal

- It's a fine, black, odorless, tasteless powder made from burning wood, coconut shell, bone, sucrose or rice starch, followed by treatment with an activating agent (steam, CO_2).
- The resultant particles are very small, but have an extremely larger surface area of adhesion; each gram works out to a surface area of 1000 square meters.
- Super activated charcoal which adheres to more surface area is available in US.

Mode of action:
- Decrease the absorption of various poisons by adsorbing to them on its surface.
- **Dose:** 1 g/kg body weight; usually 100 g in adults and 10 to 30 g in children.
- **Procedure:** Add 4 to 8 times the quantity of water to the calculated dose of activated charcoal, and mix to produce a slurry solution, and given to patient after emesis or lavage.

Disadvantages:
- Unpleasant taste
- Provocation of vomiting

- Constipation/diarrhea
- Pulmonary aspiration
- Sometimes, causes intestinal obstruction; especially with multiple doses.

Contraindications:
- Absent bowel sounds or proven ileus
- Small bowel obstruction
- Caustic ingestion
- Ingestion of petroleum distilleries

Elimination of absorbed poison:
- Forced diuresis is commonly employed method for elimination of absorbed poisons.
- Extracorporeal techniques like hemodialysis, hemoperfusion, peritoneal dialysis, hemofiltration, plasmapheresis, plasma perfusion, and cardiopulmonary bypass are also in use to eliminate the poison.

Antidote Administration

- **Antidotes** are substances which directly counteract the action of a poison; there are various modes of action of antidotes.
- Once the nature of poison is diagnosed, specific antidotes are administered to save the life of the patient. The outcome of the case depends on how much time elapsed after exposure to the poison and how much early we diagnose and administer the specific antidotes.

DESCRIBE THE PROCEDURE OF STOMACH WASH WITH A NEAT LABELED DIAGRAM; ADD A NOTE ON VARIOUS SOLUTIONS USED FOR GASTRIC LAVAGE? (FM8.8)

Gastric Lavage (Stomach Wash)

- Gastric lavage is the preferred method of emptying the stomach and should follow the instillation of one dose of activated charcoal.

TABLE 25.1: Solutions used for gastric lavage.

Poison	Solutions
Most poisons–known or unknown	Water or saline
Oxidizable poisons (alkaloids and salicylates)	Potassium permanganate—($KMnO_4$) (1:5000 or 1:10000 solution)
Cyanides	Sodium thiosulfate 25%
Carbolic acid	Castor oil and warm water
Oxalates	Calcium gluconate
Iron	Deferoxamine (2 g in 1 liter of water)

- It is effective if performed within about 4 hours of ingestion. However, in cases of ingestion of phenothiazines, antihistamines, tricyclic antidepressants or salicylates, a good amount of poison can still be recovered after several hours of ingestion because all these drugs delay gastric emptying.
- Solutions used for Gastric lavage described in **Table 25.1**.

Procedure

- Gastric lavage may have dangerous sequelae if performed clumsily.
- The patient should be prone or semiprone on his left side with head hanging over the edge of the bed and face down, supported by an assistant so that the mouth is at a lower level than larynx (trendelenburg and left lateral decubitus position) to prevent aspiration.
- The dentures, if any, must be removed. The airway must be clear and a mouth gag with a central hole is necessary especially in unconscious patients to prevent the rubber tube being bitten by the teeth.
- **In adults**, gastric lavage may be done by stomach wash tube (**Boa's tube**).

- It is a flexible rubber tube about 12.7 mm in external diameter and about a one and a half meter in length. It is sufficiently stiff to pass without kinking. A funnel is provided at the upper end and a suction bulb to suck out fluids is also provided at about the middle of the tube. The lower end is blunt and rounded to avoid any injury when it is being passed and is perforated by more than one opening on its sides to allow the administered fluid to enter the stomach easily.
- The distance between teeth and the cardiac end of the stomach is about 45 cm in adults. Therefore, at a point about 50 cm from the lower end, the tube is marked so that the operator may have some indication when the lower end of the tube has reached the stomach.
- The tube should be lubricated with liquid paraffin/glycerine and passed through the hole in the middle of mouth gag, over the tongue and down the esophagus. At about the mark, the tip of the tube should be lying in the stomach and one must make sure of this by dipping the funnel end in water. If the tip is in the air passage, bubbles of air will be found coming out of the funnel end in the water.
- After confirming the tube is inside the stomach and had not wrongly entered into the respiratory passage, about half a liter of plain water is run into the funnel, which is held above the level of patient's mouth. The fluid enters the stomach by gravity. The funnel is then lowered below the level of patient's stomach over a receptacle to allow gastric contents to siphon off.
- The contents of the first washing should be preserved for chemical analysis without any preservative. The process is then repeated with warm water or other fluid preferably containing an appropriate antidote until the returning fluid is of the same color as the lavage fluid.
- Some amount of the antidote or other suitable solution may be left in the stomach to deal with the effect and after effects of whatever small quantities may have escaped lavage or are later excreted in the stomach.
- Before the stomach tube is withdrawn, it should be pinched to prevent aspiration of material into the lungs.
- **In children,** a tube of narrower caliber and shorter length is used. A Ryle's tube may serve the purpose. About 25 cm length is necessary to reach the stomach and this distance should be marked. When the tube has reached the stomach 20 or 50 mL glass syringe is attached to the upper end of the tube and the stomach contents aspirated. Tap water containing antidote (if available) is then introduced.
- The stomach should be washed repeatedly to increase the total quantity of poison removed. Before the tube is withdrawn, it should be pinched to prevent aspiration of material into the lungs.
- During the lavage, the child should be lying prone, the foot-end of the bed elevated and the head slightly extended, turned to one side and supported by some assistant.
- Indicated for all ingested poisons and useful and effective within 2 to 4 hours (max 6–8 hours).
- **Contraindications** to gastric lavage include corrosives (except carbolic acid), convulsant, foreign body ingestion, petroleum distillates, esophageal varices, etc.

WHAT IS AN ANTIDOTE? WHAT ARE THE MECHANISM OF ACTION OF VARIOUS ANTIDOTES?

What is Universal Antidote? (FM8.6)

Antidotes are substances which directly counteract the action of a poison. The various mechanism of action of the antidotes are:

TABLE 25.2: Mechanism of action of antidotes.

Mechanism	Example
Inert complex formation	Chelating agents for heavy metals
Accelerated detoxification	Thiosulfate for cyanide
Reduced toxic conversion	Ethanol inhibits metabolism of methanol
Receptor site competition	Naloxone for opiates
Receptor site blockade	Atropine for organophosphates
Toxic effect bypass	100% oxygen for cyanide poisoning

The mechanism of action of various antidotes are depicted in **Table 25.2**.

According to their mode of actions, antidotes are classified as:
- Mechanical or physical antidotes
- Chemical antidotes
- Physiological or pharmacological antidotes.

Mechanical or Physical Antidotes

- They physically adsorb to the poison and prevent the absorption of the poison and hence called "mechanical antidotes".
- Example: Activated charcoal, demulcents (milk, egg white), bulk food (like rice for ingestion of mechanical irritants like powdered glass or solids like coins).

Chemical Antidotes

- They act chemically with the poison and forms inert complexes which are excreted by the body.
- **Example:** Acids neutralized by mild alkalis, potassium permanganate oxidizes opium, calcium compounds used to precipitate oxalic acid poisoning, etc.

Physiological Antidotes

- These are substances which produce direct opposite effect of the poison by their pharmacological action.
- **Example:** Physostigmine for atropine, amyl nitrate for cyanide poisoning, atropine for OPC, etc.

Universal Antidote

When the nature of the poison is not known or a mixture of poisons is suspected then universal antidote can be used, which consists of (i) Activated charcoal, (ii) Magnesium oxide and (iii) Tannic acid. Of course the use of such universal antidote is not in use nowadays.

WRITE SHORT NOTES ON CHELATING AGENTS? (FM8.8)

- Chelating agents are a group of chemical substances, which are used as antidotes in heavy metal poisoning.
- The heavy metals combine with the sulfhydryl group of mitochondrial enzyme system, and there by interferes with the cellular respiration.
- Chelating agents have a greater affinity for the metals, compared to the endogenous enzyme systems. They strongly bind with the heavy metals and forms inert complexes.
- The complex agents formed with the metal is relatively more water soluble and the complex is excreted through urine.
- The commonest used chelating agents are:
  - BAL (British Anti Lewisite) or Dimercaprol; Dimercaptopropanol.
  - EDTA (Ethylene Diamine Tetra acetic Acid)
  - Penicillamine (Oral chelating agent)
  - DMSA, Succimer (3-DiMercapto Succinic Acid)
  - DMPS (2,3-DiMercaptoPropane 1-Sulfonate)

WHAT ARE THE DUTIES OF A DOCTOR IN SUSPECTED CASES OF POISONING? (FM8.9)

- Medical duties stand first in the order of priority in any case of poisoning; the

doctor must make all necessary efforts to save the life of the patient.
- Follow the general lines of management like stabilization, evaluation, decontamination, antidote administration and nursing care appropriately. The specific antidotes to be administered are discussed in the detail under all the poisons.

Legal Duties

- Doctors in Government hospitals have to inform every case of poisoning to the police.
- Doctors working in private hospitals need not inform the police if it is a case of accidental or suicidal poisoning. But if the patient dies the doctor should not issue a death certificate and has to inform the police and refer the body for postmortem examination.
- All cases of homicidal poisoning (definite or suspected) either in government or private hospitals must be reported to the police (Section 39 CrPC). Failure to do so will make him liable under section 176 IPC.
- When the police require some information regarding the cases of poisoning, which is accidental, suicidal or homicidal, the doctor must divulge all the information. There is no professional secrecy in this matter (175 CrPC), if any information is withheld or wrong information is provided, the doctor is culpable under 202 and 193 IPC respectively.
- Every effort must be made by the doctor to collect and preserve evidences suggestive of poisoning. Deliberate omission to do so, will attract punishment under section 201 IPC.
- Collect vomitus, feces, stomach washings, contaminated food, etc., and dispatch the same to FSL for chemical analysis, in event of death of the patient along with the body itself.
- If the patient is conscious, but on the verge of death, arrange for dying declaration.
- Detailed written records must be made with respect to every case and should be kept under safe custody by the doctor.
- When poisoning has resulted from a common eating place, the doctor is bound to inform the public authorities, failure to do so, will attract action against him for infamous conduct.

WHAT ARE THE PROCEDURES OF POSTMORTEM EXAMINATION IN A CASE OF POISONING? (FM8.5)

- Stains of vomitus on the clothing must be collected, preserved and sent to FSL.
- Evidence of corrosion, discoloration, sloughing especially around the mouth may be present, if the poison has been ingested.
- Presence of jaundice (yellowish discolration of skin, nails, conjunctiva and internal organs) indicates hepatotoxic poison, or poisons causing hemolytic anemia.
- **Odor:** Any peculiar smell must be noted, which may not be perceptible at autopsy due to the odor inside the mortuary (in spite of it some of the poisons will have peculiar odour)
- **Color of postmortem lividity:** May give a clue to the poison involved, described in **Table 25.3**.
- **Putrefaction changes:** Arsenic and organophosphates are said to delay putrefaction.

TABLE 25.3: Color of PM staining.

Carbon monoxide	Cherry red
Cyanide	Bright red
Hydrogen sulfide	Greenish blue
Phosphorus	Brown
Nitrobenzene, potassium chloride	Brownish red
Aniline	Blue, bluish brown

- **Injection marks:** Especially in snake bite, morphine and insulin poisoning, bits of skin from the sight of injection are taken with adjoining intact skin, divided into two parts and one part to the FSL and the other for HPE (especially in snake bite).

Internal Examination

- **Odor:** Some poisons have a peculiar smell, on opening the thoraco-abdominal cavity; stomach contents should be examined for the colour, volume, consistency and any visible particulate matters.
- Evidence of inflammation on the esophagus, stomach and duodenum in ingested poison.
- The odor could give a clue to the poison involved. Odor of various poisons tabulated in **Table 25.4**.

TABLE 25.4: Odor of various poisons.

Odor	Substance
Acetone (apple like)	Chloroform, ethanol, Isopropanol, lacquer
Acrid (pear like)	Chloral hydrate, paraldehyde
Bitter almond	Cyanide
Burnt rope	Cannabis (Marijuana)
Hospital smell (disinfectant)	Carbolic acid (phenol), creosote
Garlicky	Arsenic, phosphorus, selenium, thallium
Mothballs	Naphthalene, camphor
Musty (fishy)	Aluminum phosphide, zinc phosphide
Rotten egg	Carbon disulfide, hydrogen sulfide
Shoe polish	Nitrobenzene
Vinegar	Acetic acid
Wintergreen	Methyl salicylates
Kerosene like odor	Organophosphorus, petrol, kerosene

The state of other organs:
- Kidneys may show degenerative changes or even necrosis.
- Sub-pleural petechial hemorrhages on the lungs if asphyxia has resulted.
- Heart may show sub-epicardial petechiae and sub-endocardial petechio-ecchymotic hemorrhages in cases of cardiac poisons.
- Confirmation is by subjecting the viscera for chemical analysis by forwarding the viscera to the Forensic Science Laboratory.

WHAT ARE CIRCUMSTANCES WHEN VISCERA ARE SENT FOR CHEMICAL ANALYSIS? WHAT ARE THE VISCERA PRESERVED IN VARIOUS POISONING CASES? (FM8.9)

In many situations, the doctor may have to preserve the viscera for chemical analysis; it is mandatory to preserve the viscera in the following situations:
- All cases of poisoning brought dead or treated.
- In all murder cases to detect any poison and alcohol.
- In road traffic accidents to detect alcohol
- In all cases of Magistrate inquest.
- In all suspicious and sudden deaths.

Routine Viscera to be Preserved for Chemical Analysis

- Routinely five bottles are sent for analysis and is sufficient in cases where the poison is suspected to be ingested. When the mode of administration is not by ingestion, then additional viscera has to be preserved depending on the mode of exposure.
- **Bottle no. 1:** Stomach with its contents. *Inference:* The poison was ingested.
- **Bottle no. 2:** Upper 30 cm of the duodenum with its contents.

Inference: Poison has moved to the intestines due to active peristalsis, i.e. administered when alive.
- **Bottle no. 3:** 500 gm of liver and half of each Kidney.
Inference: Absorbed poison is carried to liver for metabolism and kidneys for excretion.
- **Bottle no. 4:** 100 mL of blood with sodium fluoride as preservative.
Inference: Poison absorbed into circulation.
- **Bottle no. 5:** 100 mL of the preservative used (saturated solution of sodium chloride is used as a preservative in most cases).
Inference: To confirm that the preservative is not contaminated and the poison if any detected has not been introduced from the preservative used.
- These five bottles are sealed, labeled and sent to the Forensic Science Laboratory in any case of suspected poisoning, through the police constable in-charge of the body.
- To be safe and to maintain the chain of custody, it's always preferable to handover the viscera to the Police Constable along with the body. Many a times the police may not take the viscera on the same day due to number reasons from their side. But to avoid suspicion on our side, it's better to hand over the viscera on the same day along with the body itself. We cannot have possession of the viscera after handing over the body and a charge of manipulation may be raised against the doctor at later stage.
- In addition to the routine viscera, some other additional tissues may have to be preserved for specific poisons:

Additional Viscera in Special Circumstances

See **Table 25.5**.

TABLE 25.5: Additional viscera in special circumstances of poisoning.

Viscera	Poison
Brain	Volatile and anesthetic poisons
CSF and brain	Alcohol
Heart	Cardiac poisons (aconite, digitalis, etc.)
Spinal cord	Nervous poisons (strychnine)
Bile	Morphine and salicylates poisoning
Hair, nail and long bones	Heavy metal poisoning (arsenic)
Skin and sc tissues	Injected poisons, drugs and venoms
Blood with liquid paraffin on the top	Volatile poisons, mainly CO and sewer gas

WHAT IS ENTOMO-TOXICOLOGY?

- Entomo-toxicology is the combined application of entomology and toxicology in forensic investigation. It refers to analysis of poisons from the insects which feed on the dead bodies.
- In advanced putrefaction and skeletonization it is very difficult to extract and analyze the poisons from dead body. In those circumstances the maggots and flies present on the body can be collected and used for finding out the nature of the poison involved in causing death.

Analytical Toxicology

DESCRIBE THIN LAYER CHROMATOGRAPHY? (FM8.10)

- Thin layer chromatography is a technique used to isolate nonvolatile mixtures, the technique depends on the principle of separation.

Principle

- The experiment is conducted on a sheet of aluminum foil, plastic, or glass which is coated with a thin layer of adsorbent material. The material usually used is aluminum oxide, cellulose, or silica gel. The separation of various particles depends on movement of particles in the mobile phase over the stationary phase.
- The compounds in the mobile phase move over the surface of the stationary phase. The movement occurs in such a way that the compounds which have a higher affinity to the stationary phase move slowly while the compounds which have lower affinity to the stationary phase travel fast. Therefore, the separation of the mixture is attained.
- On completion of the separation process, the individual components from the mixture appear as spots at respective levels on the plates. Their character and nature are identified by suitable detection techniques. On completion of the separation, each component appears as spots separated vertically. Each spot has a retention factor (Rf) expressed as:
  R_f = distance travelled by sample/distance travelled by solvent
- The factors affecting retardation factor are the solvent system, amount of material spotted, adsorbent and temperature. TLC is one of the fastest, least expensive, simplest and easiest chromatography technique.

Components

- **Thin layer chromatography plates:** Ready-made plates are used which are chemically inert and stable. The stationary phase is applied on its surface in the form of a thin layer. The stationary phase on the plate has a fine particle size and also has a uniform thickness.
- Thin layer chromatography chamber is used to develop plates. It is responsible to keep a steady environment inside which will help in developing spots. Also, it prevents the solvent evaporation and keeps the entire process dust-free.
- **Thin layer chromatography mobile phase:** Mobile phase is the one that moves and consists of a solvent mixture or a solvent. This phase should be particulate-free. The higher the quality of purity the better the development of the spots
- **Thin layer chromatography filter paper:** It has to be placed inside the chamber. It is moistened in the mobile phase.

Applications of TLC

- The qualitative testing of various medicines such as sedatives, local anesthetics, anticonvulzant tranquilisers, analgesics, antihistamines, steroids, hypnotics is done by TLC.
- TLC is extremely useful in biochemical analysis such as separation or isolation of biochemical metabolites from its blood plasma, urine, body fluids, serum, etc.
- Thin layer chromatography can be used to identify natural products like essential oils or volatile oil, fixed oil, glycosides, waxes, alkaloids, etc.
- It is widely used in separating multi-component pharmaceutical formulations.
- It is used for the purification of samples and direct comparison is done between the sample and the authentic sample.
- It is used in the food industry, to separate and identify colors, sweetening agent, and preservatives.

Disadvantages of TLC

- Thin TLC plates do not have longer stationary phase.
- When compared to other chromatographic techniques the length of separation is limited.

- The results generated from TLC are difficult to reproduce.
- Since TLC operates as an open system, some factors such as humidity and temperature can affect the final outcome of the chromatogram.
- The detection limit is high and therefore if you want a lower detection limit, you cannot use TLC.
- It is only a qualitative analysis technique and not quantitative.

DESCRIBE COLUMN CHROMATOGRAPHY? (FM8.10)

Liquid chromatography is a technique used to separate a sample into its individual components. This separation occurs based on the interactions of the sample with the mobile and stationary phases.

General Scheme

- Components within a mixture are separated in a column based on each component's affinity for the mobile phase. So, if the components are of different polarities and a mobile phase of a distinct polarity is passed through the column, one component will migrate through the column faster than the other.
- Since, the molecules of the same compound will generally move in groups, the compounds are separated into distinct bands within the column. If the components being separated are colored, their corresponding bands can be seen. Otherwise as in high performance liquid chromatography (HPLC), the presence of the bands are detected using other instrumental analysis techniques such as UV-VIS spectroscopy.

Column Chromatography

- The stationary phase in column chromatography is most typically a fine adsorbent solid; a solid that is able hold onto gas or liquid particles on its outer surface.
- The column typically used in column chromatography looks similar to a Pasteur pipette (pasteur pipettes are used as columns in small scale column chromatography). The narrow exit of the column is first plugged with glass wool or a porous plate in order to support the column packing material and keep it from escaping the tube.
- Then the adsorbent solid (usually silica) is tightly packed into the glass tube to make the separating column. The packing of the stationary phase into the glass column must be done carefully to create a uniform distribution of material. A uniform distribution of adsorbent is important to minimize the presence of air bubbles and/or channels within the column.
- To finish preparing the column, the solvent to be used as the mobile phase is passed through the dry column. Then the column is said to be "wetted" and the column must remain wet throughout the entire experiment. Once the column is correctly prepared, the sample to be separated is placed at the top of the wet column. A photo of a packed separating column can be found in the links.

HIGH-PERFORMANCE LIQUID CHROMATOGRAPHY (HPLC) (FM8.10)

- Formerly referred to as **high-pressure liquid chromatography**, is a technique used in analytical toxicology to separate, identify, and quantify each component in a mixture.
- HPLC relies on pumps to pass a pressurized liquid solvent containing the sample mixture through a column filled with a solid adsorbent material.

- Each component in the sample interacts slightly differently with the adsorbent material, causing different flow rates for the different components and leading to the separation of the components as they flow out of the column.
- HPLC is used for detecting performance enhancement drugs in urine, in separating the components of a complex biological sample, or of similar synthetic chemicals from each other and in detecting vitamin D levels in blood serum.

DESCRIBE GAS CHROMATOGRAPHY? (FM8.10)

- Gas chromatography (GC) is an analytical technique used to separate and detect the chemical components of a sample mixture to determine their presence or absence and/or quantities. These chemical components are usually organic molecules or gases.
- For GC to be successful in their analysis, these components need to be volatile. Gas chromatographs are frequently hyphenated to mass spectrometers (GC-MS) to enable the identification of the chemical components.

Principle

- GC uses a carrier gas for the separation process; this plays the part of the mobile phase. The carrier gas transports the sample molecules through the GC system, ideally without reacting with the sample or damaging the instrumental components.
- The sample is first introduced into the gas chromatograph (GC), either with a syringe or transferred from an auto-sampler that may also extract the chemical components from solid or liquid sample matrices.
- The sample is injected into the GC inlet through a septum which enables the injection of the sample mixture without losing the mobile phase.
- The analytical column is held in the column oven which is heated during the analysis to elucidate the less volatile components.
- The outlet of the column is inserted into the detector which responds to the chemical components eluting from the column to produce a signal.
- The signal is recorded by the acquisition software on a computer to produce a chromatogram.

DESCRIBE ABOUT MASS SPECTROMETRY? (FM8.10)

- Mass spectrometry is an analytical tool useful for measuring the mass-to-charge ratio (m/z) of one or more molecules present in a sample. These measurements can often be used to calculate the exact molecular weight of the sample components as well.
- Hence in forensic scientists analyze the smallest of ounces of evidence they find in a crime scene can be identified with the help of mass spectrometry, also can even find out about the different isotopes associated with that element.
- Mass spectrometry is employed to analyze combinatorial libraries, sequence biomolecules and help explore single cells or objects from outer space.
- Structure elucidation of unknown substances, environmental and forensic trace evidences, quality control of drugs, foods and polymers.
- Mass spectrometers can be used to classify unknown substances by molecular weight measurement, to measure known compounds, and to determine the structure and chemical properties of molecules.
- The advantage of mass spectrometry is that it is incredibly sensitive (parts per million) over many other techniques. It is an excellent tool for identifying or confirming the presence of unknown components in a sample.

MULTIPLE CHOICE QUESTIONS

1. Stomach wash is absolutely contra-indicated in the following, except:
   a. Sulfuric acid
   b. Liquid hydrocarbons
   c. Carbolic acid
   d. Caustic soda
2. The following are normal constituents of 'coma cocktail', except:
   a. Thiamine
   b. Physostigmine
   c. Naloxone
   d. Dextrose
3. Gastric lavage is contraindicated in poisoning with:
   a. Carbolic acid
   b. OPC
   c. Salicylates
   d. Kerosene
4. Universal antidote includes all the following, except:
   a. Activated charcoal
   b. Magnesium oxide
   c. Sodium sulphate
   d. Tannic acid
5. True about formalin:
   a. Used as preservative in alcohol poisoning
   b. Never used as preservative for chemical analysis
   c. Used as preservative only in digitalis poisoning
   d. Used as preservative for any plant poisoning
6. Minimum quantity of blood to be preserved for chemical analysis is:
   a. 10 mL
   b. 25 mL
   c. 50 mL
   d. 100 mL
7. In suspected Nux Vomica poisoning the following is required to be preserved:
   a. Muscle
   b. Heart
   c. Spinal cord
   d. Long bones
8. Smell of bitter almonds is noticed in poisoning due to:
   a. HCl
   b. HCN
   c. H_2SO_4
   d. HNO_3
9. The functions of FSL includes:
   a. Examination and evaluation of physical evidence to identify the criminal
   b. Protection of innocent people
   c. Training police officers
   d. All of the above
10. The organ to be preserved in volatile organic poisons:
    a. Bone
    b. Brain
    c. Lung
    d. Heart
11. On autopsy shows signs of asphyxia in which of the following poisons:
    a. Strychnine
    b. Aconite
    c. Nicotine
    d. All of the above
12. In which of the following poisoning hemodialysis is useful:
    a. Salicylates
    b. Lithium
    c. Diazepam
    d. Organophosphorus compounds
13. Specimen for toxicological (chemical) analysis are preserved using:
    a. Rectified spirit
    b. Alcohol
    c. 10% formaldehyde
    d. Saturated solution of sodium chloride
14. Bluish green postmortem staining is present in:
    a. Hydrogen sulfide
    b. Carbon monoxide
    c. Cyanide
    d. Phosphorus
15. Father of toxicology is:
    a. Paracelsus
    b. Galen
    c. Galten
    d. Orfila
16. A dead body is having cadaveric lividity of bluish green color. The most likely cause of death is by poisoning due to:
    a. Hydrogen sulfide
    b. Carbon monoxide
    c. Cyanide
    d. Ammonia

17. A dead body with suspected poisoning is having hypostasis of red brown in color. It is suggestive of poisoning due to:
   a. Nitrites
   b. Hydrogen sulfide
   c. Carbon monoxide
   d. Cyanide
18. Doctor suspects homicide poisoning. Section under which he needs to inform police:
   a. 174 CrPC
   b. 176 CrPC
   c. 39 CrPC
   d. 302 IPC
19. Gastric lavage can be done in poisoning with:
   a. Kerosene
   b. Carbolic acid
   c. Sulfuric acid
   d. Caustic potash
20. True about household emetics are all, *except*:
   a. Ipecac syrup is potent and safe
   b. NaCl solution in warm water is the safest
   c. Apomorphine is effective orally
   d. Tickling the fauces with a tongue depressor is the best method
21. BAL is useful in treating poisoning due to all, *except*:
   a. Lead
   b. Mercury
   c. Cadmium
   d. Arsenic
22. Drug containing two sulfhydryl groups in a molecule:
   a. BAL
   b. EDTA
   c. Penicillamine
   d. None
23. Disodium EDTA is used as an antidote for ___ poisoning.
   a. Mercury
   b. Belladona
   c. Mushroom
   d. OPC
24. Chelating agent for copper, mercury, lead which is given by oral route:
   a. BAL
   b. Succimer
   c. Penicillamine
   d. EDTA

ANSWERS

1. c	2. b	3. d	4. c	5. b	6. d	7. c	8. b	9. d	10. b
11. d	12. a	13. d	14. a	15. d	16. a	17. a	18. c	19. b	20. c
21. c	22. a	23. a	24. c						

26
CHAPTER

Agricultural Poisons

KEY WORDS

Organophosphorus, insecticide, alkyl phosphates, aryl phosphates, muscarinic action, nicotinic action, acetylcholine, SLUDGE, intermediate syndrome, delayed symptoms, TLC, p-nitrophenol test, atropine, pralidoxime, kerosene odor, endrin, pyrethroids, paraquat lung, aluminum phosphide, zinc phosphide.

| FM9.5 | Describe general principles and basic methodologies in treatment of poisoning: decontamination, supportive therapy, antidote therapy, procedures of enhanced elimination with regard to organophosphates, carbamates, organochlorines, pyrethroids, paraquat, aluminum and zinc phosphide. |

INTRODUCTION

Agricultural poisons are insecticides, rodenticides, herbicides or fungicides as classification of classification of agro-chemicals and pesticides shown in **Flowchart 26.1.**

- Organophosphorus compounds are the most popular and widely used insecticides in India and they form the most important group of suicidal poisons in India.
- Organophosphorus compounds are of two groups:
  1. *Alkyl phosphates:* HETP, TEPP (tetron), OMPA, dimefox, isopestox, malathion, sulfotep, demeton, trichlorfon.
  2. *Aryl phosphates:* Parathion (folidol), paraoxon, methyl parathion (metacid), chlorthion, diazinon (diazion; Tik 20).

WHAT IS THE TOXICOKINETICS, MECHANISM OF ACTION, CLINICAL FEATURES, DIAGNOSIS AND MANAGEMENT OF OPC POISONING? (FM9.5)

Toxicokinetics

Organophosphorus compounds are absorbed through all the portals of entry, through the skin, conjunctiva, inhalation, through gastrointestinal tract, through injection and well absorbed even when poured into the nose or ears.

Mode of Action

Organophosphates are powerful inhibitors of acetylcholinesterase which is responsible for hydrolyzing acetylcholine to choline and

SECTION 7: Medical Toxicology

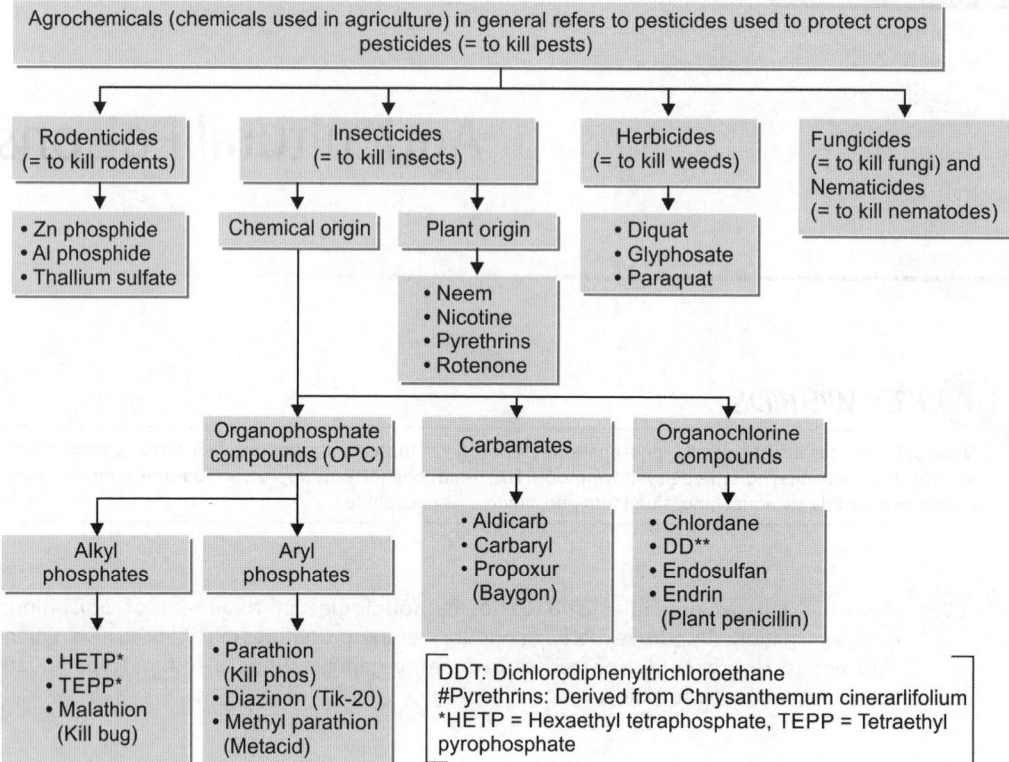

Flowchart 26.1: Classification of agrochemicals and pesticides.

acetic acid. As a result, there is continued accumulation of acetylcholine, eventually leading to paralysis of the nerves or muscle.

Clinical Features

Cholinergic excess: Due to accumulation of acetylcholine.
- **Muscarinic effect:** Hollow organ parasympathetic manifestations.
  - Bronchoconstriction with dyspnea, cough, pulmonary edema, vomiting, diarrhea, abdominal cramps, increased salivation, lacrimation and sweating, bradycardia, hypotension, meiosis and urinary retention.
  - The symptoms can be remembered using acronym "**SLUDGE**" denoting salivation, lacrimation, urination, defecation, gastrointestinal cramps and emesis.
- **Nicotinic effects:** Due to autonomic ganglion and somatic motor effects, resulting in fasciculation, weakness, hypertension, tachycardia and paralysis.

CNS effects: Restlessness, headache, tremors, drowsiness, delirium, slurred speech, ataxia and convulsions. Death is usually due to respiratory failure (paralysis of respiratory center).

Other useful signs: Characteristic kerosene odor is often present in the vicinity of the patient, since the solvent used are some petroleum derivatives like aromax.
- Pin point pupil (**miosis**) is a characteristic feature.

- Ocular exposure can result in systemic toxicity. It causes persistent miosis, in spite of appropriate systemic therapy. Topical atropine (or scopolamine) installation may be necessary.
- Respiratory failure is the commonest cause of death, but other causes like hypoxia due to seizures, hypothermia, renal failure and hepatic failure may also contribute in causing death.

Table 26.1 is depicted the clinical manifestations of OPC.

Diagnosis

- **Depression of cholinesterase activity:**
    - RBC cholinesterase level of <50% is indicative of organophosphorus toxicity.
    - Depression of plasma cholinesterase level to <50% is a less reliable indicator of organophosphorus toxicity.
    - For the purpose of estimation of cholinesterase levels, blood should be collected in heparinized tubes or alternatively the samples can be frozen.
- Thin layer chromatography (TLC)
- P-nitrophenol test:
    - P-nitrophenol is a metabolite of organophosphates and is excreted in urine.
    - 10 mL of urine is steam distilled and the distillate is collected. Add 2 pellets of sodium hydroxide to the distillate and heat on a water bath for 10 minutes. Production of yellow color indicates the presence of P-nitrophenol.

Treatment

- **Decontamination:**
    - In case of skin involvement, the patient is stripped and washed thoroughly with soap and water.
    - If there is ocular exposure, copious eye irrigation with saline, ringer's solution or water.
    - In case of ingestion, stomach wash is done. Activated charcoal is beneficial.
- **Antidote administration:**
    - *Atropine:*
        - Atropine is a competitive inhibitor of acetylcholine at the muscarinic postsynaptic membrane and CNS, and will block the muscarinic effects of OPC. Atropine acts only at postsynaptic muscarinic

TABLE 26.1: Clinical manifestations of OPC.

Muscarinic symptoms (DUMBBELS)	Nicotinic symptoms (MATCH)	CNS effects (RASH ACT)
Diarrhea	Muscle fasciculation	Restlessness
Urinary incontinence	Arrhythmias	Arrhythmias
Miosis	Tachycardia	Slurred speech
Broncho spasm	Cramps (muscle cramps)	Headache
Bradycardia	Hypertension	Confusion
Emesis		Ataxia
Lacrimation		**Late effects:**
Secretions–increased salivation, sweating		Respiratory depression, Convulsion and coma

receptors and has no effect on muscle weakness and paralysis.
- ♦ Dose: 1 to 2 mL IV or IM (0.5 mg/kg in children) every 15 minutes, till the endpoint is reaches, as indicated by drying of bronchial secretions and pupillary dilatation. Once the endpoint is reached, then the dose is adjusted to maintain the effects for 24 hours.
- *Pralidoxime:*
  - ♦ This is a nucleophilic oxime which helps to **rejuvenate** (regenerate) acetylcholinesterase at the muscarinic, nicotinic and CNS sites.
  - ♦ Dose: 1 to 2 g IV given over 30 minutes; repeated after one hour and subsequently after 6 hours to 12 hours, for 24 to 48 hours. Maximum 12 g in 24 hours.
- *Supportive measures:*
  - ♦ IV fluids to compensate fluid loss.
  - ♦ Oxygenation/intubation/positive pressure ventilation.
  - ♦ Parasympathomimetics, phenothiazines, antihistamines and opiates are contraindicated.

Prevention of further exposure and complications:
  - ♦ After the recovery, the person should not be exposed to organophosphates for atleast a few weeks, since he is likely to suffer serious harm from a dose normally harmless and result in complications like intermediate or delayed syndromes. These are due to the alteration in the body chemistry.

WHAT ARE THE DELAYED SYMPTOMS OF OPC POISONING?

Intermediate Syndrome

- Occurs 1 to 4 days after poisoning, due to long-lasting cholinesterase inhibition and muscle necrosis.
- The main features include muscle weakness and paralysis, weakness of flexor muscles of the neck and proximal limb muscles, and acute respiratory paresis.
- This intermediate syndrome may be due to inadequate treatment of the acute episode, involving sub-adequate administration of oximes or inadequate assisted ventilation.
- Management of this intermediate syndrome is by supportive measures, since it does not respond to oximes or atropine.

Delayed Syndrome

Occurs after 1 to 4 weeks after poisoning, due to nerve demyelination; characterized by flaccid weakness and atrophy of distal limb muscles or spasticity and ataxia. This syndrome also does not respond to oximes and atropine.

Chronic Poisoning

- Usually occurs as an occupational hazard in agriculturalists engaged in pesticide spraying.
- Route of exposure is inhalation or skin contamination. Chronic poisoning manifests as:
  - *Polyneuropathy:* Paresthesia, muscle cramps, weakness and gait disorders.
  - *CNS effects:* Drowsiness, confusion, irritability, anxiety and psychiatric manifestations.

WHAT ARE THE POSTMORTEM FINDINGS IN CASE OF OPC POISONING? (FM9.5)

Autopsy Findings

- Characteristic odor of kerosene or garlicky odor
- Froth at mouth and nostrils
- Cyanosis of extremities
- Contracted pupil

Internal Findings

- Congestion of GI tract and visceral congestion
- Pulmonary and cerebral edema
- If the body is attached by insects, they may die of poisoning. OPC delays putrefaction and hence can be detected even in decomposed bodies.

Forensic Significance

- Acute insecticide poisoning is a global problem and deaths due to OPC accounts for a large number of deaths throughout the world.
- Since insecticides are easily available and cheap, suicidal poisoning is very common.

WRITE SHORT NOTES ON CARBAMATES?

- Carbamates are derivatives of carbolic acid. They are marketed in the form of dusts or solutions, such as aldicarb (temix), aminocarb (metacil), aprocarb (baygon), carbofuran (furaxdan).
- Absorbed through all the portals of entry and they are also anticholinergic in action. They inhibit carboxylic esterase enzymes by carbamylation.
- Signs and symptoms begins in 15 minutes to 2 hours. Even though they have the same action as OPC, carbamates differ from OPC as they spontaneously hydrolyse from the cholinesterase enzyme site within 24 to 48 hours.
- Carbamates do not effectively penetrate into the CNS and so they are less toxic to CNS. All other clinical features are same as OPC.
- Atropine is the specific antidote and pralidoxime may help to diminish the severity of symptoms and prevent mortality.

WRITE SHORT NOTES ON ORGANOCHLORINES? WHAT IS ENDRIN? WHAT IS "PLANT PENICILLIN"?

- Endrin is a cyclodiene insecticide belongs to chlorinated hydrocarbons (organochlorines).
- It is soluble in aromatic hydrocarbon, insoluble in water and melts at 245°C.
- Endrin is also called as "**plant penicillin**" because of its broad spectrum activity against various insect pests.
- It is commonly used as sprays mixed with petroleum hydrocarbons like aromax and hence smells like kerosene.
- Poisoning is by occupational or accidental exposure.
- Symptoms of poisoning starts in one to 6 hours. Common symptoms are nausea, vomiting, abdominal pain, diarrhea, hoarseness of voice, cough, froth in mouth and nostrils, restlessness, headache, irritability, dilated pupils, inco-ordination, ataxia, mental confusion, convulsions, coma and death due to respiratory failure.

Treatment

- Gastric lavage and activated charcoal.
- Cholestyramine which is a nonabsorbable, bile acid binding anion exchange resin, is given to increase the fecal excretion of organochlorides. Given in the dose of 16 grams per day in divided doses.

- No specific antidote is available; maintain good airway, breathing and circulation.
- Mental state if altered give dextrose, thiamine and naloxone (coma cocktail).
- Convulsions are controlled using injection diazepam.
- Calcium gluconate is useful adjuvant therapy.

WRITE SHORT NOTES ON PARAQUAT POISONING? WHAT IS "PARAQUAT LUNG"? (FM 9.5)

Paraquat is a bipyridium compound used as herbicide and weed killer.

Action

- Paraquat undergoes nicotinamide adenine dinucleotide phosphate dependent reduction to form free radical. This free radical reacts with molecular oxygen and forms a superoxide free radicals and hydroxyl radicals. They disrupt the cellular function and causes cell death. Concentrated solution of paraquat corrodes the Gastrointestinal tract.
- Paraquat is absorbed through all the portals of entry. Only 10% is absorbed and the rest is excreted in feces.
- After absorption distributed to all the organs, but mainly concentrated in lungs, kidneys and muscles. More than 90% of absorbed paraquat is excreted unchanged in urine in 24 hours.

Signs and Symptoms

- Irritation and inflammation of skin, eyes and nasal mucosa.
- Oropharyngeal ulceration, gastrointestinal corrosion, vomiting, diarrhea, hematemesis, dysphagia and esphagus perforation may occur.

Lungs

- Cough, hemoptysis, dyspnea, pulmonary edema, hemorrhage in the lung parenchyma and fibrosis occur. In fatal cases at autopsy, damage to the pneumocytes with vacuolization, desquamation and necrosis of lung parenchyma is seen. Diffuse pulmonary edema and hemorrhages in the lung parenchyma are often present. On microscopy, a hyaline membrane is often appreciated. This lung symptoms and findings are called as "**paraquat lung**".
- **Kidneys:** Oliguria, renal failure due to acute tubular necrosis and proximal tubular dysfunction are present.
- Death usually results from multi-organ failure.

Treatment

- Gastric lavage within 1 hour of exposure is useful; emesis and cathartics are contraindicated. Activated charcoal can be given.
- Hemodialysis and hemoperfusion are useful within 12 hours of ingestion.

WRITE SHORT NOTES ON PYRETHRINS AND PYRETHROIDS?

- Pyrethrins are extracted from chrysanthemum plant and pyrethroids are synthetic analogues.
- They are used as insect repellants, insecticides and pesticides. They are available in the market in the form of sprays, dusts, powders, mats and coils.
- Toxicity is very low as these compounds are rapidly metabolized in the body. 1 g/kg is the usual fatal dose.
- **Action:** They prolong the inactivation of sodium channel by binding it in the open state.

Signs and Symptoms

- Skin contact causes dermatitis, blistering and paresthesia.
- Nausea, vomiting, vertigo, fasciculations, hyperthermia, altered mental state, convulsions and coma.
- Inhalation causes rhinorrhea, sore throat, bronchoconstriction, wheezing, pulmonary edema and dyspnea.

Treatment

- Stomach wash and activated charcoal.
- Atropine and oximes are contraindicated.
- Skin contact is washed with soap and water.
- For allergic reactions injection adrenaline 0.5 to 1 mL can be given; injection chlorphenamine or promethazine can be given slow IV.

WRITE SHORT NOTES ON ALUMINIUM PHOSPHIDE POISONING? (FM9.5)

Alumnium phosphide is solid fumigating pesticide, insecticide and rodenticide. It is marketed in India under many trade names (alphos, celphos, chemfine, quickphos, etc.) and available as green tablets of 3 g each, mixed with urea and ammonium carbonate, in airtight containers of 10 or 20 tablets.

Uses

- Grain preservative:
- On exposure to air, phosphine is released, when fumigated phosphine evaporates leaving no residues on the leaves.
- **Usual fatal dose:** 1 to 3 tablets (3 to 9 g).

Mode of Action

On exposure to air phosphine is liberated, which causes multi-organ failure.

Clinical Features

- Metallic taste, vomiting, garlicky or fishy odor in breath, burning pain, intense thirst and diarrhea.
- In severe cases CVS manifestations occur leading to hypotension, ECG changes and heart block.
- Coma precedes death, respiratory distress, cyanosis and cold clammy skin are present.
- Aluminum phosphide poisoning mortality is as high as 90 to 100%.

Diagnosis

- Garlicky or fishy odor in breath.
- LFT often abnormal; ECG shows ST-T wave changes.
- **Silver nitrate test:** A filter paper is impregnated with 1% silver nitrate and the patient is asked to breathe through it for 5 to 10 minutes; blackening indicates presence of phosphine in breath (silver nitrate is reduced to silver); similar reaction occurs to H_2S also.

Treatment

- Circulatory shock treated with IV fluids and dopamine.
- Respiratory distress with 100% oxygen, intubation or assisted ventilation.
- Metabolic acidosis with sodium carbonate.
- **Magnesium sulfate therapy:** Beneficial for cardiac arrhythmias.
- Intense thirst is present, but do not give water orally, since aluminum phosphide present in the stomach combines with water and releases phosphine again.

Autopsy Findings

- **Stomach:** Sub-mucosal haemorrhages with mucosal shedding and garlicky odor.

- **Heart:** Myocarditis and fibrillar necrosis; lungs: pulmonary oedema and ARDS.

Forensic Significance

No case of death due to aluminum phosphide was recorded in India, before 1980; today it has emerged as one of the leading cause of suicidal and accidental deaths.

WRITE SHORT NOTES ON ZINC PHOSPHIDE? (FM9.5)

- It is grey crystalline powder with a garlicky odor. It is used as a grain preservative and as a rat poison.
- Signs and symptoms are similar to aluminum phosphide but the symptoms start slowly because of the time taken to release phosphine gas.
- Patients may die within a few hours due to pulmonary edema; most persons die within 36 hours of exposure due to direct myocardial toxic effects.
- Fatal dose is 5 g and average fatal period is 24 hours.

Treatment

- Move the patient to fresh air.
- If ingested stomach wash followed by milk or starch solution lavage; 3 to 5% of sodium bicarbonate can be used to neutralize the gastric acids.
- **Postmortem findings:** Garlicky odor in stomach contents, cherry red blood, congestion and edema of lungs and necrosis and fatty degeneration of liver may be found at autopsy.

MULTIPLE CHOICE QUESTIONS

1. **The complication usually observed on 3rd day with organophosphate poisoning is:**
   a. Ventricular arrhythmias
   b. Intermediate syndrome
   c. Peripheral neuropathy
   d. Guillain-Barre syndrome
2. **OPC poisoning is characterized by all, except:**
   a. Pulmonary edema
   b. Pin point pupil
   c. Constipation
   d. Vomiting
3. **Aryl group of organophosphorus is:**
   a. Folidol
   b. Malathion
   c. Diazinon
   d. Parathion
4. **Zinc phosphide is a**
   a. Respiratory poison
   b. Cardiac poison
   c. GI poison
   d. CNS poison

ANSWERS

1. b   2. c   3. b   4. a

CHAPTER 27

Corrosive Poisons

KEY WORDS

Corrosive, necrosis, sulfuric acid, vitriolage, nitric acid, xanthoprotein reaction, hydrochloric acid, carbolism, carboluria, ochronosis, oxaluria, ink remover, hypocalcemia, Accouchers hand, trousseau's sign, Chvostek's sign, ammonia.

FM9.1 Describe general principles and basic methodologies in treatment of poisoning: decontamination, supportive therapy, antidote therapy, procedures of enhanced elimination with regard to: Caustics: inorganic-sulfuric, nitric, and hydrochloric acids; organic-carbolic acid (phenol), oxalic and acetylsalicylic acids.

INTRODUCTION

- Corrosive is any substance which corrodes, causes burning, erosion and necrosis.
- Both acids and alkalies are corrosive in nature; acids are mineral acids (inorganic) and organic acids. Alkalies are less corrosive than acids.
- **Acids:** Acids are hydrogen containing substances that on dissociation in water produce hydrogen ions. They are potent desiccants and when comes into contact with the body produce coagulation necrosis of the tissues.
- **On ingestion:** Esophagus is less vulnerable to damage compared with the stomach; because esophagus is lined by squamous epithelium, which are relatively resistant to acids and also the acid travels down faster into the stomach due to gravity. Whereas, the columnar epithelium of the stomach is more resistant to alkalies.
- **Mineral acids** have local corrosive action and usually no remote action after absorption; since, they dissociate into their respective ions, which are normal constituents of plasma.
- Whereas **organic acids** have less local corrosive effect and have pronounced remote systemic effect after absorption.

MINERAL ACIDS

WHAT IS SULFURIC ACID? WHAT ARE THE CLINICAL FEATURES, DIAGNOSIS, MANAGEMENT AND AUTOPSY FINDINGS OF SULFURIC ACID POISONING? (FM9.1)

Sulfuric Acid

- It is a highly corrosive mineral acid and is also called as **"oil of vitriol"**.

- Heavy, oily, colorless, odorless, nonfuming liquid and is hygroscopic in nature.
- **Hygroscopic** means has greater affinity for water, reacts violently, giving off intense heat.
- Usual fatal dose is 20 to 30 mL of concentration sulfuric acid; produces coagulation necrosis.

  Uses of sulfuric acid
  - Industrial chemical (concentration is 95-98%).
  - Storage batteries (concentration is 30-35%).
  - Domestic use as drain cleaners (concentration is 8-10%).

Clinical Features

- Burning pain from mouth to stomach.
- Intense thirst, drinking water provokes vomiting.
- Vomitus is brownish black in color (due to altered blood).
- Teeth chalky white in color; tongue swollen and black in color, with constant drooping of saliva from the mouth shown in **Figure 27.1**.
- Usually acid spillage around the mouth, hence corrosion of face is present.

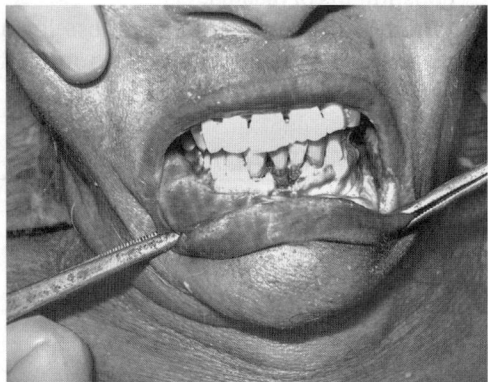

Fig. 27.1: Chalky white teeth in sulfuric acid poisoning *(For color version see Plate 17).*

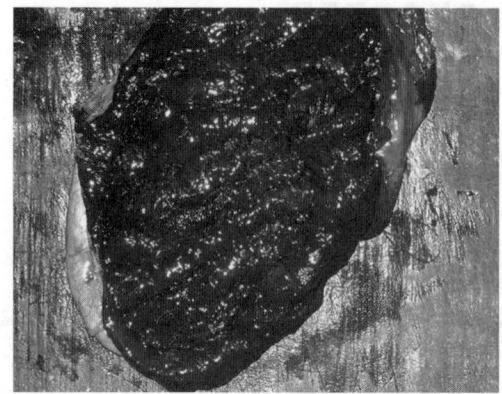

Fig. 27.2: Erosion and necrosis of stomach mucosa in case of sulfuric acid poisoning *(For color version see Plate 17).*

- Perforation of stomach is more common with sulfuric acid ingestion, with resultant chemical peritonitis shown in **Figure 27.2**.
- If the patient recovers, there are long term sequelae, such as stricture formation, pyloric obstruction and stenosis (hour glass deformity of the stomach).
- Contact with the eyes, results in conjunctivitis, corneal edema, necrosis and blindness.

Diagnosis

- **Litmus test:** Saliva can be tested with litmus paper to find out acid or alkali ingestion.
- Fresh stains on the clothing can be tested by adding a few drops of sodium carbonate, results in production of effervescence (bubbles).

Treatment

- Intense laryngeal spasm is treated with 100% oxygen and crico-thyroidectomy.
- No attempt to neutralize the ingested acid, since it results in exothermic reaction with liberation of excessive heat and easy chances of perforation of stomach.

- Water or milk (demulcent) can be given to dilute the acid.
- Remove all contaminated clothes, and exposed skin is washed with saline.
- Eye contact, by prolonged irrigation with water.
- Use of oral feeds, activated charcoal and induced vomiting are contraindicated.
- Steroids are helpful to delay stricture formation but may increase the chance of perforation.
- Powerful analgesics, such as morphine is helpful.
- Flexible fiberoptic endoscopy is done to assess the damage; if 2nd or 3rd degree burns and necroses are present, then esophago-gastrectomy may have to be done.
- If perforation is present, an emergency laparotomy is mandatory; perforation closure done.

Autopsy Findings

- Corroded areas of skin and mucus membrane; tongue, gums and lips are swollen and black in color; teeth are chalky white in color.
- Stomach; inflammation, erosion, necrosis, hemorrhage and blackening of the mucosa are present and perforation are also common—"**wet blotting paper appearance of stomach**".
- In addition to routine viscera, corroded skin can also be sent for analysis and also for HPE.
- Usually, the results are negative and opinion is finalized on the basis of autopsy findings (the classical stomach picture is not present in any other type of poison).

WHAT IS VITRIOLAGE? (FM9.1)

- Throwing of acid on a person is called as vitriolage. It is mainly thrown on the face, to disfigure the individual; there is an obvious motive of revenge or jealousy.
- Sulfuric acid is commonly used for this purpose, any other acid or any other corrosives can also used for this purpose. They may fill the acid into the egg shell after carefully evacuating the contents of the egg through a small opening and seal the shell after filling with the acid, hence can be carried in the hand without suspicion and through on the victim from an accessible distance. Acid is also carried inside small bottles for this purpose of vitriolage.
- When face is involved there is permanent disfiguration, eye contact with the acid results in blindness and both amounts to grievous hurt (Section 320 IPC).

Treatment

Wash the areas of contact with water; eyes when involved are irrigated with plenty of water; antiseptic and local anesthetic ointments can be used. Morphine can be given to control pain.

WRITE SHORT NOTES ON NITRIC ACID POISONING? (FM9.1)

What is Xanthoprotein Reaction?

- Nitric acid is also known as "**aqua fortis**".
- Nitric acid is yellowish fuming liquid, with acrid pungent odor.
- **Uses:** Electroplating, manufacture of fertilizers and metal refinery.
    - *Mode of action:* Xanthoprotein reaction.
- Nitric acid is a powerful oxidizing agent, reacts with organic matter and produce trinitrophenol, liberating nitrogen monoxide and the tissues are stained yellow in color and this is called as "***xanthoprotein reaction***".
- It is less corrosive than sulfuric acid, but leaves back a yellow color.

Clinical Features

- More severe eructation and abdominal distension, due to gas formation.
- Perforation of the stomach is less common.
- Inhalation of the fumes produces coughing, rhinorrhea, lacrimation and dysponea.

Treatment

Similar to sulfuric acid poisoning; respiratory distress is severe and needs special attention.

Autopsy Findings

Stains on the clothes, corroded areas on the skin, mucus membrane and teeth appear yellow in color, which is diagnostic of nitric acid poisoning.

WRITE SHORT NOTES ON HYDROCHLORIC ACID? (FM9.1)

HCl is called as sprit of salts; it is a colorless fuming liquid, which may acquire a yellow color on exposure to air.

Uses

- Bleaching agent, dying industry, metal refinery, flux for soldering, and metal and drain cleaner.
- All the features are same as for sulfuric acid, except:
    - Corrosion less severe and appear grayish and not black shown in **Figure 27.3** in case of lung inhalation.
    - **Figures 27.4 and 27.5** depicts kerosene poisoning.
    - All the symptoms are less severe compared to sulfuric acid.
    - Respiratory complications are more pronounced than corrosive effects due to the fuming effect and needs special attention.

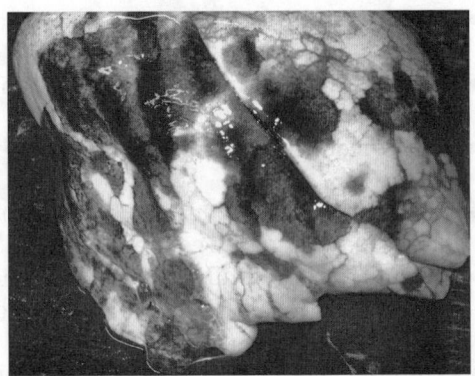

Fig. 27.3: Lung—inhalation of mixture of acids (cleaning acid): Alternative areas of bleeding (corrosion and rupture of arteries) and pale lung parenchyma caused by inhalation while the victim consumed the cleaning acid to commit suicide—a treated case died after 20 days of poisoning near the recovery period; CT could not pick up the lung finding and the patient suddenly collapsed and died after a heavy bout of hemoptysis *(For color version see Plate 18).*

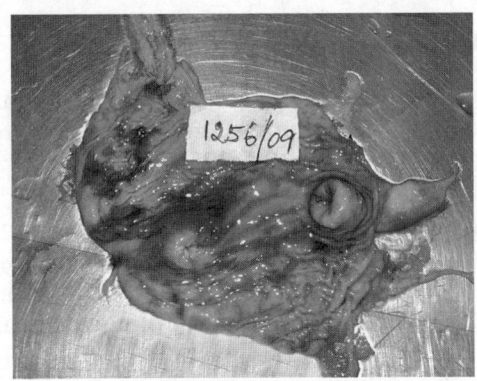

Fig. 27.4: Kerosene poisoning—diffuse submucosal hemorrhages in stomach *(For color version see Plate 18).*

ORGANIC ACIDS

DESCRIBE THE PROPERTIES, USES, CLINICAL FEATURES, DIAGNOSIS AND TREATMENT OF CARBOLIC ACID POISONING? (FM9.1)

Carbolic acid is hydroxybenzene (phenol).

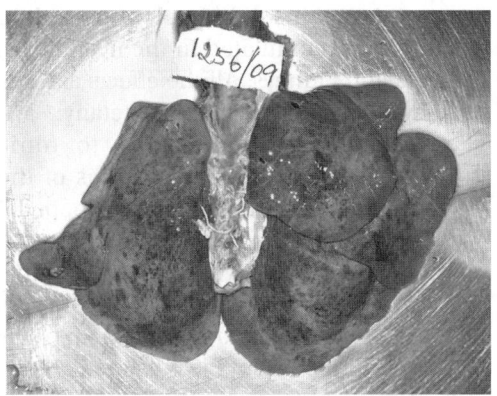

Fig. 27.5: Lung in kerosene poisoning—petechio-ecchymotic hemorrhages more concentrated on the upper lobe; the child died of aspiration pneumonitis *(For color version see Plate 18).*

Physical Properties

- Colorless, needle like crystals, and turn into pink color and liquefy when exposed to air.
- Commercial phenol is brownish in color which contains impurities like cresol, and used as 5% solution (becomes white in color on dilution with water) for household disinfection purpose which has a typical hospital odor.

Uses

- Introduced in the 19th century and was popular disinfectant for both hospital and domestic purposes, but lost importance of use in the operation theatres due to invention of safer antiseptics like certimide, chlorhexidine, cresol and povidine iodide.
- Still in use as floor and toilet cleaner in hospitals and homes antiseptic and disinfectant.
- **Preservative:** For commonly used injections like glucagon, pethidine, neostigmine, etc.
- Manufacture of plastics.
- **Medical use:** 'Face peel' in plastic surgery and neurolysis of spaticity (phenol is injected into the neuromuscular junction).
- **Fatal dose:** 10 to 30 g; 25 to 50 mL of household phenol may prove fatal.
- **Absorption:** Phenol is rapidly absorbed through intact skin, lungs and GI tract (dilution increases absorption).
- **Mode of action:** Mild corrosive action locally and after absorption results in CNS depression, metabolic acidosis and renal damage.

Clinical Features

Acute poisoning with phenol is known as "**carbolism**".

Locally it has a mild corrosive effect; hardening and grayish white discoloration of the skin is present on exposure; there may be burning pain, followed by tingling, numbness and anesthesia (the white escher on the skin may fall away in a few days and looks brown).

Systemic Features

- **GIT:** Burning pain, vomiting and the stomach mucosa turns into whitish, hard and rubbery in consistency, and hence stomach wash is very well indicated (the only corrosive where stomach wash can be done).
- **CNS:** Vertigo, convulsions and coma (pupils usually constricted).
- **RS:** Slow labored breathing, progressing to respiratory failure.
- **Metabolic:** Hypothermia with cold clammy skin and metabolic acidosis.
- **Hepato-renal:** Phenol is metabolized in the liver and the metabolites hydroquinone and pyrocatechol are excreted in urine; urine turns green on exposure to air due to these metabolites and this condition is called "**carboluria**"; oliguria is present and progressing on to acute renal and hepatic failure.

Chronic Poisoning (Phenol Marasmus)

This was common in olden days, in medical professional when phenol was routinely used as skin disinfectant. Chronic exposure to phenol results in phenol marasmus characterized by anorexia, weight loss, vertigo, dark colored urine and pigmentation of skin and sclera (**ochrnosis**).

Diagnosis

- Typical odor in the vicinity of the patient.
- **Bed side test:** Collect urine in a transparent container and expose to sunlight, gradual color change from brown to green.
- Add 1 mL of 10% ferric chloride solution to 10 mL of urine, a purple or blue color develops and persists even after heating, indicates phenol poisoning.

Treatment

- Decontamination with copious amount of water, if there is skin contact.
- Stomach wash with sodium or magnesium sulfate.
- Activated charcoal and other supportive measures.

Autopsy Findings

- Distinct odor around mouth and stomach contents.
- Stomach mucosa is grayish white in color, swollen, hard and leathery; if death is delayed the color may change to brown.

DESCRIBE THE SYSTEMIC EFFECTS OF OXALIC ACID POISONING? (FM9.1)

- Oxalic acid is also called as "salts of sorrel"; it reacts with calcium in the plasma and precipitates insoluble **calcium oxalate** and gets accumulated in the liver, heart, lungs and kidneys. All the effects are due to **hypocalcaemia** leading to tetany:
  - **Acconcher's hand** due to tonic muscular spasm and cramps of the muscles of the upper limb (carpopedal spasm).
  - **Trousseau's sign** is often positive when pressure is applied on the nerves and vessels of upper arm there is sudden spasm of the muscles.
  - **Chvostek's sign:** When the facial nerve is tapped, there is spasm of facial muscles.
- The excretion of oxalate crystals in urine is called as **oxaluria.**
- Diagnosis is by demonstration of oxalate crystals in the urine as monohydrates (needle like or prism shaped crystals) or dihydrates (tent or envelope shaped crystals).

Ink Remover

Criminals use oxalic acid for altering the signature or even by anyone to change the contents of the documents (tampering of records) and produce fake documents, but which can be detected by analysis at FSL.

WHAT IS SHOCK LUNG?

Formic Acid

- In formic acid poisoning there is coagulative necrosis and corrosion of the GI mucosa.
- There is damage to the clotting factors which leads to hemolysis and renal failure.
- Formic acid inhibits aerobic respiration and results in diminution of ATP.
- Aspiration pneumonitis and respiratory distress leads to '**shock lung**'.

WHAT ARE THE USES, CLINICAL FEATURES, TREATMENT AND POSTMORTEM FINDINGS OF ALKALIES?

Alkalies

- Commonly encountered alkalies are ammonia (ammonium hydroxide), carbonates (of sodium, potassium and calcium) and sodium hypochlorite.
- Most of these alkalies appear as white powders or colorless solutions; ammonia gas is colorless, with a pungent choking odor.

Uses

- **Ammonium hydroxide:** Used in paints, dirt remover and as refrigerant.
- **Sodium hydroxide (caustic soda):** Drain cleaner and oven cleaner.
- **Potassium hydroxide (caustic potash):** Drain cleaner and hearing aid batteries.
- **Sodium carbonate (washing soda):** Household cleaner and detergent.
- **Sodium hypochlorite:** Household bleach.
- **Usual fatal dose:** 10 to 15 g; 15 to 20 mL for ammonia.

Mode of Action

Locally, alkalies produce liquefaction necrosis and saponification of fats; ulcer formation is common and takes several weeks to heal; esophagus is more vulnerable than stomach.

Clinical Features

- Corrosion of GIT with grayish discoloration; dysphagia, vomiting and hematemesis.
- Abdominal pain and diarrhea.
- **Skin:** Grayish, soapy, necrotic areas without charring.
- Eye involvement causes serious ophthalmologic emergencies.
- Ammonia inhalation results in respiratory problems.

Treatment

- **Inhalation of ammonia:** Needs endotracheal intubation or tracheostomy and oxygen.
- **When alkalies are ingested:** Dilution with milk or water.
- Emesis, gastric lavage, catharsis and activated charcoal are contraindicated.
- Early surgical intervention and use of intraluminal stent in the esophagus is also recommended (esophageal perforation could be missed at latter stage).
- If gastric necrosis is found out, then an exploratory laparotomy followed by gastric resection and oesophagectomy is done.
- Corticosteroids for prevention of stricture formation (but increases the chance of perforation and infections).
- Prophylactic antibiotics not necessary, unless there is perforation.
- **Injuries to eyes and skin:** Should be irrigated with plenty of water; topical steroids and antibiotics are helpful.

Autopsy Findings

- Characteristic odor (especially in ammonia).
- Brownish or grayish discoloration of the skin and mucosa.
- Corrosion and inflammatory edema; slimness of the mucosa of esophagus and stomach.
- Congestion of respiratory tract and pulmonary edema (ammonia inhalation).

MULTIPLE CHOICE QUESTIONS

1. **The following terms denotes chronic poisoning syndrome,** *except*:
   a. Iodism
   b. Bromism
   c. Plumbism
   d. Carbolism

SECTION 7: Medical Toxicology

2. **Antidote for oxalic acid poisoning is:**
   a. BAL
   b. Animal charcoal
   c. Calcium gluconate
   d. Magnesium
3. **Perforation of stomach is more common in:**
   a. Nitric acid
   b. Sulfuric acid
   c. Hydrochloric acid
   d. Acetic acid
4. **One of the following is used as ink remover solution:**
   a. Carbolic acid
   b. Acetic acid
   c. Sulfuric acid
   d. Oxalic acid
5. **The antidote for mineral acid poisoning:**
   a. Sodium bicarbonate
   b. Sodium hydroxide
   c. Sodium chloride
   d. Magnesium oxide
6. **In sulfuric acid poisoning all the following are seen, *except*:**
   a. Dryness of mouth
   b. Damaged tongue
   c. Chalky white teeth
   d. Swollen tongue with white coating
7. **Which of the following corrosive poisoning causes brown discoloration of gastric mucosa?**
   a. Sulfuric acid
   b. Nitric acid
   c. Hydrochloric acid
   d. All of the above
8. **Poison having local action only:**
   a. Sulfuric acid
   b. Carbolic acid
   c. Oxalic acid
   d. Acetic acid
9. **Yellow discoloration of skin and mucosa is seen inpoisoning with:**
   a. Nitrous oxide
   b. Nitric acid
   c. Sulfuric acid
   d. Phosphoric acid
10. **Magenstrasse refers to:**
    a. Signs of magnesium poisoning
    b. Marks of violence in case of poisoning
    c. Route of acidic poisons in stomach
    d. Color change of mucosa seen in corrosives
11. **Vitriolage is punishable under which section of IPC:**
    a. 302
    b. 320 A
    c. 326
    d. 326 A
12. **Boiled lobster' appearance is seen in poisoning with:**
    a. Carbolic acid
    b. Boric acid
    c. Oxalic acid
    d. Sulphuric acid
13. **Common toxin through vegetables:**
    a. Boric acid
    b. Carbolic acid
    c. Oxalic acid
    d. Tartaric acid
14. **Tetany is caused by poisoning with:**
    a. Carbolic acid
    b. Oxalic acid
    c. Tartaric acid
    d. Sulphuric acid
15. **Trousseau sign is positive in which poisoning:**
    a. Boric acid
    b. Carbolic acid
    c. Oxalic acid
    d. Sulphuric acid
16. **Green colored urine is seen after ingestion of:**
    a. Copper sulphate
    b. Phenol
    c. Organophosphorus compound
    d. Cyanide

ANSWERS

1. d	2. c	3. b	4. d	5. d	6. d	7. a	8. a	9. b	10. c
11. d	12. b	13. c	14. b	15. c	16. b				

CHAPTER 28

Metallic and Inorganic Irritants Poisons

KEY WORDS

Arsenic, aldrich-mees lines, raindrop pigmentation, black foot disease, plumbism, burtonian lines, punctate basophilia, basophilic stippling, hydrargyrism, danbury's tremors, hatter's shake, acrodynia, iron, desferrioxamine, copper sulfate, thalium, white phosphorus, phossy jaw, phosphine, barium.

FM9.2 Describe general principles and basic methodologies in treatment of poisoning: decontamination, supportive therapy, antidote therapy, procedures of enhanced elimination with regard to phosphorus, Iodine, barium.

FM9.3 Describe general principles and basic methodologies in treatment of poisoning: decontamination, supportive therapy, antidote therapy, procedures of enhanced elimination with regard to arsenic, lead, mercury, copper, iron, cadmium and thallium.

HOW DO WE CLASSIFY IRRITANTS?

- Irritants can be classified as:
    - *Heavy metals:* Arsenic, lead, mercury, copper, thallium and iron.
    - *Inorganic irritants:* Phosphorus, aluminum phosphide, iodine and chlorine.
    - *Organic irritants:* Plants, animals, and mechanical irritants.
        ♦ Plants: *Abrus precatorius, Calotropis, Semecarpus anacardium, Ricinus communis, Croton tiglium* and *Capsicum annuum.*
        ♦ Animals: Snakes, Scorpion, Cantharides and Bees and Wasp stings.

WHAT ARE THE ENVIRONMENTAL SULFIDES OF ARSENIC? (FM9.3)

- Arsenic is a naturally occurring element widely distributed in the earth's crust.
- Arsenic combines with oxygen, chlorine, and sulfur to form **inorganic** arsenic compounds.
- In animals and plants combines with carbon and hydrogen to form **organic** arsenic compound.
- **Inorganic** arsenic compounds are mainly used to preserve wood.
- **Organic** arsenic compounds are used as pesticides, primarily on cotton plants.

Environmental Sulfide of Arsenic

- **Realgar:** Yellow (As_2S_2)
- **Orpiment:** Red (As_2S_3)
  - On heating of these ores, arsenic sublimes and oxidizes to form arsenic trioxide (As_2O_3) fine granular white powder also known as white arsenic.
- **Copper Arsenite** (Scheele's green)
- **Copper Acetoarsenite** (Paris green or Emerald green)
- **Arsine gas:** Arsine gas (AsH_3), formed by the hydrolysis of metal arsenide and by the reduction of metals of arsenic compounds in acidic solutions.

WHAT ARE THE MEDICINAL USES OF ARSENICALS? WHAT IS THE USUAL LEVEL OF EXPOSURE IN HUMANS?

Medicinal Uses

- **Fowler solution:** (1% potassium arsenite) used for psoriasis; hepatic angiosarcoma is commonest complication.
- Regular, long-term arsenic exposure, results in cutaneous carcinomas as well as internal malignancies including bronchogenic carcinoma and hepatocellular carcinoma.

Human Exposure

- Average 20 µg/day from food and water
- Background air is less than 0.1 µg/m³
- Drinking water usually less that 5 µg/L
- Food is usually less that 10 µg/day

HOW ARSENIC IS METABOLIZED AND DISTRIBUTED IN THE HUMAN BODY?

Metabolism

- As^{3+} (Arsenite) is metabolized into Methylarsenite (in liver).
- Dimethylarsenite (readily eliminated in urine).
- Half-life is 3 to 5 days; excretion is mainly through urine and also through skin in sweat.

Distribution

- Bound to red blood cells.
- Distributes to liver, lungs, and spleen.
- Binds to sulfhydryl group of mitochondrial enzymes especially, pyruvate oxidase and gets concentrated in the hair and fingernails (Mees' lines).

WHAT ARE THE TYPES OF ARSENIC POISONING? (FM9.3) WRITE SHORT NOTES ON: ACUTE ARSENIC POISONING?

- **Acute poisoning:**
  - Fulminant and
  - Gastroenteritis type
- Inhalation of arsine gas
- Sub-acute
- Chronic poisoning.

Mode of Action

- Locally acts as an irritant of the gastric and mucus membrane.
- **Remote:** Arsenic acts as a depressant of nervous system, heart, and respiration.

Mechanism of Action

- Arsenic combines with the sulfhydryl group of mitochondrial enzyme system, mainly pyruvate kinase and thereby, interferes with the cellular respiration.
- It gets deposited in bones, hair, and nails.

Toxicity Depends on

- Compound ingested and its physical form (soluble or insoluble).
- Stomach empty or full: Actions starts within 10 minutes when the stomach is empty and more than half an hour if full.

- Inherent tolerance of the patient to arsenic is also an important factor in the development of symptoms; on an average tolerance of arsenic trioxide is 70 to 180 mg.
- The fatal period is 12 to 48 hours of ingestion.

Acute Poisoning

- **Narcotic form of acute poisoning (fulminant poisoning):**
  - Rare and occurs when massive dose is taken in empty stomach.
  - There are no symptoms of gastroenteritis, CNS symptoms predominate.
  - Delirium, tenderness of muscles and convulsion leading to complete paralysis of muscles, followed by coma and death.
- **Signs and symptoms of acute poisoning: (gastroenteritis type)**
  - Occur within 30 minutes of exposure.
  - Metallic taste and slight garlicky odor to the breath.
  - Xerostomia (dry mouth) and dysphasia.
  - Burning pain in stomach and throat; intense thirst and salivation.
  - The tongue is coated with thick white fur.
  - Nausea and projectile vomiting (characteristic symptom)
  - Heart burn, with colicky abdominal pain and distention.
  - Profuse diarrhea, usually rice water stools (mimic cholera) and in some cases mixed with blood; tenesmus and anal pain are present.
  - Urine output is suppressed, and urination is painful.
  - Non-cardiogenic pulmonary edema develops.
  - *Cardiac manifestations:* Acute cardiomyopathy and sub-endocardial hemorrhages (decreased cardiac output due to hypovolemia and due to the direct toxic effect of arsenic on cardiac muscles)
  - *ECG changes:* Prolonged QT interval and nonspecific ST-T changes.
- **Inhalation of arsine gas:**
  - Instantaneous development of symptoms of formication, frothy sputum, and pulmonary edema.
- **Cause of death:**
  - Acute arsenic poisoning: Irreversible circulatory insufficiency.
  - Chronic arsenic poisoning: Failure of heart muscle.

WHAT IS THE TREATMENT FOR ACUTE ARSENIC POISONING? (FM9.3)

Treatment

Acute Arsenic Poisoning

- **Nonspecific measures:**
  - Gastric lavage to remove residual arsenic from the stomach using 1% sodium thiosulfate solution. Recently 2,3-dimercaptosuccinic acid orally have been tried useful.
  - Activated charcoal/$MgSO_4$ to decrease further intestinal absorption.
  - Intravenous fluids to maintain intravascular volume and prevent circulatory collapse.
  - The vital organs must be monitored, and specific measures are to be taken.
  - Hemodialysis is useful to remove arsenic in the presence of renal failure.
  - Narcotic analgesics can be given to combat pain.
- **Specific therapy:**
  - Antidote: **Freshly prepared hydrated ferric oxide** is given which converts arsenic to ferric arsenite.
  - British antilewisite (**BAL dimercaprol**) are given which reverses the hematologic effects of arsenic, it does not appear to reverse the neurologic effects caused by chronic poisoning. Therefore, before any treatment with

dimercaprol is started in chronic poisoning cases the benefits must be weighed against the side effects.
- *Tests:* Reinsch test and Marsh Berzelius test are done.

WHAT IS SUB-ACUTE FORM OF ARSENIC POISONING?

- Symptoms of neuritis are more pronounced.
- Liver shows fatty degeneration resulting in Jaundice.
- Pigmentation of skin and rashes may appear.
- Muscular weakness ending in paralysis; convulsion and delirium may be present.

WHAT ARE THE EFFECTS OF ARSENIC ON PREGNANCY?

- Inorganic arsenic cross placenta and causes Intrauterine death.
- In 3rd trimester: Premature labor, pulmonary hemorrhage and hyaline membrane disease occurs, may lead to death of the fetus due to respiratory distress.

WRITE SHORT NOTES ON CHRONIC ARSENIC POISONING? (FM9.3) WHAT IS ALRICH MEE'S LINE AND BLACK FOOT DISEASE?

Chronic Toxicity

- **After ingestion:**
  - 2 to 4 weeks after ingestion: Incorporated into hair, nails, and skin.
  - 4 weeks after ingestion: localize in the bone, where it substitutes phosphate.
  - Arsenic is associated with causing cancer of the lung, skin, liver, kidney, and bladder.
- **Chronic exposure:** (usually through drinking water)
  - Skin cancer (recognized 100 years ago)

- Garlic odor on breath and excessive perspiration
- Muscle tenderness and weakness
- Skin pigmentation and paresthesia in hands and feet
- Sub endocardial hemorrhage in the left ventricle of heart.
- Hyperkeratosis (wart like lesion) of the palms and soles
- Symmetrical sensory motor polyneuropathy, often resembling Guillain-Barre syndrome.

Rain Drop Pigmentation

Hyperpigmentation of skin of the face or extremities, with classical picture of "dew drops on a dusty road" brownish in color, which resembles **Addison's disease**.

Blackfoot Disease

Due to chronic exposure to arsenic there is peripheral vascular disease resulting in **gangrene of feet** is known as "blackfoot disease".

Aldrich Mee's Lines

Nails become brittle with transverse whitish striate (lines) of 1 to 2 mm in breath on the fingernails is called as "Mee's lines.

WHAT ARE THE EFFECTS OF CHRONIC EXPOSURE TO ARSINE GAS?

- **Chronic exposure to arsine gas manifests as:**
  - Acute hemolytic anemia, jaundice and striking chills.
  - Noncardiogenic pulmonary edema with bilateral basal crepitation.
  - Hemoglobinuria, urine appears black in color.
  - Heart failure; delirium and coma.
  - Arsine dust causes pulmonary edema, corneal ulcer and conjunctivitis.

WHAT ARE THE METHODS OF DIAGNOSIS OF ARSENIC POISONING? (FM9.3)

- Definitive diagnosis of arsenic poisoning is difficult because of natural presence of trace amounts of arsenic in the body.
- Clinical manifestations simulate many other diseases: Acute poisoning simulates cholera and chronic poisoning simulates addison's disease, guillian barre syndrome and black foot disease as gangrene of foot.

Lab Diagnosis

Urine test: Monomethylarsine and dimethylarsine

- Arsenic in urine more than 100 to 200 mg/24 hour is regarded as indicative of exposure to a potentially toxic amount of arsenic (be sure the patient has not consumed shellfish for at least 3 days before collection of the sample).
- Coproporphyrin test is positive; gastric contents are useful in acute ingestion.

Blood Test

- Anemia and leucopenia (acute hemolytic anemia is the rule with arsine exposure).
- Blood arsenic concentrations should not exceed 50 µg/L.
- **LFT:** Increased serum alkaline phosphatase and bilirubin.

Chronic Arsenic Ingestion

Body tissues, nails and hair are useful in diagnosis.

Methods

- Colorimetry, polarography, atomic absorption spectroscopy and neutron activation analysis.
- Hair and nail samples containing >3 ppm or 100 mg or arsenic per 100 g of specimen are diagnostic of arsenic poisoning.
- **Napoleon bonaparte** was determined to have died of arsenic poisoning after 140 years of his death (Weirder, 1999).

WHAT ARE THE POSTMORTEM FINDINGS OF ARSENIC POISONING? (FM9.3)

External

- Pinched face with sunken eyes.
- Cyanosis of lips and fingernails, associated with jaundice if liver is involved.

Internal

- Stomach and mucosa are inflamed.
- **Red velvety appearance** is the classical picture of stomach in acute arsenic poisoning; with scattered sub-mucosal hemorrhages on the surface of the mucosa.
- Stomach contents are black, green or dark brown in color; intestine shows inflammation.
- **Heart:** Sub-endocardial hemorrhage on the left ventricle.
- **Lungs:** Deeply congested, edematous and sub pleural petechial hemorrhage.
- **Liver and spleen:** Enlarged, congested and fatty infiltration.
- **Kidney:** Enlarged, congested, fatty infiltration and cloudy swelling of the kidneys.
- **Rectum:** Inflammatory changes are present.

WHAT ARE THE MEDICO-LEGAL ISSUES RELATED TO ARSENIC POISONING?

Arsenic is an ideal homicidal poison.

Advantage

- Tasteless and odorless; effects are not immediate.

- Acute poisoning mimic **cholera** and chronic poisoning mimic Addison's disease.
- Successful homicidal cases have been reported and the individual is killed without any suspicion.

Disadvantage

Delays putrefaction; detected even if the body is decomposed; even after many years arsenic can be detected from the nails, hairs and bones.

Medico-legal Significance

- Rarely suicidal
- **Accidental:** Consumption of more Seafoods and also by mistake for baking soda.
- **In exhumed bodies:** If nails, hairs and bones contain more arsenic than that of the soil present around the body, indicates poisoning by arsenic.
- WHO recommended levels of arsenic in water, should be less than 5 mg/100 mL.

Other Criminal Uses

Cattle poisoning, abortifacient and as aphrodisiac.

HOW WILL DIFFERENTIATE CHOLERA FROM ARSENIC POISONING? (FM9.3)

Table 28.1 is depicted the differences between acute arsenic poisoning and cholera.

TABLE 28.1: Difference between acute arsenic poisoning and cholera.

Trait	Arsenic	Cholera
Throat pain	Before vomiting	After vomiting
Purging	After vomiting	Before vomiting
Stools	Rice water, later bloody	Rice water
Tenesmus	Present	Absent
Vomitus	Mucus, bile and blood	Watery
Voice	Not affected	Rough and whistling
Conjunctiva	Inflamed	Not
Analysis	Arsenic	Vibrio cholera

- Its high resistance to corrosion makes it ideal for weatherproofing buildings and for equipment used in the manufacture of acids.
- It is a heavy steel gray metal; metallic form and all salts are poisonous.
- Toxic forms are:
    - Lead acetate (Sugar of lead)
    - Lead carbonate (Safeda)
    - Lead monoxide (Litharge)
    - Lead tetroxide (Red lead, sindur, vermillion)
    - Lead sulfide.

WHAT IS THE MECHANISM OF ACTION OF LEAD?

- Lead interacts with sulfhydryl group of enzymes and interferes with haem synthesis and cytochrome production, thus leads to hemolysis.
- Acute poisoning is not common and clinically shows metallic taste, burning pain in mouth and abdomen, thirst, vomiting, circulatory collapse, etc.
- Characteristic finding is cerebellar ataxia in children.

LEAD

WHAT ARE THE PROPERTIES AND TOXIC COMPOUNDS OF LEAD?

Properties

- Lead is a versatile metal; its softness and low melting point make lead very easy to handle.

SHORT NOTES ON PLUMBISM? (FM9.3)

- Chronic lead poisoning is called as **plumbism** or saturnism.
- Poisoning occurs due to inhalation of lead dust and fumes in factories, from drinking water stored in lead vessels, food contaminated with lead oleate present in tin lined food packets.
- Other ways are absorption from Sindur or accidental poisoning in children due to ingestion of toys painted with lead paint.

Signs and Symptoms

- Lead affects almost all the systems of the body.
    - *Facial pallor:* Earliest symptom, seen around the mouth; present in almost 90% of cases.
    - Anemia with punctate basophilia, reticulocytosis and basophilic stippling of RBC.
    - *Lead lines:* Called '**burtonian line**' which is seen on the gums; due to sub-epithelial deposits of lead granules near caries tooth; this is due to the formation of lead sulfide.
    - *Lead palsy:* Presents with tremors, numbness, hyperesthesia and cramps occurs; there may be wrist drop, or foot drop.
    - *Lead encephalopathy:* Present in most cases of chronic poisoning, common in children; characterized by headache, insomnia, visual disturbances, irritability and delirium.
    - *Colic and constipation:* This is a late symptom and occurs at night.
    - *CVS:* Vascular constriction and arteriolar degeneration.
    - Renal involvement leading to hypertension and interstitial nephritis.
    - Reproductive system leading to menstrual irregularities and infertility.
    - *Lead osteopathy:* Deposition of lead in growing ends of long bones.

Diagnosis

Serum Lead >0.1 mg/100 mL; urinary lead >0.25 mg/100 mL.

Treatment

- **In severe poisoning with encephalopathy:**
  BAL: 4 mg/kg 4 hourly, till blood lead level falls to <40 mcgm%.
  Calcium sodium EDTA: 75 g/kg/day IV.
  Then, followed by D-Penicillamine.
- **Severe poisoning but no encephalopathy:**
  BAL: 12 mg/kg/day.
  EDTA: 50 mg/kg/day.
  Continue oral chelation till blood level is <15 mcgm%
- **Moderate poisoning:** EDTA therapy followed with oral chelation.
- **Mild poisoning:** D-Penicillamine therapy.
- **Supportive:** Thiamine, calcium gluconate, $MgSO_4$, and calcium disodium versenate.

WHAT ARE THE POSTMORTEM FINDINGS AND MEDICO-LEGAL SIGNIFICANCE OF LEAD?

Postmortem Findings

- Blue line on the gums.
- Fatty degeneration of muscles.
- Ulcerative and hemorrhagic changes in stomach and intestines.
- Liver and kidneys are contracted.
- Brain looks pale with PAS positive material in perivascular spaces.
- Bone marrow shows hyperplasia of leucoblasts and erythroblasts.

Medico-legal Aspects

Cause of Death

In chronic poisoning death occurs due to gastroenteritis and shock, malnutrition, intercurrent infection or hepatic failure, etc.

Circumstances of Poisoning
- Chronic poisoning is more common among people who work in plumbing industries. Any individual who develops plumbism is more of occupational hazard; the victim is eligible for compensation as per workman's compensation act.
- **Abortifacient:** Lead oleate mixed with juices of plant irritants and used in "abortion stick".
- **Cattle poison:** Red lead is used to mix with seeds of *Abrus precatorius* and used as cattle poison in the form of "SUI".
- **Fire-arm injuries:** Death due to chronic lead poisoning rarely occurs from imbedded missiles (pellet or bullets) from firearms.

Mercury

Introduction
- After inhalation, mercury is readily absorbed into circulation through the alveolar membranes and rapidly converted into mercuric ions; absorbed through skin also.
- **Kidneys:** Target organ for mercury are the kidneys. Acute tubular necrosis occurs in the kidneys; CNS: Acts mainly on the cerebellum and corpus callosum.

WHAT IS MERCURIALISM?
- SC or IM injections of mercury results in abscess formation with ulceration, exuding tiny droplets of mercury.
- Intravenous injection causes '**mercurialism**' characterized by thrombophlebitis, granuloma formation and pulmonary embolism; repeated hemoptysis is characteristic feature.

WRITE SHORT NOTES ON HYDRARGYRISM? (FM9.3)
- Chronic poisoning with mercury is called as "**hydrargyrism**".
- Inhalation of the fumes is the usual mode of contact and is more of an occupational hazard.

Danbury's Tremors
- Due to chronic inhalation of mercury vapors there is Coarse tremors, begins in the hands, intentional type, interspersed with jerky movements is Danbury's tremors, this is also called as **Glassblowers tremors**.
- These coarse tremors later on progresses to lips, tongue, arms and legs and is called as "**Hatter's Shake**".
- Tremors gradually become severe and interfere with all normal daily activities, like shaving, holding a glass, etc., and the advanced condition is called '**concussion mercurialis**' where literally no activity is possible.
- Gingivitis, increased salivation, halitosis, blue lines on the gums (similar to plumbism).

Mercurial Erythrism
- Cluster of psychiatric symptoms, including abnormal shyness, loss of self confidence, depression, irritability, amnesia, progressing to delirium and hallucinations. Maniac depressive psychosis (**Mad Hatter**).
- **Acrodynia:** (Acro: Extremity; dynia: Pain)
  - Also known as "**pink disease**" or "Erythroderma".
  - This is commonly seen in children and is due to idiosyncratic hypersensitivity.
  - The prime features are painful, pink, puffy, paresthetic, pruritic hands and feet, which are accompanied by polyneuritis, desquamating rashes, behavioral changes, insomnia, and irritability.
  - Renal involvement results in membranous glomerulonephritis, with hyaline casts and fatty casts in urine.

Mercuria Lentis

Deposition of mercuric vapors on the anterior lens capsule of the eye. Characterized by brown reflex and fine punctate opacities.

HOW TO DIAGNOSIS MERCURY POISONING? (FM9.3)

- **X-ray:** Progressive movement of mercury by X-ray at regular intervals.
- **Blood mercury level:** Flameless atomic absorption spectrometry (AAS).
- Urine mercury level.
- **Hair analysis:** Cold vapors AAS.

IRON

WRITE SHORT NOTES ON IRON POISONING? (FM9.3)

- Iron is an Essential element, deficiency states results in anemia.
- In some individuals due to inborn error, normal dietary requirement may lead to toxicity due accumulation. **Example:** Hemochromatosis (**bronze diabetes**).
- Various iron salts are used for therapeutic purpose to treat anemia; most instances of iron poisoning are due to over dosage.
- **Usual fatal dose:** 200 to 250 mg of elemental iron per kg body weight.
- Iron poisoning results when serum iron level exceeds the total iron binding capacity (TIBC). Resulting in free circulating iron in the bloodstream.

Clinical Features

- **Stage I:** (30 minutes to 6 hours): Vomiting, diarrhea, abdominal pain, pallor, lethargy, metabolic acidosis, leukocytosis and hypoglycemia.
- **Stage II:** (6 to 24 hours): Hypotension and severe metabolic acidosis.
- **Stage III:** (24 to 48 hours): Multiple organ failure involving GIT, hepatorenal, CNS, CVS with metabolic coagulopathies, hypoglycemia, convulsions, disorientation, coma and death due to hepatic failure.
- **Stage IV:** Recovery is often associated with late complications such as gastric scarring and pyloric obstruction.

Diagnosis

- **X-Ray**
- **Serum iron level:** 150 mg/100 mL; beyond 500 mg/100 mL indicates serious toxicity.
- **Chelation challenging test:** Desferrioxamine 25 mg/kg (maximum 1 g) is given IM; if TIBC has exceeded then excess iron is chelated and the compound excreted is pinkish (vin rose) in color; negative result does not rules out iron toxicity.
- **Quantitative desferrioxamine color test:** Confirmatory test.

Treatment

- Stomach wash with normal saline.
- Magnesium hydroxide (1%) solution given orally may reduce absorption, by precipitating the formation of ferrous hydroxide.
- Correction of hypovolemia and metabolic acidosis.
- **Chelation therapy:** Desferrioxamine 1 g IM; followed by 500 mg every 4th hourly for 2 doses, and finally 500 mg every 12th hourly up to a maximum of 6 g in 24 hours. It can also be given as IV infusion normal saline, glucose water or ringer's lactate.
- Liver transplant may be required in Fulminant hepatic failure.

Autopsy Findings

- Hemorrhagic necrosis of GI mucosa; gastric contents may appear bluish green.
- Hepatic and renal necrosis.

Forensic Significance

Acute accidental poisoning due to therapeutic over dosage is frequently reported in children.

COPPER

DESCRIBE COPPER SULFATE POISONING (FM 9.3)

Copper is a brown colored metal, several salts of copper are poisonous; copper sulfate is blue colored salt. Because of the irritant action it is also used for vitriolage and is called "blue vitriol".

Copper sulphate shown in **Figure 28.1**.

Clinical Features

Acute Poisoning

Burning pain in the stomach, abdominal pain, vomiting, diarrhea, acidosis, pancreatitis, hemolysis, myalgia, jaundice, renal failure, delirium, seizures and coma.

Chronic Poisoning

- Chronic inhalation of copper sulfate spray used as insecticide causes 'vineyard sprayer's lung disease' characterized by histocytic granulomatous lung; liver damage is also common.
- Chronic contact in swimming pools causes greenish discoloration of hair.
- Chronic copper toxicity is the hallmark of 'Wilson's disease' an autosomal recessive genetic disorder due to deficiency of caeruloplasmin.

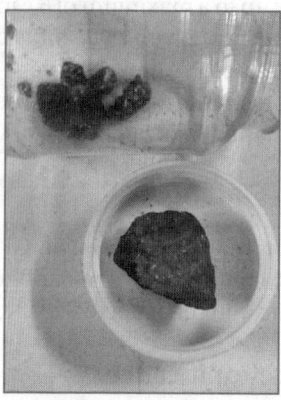

Fig. 28.1: Metallic irritant poison (copper sulphate) (For color version see Plate 18).

Diagnosis

- Serum caeruloplasmin level less than 35 mg% at 24 hours, indicate severe toxicity.
- **Blood copper level:** Elevated more than 1.5 mg/100 mL indicates severe toxicity.

Treatment

- Induced emesis is contra-indicated.
- Stomach wash using potassium ferrocyanide converts copper into cupric ferrocyanide.
- Administration of **egg white or milk** orally, helps in detoxifying copper.
- Hemodialysis is useful in early stages.
- Severe cases need chelation with dimercaprol 2.5 mg/kg, 4th hourly; followed by oral penicillamine.

Autopsy Findings

- Greenish blue discoloration of GI mucosa.
- Jaundice, hepatic and renal necrosis.

THALLIUM

SHORT NOTES ON THALLIUM POISONING? (FM9.3) WHAT IS THALLIUM TRIAD?

- Thallium is a soft, pliable metal, acquiring notorious reputation as an ideal homicidal poison.
- Absorption occurs through inhalation, ingestion and through intact skin.
- Usual fatal dose is 12 to 15 mg/kg.

Acute Poisoning

- Abdominal pain, gastroenteritis with hematemesis, tachycardia, confusion and headache; hallucination, convulsion, retrobulbar neuritis and ophthalmoplegia.
- Death results from respiratory failure; there is usually bone marrow depression.

- A characteristic dark pigment band is often noticed in the scalp hair in about 3 to 4 days.

Chronic Poisoning

- Alopecia is diagnostic of chronic poisoning; begins in 10 days, and may lead to total loss of scalp hair within a month; lateral half of eyebrows are also peculiarly affected.
- **Skin rash:** Papulomacular rash often assumes a 'butterfly' shape distribution on the face.
- Dystrophy of nails 'Mees stripes'.
- Painful ascending peripheral sensory motor neuropathy; more pronounced in lower limbs.
- **Ataxia and other cranial nerve palsies:** Optic neuropathy, tremors and encephalopathy; psychotic behavior may also be present.
- **CVS and blood:** Hypertension, cardiomyopathy, ECG changes and thrombocytopenia.
- **Miscellaneous:** Autonomic dysfunction, testicular toxicity, hypokalemia and renal failure.

Thallium Triad

- If symptoms of alopecia, skin rash, painful peripheral neuropathy, lethargy and mental confusion are present, one should suspect chronic thallium poisoning.
- Symptoms mimic Guillain Barre syndrome, acute porphyria, psychosis and thiamine deficiency.

Diagnosis

- **X-ray:** Opacities in GIT and liver.
- Tests for contrast sensitivity and color vision in early stages
- Abnormal ECG and delayed peripheral nerve conduction.
- **Microscopy of hair:** Reveals black pigmentation of hair roots

Treatment

- **Stomach wash:** Using potassium ferric ferrocyanide (Prussian blue).
- Activated charcoal may be useful.
- Forced diuresis in conjugation with potassium chloride.
- Hemodialysis and hemoperfusion.
- Chelation therapy not much useful (previous days done with dithiocarb).
- Oral hygiene to prevent stomatitis.
- Physiotherapy to prevent muscle contracture.

Autopsy Findings

- Alopecia and stomatitis.
- Fatty degeneration of heart ('tabby cat striations' on the ventricles).
- Fatty degeneration of liver and renal damage.
- Pulmonary and cerebral edema, with degeneration of nerve cells and axons.

Forensic Significance

- Accidental and occupational exposure is common.
- There is increase in the use of thallium as a homicidal poison.

DESCRIBE ABOUT METAL FUME FEVER? (FM9.3)

Synonyms: Brass chills, brazier disease, foundry fever, monday fever, smelter's shake, welder's ague.

Occupations Affected

Welding, galvanizing, smelting, metal refining, electroplating, alloy making, ship breaking

Metals Involved

Caused by inhalation of fumes produced when these metals are heated above their melting point; zinc, copper, magnesium, iron, chromium, cadmium, nickel, manganese, mercury, cobalt, lead, antimony, selenium, beryllium, vanadium, silver and aluminum.

Clinical Presentation

- Resembles flu like illness; beginning 4 to 6 hours after exposure to the fumes.
- Characterized by chills, fever, myalgia, cough, thirst, sweating, fatigue, dyspnea, leukocytosis; cyanosis and reduced pulmonary tests.
- Resolution of symptoms occurs in 36 hours after withdrawing from the source of exposure.

Treatment

Symptomatic; chelation therapy may be required in chronic recurrent cases.

Prevention

- Implementation of proper automatic engineering control
- Good ventilation and exhaust ventilation
- Use of fume extractors.

Related Syndromes

Condition closely resembling metal fume fever is 'polymer fume fever' results from inhalation of gases produced by burning of polytetrafluoroethylene.

PHOSPHORUS

WHAT ARE THE TWO VARIETIES OF PHOSPHORUS AND USES OF PHOSPHORUS? (FM9.2)

There are two main varieties of phosphorus: White and red phosphorus.
- **Yellow or white phosphorus:**
  - Yellowish, waxy, crystalline solid with garlicky odor.
  - On exposure to air, it oxidizes into white fumes of phosphorus pentoxide, and hence stored under water. It's highly combustible and ignites into flames at 34°C.
  - It is luminescent in dark (phosphorescence).
- **Red phosphorus:** Reddish, amorphous, odorless substance; it's insoluble and is harmless.

Uses

- It was widely used in the manufacture of friction matches; but due to its chronic toxicity replaced by potassium chlorate and antimony sulfide. The igniting surface of the match box is coated with powdered glass and red phosphorus.
- **Fireworks:** Important ingredient in manufacture of fireworks (crackers) in India.
- **Military use:** Yellow phosphorus is an important ingredient in tracer bullets, smoke screams and air-sea rescue flares.
- Insecticide and rodenticide, and as fertilizers.
- Many pastes and powders used for killing cockroaches and rats (zinc phosphide).
- **Usual fatal dose:** 60 mg (1 mg/kg body weight).

WHAT IS THE MODE OF ACTION AND SYMPTOMS OF ACUTE PHOSPHORUS POISONING? (FM9.2)

Mode of Action

- Phosphorus is a protoplasmic poison and is a potent hepatotoxic.
- In large doses cause shock and cardiovascular collapse.
- Locally it produces severe irritation of skin and mucosa.
- Absorption is enhanced by administering in an oily vehicle.

Clinical Features

Fulminant poisoning: Massive dose of 1 to 2 g results in fulminant poisoning; peripheral vascular collapse and death occurs in 12 to 24 hours.

Acute Poisoning

- Symptoms of acute poisoning are divided into three stages.
- **1st stage (up to 3 days):** Severe burning pain, vomiting, diarrhea, abdominal pain and breath smell's garlic; vomitus and stools are luminescent in dark; and eliminate faint fumes (**Smoky Stool syndrome**).
- **2nd stage (up to several days after the symptoms of 1st stage subsides):** essentially symptomless.
- **3rd stage:** Due to systemic effects; there is return of GI symptoms with increased severity; hepatomegaly, pruritis and jaundice, progressing to olive green hue; finally leading hepatic encephalopathy, stupor and coma; at this stage there is mousy odor in the breath (**fetor hepaticus**). Renal damage, oliguria, hematuria, albuminuria and acute renal failure.
- Dermal contact results in acute painful corrosion.

Diagnosis

- Garlicky odor in breath and vomitus.
- Fuming and luminous vomitus and stools.
- Hepatic and renal failure.

WHAT IS PHOSSY JAW?

- Due to long term occupational inhalation of phosphorus fumes results in sequestration, necrosis and osteomyelitis of the jaw (usually lower jaw) and occurs in place of an extracted carries tooth. This is called as "**phossy jaw**" or "**glass jaw**".
- It is also more of an occupational hazard among workers of match industry.
- Chronic inhalation of phosphorus fumes first results in tooth ache in the already decaying teeth, which is followed by swelling of the gums, leading to loosening of the tooth. Later on leads to osteomyelitis of the jaw, progressing on to multiple sinuses discharging foul smelling pus resulting in sequestration of the jaw bone.

WHAT IS THE TREAT OF PHOSPHORUS POISONING? (FM9.2)

Treatment

Acute Poisoning

- **Gastric lavage:** Using potassium permanganate (1:5000 solution); copper sulfate can also be used (converts phosphorus into nontoxic copper phosphide).
- Milk or oily food is contraindicated (as it enhances absorption of phosphorus).
- Vitamin K (65 mg) slow IV drip, to combat hypoprothrombinemia.
- Whole blood or frozen plasma transfusion for coagulation defects.
- Steroids to combat shock.
- Dermal burns with is treated with 1% copper sulfate solution.

Chronic Poisoning

- Remove the patient from the source of exposure.
- Dental treatment, symptomatic treatment and follow up care.

WHAT ARE THE CHARACTERISTIC AUTOPSY FINDINGS IN PHOSPHORUS? (FM9.2)

- Garlicky odor in the vicinity of the mouth and gastric contents.
- Jaundice and subcutaneous hemorrhages (bleeding points).
- Luminous gastric contents.
- Enlarged fatty liver, as time passes on acute yellow atrophy of the liver may be present.
- Viscera preserved in saturated saline and not alcohol (luminance is lost if preserved in alcohol).

Forensic Significance

- Accidental poisoning is quite common in children.
- Suicidal poisoning is less common; rat poisons containing phosphorus are used for suicide.
- **Homicidal poisoning:** Formerly, many murders have been successfully accomplished by mixing phosphorus with any beverage like beer, rum, soup and jam.

WRITE SHORT NOTES ON BARIUM POISONING? (FM9.2)

Barium compounds are barium chloride, barium nitrate, barium sulfate and barium sulfide. Barium acts as irritant and after absorption acts especially on muscles and also on heart muscles.

Signs and Symptoms

- Acts as irritant on the GIT causes nausea, vomiting and diarrhea.
- After absorption causes muscle cramps, paralysis of tongue and larynx.
- Pulse rate slows down and irregular and heart may stop function in systole.
- Fatal dose about one gram; fatal period within 12 hours.

Treatment

Stomach wash using magnesium sulfate to precipitate barium sulfate which is insoluble. Followed by 10 mL of sodium sulfate IV every 15 minutes. Purging with magnesium sulfate and rest are symptomatic treatment.

MULTIPLE CHOICE QUESTIONS

1. The following type of poisoning retards the decomposition of the body:
   a. Arsenic
   b. Copper
   c. Mercury
   d. Nux vomica
2. Which one of the following poisoning causes basophilic stippling of RBC?
   a. Arsenic
   b. Lead
   c. Mercury
   d. Phosphorus
3. The earliest sign of chronic lead poisoning:
   a. Lead lines
   b. Lead palsy
   c. Anemia and facial pallor
   d. Lead encephalopathy
4. Changes in the anterior lens capsule, coarse tremors and skin eruptions are diagnostic of chronic poisoning by:
   a. Mercury
   b. Lead
   c. Antimony
   d. Copper
5. "Possy jaw" is caused by
   a. Lead
   b. Mercury
   c. White phosphorus
   d. Red phosphorus
6. One of the poisons can be detected even from burnt bones:
   a. OPC
   b. Antimony
   c. Lead
   d. Arsenic
7. Arsenic acts by:
   a. Inhibition of choline esterase enzyme
   b. Preventing action of cytochrome oxidase
   c. Combining with sulfhydryl enzymes
   d. None of the above
8. Burtonian line is seen in chronic poisoning with:
   a. Arsenic
   b. Lead
   c. Mercury
   d. Copper
9. Black foot disease is due to chronic exposure due to:
   a. Arsenic
   b. Antimony
   c. Copper
   d. Zinc
10. Smoky stool syndrome is characteristically seen in poisoning with:
    a. Iodine
    b. Bromine

c. Fluorine
d. Phosphorus
11. **The triad of alopecia, neuropathy and diarrhea results from:**
    a. Thallium
    b. Mercury
    c. Datura
    d. Opium
12. **The most common symptom of thallium poisoning is:**
    a. Headache
    b. Neuropathy
    c. Visual disturbance
    d. Abdominal pain
13. **Marsh test is done to detect:**
    a. Nickel
    b. Mercury
    c. Arsenic
    d. Lead
14. **Cholera like diarrhea is seen in poisoning with:**
    a. Copper
    b. Mercury
    c. Lead
    d. Arsenic
15. **Mee's lines are seen in chronic poisoning with:**
    a. White phosphorus
    b. Mercury
    c. Arsenic
    d. Lead
16. **Which of the following findings is more specific for arsenic poisoning?**
    a. Red velvety appearance of stomach mucosa
    b. Tremors
    c. Anemia
    d. Blue lining of gums
17. **All the following are symptoms of acute arsenic poisoning, *except*:**
    a. Tenesmus
    b. Red velvety gastric mucosa
    c. Acute tubular necrosis
    d. Rain drop pigmentation
18. **Antidote for arsenic is:**
    a. Nickel oxide
    b. Ferric oxide
    c. Aluminum oxide
    d. Magnesium oxide
19. **Abdominal colic is a symptom of poisoning with:**
    a. Arsenic
    b. Lead
    c. Opium
    d. Mercury
20. **Ochronosis is seen in poisoning with:**
    a. HCl
    b. Boric acid
    c. Carbolic acid
    d. Oxalic acid
21. **Ferric chloride test is used in diagnosis of:**
    a. HCl
    b. Acetic acid
    c. Carbolic acid
    d. Alcohol
22. **Leathery stomach is seen in poisoning with:**
    a. HCl
    b. Sulfuric acid
    c. Carbolic acid
    d. Oxalic acid
23. **Maximum damage to esophagus is with:**
    a. Acetic acid
    b. Sulfuric acid
    c. Sodium hydroxide
    d. Nitric acid
24. **Chronic arsenic poisoning does not cause:**
    a. Mixed sensory and motor neuropathy
    b. Mesothelioma
    c. Hyperkeratosis of skin
    d. Anemia
25. **Fatal dose of arsenic trioxide in adults:**
    a. 20–30 mg
    b. 50–60 mg
    c. 60–80 mg
    d. 120–200 mg
26. **Reinsch test is used in diagnosis of poisoning due to:**
    a. Arsenic
    b. Lead
    c. Iron
    d. Copper sulfate
27. **In a suspected death due to poisoning where cadaveric rigidity is lasting longer than usual, it may be a case of poisoning due to:**
    a. Arsenic
    b. Lead
    c. Mercury
    d. Copper sulfate
28. **Arsenic causes all, *except*:**
    a. Raindrop pigmentation
    b. Alopecia
    c. Palmar hyperkeratosis
    d. Blue line in gums

SECTION 7: Medical Toxicology

29. Fatty yellow liver is seen in poisoning with:
    a. Arsenic
    b. Aconite
    c. Oxalic acid
    d. Mercury
30. Mercury pollution is caused by all, *except:*
    a. Compact fluorescent lamp
    b. Incandescent bulb
    c. LED bulb
    d. Fluorescent lamp
31. A factory worker presented with tremors, personality change and a blue line in gums. Probable diagnosis is chronic poisoning with:
    a. Lead
    b. Arsenic
    c. Mercury
    d. Cadmium
32. In mercury poisoning, brown reflex is from:
    a. Anterior cornea
    b. Posterior cornea
    c. Anterior lens capsule
    d. Posterior lens capsule
33. Acrodynia/pink disease occurs in poisoning with:
    a. Thallium
    b. Arsenic
    c. Barium
    d. Mercury
34. Minamata bay disease refers to chronic toxicity with:
    a. Ergot
    b. Datura
    c. Mercury
    d. Organophosphorus
35. Pica is associated with poisoning:
    a. Mercury
    b. Lead
    c. Thallium
    d. Arsenic
36. Not a symptom of inorganic chronic lead poisoning:
    a. Insomnia
    b. Anorexia
    c. Constipation
    d. Colic
37. Seen in lead poisoning:
    a. Normoblasts
    b. Sideroblasts
    c. Lymphoblasts
    d. Myeloblasts
38. Lead inhibits which enzymes in the heme synthesis pathway:
    a. Aminolevulinate synthase
    b. Ferrochelatase and δ-ALA dehydratase
    c. Porphobilinogen deaminase
    d. Uroporphyrinogen decarboxylase
39. A car repair worker presented with abdominal pain, weakness in hand and constipation since 2 years. He has anemia and neurological deficits. Probable diagnosis is:
    a. Lead toxicity
    b. Gastric carcinoma
    c. Chronic pancreatitis
    d. Mercury poisoning
40. In case of chronic lead poisoning, the levels of which of the following is elevated:
    a. Porphobilinogen
    b. Aminolevulinic acid
    c. Bilirubin
    d. Urobilinogen
41. Acts both as poison and antidote:
    a. Copper sulfate
    b. Mercuric chloride
    c. Silver chloride
    d. Thallium arsenate
42. Copper sulfate poisoning manifests with:
    a. Acute hemolysis
    b. High anion gap acidosis
    c. Peripheral neuropathy
    d. Rhabdomyolysis
43. Instead of penicillamine, following can be used in copper poisoning:
    a. EDTA
    b. Desferrioxamine
    c. Succimer
    d. $KMnO_4$
44. A person was found dead with bluish green frothy discharge at the angle of mouth and nostrils. Probable cause can be:
    a. Arsenic poisoning
    b. Copper poisoning
    c. Mercury poisoning
    d. Lead poisoning
45. Cadmium causes:
    a. Proximal tubular necrosis
    b. Distal tubular necrosis
    c. Polyneuritis
    d. Cirrhosis
46. A housewife ingests a rodenticide white powder accidentally. Her examination

showed generalized flaccid paralysis and an irregular pulse. ECG shows multiple ventricular ectopic, generalized changes within ST-T. Serum potassium is 2.5 mEq/L. The most likely ingested poison is:
a. Barium carbonate
b. Superwarfarin
c. Zinc phosphide
d. Aluminum phosphide

47. Barium carbonate poisoning causes:
a. Respiratory distress
b. Gastrointestinal irritation
c. Muscular weakness
d. Cyanosis

48. A person presents with acute poisoning, with chill sand rigors similar to malaria. Most likely poisoning is with:
a. Mercury
b. Zinc
c. Red phosphorus
d. Arsenic

49. Patient with BP 90/60 mm Hg, lips and peripheries are cyanosed; blood drawn was chocolate color. Diagnosis is:
a. Methemoglobinemia
b. Hypovolemic shock
c. Metal fume fever
d. Alphos poisoning

50. A poison which is luminescent and waxy and have a garlic smell:
a. Alphos
b. Ammonium bromide
c. Opium
d. Yellow phosphorous

51. $CuSO_4$ was used as an antidote for:
a. Datura poisoning
b. Cocaine poisoning
c. Phosphorus poisoning
d. Opium poisoning

52. A body is brought for autopsy. On postmortem, there is dark brown postmortem staining and garlic odor in stomach. The poisoning is most likely due to:
a. Hydrocyanic acid
b. Carbon dioxide
c. Aniline dye
d. Phosphorus

53. Yellow/fatty liver is characteristically seen in:
a. Datura poisoning
b. Cocaine poisoning
c. Phosphorus poisoning
d. Opium poisoning

ANSWERS

1. a	2. b	3. c	4. a	5. c	6. c	7. c	8. b	9. a	10. b
11. a	12. c	13. c	14. d	15. c	16. a	17. d	18. b	19. b	20. c
21. c	22. c	23. c	24. a	25. d	26. a	27. a	28. d	29. a	30. c
31. c	32. c	33. d	34. c	35. b	36. a	37. b	38. b	39. a	40. b
41. a	42. a	43. c	44. b	45. a	46. d	47. c	48. b	49. c	50. d
51. c	52. d	53. c							

29

CHAPTER

Organic Irritant Poisons

KEY WORDS

Abrus precatorius, toxalbumin, glucoside, SUI, cattle poison, semicarpus, artificial bruise, calotropis, ricin, hemolytic, cotton, capsicum, neem, lilly, eucalyptus, purging nut, cobra, neurotoxic venom, viper, hemotoxic venom, krait, sea snakes, myotoxic, scorpion sting, cantharides, aphrodisiac.

FM11.1	Describe features and management of snake bite, scorpion sting, bee and wasp sting and spider bite.
FM14.7	To identify and draw medico-legal inference from common poisons, e.g., datura, castor, cannabis, opium, aconite copper sulphate, pesticides compounds, marking nut, oleander, nux vomica, abrus seeds, snakes, capsicum, calotropis, lead compounds and tobacco.

INTRODUCTION

Organic irritants comprise of plant and animal irritants.

Plant Irritants

- There are a wide variety of plant irritants; only *Abrus Precatorius, Calotropis, Ricinus communis,* Croton, *Semecarpus, Capsicum,* Glory lily, Neem, *Eucalyptus,* Jatropha and Ginseng will be discussed.
- Animal irritants snakes, scorpion and cantharides.

WHAT IS ABRUS PRECATORIUS? WHAT ARE CLINICAL FEATURES OF POISONING? (FM14.7) WHAT ARE ITS CRIMINAL USES? WHAT IS SUI?

Abrus precatorius is called as Jequirity, Rosary bead, Indian Liquorice **(Fig. 29.1)**.

Characteristics

Slender, climbing vine, with compound leaves, small pinkish flower and seed pods containing 4 to 6 seeds of 1 cm in circumference; the

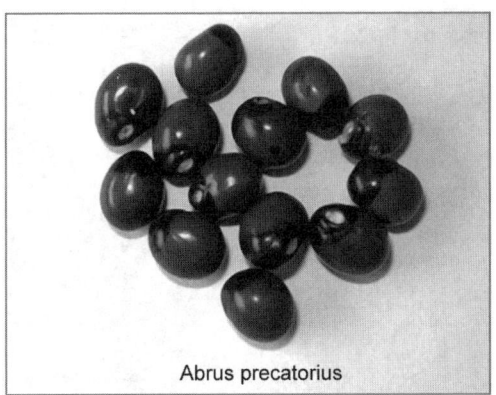

Fig. 29.1: Abrus precatorius
(For color version see Plate 18).

seeds are scarlet red in color with a black spot on one side.

Active Principles

Abrin (toxalbumin), abrine (amino acid), Abralin (glucoside) and abric acid.

Clinical Features

- Hemorrhagic gastritis and cardiac manifestations similar to viperine snake bite (cardiac arrhythmias and convulsions) leading to death.
- **Usual fatal dose:** 60 to 120 mg (1 to 2 seeds) "**super toxic**".
- **Treatment:** Decontamination and supportive measures.

Autopsy Findings

Sub-mucosal hemorrhages on stomach mucosa and congestion of the internal organs.

If injected: Local signs of inflammation, edema and necrosis are present, which mimics "**viperine snake bite**".

Medico-legal Significance

Accidental poisoning common in children, as they are attracted towards the color.

"Sui" Poison

Seeds are crushed and added with pastes of arsenic, lead and *Calotropis* and made into injecting needs and used to kill the enemy from a distance by blowing using a bamboo stick; also used to kill cattle by this method, death of the cattle will appear to be due to viperine snake bite.

WHAT ARE ACTIVE INGREDIENTS, CLINICAL FEATURES AND CRIMINAL USE OF *CALOTROPIS*? (FM14.7)

- *Calotropis* is madar. It is a tall shrub, with yellowish white bark, oblong thick leaves, with purplish or white flowers; stem and leaves when incised yield a whitish, milky acrid juice.
- *Calotropis gigantea* (purple flowers); *Calotropis procera* (white flowers) Calotropis shown in **Figure 29.2**.

Active Principles

All parts of the plant are poisonous and contain the active principles in the milky juice. There are four main active ingredients present in the milky juice: (i) Caloptropin, (ii) Calotoxin, (iii) Calactin and (iv) Uscharin.

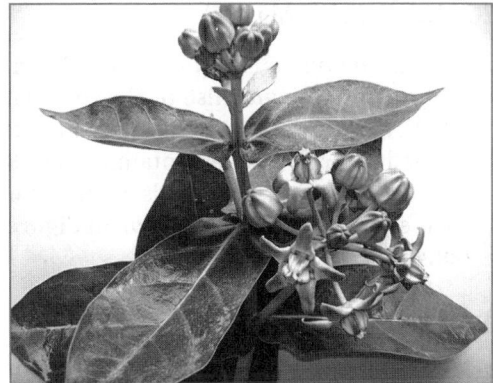

Fig. 29.2: Calotropis
(For color version see Plate 19).

Clinical Features

- When the juice is ingested there is burning sensation in throat and abdomen. Vomiting, diarrhea and abdominal pain, followed by mydriasis, convulsion and delirium.
- Skin contact produces inflammation and vesication.
- Eye contact produces severe conjunctivitis.

Treatment

- Gastric lavage
- Demulcents
- IV fluids
- Diazepam for convulsions
- Skin and eyes are irrigated with saline water.

Medico-legal Significance

- Juice is used as an abortifacient; the stem is used as "**abortion stick**".
- Accidental poisoning due to quackery.
- Juice is given orally for female infanticide.
- Used as cattle poison.
- Artificial bruise (false bruise) on skin and conjunctivitis.

WRITE SHORT NOTES ON RICINUS COMMUNIS? (FM14.7)

- *Ricinus communis* is **castor or mole bean.**
- Long shrub with greenish red leaves (**Fig. 29.3**); fruits are borne in clusters, with soft spined brown capsule containing 2 or 3 mottled grayish brown seeds, with linear stripes on the surface, as shown in **Figure 29.4.**

Active Principle

- Seeds yield a pale yellow oil with faint acrid odor.
- Pressed cake retains the toxic principle, ricin a toxalbumin which causes hemolysis and is a super toxic, even superior to cobra venom and hence also called "terrorist weapon".
- **Toxalbumin: (Phytotoxin)**
- Toxalbumin is a toxic protein, which acts like a bacterial toxin; it causes agglutination and lysis of RBC and has antigenic properties.
- **Action:** Ricin blocks the protein synthesis through the inhibition of RNA polymerase.
- **Uses:** Castor oil is used as a purgative and also used as a lubricant.

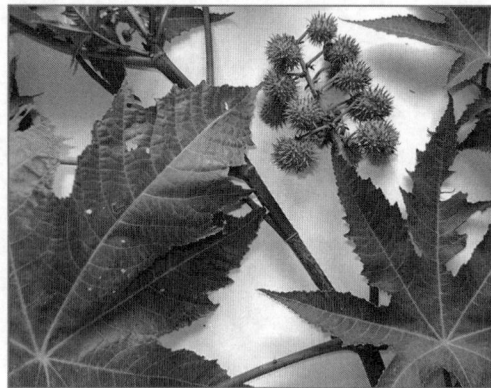

Fig. 29.3: Castor plant (ricinus communis) *(For color version see Plate 19).*

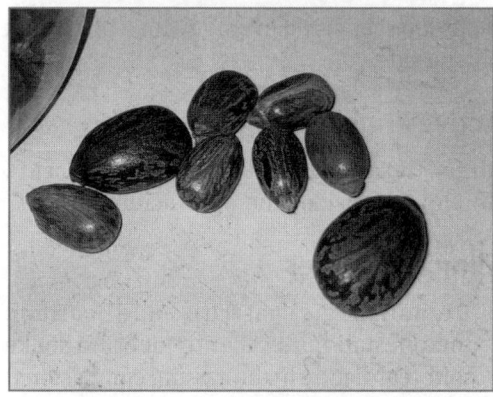

Fig. 29.4: Ricinus communis/castor seeds *(For color version see Plate 19).*

Clinical Features

- Vomiting, diarrhea, abdominal pain
- Hypotension and dehydration
- Fever with chills

- Hemolysis and renal failure
- **Usual fatal dose:** 1 mg/kg; 5 to 10 seeds.

Treatment

- Decontamination (gastric lavage and activated charcoal).
- Correct fluid and electrolyte imbalance.
- Supportive measures.

Autopsy Findings

GI congestion and erosion, with marked renal congestion.

Medico-legal Aspects

- Accidental ingestion in children and rarely homicidal.
- Over dosage of castor oil causes severe diarrhea.
- It is also called "**terrorist weapon**" if the ricin injected into the body, it causes death by agglutination of RBC and hemolysis.

WRITE SHORT NOTES ON CROTON TIGLIUM?

- Evergreen tree with smooth ash colored bark; ovate-lanceolate leaves with small flowers; oblong three lobed fruits containing oval, dark brown seeds (looks like castor seeds but are slightly larger in size, darker and the linear striations are not so marked). Oil extracted from the seed is highly toxic. Seeds of castor and croton depicted in **Figure 29.5.**
- **Active principles:** Croton (toxalbumin) and crotonoside (glycoside).
- **Clinical features:** Similar to castor seeds; skin contact produces inflammation.
- **Usual fatal dose:** 1 to 2 mL of oil; 5 to 6 seeds.
- **Treatment:** Same like castor.

Medico-legal Aspects

Oil is used as an abortifacient; accidental ingestion mistaken for castor oil.

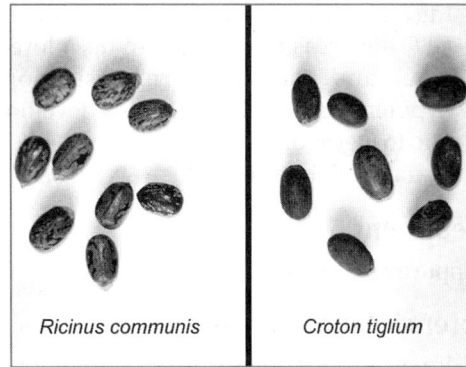

Fig. 29.5: Castor and croton seeds
(For color version see Plate 19).

WHAT IS MARKING NUT? WHAT ARE THE CRIMINAL USES? (FM14.7)

- **Semecarpus anacardium** is marking nut.
- Tree bearing hard nut like fruits, the acrid blackish juice extracted from the seeds is used by the washer men (dhobis) for marking on the clothes, hence the name marking nut. Images of Semecarpus shown in **Figure 29.6.**
- **Active principles:** Semecarpol and bhilawanol.
- **Uses:** Laundry marker and quackery remedies.

Clinical Manifestations

- Skin contact with the juice results in inflammation and vesication.

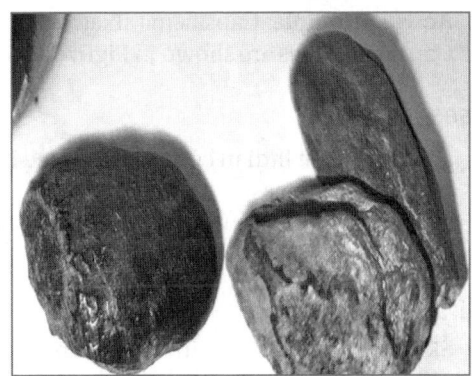

Fig. 29.6: Semecarpus anacardium (marking nut)
(For color version see Plate 19).

- Ingestion causes burning sensation in GIT, the areas of contact are discolored black and may also form vesication; hypotension and delirium also develops due to ingestion.
- **Usual fatal dose:** 10 g.

Treatment
Supportive measures.

Forensic Significance
- Juice is used as an abortifacient and accidental poisoning by quackery.
- **Malingering: Artificial bruise** and conjunctivitis are produced by juice of marking nut. It is differentiated from true bruise by color changes, itching and vesication (Refer chapter on Injuries—Contusion).

WHAT IS CAPSICUM ANNUM? WHAT ARE THE FORENSIC SIGNIFICANCE?
- Capsicum annum is chilly/red pepper.
- Small herb bearing long tapering fruits, which become red when ripe; possesses a pungent odor and taste. The fruit contains a number of small flat, yellowish seeds which resembles datura seeds.
- Chilly seeds are small, yellow, rounded, smooth and pungent in odour and taste.
- Datura seeds are large, brown, reniform, pitted, odorless and bitter in taste.
- **Active principle:** Capsaicin (alkaloid).
- Capsicum seeds are shown in **Figure 29.7**.

Uses
- Continental in Indian cuisine, also used in pickles and sauces.
- Carminative and appetite stimulant; as counterirritant in balms.

Clinical Features
- Skin contact results in irritation and reddening.

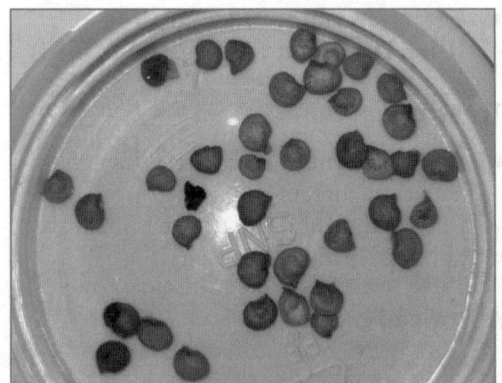

Fig. 29.7: Capsicum seeds *(For color version see Plate 19).*

- Eye contact causes intense burning, lacrimation and reddening.
- Ingestion of large quantities causes burning sensation in the mouth, salivation, abdominal pain, vomiting and diarrhea; sweating is common; urine may turn dark.

Treatment
- Wash and bath the affected area with vinegar or ice-cold water.
- In case of ingestion, give ice cubes to suck and sips of ice cold water.
- Supportive measures.

Forensic Significance
- Workers in pickle manufacturing units often suffer from dermatitis and burning lesions of fingers (human hand: vascular and sensory responses of human skin to topical treatment with capsaicin).
- Robbery, assault, rape, etc. can be facilitated easily by throwing chilly powder on the eyes of the victim.
- Can be used for torture or extortion, by forcing chilly powder into rectum or vagina.
- Datura seeds can be mistaken for chilly and eaten, resulting in serious complications.

CHAPTER 29: Organic Irritant Poisons

WHAT IS GLORY LILY?

- Gloriosa superb is climbing lily, superb lily.
- Large herb, climbing plant with terminate leaves in with tendril, long, curling tips. flowers are large, solitary and long stalked.

Uses

- Juice from the leaves is used as a pediculicide (to kill head lice).
- Root is used for folk remedies.
- **Toxic parts:** Leaves and root.
- **Toxic principles:** Root contains colchicine and superbine.

Clinical Features

- Acute poisoning results in severe vomiting, diarrhea, abdominal pain, hypotension and respiratory failure.
- **Treatment:** Decontamination; symptomatic and supportive measures.

WHAT IS PURGING NUT?

- **Jatropha curcas** is purging nut; also known as "**physic nut**".
- Seeds have a powerful purgative action.
- **Toxic principles:** Ricin and tannic acid.

Clinical Features

- Salivation, abdominal pain, diarrhea, weakness, and muscle twitching.
- **Treatment:** Supportive therapy.

Animal Irritants

Snakes, scorpion, cantharides, bees and wasps will be discussed.

WHAT ARE THE TWO IMPORTANT FAMILIES OF POISONOUS SNAKES? (FM11.1) HOW TO DIFFERENTIATE POISONOUS SNAKES FROM NON-POISONOUS SNAKES? (TABLE 29.1)

- There are thousands of snake species of which more than 200 are venomous species.
- In India, there are more than 200 species of which 50 are poisonous.
- There are two important groups (families) of venomous snakes: Elapidae and viperidae.

Elapidae

Elapidae have short permanently erect fangs; this family includes the cobra, king cobra, kraits, coral snakes and the sea snakes). Common cobra—the "hood" unique identity of cobra depicts in **Figure 29.8.**

Viperidae

- Viperidae have long and canalized fangs, grooved or hypodermic needles like fangs. This family includes russell's vipers, saw-scaled (carpet) vipers, pit vipers, green pit vipers (bamboo vipers). Viper—hemotoxic depicts in **Figure 29.9.**

TABLE 29.1: Difference between venomous snakes and nonvenomous snakes.

Characteristics	Venomous snakes	Nonvenomous snakes
Head	Triangular or diamond shaped	Smooth and tapered head
Pupils	Elliptical or "cat like" pupil	Rounded pupil
Fangs	Long and movable fangs	No fangs, have small teeth
Facial pits	Located below the eyes	No facial pits
Bite marks	Two or one puncture wounds	Multiple teeth marks

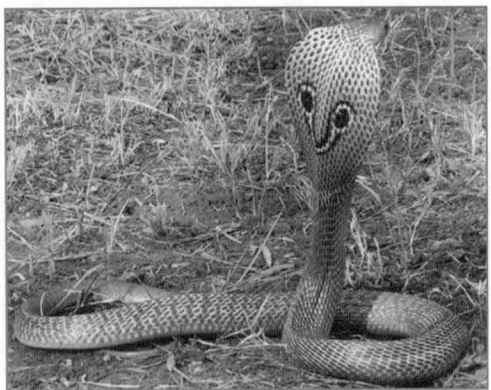

Fig. 29.8: Cobra (Elapidae)
(For color version see Plate 20).

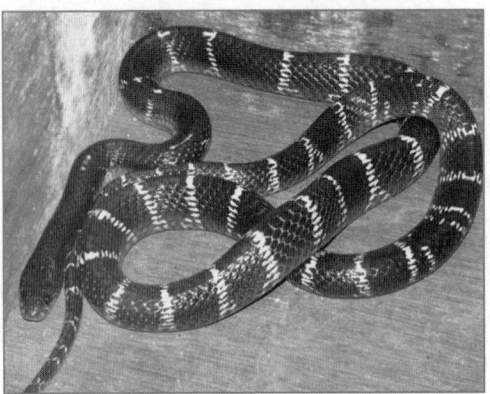

Fig. 29.9: Viperidae
(For color version see Plate 20).

- Venomous snakes of medical importance have a pair of enlarged teeth (the fangs), at the front of their upper jaw. These fangs contain a venom channel (like a hypodermic needle) or groove, along which venom can be introduced deep into the tissues of their natural prey.
- If human beings are bitten, venom is usually injected subcutaneously or intramuscularly.
- Spitting cobras can squeeze the venom out of the tips of their fangs producing a fine spray directed towards the eyes of an aggressor.

WHAT ARE THE BASIC CONSTITUENTS OF SNAKE VENOM AND WHAT ARE THE ACTIONS ON HUMAN BODY?

Snake venoms contain more than 20 different constituents, mainly proteins, including enzymes and polypeptide toxins. The following venom constituents cause important clinical effects:

- **Procoagulant enzymes (viperidae):**
  - That stimulates blood clotting but result in noncoagulation of blood. Venoms such as Russell's viper venom contain several different procoagulants which activate different steps of the clotting cascade. The result is formation of fibrin in the blood stream.
  - Most of these components are immediately broken down by the body's own fibrinolytic system.
  - Eventually, and sometimes within 30 minutes of the bite, the levels of clotting factors have been so depleted ("**consumption coagulopathy**") that the blood will not clot at all.
- **Hemorrhagins: (zinc metalloproteinases)**
  - Damage the endothelial lining of the blood vessel walls causing spontaneous systemic haemorrhage.
- **Cytolytic or necrotic toxins:**
  - These digestive hydrolases (proteolytic enzymes and phospholipases A) polypeptide toxins and other factors increase permeability resulting in local swelling. They may also destroy cell membranes and tissues.
- **Hemolytic and myolytic phospholipases A2:**
  - These enzymes damage cell membranes, endothelium, skeletal muscle, nerve and red blood cells.
- **Presynaptic neurotoxins** (elapidae and some viperidae).

- These are phospholipases A2 that damage nerve endings, initially releasing acetylcholine transmitter, later interfering with release.
- **Postsynaptic neurotoxins (elapidae):**
  - These polypeptides compete with acetylcholine for receptors in the neuromuscular junction and lead to curare-like paralysis.

WHAT COULD BE THE QUANTITY OF VENOM INJECTED IN A BITE?

- This is very variable, depending on the species and size of the snake, the mechanical efficiency of the bite, whether one or two fangs penetrated the skin and whether there were repeated strikes.
- Although large snakes tend to inject more venom than smaller specimens of the same species, the venom of younger vipers may be richer in some dangerous components, such as those affecting hemostasis.

WHO ARE THE PEOPLE COMMONLY BITTEN BY SNAKES?

- Farmers (rice)
- Plantation workers (rubber, coffee)
- Herdsmen
- Hunters
- Snake handlers (snake charmers, in snake restaurants and traditional Chinese pharmacies)
- Fishermen and fish farmers
- Sea snake catchers (for sea snake skins, leather).

DESCRIBE THE SIGNS AND SYMPTOMS OF A VENOMOUS SNAKE BITE? (FM11.1)

What is Ophitoxaemia?

- Venomous snake bite is called as 'ophitoxaemia'.

Early Symptoms and Signs

- Following the immediate pain of mechanical penetration of the skin by the snake's fangs, there may be increasing local pain (burning, bursting, throbbing) at the site of the bite, local swelling that gradually extends proximally up the bitten limb and tender, painful enlargement of the regional lymph nodes draining the site of the bite (in the groin—femoral or inguinal, following bites in the lower limb; at the elbow (epitrochlear) or in the axilla following bites in the upper limb).
- Bites by kraits, sea snakes and Philippine cobras may be virtually painless and may cause negligible local swelling. Someone who is sleeping may not even wake up when bitten by a krait and there may be no detectable fang marks or signs of local envenoming.

Local Symptoms and Signs in the Bitten Part

- **Fang marks:** Bite mark of cobra snake. No local signs except for the fang mark shown in **Figure 29.10**.
- Local pain and bleeding
- Bruising, lymphangitis and lymph node enlargement depicts in **Figure 29.11**.

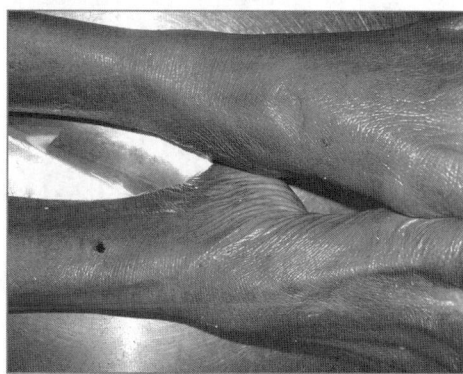

Fig. 29.10: Bite mark of cobra snake. No local signs except for the fang mark.

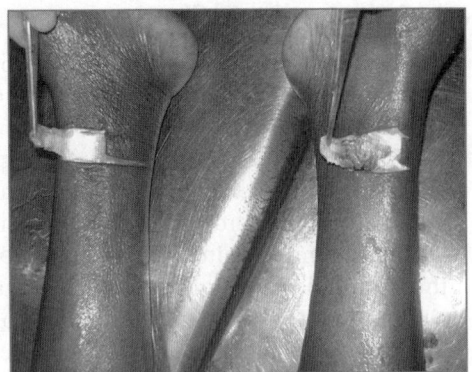

Fig. 29.11: Dissection of the bitten area demonstrating bruising of the underlying subcutaneous tissues. The opposite limb is also dissected as a control, which shows no bruising *(For color version see Plate 20)*.

- Inflammation (swelling, redness, heat) and sometimes blistering.
- Local infection, abscess formation and necrosis. Gangrene of foot in viper snake bite shown in **Figure 29.12**.

Generalized (Systemic) Symptoms and Signs

General

Nausea, vomiting, malaise, abdominal pain, weakness, drowsiness, prostration.

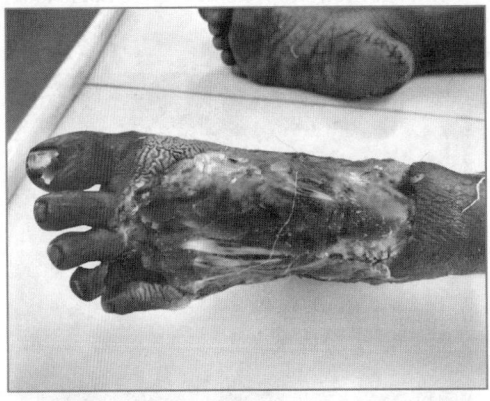

Fig. 29.12: Gangrene of foot in viper snake bite.

Cardiovascular (Viperidae)

- Visual disturbances, dizziness, faintness, collapse, shock, hypotension, cardiac arrhythmias, pulmonary edema, conjunctival edema.
- **Bleeding and clotting disorders:** Bleeding from recent wounds, including fang marks, venepunctures, etc., and from old partly-healed wounds; spontaneous systemic bleeding from gums, epistaxis, hemoptysis, hematemesis, rectal bleeding or melaena, hematuria, vaginal bleeding, bleeding into the skin (petechiae, purpura, ecchymoses) and mucosa (example: conjunctivae, intracranial hemorrhage); meningism from subarachnoid hemorrhage, lateralizing signs and/or coma from cerebral hemorrhage.

Neurological (Elapidae)

Drowsiness, paresthesia, abnormalities of taste and smell, "heavy" eyelids, ptosis, external ophthalmoplegia, paralysis of facial muscles and other muscles innervated by the cranial nerves, aphonia, difficulty in swallowing secretions, respiratory and generalized flaccid paralysis.

Skeletal Muscle Breakdown (Sea Snakes)

Generalized pain, stiffness and tenderness of muscles, trismus, myoglobinuria, hyperkalemia, cardiac arrest and acute renal failure.

Renal (Viperidae, Sea Snakes)

- Loin (lower back) pain, hematuria, hemoglobinuria, myoglobinuria, oliguria/anuria.
- Symptoms and signs of uremia like acidotic breathing, hiccups, nausea, pleuritic chest pain, etc.

Endocrine (Acute Pituitary/Adrenal Insufficiency) (Russell's Viper)

- **Acute phase:** Shock and hypoglycemia.
- **Chronic phase (months to years after the bite):** Weakness, loss of secondary sexual hair, amenorrhea, testicular atrophy, hypothyroidism, etc.

DISCUSS THE GENERAL LINES OF MANAGEMENT OF SNAKE BITE? (FM11.1)

The scheme of management should be:
- First aid treatment
- Transport to hospital
- Rapid clinical assessment and resuscitation.
- Detailed clinical assessment and species diagnosis.
- Investigations/laboratory tests.
- Antivenom treatment and observation of the response to antivenom.
- Treatment of the bitten part and rehabilitation.
- Treatment of chronic (late) complications.

Aims of First Aid

- Attempt to retard systemic absorption of venom.
- Preserve life and prevent complications before the patient can receive medical care (at a dispensary or hospital).
- Control distressing or dangerous early symptoms of envenoming.
- Arrange the transport of the patient to a place where they can receive medical care.

Recommended First Aid Methods

- Reassure the victim who may be very anxious.
- Immobilize the bitten limb with a splint or sling (any movement or muscular contraction increases absorption of venom into the bloodstream and lymphatics).
- Consider pressure-immobilization for some elapid bites.
- Avoid any interference with the bite wound as this may introduce infection, increase absorption of the venom and increase local bleeding.

Pressure Immobilization Method

Recommended first-aid for bites by neurotoxic elapid snakes:
- Pressure immobilization is recommended for bites by neurotoxic elapid snakes, including sea snakes but should not be used for viper bites because of the danger of increasing the local effects of the necrotic venom.

Tight (Arterial) Tourniquets are not Recommended

This method is extremely painful and very dangerous if the tourniquet was left on for too long (more than about 40 minutes), as the limb might be damaged by ischemia, followed by gangrene formation.

Early Clues that a Patient has Severe Envenoming

- Snake identified as a very dangerous one.
- Rapid early extension of local swelling from the site of the bite.
- Early tender enlargement of local lymph nodes, indicating spread of venom in the lymphatic system.
- **Early systemic symptoms:** Collapse (hypotension, shock), nausea, vomiting, diarrhea, severe headache, "heaviness" of the eyelids, inappropriate (pathological) drowsiness or early ptosis/ophthalmoplegia.
- Early spontaneous systemic bleeding.
- Passage of dark brown urine.

Physical Examination

- **Examination of the bitten part**
  - The extent of swelling and tenderness to palpation should be recorded. Lymph nodes draining the limb should be palpated for ecchymoses and lymphangitis.
- **General examination**
  - Measure the blood pressure (sitting up and lying to detect a postural drop indicative of hypovolemia) and heart rate. Examine the skin and mucous membranes for evidence of petechiae, purpura and ecchymosis in the conjunctivae.
- **Neurotoxic envenoming**
  - To exclude early neurotoxic envenoming, ask the patient to look up and observe whether the upper lids retract fully. Test eye movements for evidence of early external ophthalmoplegia. Check the size and reaction of the pupils.
- **Bulbar and respiratory paralysis**
  - Can the patient swallow or whether any secretions accumulated in the pharynx, which is the early sign of bulbar paralysis. Ask the patient to take deep breath in and out. "**Paradoxical respiration**" (abdomen expands rather than the chest on attempted inspiration) indicates that the diaphragm is still contracting but that the intercostal muscles and accessory muscles of inspiration are paralyzed.
  - Do not assume that patients have irreversible brain damage because they are unresponsive to painful stimuli, or have fixed dilated pupils.
  - Inability to open the mouth and protrude the tongue in patient.

Investigations/Laboratory Tests

- **20 minute whole blood clotting test (20WBCT)**
  - Place a few mL of fresh sample of venous blood in a small glass vessel, leave undisturbed for 20 minutes at ambient temperature. Tip the vessel once, if the blood is still liquid (unclotted) and runs out, the patient has hypofibrinogenemia (incoagulable blood) as a result of venom-induced consumption coagulopathy
- **Hemoglobin concentration/hematocrit:**
  - A transient increase indicates: Hemoconcentration resulting from a generalized increase in capillary permeability.
- Platelet count may be decreased in victims of viper bites.
- **White blood cell count:**
  - An early neutrophil leukocytosis is evidence of systemic envenoming from any species.
- **Blood film:**
  - Fragmented red cells ("**helmet cell**" schistocytes) are seen when there is microangiopathic hemolysis.
  - Plasma/serum may be pinkish or brownish if there is gross hemoglobinemia or myoglobinemia.
- **Urine examination:**
  - The urine should be tested by dipsticks for blood/hemoglobin/myoglobins.

WHAT IS THE COMPOSITION OF ANTIVENOM? (FM11.1)

What are the Indications for Antivenom Treatment?

- Antivenom is the only specific antidote to snake venom. The most important

decision in the management of a snake bite victim is whether or not to give antivenom.
- **Antisnake venom** available in India is prepared by hyper-immunizing horses, against the four common poisonous snakes: (i) common cobra, (ii) common krait, (iii) russell's viper, (iv) saw scald viper.

Indications for Antivenom

Antivenom treatment is recommended if and when a patient with proven or suspected snake bite develops one or more of the following signs.

Systemic Envenoming

- **Hemostatic abnormalities:** Spontaneous systemic bleeding or thrombocytopenia.
- **Neurotoxic signs:** Ptosis, external ophthalmoplegia, paralysis, etc.
- **Cardiovascular abnormalities:** Hypotension, shock, cardiac arrhythmia or abnormal ECG.
- **Acute renal failure:** Oliguria/anuria, rising blood creatinine/urea.
- **Hemoglobin/myoglobin uria:** Dark brown urine, urine dipsticks, other evidence of intravascular hemolysis or generalized rhabdomyolysis (muscle aches and pains, hyperkalemia).

Local Envenoming

- Local swelling involving more than half of the bitten limb.
- Rapid extension of swelling (for example beyond the wrist or ankle within a few hours of bites on the hands or feet).
- Development of an enlarged tender lymph node draining the bitten limb.

WHAT IS DOSAGE SCHEDULE OF ANTIVENOM INJECTION? (FM11.1)

- **Intravenous "push" injection:**
  - Reconstituted freeze-dried antivenom or near liquid antivenom is given by slow intravenous injection (not more than 2 mL/min).
- **Intravenous infusion:**
  - Reconstituted freeze-dried or near liquid antivenom is diluted in approximately 5-10 mL of isotonic fluid per kg body weight (i.e., 250-500 mL of isotonic saline or 5% dextrose in the case of an adult patient) and is infused at a constant rate over a period of about 1 hour. Snakes inject the same dose of venom into children and adults. Children must therefore be given exactly the same dose of antivenom as adults.

WHAT IS ANTIVENOM REACTION? (FM11.1)

How to Manage Such Cases?

- **Early anaphylactic reactions:**
  - Occurs usually within 10-180 minutes of starting antivenom.
- **Pyrogenic (endotoxin) reactions:**
  - Usually develop 1-2 hours after treatment. Symptoms include shaking chills (rigors), fever, vasodilatation and a fall in blood pressure; serum sickness type of late reactions develops 1 to 12 (mean 7) days after treatment.
  - Clinical features include fever, nausea, vomiting, diarrhea, itching, recurrent urticaria, arthralgia, myalgia, lymphadenopathy and periarticular swellings.

Management of Antivenomreaction

- **At the earliest sign of a reaction:**
  - Antivenom administration must be temporarily suspended. Epinephrine (adrenaline) 0.1% solution (1 in 1,000; 1 mg/mL) is the effective treatment for early anaphylactic reactions.
- **Additional treatment:**
  - After epinephrine (adrenaline), an anti H1 antihistamine such as chlorpheniramine maleate (adults 10 mg, children 0.2 mg/kg by intravenous injection over a few minutes).
  - Hydrocortisone (adults 100 mg, children 2 mg/kg body weight). The corticosteroid is unlikely to act for several hours, but may prevent recurrent anaphylaxis.

DISCUSS THE CLINICAL FEATURES OF A COMPARTMENTAL SYNDROME?

- Disproportionately severe pain.
- Weakness of intracompartmental muscles.
- Pain on passive stretching of intracompartmental muscles.
- Hypoesthesia of areas of skin supplied by nerves running through the compartment.
- Obvious tenseness of the compartment on palpation.

Criteria for Fasciotomy in Snake-Bitten Limbs

After the hemostatic abnormalities have been corrected, when there is clinical evidence of an intracompartmental syndrome, fasciotomy may be necessary.

Rehabilitation

Conventional physiotherapy in patients with severe local envenoming. The limb should be maintained in a functional position. For example, in the leg, equinus deformity of the ankle should be prevented by application of a back slab.

WRITE SHORT NOTES ON SCORPIONS? (FM11.1)

- They are eight legged arthropods and have a hollow sting in the last joint of their tail, which communicates by means of a duct with the poisonous gland.
- The venom is clear colorless toxalbumin, can be classified as either neurotoxic or hemotoxic; the toxicity is more than that of snakes but only a very small quantity is injected.
- Venom is a potent autonomic stimulator, releasing massive amounts of catecholamines from the adrenals.
- In majority of cases the mortality is negligible except in children and rarely in women.

Signs and Symptoms

- Scorpion sting usually has only one hole in the center of the reddened area.
- Symptoms usually localized; but sometimes results in systemic toxicity leading to restlessness, cardiac arrhythmias, paralysis, convulsions, respiratory depression and death, within an hour due to pulmonary edema and peripheral vascular collapse.

Treatment

- Immobilize the limb; a tourniquet can be applied above the level of the sting.
- Pack the area of sting with ice.
- Local anesthetic is injected at the site; if the sting is left in-situ, then an incision can be made with sterile blade and excise the broken fragment of the sting left inside the body.
- Calcium gluconate IV is of some value to control local swelling.
- Barbiturates can be given to reduce excitement and convulsions, but morphine is not indicated.
- Atropine is used to control pulmonary edema.

WHAT ARE CANTHARIDES? WHAT ARE THE CIRCUMSTANCES OF POISONING? (FM11.1)

- Cantharides are Spanish fly; also called as "**blister beetle**".
- The fly is 2 cm long and 0.6 cm broad.
- The powder of the dried body of the fly is brown in color.
- Active principle is cantharidin. It is readily absorbed through all the surfaces including the skin; locally it acts as an irritant.

Signs and Symptoms

- Contact with the skin produces burning pain and redness followed by vesication in 1 to 2 hours.
- **When ingested:** Causes severe burning pain in the mouth and throat, followed by pain in stomach, nausea, vomiting, severe thirst followed by difficulty in swallowing and speech.
- Urine is scanty and blood stained.
- Priapism (painful erection of penis) is a persistent symptom of cantharides poisoning.
- Abortion may occur in a pregnant woman.
- In severe cases, the patient become prostrated, convulsions occur followed by coma and death.
- **Fatal dose:** 15 to 50 g of the powder; fatal period: 24 to 48 hours.

Treatment

Stomach wash, demulcents and symptomatic treatment.

MULTIPLE CHOICE QUESTIONS

1. **The following plant poisons do not have specific antidote, *except*:**
   a. Calotropis
   b. Ricinus communis
   c. Datura
   d. Croton

2. **One of the following toxalbumin is used as terrorist weapon:**
   a. Ricin
   b. Abrin
   c. Croton
   d. Chilly

3. **One of the following plant is an ideal cattle poison:**
   a. Nerium odorum
   b. Calotropis
   c. Abrus precatorius
   d. Cerbera thevetia

4. **The active principle in calotropis is all, *except*:**
   a. Calotoxin
   b. Calactin
   c. Uscharin
   d. Bhilawanol

5. **Artificial bruise is commonly seen in which of the following irritant poison:**
   a. Calotropis
   b. Semecarpus anacardium
   c. Abrus precatorius
   d. Capsicum annum

6. **The antisnake venom available in India is effective against the following snakes, *except*:**
   a. Russell viper
   b. Cobra
   c. Krait
   d. Coral snake

7. **Russel's viper snake venom is similar to the poisoning of:**
   a. Abrus precatorius
   b. Semecarpus anacardium
   c. Ricinus communis
   d. Datura stramonium

8. **All of the following poisons are neurotoxic *except*:**
   a. Cobra
   b. Krait
   c. Viper
   d. Scorpion

9. **A toxalbumin similar to viperine snake venom is present in the seeds of:**
   a. Abrus precatorius
   b. Datura
   c. Ergot
   d. Croton tiglium

10. **'Sui' needle used to kill animals are made of:**
    a. Datura seeds
    b. Rati seeds
    c. Lead peroxide
    d. Arsenic

11. **Capsicum seed can be confused with:**
    a. Strychnine
    b. Datura
    c. Ricinus
    d. Opium
12. **Hunan hand occurs due to:**
    a. Abrus precatorius
    b. Capsicum
    c. Datura
    d. Strychnine
13. **Oduvanthalai poisoning is associated with:**
    a. Hypokalemia
    b. Hyponatremia
    c. Respiratory acidosis
    d. Metabolic alkalosis
14. **Cobras belong to:**
    a. Viperidae
    b. Elapidae
    c. Colubridae
    d. Crotalidae
15. **All are true about poisonous snakes, *except*:**
    a. Nocturnal in habit
    b. Have compressed tail
    c. Have solid and stout fangs
    d. Have large scales on head
16. **Snake that causes muscle paralysis with convulsions:**
    a. Vipers
    b. Sea snakes
    c. Cobra
    d. Krait
17. **Neurotoxin venom seen in which snake:**
    a. Viper
    b. Krait
    c. Sea snake
    d. None
18. **Snakebite causing hematologic abnormalities:**
    a. Cobra
    b. Krait
    c. Viper
    d. Sea snake
19. **Cholinesterase is seen in venom of:**
    a. Elapids
    b. Vipers
    c. Sea snakes
    d. All
20. **Lethal dose of krait venom:**
    a. 3 mg
    b. 6 mg
    c. 12 mg
    d. 15 mg
21. **Ophitoxaemia is:**
    a. Snakebite poisoning
    b. Phenol poisoning
    c. Chronic lead poisoning
    d. Opium poisoning
22. **Most characteristic feature of elapid snake envenomation:**
    a. Bleeding manifestation
    b. Neuro-paralytic symptoms
    c. Rhabdomyolysis
    d. Cardiotoxicity
23. **A patient presented with history of snakebite along with ptosis, paralysis and external ophthalmoplegia. Most probable species implicated:**
    a. Sea snake
    b. Krait
    c. Viper
    d. Cobra
24. **A girl, otherwise healthy, sleeping on the floor suddenly develops nausea, vomiting, abdominal pain quadriplegia at night. Diagnosis is:**
    a. Guillain Barre syndrome
    b. Poliomyelitis
    c. Krait bite
    d. Periodic paralysis
25. **Treatment of snakebite all, *except*:**
    a. Firm bandage to occlude lymphatic
    b. Incision over wound
    c. Reassure the patient
    d. Immobilization of bitten part
26. **Polyvalent snake vaccines contains immunoglobins against all, *except*:**
    a. Ophiophagus hannah
    b. Naja naja
    c. Daboia russelii
    d. Bungarus caeruleus
27. **In a snake envenomation, antivenom is started by giving a dose of:**
    a. 2 vials
    b. 4 vials
    c. 10 vials
    d. 20 vials
28. **Ligature pressure that should be used to resist spread of poison in elapidae poisoning:**
    a. <10 mm Hg
    b. 20–30 mm Hg
    c. 50–70 mm Hg
    d. >100 mm Hg

29. **Antisnake venom may cause:**
    a. Type II hypersensitivity reactions
    b. Type III hypersensitivity reactions
    c. Type IV hypersensitivity reactions
    d. Type V hypersensitivity reactions
30. **Drug used for muscarinic symptoms seen in cobra envenomation:**
    a. Neostigmine
    b. Pralidoxime
    c. Prazosin
    d. Naloxone
31. **Priapism occurs in:**
    a. Snake bite
    b. Rati poisoning
    c. Cantharide poisoning
    d. Arsenic poisoning
32. **Scorpion venom resembles venom of:**
    a. Cobra
    b. Viper
    c. Krait
    d. All of the above
33. **A 3-year-old child sleeping in a hut woke up in the middle of the night screaming. Her mother thought the child had a nightmare and tried to pacify her. After some time, she noticed that the child was sweating profusely and the hands were becoming cold. She vomited a couple of times. The mother immediately rushed her to the emergency services. Her pulse was 150/minute and her BP 90/60 mm Hg. This child is likely to have:**
    a. Snake bite
    b. Scorpion bite
    c. Septic shock
    d. Food poisoning
34. **Drug used in scorpion bite:**
    a. EDTA
    b. Neostigmine
    c. N-acetylcysteine
    d. Prazosin

ANSWERS

1. c	2. a	3. c	4. d	5. b	6. d	7. a	8. c	9. a	10. b
11. b	12. b	13. a	14. b	15. d	16. b	17. b	18. c	19. a	20. b
21. a	22. b	23. b	24. c	25. b	26. a	27. c	28. c	29. b	30. a
31. c	32. a	33. b	34. d						

30 CHAPTER

Neurotoxic Poisons

KEY WORDS

Somniferous poisons, opium, morphine, naloxone, cocaine, speed balls, body packers, inebriants, ethanol, McEwan's sign, nystagmus, alcoholism, Widmark's formula, methanol, formic acid, barbiturates, automatism, deliriants, *Datura*, cannabis, bhang, hashish, run amok, drug dependence, drug habituation, drug abuse, nux vomica, strychnine, anterior horn cells, convulsions, tetanus.

FM10.1 Describe general principles and basic methodologies in treatment of poisoning: Decontamination, supportive therapy, antidote therapy, procedures of enhanced elimination with regard to:
  ➤ Neuropsychotoxicology barbiturates, benzodiazepines
  ➤ Phenytoin, lithium, haloperidol, neuroleptics, tricyclics
  ➤ Narcotic analgesics

FM12.1 Describe features and management of abuse/poisoning with following chemicals: Tobacco, cannabis, amphetamines, cocaine, hallucinogens, designer drugs and solvent.

FM9.4 Describe general principles and basic methodologies in treatment of poisoning: Decontamination, supportive therapy, antidote therapy, procedures of enhanced elimination with regard to ethanol, methanol, ethylene glycol.

CLASSIFY NEUROTOXIC POISONS? (FM10.1)

Poisons which act on the nervous system are collectively called as neurotoxic poisons. Based on their effect on the three divisions of the nervous system the neurotoxic poison are classified into:
1. Cerebral poisons
2. Spinal poisons
3. Peripheral poisons

Cerebral Poisons

Poisons which acts on the brain are called as cerebral poisons. Based on their effects on brain function the cerebral poisons are grouped into:
- **Somniferous:** Sleep producing substances: Morphine.
- **Inebriant:** Producing euphoria (intoxicates): Alcohol, barbiturates, chloral hydrate.

- **Deliriant:** Causing excitation: Datura and cannabis.
- **Psychotropic:** Mind altering substances: LSD.

Spinal Poisons

- Substances altering or affecting the spinal cord functioning:
  - *Excitatory:* Strychnine
  - *Depressant:* Gelsemium

Peripheral Poison

Substances interrupting the function of peripheral nerves curare and conium.

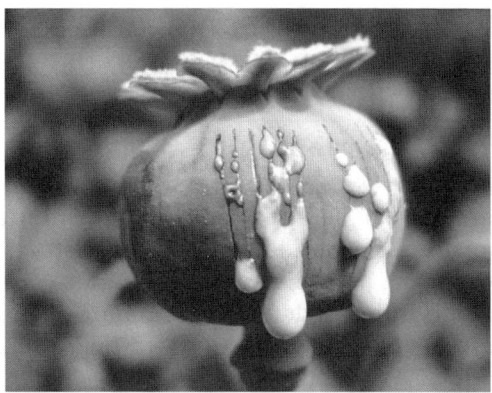

Fig. 30.2: Poppy capsule
(For color version see Plate 20).

WHAT IS OPIUM? WHAT ARE THE ALKALOIDS DERIVED FROM OPIUM? (FM10.1)

- Opium is a somniferous poison (induces sleep), as shown in **Figure 30.1**.
- Opium is the natural source for many drugs which are prescribed mainly to relieve the pain with an additional pleasure of sleep.
- Opium is extracted from the unripped fruit of papaver somniferum which is being cultivated under strict regulations.

Opium plant with unripe fruit **(Fig. 30.2)**; on incising exudes milky white juice, it is dried up into brown powder which is crude morphine.

Extraction

- Upon incision over the unripe fruit yields a milky white fluid which becomes dark and dry on exposure to a number of alkaloids. On their chemical basis these alkaloids are divided into two groups:
  - *Phenanthrene group:* 1. Morphine 2. Codeine 3. Thebaine
  - *Benzylisoquinoline group:* 1. Papaverine 2. Noscapine [narcoting].
- The ripped fruit capsule becomes brown and dry containing the brownish or pale brown fine granular seeds **(Fig. 30.3)**. Seeds are nonpoisonous used as condiments in preparation of condimental food.

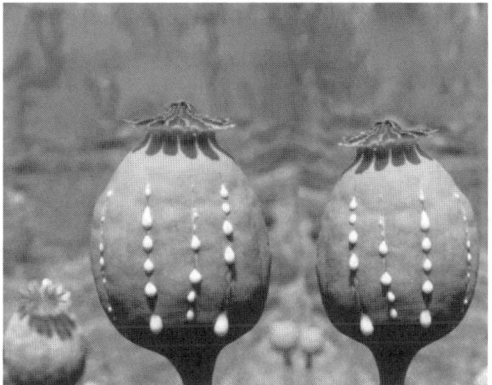

Fig. 30.1: Papaver somniferum/poppy
(For color version see Plate 20).

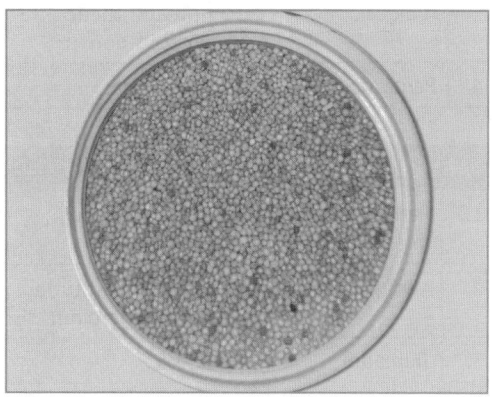

Fig. 30.3: Poppy seeds
(For color version see Plate 20).

WHAT ARE OPIATES AND OPIOIDS? WHAT IS THEIR ACTION AND USES? (FM10.1)

The naturally occurring opium and the derivatives of opium (semisynthetic) are called as **opiates**. Pure synthetic analogues are called as **opioids**. Natural-occurring opioids tabulated in **Table 30.1**. Semisynthetic derivatives (opiates) and synthetic derivatives tabulated in **Tables 30.2 and 30.3** respectively.

TABLE 30.1: Natural alkaloids and their action.

	Natural alkaloids	Action
1.	Morphine	Analgesic
2.	Codeine	Antitussive
3.	Thebaine	Analgesic
4.	Papaverine	Smooth muscle
5.	Noscapine	Narcosis

TABLE 30.2: Semisynthetic derivatives (opiates).

1.	Apomorphine	Used as emetic
2.	Diacetyl morphine (heroin)	Brown sugar—addiction
3.	Buprenorphine (tidigesic)	Analgesic and preanesthetic medication
4.	Pentazocine	Analgesic

TABLE 30.3: Synthetic derivatives (opioids).

1.	Pethidine (meperidine)	Analgesic
2.	Methadone	Analgesic (substitution therapy for heroine)
3.	Tramadol	Analgesic
4.	Loperamide	Antidiarrhea

WHAT IS THE MECHANISM OF ACTION OF MORPHINE? (FM10.1)

- The effect of opiates and opioids depends upon the receptors in the brain which are recognized as Mu (μ) Kappa (κ) and Delta (δ) primarily and the alkaloids and analogues are having agonistic antagonistic and combine agnostic and antagonistic properties.
- Mu receptor is responsible for euphoria, analgesia, respiratory depression and reduced gastrointestinal mobility.
- Kappa receptor is responsible for CNS depression, miosis and analgesia.
- Delta receptor is responsible for analgesic effect.

WHAT IS THE PHARMACOKINETICS AND CLINICAL SYMPTOMS OF MORPHINE? (FM10.1)

Pharmacokinetics

- **Absorption:** Opiates and opioids are absorbed from gastrointestinal tract, lungs and muscles. They are usually taken orally, parentally and by inhalation.
- **Metabolism:** Mostly in the liver by conjugation with glucuronic acid.
- Excretion is mainly through urine and faces.
- Pharmacodynamically opiates and opioids are known for their **three classical effects**.
  1. CNS depression
  2. Respiratory depression
  3. Miosis

Clinical Features

- The three stages of opium toxicity greatly depend upon the amount (dosage) and tolerance (duration) hence may not be classically seen always.
  - *Stage of excitement:* A brief period of euphoria due to effects on limbic system.

- *Stage of stupor:* The pleasurable mental excitement soon taken over by anorexia, nausea, vomiting constipation constricted pupil loss of sex desire and intense desire to sleep. Progressing to stupor but arousable.
- *Stage of narcosis:* Patient becomes deeply comatose and unarousable, insensible with abolished reflexes.
- Cyanotic face, cheyne-stoke breath, pinpoint pupil, bradycardia, hypotension, hypothermia, foaming over nose due to pulmonary congestion and edema and death due to **respiratory paralysis** may be preceded by convulsions.

DESCRIBE THE TREATMENT OF ACUTE MORPHINE POISONING? (FM10.1)

- **Airway:** Clear the airway by removing the froth or particulate matter taken by the individual by snorting or inhalation.
- **Breathing:** Adequate ventilatory support.
- **Circulation:** Cardiovascular support and monitoring.
- **Decontamination:**
  - Gastric lavage with cuffed Endotracheal intubation with potassium permanganate (1:5000) solution till the returning fluid is clear. Since, opium derivatives markedly reduce gastric motility, stomach wash should be given even in delayed detection. Since, opium derivatives are resecreted into the bile, stomach wash is indicated even in cases of parental administration.
  - Promote fecal excretion by purgatives.
- **Antidote administration:** Naloxone is the specific antidote for opium derivatives. Naloxone is an opioid antagonist competes with them at the receptor site. Dose is 0.4 mg to 2 mg IV can be repeated every 10–15 minutes up to 10 mg.
- Prevention of respiratory infection by antibiotics.
- Correction of electrolytic imbalance by IV fluids.
- General supportive measure.
- Psychiatric counseling.
- Periodic evaluation to prevent addiction.

WHAT ARE THE POSTMORTEM APPEARANCES AND VISCERA TO BE PRESERVED IN MORPHINE POISONING? (FM10.1)

External

- Cyanosis of face, lips, earlobes and fingernails.
- Foam cone over nose and mouth.
- Needle puncture marks in classical sites if administered parentally.

Internal

- Dark fluid blood, with intense congestion of internal organs.
- Remnants of poison in stomach.
- Respiratory passage and lungs are filled with frothy fluid.

Specimens to be Collected for Toxicological Analysis

Routine Specimens

- **Stomach:** Half stomach with half of its contents.
- **Intestine:** Proximal 100 cm.
- **Liver:** Not <500 g.
- **Kidney:** Half of each kidney.
- **Blood:** From peripheral vessel 30 mL preserved with sodium fluoride.
- **Urine:** Not <30 mL (No preservative)

Special Specimens

- Gallbladder (intact)
- Half of brain.

WHAT ARE THE MEDICO-LEGAL IMPORTANCE OF MORPHINE?

- Accidental death is commonly seen among drug addicts.
- Suicide is also common because of painless and pleasurable (devine death) but only to those who have accessibility to the drug.
- Homicide is rare because of the bitter taste and dark color. But infanticide is possible by smearing opium over breast.
- It is a powerful drug of addiction.

WRITE SHORT NOTES ON COCAINE? (FM12.1)

What is Speed Ball? What is Magnan's Symptom?

- Cocaine is also known as coke, snow, cadillac or white lady.
- Cocaine is an alkaloid obtained from the leaves of coco-tree erythroxylon coco and *E novogranatense*, which grows well in South America, India, Indonesia, Java, etc.
- Cocaine is colorless, odorless, crystalline substance bitter in taste, causes numbness of tongue and mucous membrane.

Common Routes of Administration

- Oral, injection, nasal and buccal membranes or by inhalation.
- Cocaine hydrochloride, the water soluble form is typically used for snorting and injection.
- Crude form of free base cocaine is suitable for smoking.

Action

- Cocaine desensitizes the terminal nerves and causes vasoconstriction at the site of application.
- It stimulates the cortex for a short time, followed by depression. Similar but less marked effect is seen on the spinal cord.

Medicinal Uses

- Formally used as topical anesthetic for corneal and ENT procedures.
- **Brampton's cocktail:** Cocaine was one of the constituents of this mixture, which was popular as a pain reliever in terminal cancer.

Signs and Symptoms

- **Stage of early stimulation:**
  - Euphoria, excitement, mydriasis, tachycardia, vertigo and nausea.
- **Stage of advanced stimulation:**
  - Vomiting, muscle twitching, convulsions, dyspnea, hyperthermia (cocaine fever), hallucination (tactile—cocaine bugs), circulatory and respiratory failure.
- **Stage of depression:**
  - Paralysis of muscles, loss of reflexes, coma and death.

Speed Balls

A combination of cocaine and heroin taken by injection is known as "speed balls".

Cocaine Bugs

- Also known as Magnan's symptom/tactile hallucination/formication.
- It is a withdrawal symptom of chronic cocaine poisoning. Where is a feeling of insects crawling all over the body (tactile hallucination).

WRITE SHORT NOTES ON BODY PACKER SYNDROME? (FM12.1)

- This condition is also called as "mini packer syndrome" or "body stuffing".
- It is a method used to smuggle drugs of abuse (mainly cocaine) across the international borders. The people involved are referred to as "mules".
- The mode of smuggling is by packing the drug (cocaine) in small plastic bags,

balloons or condoms of size 2.5 × 1 cm and swallowing them; rectal suppositories or disposable enemas are also used in these methods.
- Retrieval of these drug packets is by self-administration of purgative, followed by defecation.

Acute Poisoning

Acute poisoning is due to the complication of bursting of the packets during their transit through GIT thus releasing massive amounts of cocaine resulting in rapid collapse and death.

Diagnosis

Diagnosis is easy by abdominal X-ray, ultrasound or CT scan; the packets are visualized as radio-opaque shadows on X-ray.

Treatment (in Asymptomatic Patients)

- Whole bowel irrigation using polyethylene glycol.
- Alternatively, after waiting for a period of time till the drug reaches the colon; low volume phospho soda enemas/high volume saline enemas are administered.
- Food intake is not permitted till the drug is taken out.
- Bowel obstruction is to be ruled out before trying to evacuate the drug packets.
- Emptying of rectum by bisacodyl (Dulcolax) suppository and metoclopramide 10 mg, 8th hourly for gastric emptying are also useful.

Acute Poisoning: Symptomatic People

- Whole bowel irrigation and activated charcoal.
- Supportive measures like assisted ventilation.

- Benzodiazepines for convulsions.
- **Antidote:** Amyl nitrite inhalation, thiamine 100 mg IV, naloxone 2 mg IV.
- Administration of specific drugs depending on the symptoms.

Complication

Intestinal obstruction and rarely, intestinal perforation may occur, which requires surgical intervention.

WHAT ARE INEBRIANTS? WHICH ALL POISONS FALL INTO THIS CATEGORY? (FM9.4)

- Inebriant refers to any substance which intoxicates, i.e., causes mental confusion, light headedness, disorientation and drowsiness.
- There are several poisons and drugs which fall under this category, they are:
  - **Alcohol:** The most important representative of this group.
  - Barbiturates
  - Chloral hydrate
  - Benzodiazepines
  - Hydrocarbons
  - Formaldehyde and
  - Paraldehyde.

WHAT IS ETHANOL? HOW IT IS PRODUCED? (FM9.4)

What is Proof Spirit? What are Congeners?

Ethanol is ethyl alcohol, also referred as grain alcohol.

Physical Appearance

- Clear, colorless liquid with faint fruity odor and sweet burning taste.
- It is both water soluble and fat soluble.

TABLE 30.4: Concentration of alcohol in various beverages.

Beverage	Alcohol content (% by volume)
Light beer	3.5 to 6%
Strong beer	6 to 8%
Natural wine	10 to 15%
Fortified wine	15 to 20%
Whisky, Gin, Brandy	40 to 45%
Rum	45 to 50%

Source

Ethanol is produced by **fermentation of sugar with yeast**. The source of sugar could be cereal, vegetable or fruits. Alcoholic beverages are distilled after fermentation.

Proof Spirit

Refers to a standard mixture of alcohol and water of relative density 12/13 at 51°F, i.e., 49.28% of alcohol by weight or 57.10% by volume. Concentration of alcohol in various beverages tabulated in **Table 30.4**.

Congeners

- They are the by-products of the process of fermentation. All the alcoholic beverages contain several congeners to a varying extent. The odor of the alcoholic beverage is due to the congeners used.
- Vodka is the purest form and contains no congeners and hence virtually odorless. White rum is also relatively pure.

WHAT ARE THE USES OF ETHANOL? (FM9.4)

- **Alcoholic beverages**
- **Solvents:**
 - For after-shave lotions, colognes, mouth wash, perfumes, etc., the alcohol concentration varies from 15 to 80%.
- **Medicinal use:**
 - Several antihistamines, decongestants and cough syrups (2 to 25%).
 - **Surgical spirit:** Mixture of 90 to 95% of ethanol and 5 to 10% of methanol, is a popular antiseptic.
 - Ethanol sponging is an effective remedy for hyperthermia.
 - Injection of alcohol in close proximity to the nerve or sympathetic ganglia for trigeminal neuralgia.
 - Small doses of alcohol is useful in common cold.
- Ethanol is the antidote for methanol poisoning.
- Rectified spirit (90 to 95% ethanol) is used as a preservative.

HOW DOES ETHANOL GETS METABOLIZED IN THE BODY? (FM9.4)

What is the Usual Fatal Dose of Ethanol?

Absorption and Metabolism

- 20% is absorbed in the stomach and 80% from the intestines. Peak alcohol concentration in the blood is achieved in 30 to 90 minutes.
- More than 90% is metabolized in the body and 5 to 20% is excreted unchanged by kidneys, lungs and sweat.
- Metabolism is mainly by alcohol dehydrogenase pathway.
- In adults, the average rate of metabolism is 100 to 125 mg/kg/hour. In chronic alcoholics, it is up to 175 mg/kg/hour.
- The blood alcohol level falls at the rate of 15 to 20 mg/100 mL/hour and is higher (up to 30 mg/100 mL/hour) in chronic alcoholics.

WHAT ARE THE EFFECTS OF ETHANOL IN THE BODY? (FM9.4)

- **Intoxication:**
  - Alcohol is a well-known stimulant but is a selective depressant, especially of higher centers. Ethanol primarily depresses the reticular activating system.
  - The frontal lobes are sensitive to low concentration of alcohol resulting in mood changes, followed by the occipital lobe leading to visual disturbances and later the cerebellum resulting in loss of coordination.
  - The old Roman saying "**In Vino Veritas**" which means "in wine there is truth", i.e., the real personality of an individual will be often revealed when he is intoxicated.
- **CNS:**
  - Ethanol depresses the CNS. First affects memory and concentration, later there is emotional liability and mood swing. With severe intoxication, there is general impairment of CNS functions, passing on into coma.
- **CVS:**
  - In moderate doses ethanol produces tachycardia and vasodilation, resulting in a feeling of warmth.
- **GIT:**
  - Ethanol stimulates salivary and gastric secretions, but in high concentration they are inhibited, and mucosa becomes inflamed leading to erosive gastritis.
- **Genitor-urinary system:**
  - Ethanol induces diuresis by inhibiting ADH. Ethanol is said to be an aphrodisiac, but in chronic alcoholics it slowly leads to impotence.

WHAT ARE THE CLINICAL FEATURES OF ETHANOL POISONING? (FM9.4)

- **Stage of excitement:**
  - Loss of imbibitions, feeling of well-being, talkative, increased self-confidence and fine movements are affected. Blood alcohol 30 to 100 mg%.
- **Stage of intoxication:**
  - Emotional instability, slurred speech, impaired memory, increased reaction time and muscular in-coordination. BAC 150 to 300 mg%.
- **Stage of coma:**
  - Unconsciousness, abolished reflexes, sub-normal temperature, incontinence of urine and feces. BAC 300 to 450 mg%. Above 500 mg% the person may go into respiratory failure and death. Death from acute alcohol poisoning is usually rare. The individual goes on for a prolonged sleep coma and may recur spontaneously once the blood alcohol level goes down (16 to 24 hours).
- **Hangover:**
  - When the individual recovers from coma after a long sleep, he may present with symptoms of acute depression, nausea, abdominal discomfort, irritability, lethargy and severe headache.

McEwan's Sign (MacEwan's Sign)

- In the comatose stage, the pupils will be constricted. But, on stimulation of the patient (by pinching his face) the pupils dilate and slowly return to the original contracted size. This is called as McEwan's sign and is useful in differentiating alcoholic coma from other coma.
- Fine lateral nystagmus is usually present and is characteristic of alcoholism.

Micturition Syncope

It is a condition which occurs after heavy beer drinking. When the individual rises from bed in the middle of the night to pass urine, due to the sudden upright posture he loses consciousness during the act of urination.

Munich Beer Heart

It is a condition in which there is cardiac dilatation and hypertrophy due to excessive and prolonged beer drinking.

HOW TO DIAGNOSIS ETHANOL POISONING/CONSUMPTION? (FM9.4)

What is Widmark's Formula?

- Smell of alcohol in breath, slurred speech, muscular in-coordination, dilated and sluggish reacting pupil are helpful in diagnosing alcohol intoxication.
- Breath analyzer, urine and blood alcohol concentration are diagnostic.
- **Blood:**
  - Skin is cleaned with 1:1000 mercuric chloride and washed with soap and water. 10 mL of blood with 100 mg of sodium fluoride or 30 mg of potassium oxalate as preservative and the sample is shaken thoroughly to prevent loss of alcohol by glycolysis and bacterial action.

Widmark's Formula

- It was evolved by Widmark to find out the amount of alcohol consumed from the blood alcohol or urine alcohol concentration; $a = prc$.
- Where (a) is the weight of alcohol in gm in the body; (p) is the body weight in kg; (c) is the concentration of alcohol in blood in mg/kg and (r) is the constant, which is 0.6 for men and 0.5 for woman.
- For **urine analysis** the formula is: $a = ¾ prq$; where is (q) is alcohol concentration mg/kg.

Breath Analysis

It is bases on Henry's law 1:2100. Concentration of alcohol in 1 mL of blood is equal to concentration of alcohol in 2100 mL of alveolar air.

WHAT IS ALCOHOLISM? (FM9.4)

What are the Complications of Alcoholism?

- Chronic poisoning of ethanol is alcoholism.
- **Alcoholism** is a condition in which an individual consumes large quantities of alcohol over a prolonged period of time. Alcoholism is characterized by, pathological desire to consume alcohol and withdrawal symptoms on ceasing alcohol intake.
- Alcohol is quantified in terms of units. One unit contains 8 to 10 mg of alcohol and is equal to 30 mL of spirits.

Complications of Alcoholism

- **CNS:** Alcoholic hallucinosis, Wernike's encephalopathy and Korsakov's psychosis.
- **GIT:** Gastritis, periodic diarrhea and an increased incidence of cancers.
- **Liver:** Fatty degeneration of liver, cirrhosis and pancreatitis.
- **CVS:** Cardiomyopathy and hypertension.
- **CNS:** Polyneuropathy.

DEFINE DRUNKENNESS? HOW WILL YOU CERTIFY A CASE OF DRUNKENNESS? (FM9.4)

- **Drunkenness** is a condition produced in a person, who has consumed alcohol in sufficient quantities, so as to lose control

over his faculties to such an extent, that he is unable to execute the occupation safely, in which he is engaged at the material time.
- **Note:** Examination and certification of drunkenness are discussed under practical.

WHAT ARE THE SIGNS AND SYMPTOMS, TREATMENT AND POSTMORTEM FINDINGS OF METHYL ALCOHOL POISONING? (FM9.4)

Methyl alcohol is called as wood alcohol or methanol. It is a colorless, volatile liquid with a burning taste.

Signs and Symptoms
- Same as ethyl alcohol but inebriation is less prominent and the effects are prolonged.
- Toxicity can result following absorption through skin and respiratory tract.
- Symptoms include nausea, vomiting, pain or severe abdominal cramps, headache, neck stiffness, confusion and vertigo.
- There is marked muscular weakness and depressed cardiac action and hypothermia.
- Acute tubular necrosis in the kidneys.

Visual Disturbances
- Photophobia, blurred or misty vision, seeing spots central or peripheral scotomata, decreased light perception, concentric diminution of visual fields for color followed by fairly sudden failure of vision or complete **blindness**.
- This is due to optic neuritis and atrophy of optic nerve due to the effects of formic acid which are the end products of methanol metabolism.
- Fundoscopy reveals hyperemia of optic disc and retinal edema. The retinal ganglion cells and optic disc show degenerative changes.

Diagnosis
An increased osmolal gap accompanied by visual symptoms is suggestive of methanol poisoning.

Metabolism
Methanol is oxidized to formaldehyde in the liver, which is 33 times more toxic than methanol. Formaldehyde is then oxidized to formic acid, which is responsible for metabolic acidosis and visual toxicity.

Elimination
About 80% is excreted unchanged from the lungs and 3 to 5% is excreted unchanged through urine.

Analysis
Methyl alcohol and formic acid are readily detected from all the organs.

Treatment
- Gastric lavage using 5% bicarbonate solution and 500 mL is left inside the stomach.
- Activate charcoal is useful.

Antidote
- **Ethanol** is the antidote and is given as 10% solution in 500 mL infusion and repeated as required till the blood level falls below 25%. Serum ethanol level is frequently checked so as to maintain the level of 100 to 150 mg%.
- Hemodialysis is the treatment of choice in severe poisoning.

- Folinic acid or folic acid 50 to 75 mg every 4 hours, is useful in eliminating formic acid.
- Sodium bicarbonate to combat acidosis.
- Blood sugar is frequently monitored.
- Eyes are kept cover to protect from light.

Postmortem Appearance

- Cyanosis is marked.
- Blood could be fluid in nature.
- Skin may be purple in color due to pyridine.
- Stomach and intestines congested, inflamed and small hemorrhages may be present.
- Lungs congested and edematous.
- Brian edematous and may show hemorrhage.
- Liver shows fatty change and sometimes early necrosis.
- Kidneys show tubular degeneration.

WHAT ARE BARBITURATES? WHAT ARE THE GROUPS OF BARBITURATES? (FM10.1)

- Barbiturates are derivatives of barbituric acid.
- Barbiturates were used extensively until benzodiazepines occupied the market.
- Now, have become "museum drugs" many barbiturates are still available and are still being abused.

There are four classes of barbiturates:
1. **Ultra short acting:** Acts immediately and lasts for about 15 minutes, e.g., thiopentone sodium.
2. **Short acting:** Acts within minutes and lasts for about 3 hours, e.g., pentobarbitone.
3. **Intermediate acting:** Acts within 1–2 hours and lasts for 3–6 hours, e.g., butobarbitone.
4. **Long acting:** Acts within 2 hours and lasts for 6–12 hours, e.g., phenobarbitone.

WHAT ARE THE SIGNS AND SYMPTOMS AND TREATMENT OF BARBITURATE POISONING? WHAT IS AUTOMATISM? (FM10.1)

Acute Poisoning

Taking barbiturates (usually tablets), repeatedly to get sleep out of mental sickness, compels the person to take more and more tablets ultimately resulting in acute toxicity, the individual usually does not remember (forgets) that he has taken the dose and continues to take the drug again and again, this is called "**barbiturate automatism**".

Signs and Symptoms

- Slurred speech, ataxia, lethargy, mental confusion and headache.
- Pupils are first constricted but later dilated due to hypoxia.
- Hypersensitivity reaction, swelling over cheeks, lips, etc.
- Paradoxical excitement (especially in elderly).
- CNS depression, coma and shock.
- Finally death is due to respiratory arrest or cardiovascular collapse.
- Cutaneous bullae (**barbiturate blisters**).

Fatal Dose

- **Long acting barbiturates:** 3 to 4 g.
- **Intermediate acting:** 2 to 3 g.
- **Short acting:** 1 to 2 g.

Fatal Period

24 to 48 hours, however, patient may be in coma for several days and then die.

When Taken with Alcohol

Can bring about death easily as alcohol potentiates barbiturate action and even a sub lethal dose may prove fatal.

Treatment

- Maintain air way, breathing and circulation.
- Gastric lavage can be done up to 6 to 12 hours.
- Activated charcoal in the usual dose.
- Forced alkaline diuresis is said to be very useful in phenobarbitone poisoning.
- Hemodialysis or hemoperfusion.
- **Supportive measures:** Oxygen, intubation, assisted ventilation and IV fluid.

WHAT IS BARBITURATE ADDICTION? (FM10.1)

Chronic Poisoning (Addiction)

- Barbiturates are the most addictive drugs.
- They are often used to get a sense of euphoria and relaxation.
- Chronic use is associated with tolerance and hence, a chronic user usually requires 5 times the normal dose to obtain therapeutic effect.
- Abrupt cessation provokes a mild withdrawal reaction characterized by anxiety, headache, tremors and insomnia.

HOW TO DIAGNOSE BARBITURATE POISONING? (FM10.1)

What are the Medico-Legal Aspects?

- Thin layer chromatography (TLC) for urine, stomach contents, or scene residue.
- Gas chromatography (GC) or high pressure liquid chromatography (HPLC).
- **EEG:** Alpha coma indicates poor prognosis.

Differential Diagnosis

Other poisoning are due to carbon monoxide, meprobamate, etc.

Medico-Legal Significance

- Often used by alcoholics and opiate addicts when alcohol or opium is not available.
- **Example:** Emotional tension developed by cocaine is controlled when its intake is combined with barbiturates.
- Addiction is usually due to excessive use of barbiturates to relieve anxiety and depression.
- Death is usually suicidal by over dosage or accidental and rarely homicidal.

WHAT IS TRUTH SERUM? (FM10.1)

Sodium pentothal is often used to extract truth from criminals and is also called "truth serum". However, it actually does not cause people to tell the truth; rather, it just lowers their inhibitions and makes them talkative.

WRITE SHORT NOTES ON CHLORAL HYDRATE? (FM9.4)

What is Dry Wine and Micky Finn/Knockout Drops?

Chloral Hydrate

- **Physical properties:**
    - Crystalline, nauseating bitter sweet taste with an aromatic odor.
- **Action:**
    - Chloral hydrate in small doses it acts as a hypnotic; in large doses it paralyses the vital center of the brain.
- **Signs and symptoms:**
    - Acute poisoning:
        - Burning sensation in throat
        - Nausea and vomiting
        - Drowsiness and unconsciousness
        - Loss of reflexes and muscular relaxation
        - Depression of medullary center, resulting in fall in BP, respiratory rate, convulsions and death with pinpoint pupils.
- **Chronic poisoning:**
    - Epigastric pain, nausea, vomiting and gastritis.
    - Erythematous rashes
    - Nervous disorders.

- **Fatal dose:** 5 to 10 g; fatal period: 6 to 24 hours.

Treatment
- Withdrawal from the drug
- Gastric lavage
- Artificial respiration
- High protein and carbohydrate diet and no fatty food should be given.

Postmortem Findings
- Signs of asphyxia
- In acute poisoning the stomach contents have a peculiar smell.
- In chronic poisoning evidence of fatty degeneration of heart, liver and kidneys.
- It deteriorates rapidly form the body after death and hence viscera should be sent immediately for chemical analysis.

Medico-Legal Significance
- Therapeutic over dosage causes hypnotic effects.
- It is rarely used for suicide.
- Not used for homicidal purposes due to the taste and smell.
- "**Dry wine**" a combination of chloral hydrate and alcohol is used as liquor is some parts of Punjab to induce sleep.
- Chloral hydrate is mixed in some food or drink to make a person suddenly helpless for the purpose of robbery or rape. When mixed with alcohol, it greatly enhances the kick and the person may go in for sudden unconsciousness and is called as "**knock out drops**" or **Mickey Finn**.

WHAT ARE DELIRIANTS?
- Deliriants are drugs which act on the brain and induce altered consciousness, confusion, delusions and agitation.
- Two important drugs of this group are Datura, and Cannabis Indica. They are also called as "**stupefying agents**".

WHAT ARE THE TWO VARIETIES OF DATURA PLANT?
- There are two varieties of plants.
  i. Datura alba (white flowers) and
  ii. Datura niger (purple flowers)
- The plant grows all over India in the waste places. Flowers are bell shaped; fruits are spherical and have sharp spines on the surface (thorn apple) **(Fig. 30.4)** and contain about 500 yellowish brown seeds inside the fruit shown in **Figure 30.5**.

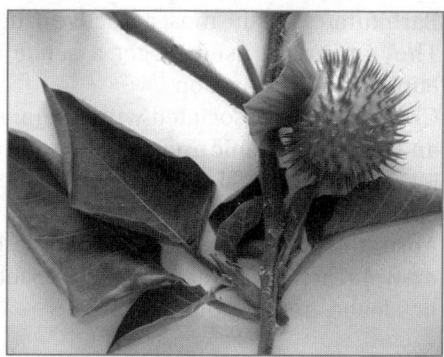

Fig 30.4: Datura plant with fruit (thorn apple)
(For color version see Plate 21).

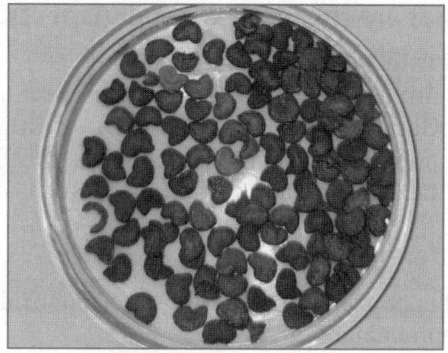

Fig. 30.5: Datura seeds
(For color version see Plate 21).

WHAT ARE THE ACTIVE PRINCIPAL AND THEIR ACTION OF DATURA SEEDS?

- The seeds contain three **alkaloids** as active principles:
  1. Hyoscine (scopolamine)
  2. Hyoscyamine, and
  3. Traces of atropine.
- **Alkaloids** are complex substances having nitrogenous base; chemically they behave as alkalis, react with acids to form salts. In plants they are not uniformly distributed, rather concentrated in certain regions such as root, leaves or fruits.
- Alkaloids atropine, hyoscine and hyoscyamine first stimulate the higher centers of the brain followed by motor neurons; finally causes depression and paralysis, especially the medulla.

WHAT ARE THE SIGNS AND SYMPTOMS OF DATURA POISONING?

- When the seeds are ingested, there is bitter taste in the mouth, dryness of mouth, difficulty in swallowing and talking, burning pain in the stomach which is followed by vomiting.
- Voice becomes hoarse; face becomes flushed; pupils are widely dilated, loss of accommodation and photophobia leading to temporary blindness.
- **Kidneys:** Urinary retention and inability to pass urine.
- **Skin:** Becomes **hot**, **dry** and scarlatinal rash may appear; pulse is rapid and bounding, but later on weak and irregular.
- **CNS:** Restlessness, agitation, confusion, giddiness and staggering gait.
- Delirium develops and the patient may try to run away from the bed.
- **Carphologia:** Tries to pull imaginary threads from the fingernails.
- Auditory and visual hallucinations and delusions may develop.
- The patient may go into deep sleep or coma and rarely may die of respiratory paralysis.
- **Fatal dose:** 0.6 to 1 g (100 to 125 seeds); fatal period: 24 hours.

WHAT IS THE TREATMENT FOR DATURA POISONING? (FM12.1)

- Emetics and/stomach wash.
- **Injection physostigmine** 1 mg, repeated hourly if necessary.
- **Injection pilocarpine** nitrate 5 mg subcutaneous, repeated every 2 hours as required to counteract the action of datura on the brain.
- Delirium is controlled using **barbiturates**, ether or chloroform.

WHAT ARE THE CIRCUMSTANCES OF DATURA POISONING? (FM12.1)

- Either alone or in combination with cannabis, it is used as a **stupefying agent**, by the robbers to facilitate robbery in trains or buses. Datura is mixed with any food or drink for this purpose; the victim falls into deep sleep and wakes up later and finds his belongings being lost.
- Datura is believed to have **aphrodisiac** effect and used as a love filter; it is also used as an **abortifacient**.
- The leaves and seeds are mixed with tobacco and ganja and smoked; it may also be mixed with toddy or liquor to increase the intoxication effect.
- Accidental poisoning occurs in children; homicide is very rare.

HOW TO DIFFERENTIATE DATURA SEEDS FROM CAPSICUM SEEDS? (TABLE 30.5 AND FIG. 30.6)

TABLE 30.5: Difference between datura seeds and capsicum seeds.

Feature	Datura seed	Capsicum seed
Size	Large and stout	Small and thin
Shape	Kidney or bean shaped	Rounded
Color	Brown or yellowish-brown	Pale-yellow
Margins	Laterally compressed convexity	Sharp convex borders
Surface	Numerous depressions on the surface	Smooth
Odor and taste	Odorless and bitter	Pungent and burning taste

Test: Mydriatic test: A drop of the sample solution to be tested is put into the eyes of a cat; the pupils dilate if datura is present (effect of atropine).

WHAT IS CANNABIS INDICA? (FM10.1)

- Cannabis Indica is Indian hemp, hashish, marihuana or ganja **(Fig. 30.7)**.

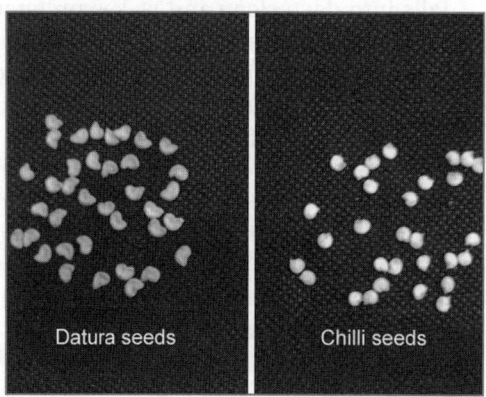

Fig. 30.6: Datura seeds and chilli seeds
(For color version see Plate 21).

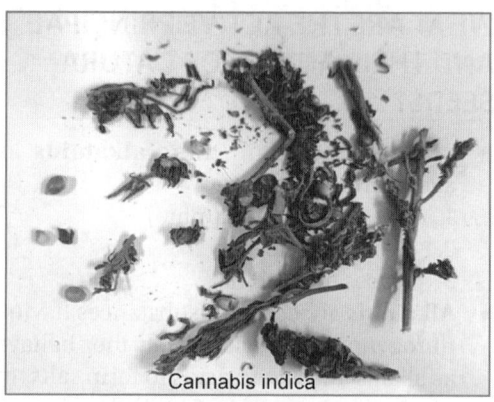

Fig. 30.7: Cannabis indica
(For color version see Plate 21).

- The plant grows wildly in India, but the cultivation is banned by the government.
- **Female plant** is tall, grows 4 to 6 meters in height and bushy; **male plant** is short and grows <4 meters in height.
- There are many names for cannabis from area to area: Pot, grass, hash, marijuana, bhang, hashish, joint, etc.
- Cannabis is the most abused drug in India by the people of low socio-economic group; mostly people habituated to cannabis would like to use it with company.

WHAT IS THE ACTIVE PRINCIPAL IN CANNABIS AND WHICH PARTS OF THE PLANT CONTAINS ACTIVE INGRDIENET?

- The active principle is contained in the resin; cannabinol is the constituent of the resin.
- Cannabinol is inert and gets converted into tetrahydrocannabinol (THC) on burning/heating.
- All parts of the plant contain the resin; the shooting flowers of the female plant (**ganja**) have the highest concentration of cannabinol, next the leaves and then the stem; the seeds do not contain the active ingredient.

- On **incising the stem,** it yields a brown thick resin called **hashish.**
- Hashish is said to be the purest form and contains maximum concentration of the active ingredient, about 40%.

WHAT ARE THE VARIOUS FORMS OF PREPARATIONS OF CANNABIS?

Bhang: Prepared from the dried leaves and flowers in the form a decoction and is consumed by mixing with any food or betel. Bhang is directly mixed to prepare sweets (**majoon**). It increases appetite and sexual desire. Bhang is the mildest form of intoxication.

Ganja: The shooting flower top of the female plant is ganja. This is the commonly abused of all forms of cannabis. It is dark green in color; it is mixed with tobacco and smoked, in cigars or pipes (hookah). On burning cannabinol gets converted into THC and has a characteristic odor (**burnt rope odor**) in the vicinity of an individual who has smoked ganja.

Charas or hashish: It is the resin (dope or shit) exuded from the stem; brown in color and smoked with tobacco in pipes.

WHAT ARE THE SIGNS AND SYMPTOMS CANNABIS?

- Appear immediately and last for 2 hours if smoked; appears in half an hour and lasts for several hours if ingested.
- Euphoria, disorientation, impaired memory, disturbed thought process and lapse of attention in the initial stages. The individual starts laughing for silly jokes; this is classically observed when the person consumes on rare occasions. But on continued smoking for a long period the individual detaches from the family members.
- Irrelevant thought process, decreased concentration, disorientation and sleepiness.
- Impaired judgment altered sexual desire and failure to meet the responsibilities.
- Death is extremely rare the individual passes of into sleep and wakes up late.
- **Fatal dose:** Charas 2 g and ganja 8 g/kg body weight.

WHAT ARE THE COMPLICATIONS OF CHRONIC CANNABIS ABUSE?

What is "Run Amok"?

- Using the drug in small dose for long periods does not cause much harm. If large doses are consumed for a prolonged period, tolerance and psychological dependence develops and sometimes, there may be degeneration of CNS and symptoms of insanity.
- Reduces serum testosterone levels and reduced sperm count associated with gynecomastia.
- Rarely the individual may develop symptoms of insanity (**hashish psychosis**).

Run Amok

- Develops in an individual who chronically abuses cannabis or rarely in an individual who consumes a high dose of ganja.
- There is development of psychiatric disturbances marked by a period of depression followed by violent impulsive behaviors.
- He may run here and there, he is impulsive in behavior; the individual may commit suicide (suicidal impulse) by inflicting injuries or may jump from a height. He may attempt to kill individuals with whom he has real or imaginary enemity (homicidal impulse) and surrender himself to the police or he may kill himself.

Medico-Legal Significance

- Circumstances of poisoning are usually accidental due to overindulgence.
- There is no physical dependence for cannabis and there is only psychological dependence to the drug.
- Prolonged consumption leads to psychiatric disturbances ranging from depression to hashish and paranoid psychosis.
- It is the most widely abused drug of a low socio-economic population.

DRUG DEPENDENCE (FM10.1)

Define: Drug Dependence, Abuse, Psychological Dependence, Drug Addiction and Habituation?

- **Drug:**
  - A drug is any substance, other than those required for the maintenance of normal health, that when taken into the living organism may modify one or more of its functions.
- **Drug dependence:**
  - It is a state of dependence on a drug which arises out of a maladaptive pattern of substance use, leading to cluster of behavioral, cognitive and physiological symptoms that develop after repeated intake.
- **Substance abuse:**
  - It is persistent excessive desire to use a drug, inconsistent with or unrelated to acceptable medical practice.
- **Substance intoxication:**
  - Involves unwanted physiological, psychological or sexual effects that cause maladaptive behavior.
  - **Example**: (i) a individual bribes a nurse of a hospital and manages to get morphine from the hospital—substance abuse; (ii) he takes in morphine and experiences the effects of the drug like euphoria and feeling of well-being—substance intoxication; (iii) he continues to visit the hospital demanding higher doses of morphine—drug dependence.
- **Physiological dependence:**
  - It is the alteration in neural system which is manifested by tolerance due to repeated doses of the drug and there is appearance of withdrawal symptoms when the drug is discontinued.
- **Psychological dependence:**
  - It is a condition in which the individual believes that an optimal state of well-being is achieved only through the intake of the drug.
  - **Example**: (i) an individual takes in heroin and wishes to take it again—psychological dependence; (ii) he now is a regular heroine abuser and experiences withdrawal symptoms when he discontinues the use of heroine—physical dependence.
- **Drug addiction:**
  - It is a chronic disorder characterized by compulsive use of a drug resulting in physical and psychological dependence; associated with social harm and continue to use the drug in spite of these harm.
- **Drug habituation:**
  - It s a condition resulting from the repeated consumption of a drug and there is psychological or emotional dependency on the drug, but there are no withdrawal symptoms on discontinuation of the drug.
  - **Example:** (i) an individual breaks up with his wife because of his constant use of cocaine but still continues to use it—drug addiction; (ii) he shouts at his wife for not bringing bed coffee on time—drug habituation.

WHAT ARE THE DIFFERENCE BETWEEN DRUG DEPENDENCE AND HABITUATION? (TABLE 30.6)

TABLE 30.6: Difference between drug dependence and habituation.

Drug dependence	Drug habituation
Compulsion to take the drug	No compulsion
Increase in the dose	No increase in dose
Physical and psychological dependence	Some degree of psychological dependence
Withdrawal symptoms present	No withdrawal symptoms

WHAT ARE THE COMMON DRUGS OF ADDICTION? (TABLE 30.7)

TABLE 30.7: Drugs of addiction.

Group	Drugs
Opiates	Heroin, morphine, codeine, methadone and pethidine
Stimulants	Cocaine and amphetamine
Hallucinogens	LSD, marijuana, mescaline and psilocybin
Depressants	Barbiturates, glutethimide, paraldehyde and methyprylon
Miscellaneous	Propoxyphene, pentazocine, amitriptyline, cough syrups, etc.

WHAT ARE WITHDRAWAL SYMPTOMS?

- A group of symptoms produced upon sudden stoppage of a drug of addiction are called **withdrawal symptoms.**
- These symptoms occur 6 to 8 hours after stoppage or sometimes may be delayed and last for 10 to 21 days. There are 3 stages of symptoms of withdrawal.

Early Symptoms

Chillness, cold, uneasiness, yawning and rhinorrhea.

Second Stage

Labored and sharp respirations, goose skin, lacrimation, gross tremors and anorexia.

Third Stage

- Prolonged sleep, fever, hypertension, pain and cramps of muscles especially calf and abdomen muscles.
- Withdrawal symptoms in new born of addicted mothers: Occurs within 1 to 56 hours of delivery and presents with symptoms of hyperactivity, convulsions and twitching.

WHAT IS DRUG DEPENDENCE? WHAT ARE THE TYPES OF DRUG DEPENDENCE? (FM12.1)

Drug Dependence

It is a state of dependence on a drug which arises out of a maladaptive pattern of substance use, leading to cluster of behavioral, cognitive and physiological symptoms that develop after repeated intake.

Types of Drug Dependence

- Morphine type
- Barbiturate type
- Cocaine type
- Cannabis type
- Amphetamine type
- **Psychedelics:** Hallucinogenic drugs: LSD (ergot) and solvent abuse.

Morphine

- Addiction to morphine, heroin, opium and methadone.

- Overpowering desire or need to continue the drug.
- Mode of abuse: IV, IM and sniffing.
- Tolerance occurs very early within 48 to 72 hours and physical dependence.
- **Cross tolerance:** Morphine and pethidine have a high degree of cross tolerance.

Withdrawal symptoms:

- **Early:** Dilated pupils, yawning, rhinorrhea, myalgia, cramps, lacrimation and anorexia.
- **Moderate:** Restlessness, insomnia, hypertension and tachycardia.
- **Severe:** Vomiting, diarrhea, hyperactive bowel syndrome and hypotension.
- **Causes of death:** Rapid death due to cardiac arrest, arrhythmia and ventricular fibrillation.

Barbiturate

- Physical dependence, tolerance and cross tolerance.
- Withdrawal symptoms develop within 2 to 3 days.
- **Early:** Tremors, hyper reflexes, diaphoresis, irritability, restlessness, anxiety, tinnitus, nausea and vomiting.
- **Late:** Profuse diaphoresis, marked disorientation, hallucination, agitation, tremors and hyperthermia.
- **Purple hearts tablet:** Combination of barbiturate and amphetamine.

Cocaine

- Psychological dependence and absence of tolerance.
- Withdrawal symptoms are mild (cocaine bugs—tactile hallucination).
- Paranoid psychosis, depression and mental dysfunction.
- **Crack:** Heating cocaine with bicarbonate and is more potent.

Cannabis Type

- Psychological dependence and no physical dependence.
- No tolerance and no withdrawal symptoms

Amphetamine Type

- Psychological dependence.
- Tolerance is present but no withdrawal symptoms.
- Severe hyper-excitement, hallucinations and psychoses develop due to prolonged use.
- Hyperpyrexia, hypertension and cerebral hemorrhages may also occur.

WRITE SHORT NOTES ON SPINAL POISONS/STRYCHNINE? (FM10.1)

- Strychnine is a powerful alkaloid, present in the seeds of strychnos nux vomica growing in the jungles of India. Fruits are orange, round and hard, and bear 3 to 5 seeds **(Fig. 30.8)**.
- Strychnine seeds are flat, circular disc shaped, 6 mm in thickness and 2.5 cm in diameter; the seeds are light brown

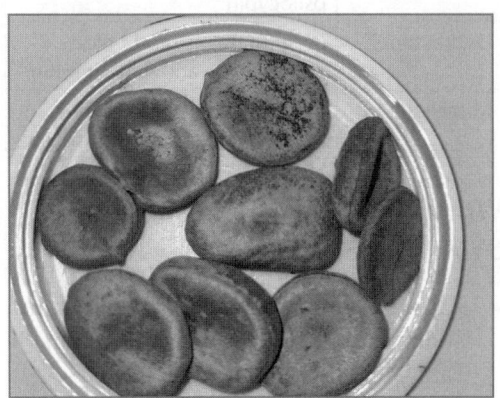

Fig 30.8: Nux vomica seeds
(For color version see Plate 21).

in color and are convex on one side and concave on the other.
- The seeds contain strychnine and brucine as active ingredients. Strychnine is many times more poisonous than brucine.
- Strychnine seeds are used as rodenticide to kill stay dogs.

Action

Acts on the **anterior horn cells of the spinal cord** and depresses the inhibitory synaptic potentials of the spinal cord. Widespread inhibition of the spinal cord results in release excitation and convulsions resembling tetanus.

Signs and Symptoms

- When the seed is swallowed as a whole, it does not cause any symptoms; if crushed and swallowed, the symptoms start in an hour.
- Bitter taste in the mouth, restlessness, difficulty in swallowing.
- Increased rigidity of muscles, muscular twitching followed by convulsions.
- Convulsions affect all the muscles at a time. Convulsion lasts for half minute to two minutes; repeated after 5 to 15 minutes; in between the convulsions the muscles remain relaxed.
- The patient is unable to breathe as the diaphragm and the thoracic muscles are fully contracted. Hypoxia causes medullary paralysis and death.
- Consciousness is not lost and the mind is clear till the death.
- **Fatal dose:** 50 mg (one crushed seed); fatal period: few hours.

Treatment

- Convulsions are controlled by: (i) diazepam or phenobarbitone; when they are ineffective (ii) succinylcholine, curare or pancuronium; in between convulsions ether may be given.
- Short acting barbiturates like pentobarbital sodium and sodium amytal are antidotes for strychnine.
- Stomach wash with warm water and dilute potassium permanganate; activated charcoal to absorb strychnine (tannic acid may be used when charcoal is not available).
- Increasing acidity of urine will increase excretion of strychnine.

Postmortem Findings

- Signs of asphyxia will be present; rigor mortis appears early; hemorhhages may be found inside the muscles and stomach.
- **Test:** Suspected solution is injected into the dorsal lymph sac of a frog, will produce convulsions if strychnine is present.

Forensic Significance

- Homicide is common, as it resembles death due to **tetanus** and may go undetected.
- Suicide is rare due to the potentially dreadful death.
- Accidental by children and over dosage of medicines in folk remedies.
- Used as cattle poison and also as arrow poison.
- Used as an aphrodisiac.
- Strychnine is said to delay putrefaction.

MULTIPLE CHOICE QUESTIONS

1. **Carphologia is seen in:**
   a. Abrus precatorius
   b. Calotropis procera
   c. Datura niger
   d. Ricinus communis
2. **One of the following is a stupefying agent:**
   a. Atropine
   b. Aconite
   c. Datura
   d. Nerium

SECTION 7: Medical Toxicology

3. **Strychnine acts at:**
   a. Anterior horn cells
   b. Posterior horn cells
   c. Reflux vagal inhibition
   d. Brain stem
4. **Automatism is typically seen in:**
   a. Barbiturates
   b. Cocaine
   c. Choral hydrate
   d. Opium
5. **Nalorphine is used as an antidote in:**
   a. Strychnine
   b. Barbiturates
   c. Opium
   d. Cocaine
6. **In suspected nux vomica poisoning the following is required to be preserved:**
   a. Muscle
   b. Heart
   c. Spinal cord
   d. Long bones
7. **One of the following is known as knock out drops:**
   a. Chloroform
   b. Chloral hydrate
   c. Methyl alcohol
   d. Cocaine
8. **The following is used for stomach wash in datura poisoning:**
   a. Potassium permanganate
   b. Lime water
   c. Glycerol
   d. Any of the above can be used
9. **Coma and pinpoint pupil are seen in poisoning due to:**
   a. Alcohol
   b. Carbolic acid
   c. Opium
   d. Parathion
10. **Optic atrophy is characteristic feature of _____ poisoning.**
    a. Lead
    b. Phosphorus
    c. Ethyl alcohol
    d. Methyl alcohol
11. **The organ to be preserved in volatile organic poisons:**
    a. Bone
    b. Brain
    c. Lung
    d. Heart
12. **Treatment of opium poisoning includes all, except:**
    a. Stomach wash
    b. Purgatives
    c. Naloxone
    d. Digitalis
13. **Datura poisoning is characterized by all, except:**
    a. Constricted pupil
    b. Dilated pupil
    c. Dysphagia
    d. Dryness of mouth and throat
14. **Drug that inhibits aldehyde dehydrogenase is:**
    a. Phenytoin
    b. Valproate
    c. Disulfiram
    d. Erythromycin
15. **Active component of ganja includes:**
    a. Tetrahydrocannabinols
    b. LSD
    c. Ethyl alcohol
    d. N methyl tryptophan
16. **Mc Ewan's sign is characteristically seen in:**
    a. Alcoholic coma
    b. Hepatic encephalopathy
    c. Carbon monoxide poisoning
    d. Classifying medico-legal aspects of wounds
17. **Tactile hallucinations are noticed in:**
    a. Parkinsonism
    b. Chronic depression
    c. Chronic cocaine poisoning
    d. Acute barbiturate poisoning
18. **In strychnine poisoning, there is the following feature of the muscles in between the convulsive seizures:**
    a. Rigidity
    b. Fasciculations
    c. Relaxation
    d. All
19. **Under the 'NDPS Act' following drugs are included, except:**
    a. Opium
    b. Amphetamine
    c. Cannabis
    d. Alcohol
20. **Smell of burnt rope due to poisoning with:**
    a. Cannabis
    b. Cyanide
    c. Hydrogen sulfide
    d. Aluminum phosphide

21. Urinary alkalization increases urine elimination of all the following drugs, *except:*
    a. Salicylate
    b. Methotrexate
    c. Amphetamine
    d. Phenobarbitone
22. Alcohol, salicylates and pilocarpine can be used as:
    a. Chelating agents
    b. Purgatives
    c. Diaphoretics
    d. Forced alkaline diuresis
23. Hemodialysis is used in all the poisonings, *except:*
    a. Kerosene oil
    b. Alcohol
    c. Barbiturate
    d. Cocaine
24. Constricted pupil is seen in all poisoning, *except:*
    a. Paracetamol
    b. Phenol
    c. OPC
    d. Opium
25. Which of these is not an opioid agonist:
    a. Heroin
    b. Ketamine
    c. Methadone
    d. Fentanyl
26. A 28-year-old male patient is brought to casualty in comatose state with pin-point pupils, reduced respiratory rate and bradycardia. Most likely diagnosis:
    a. Tricyclic antidepressant poisoning
    b. Opioid poisoning
    c. Benzodiazepine poisoning
    d. Organophosphorus poisoning
27. All are features of acute morphine poisoning:
    a. Pin-point pupil
    b. Hyperpyrexia
    c. Fall in blood pressure
    d. Slow labored breathing
28. Most common feature of opiate poisoning:
    a. Respiratory depression
    b. Hypotension
    c. Bradycardia
    d. Hypothermia
29. Marquis test is done for:
    a. Mercury poisoning
    b. Arsenic poisoning
    c. Morphine poisoning
    d. Cyanide poisoning
30. Safe limit of alcohol consumption in males and females are:
    a. 15 and 10 units/week
    b. 18 and 15 units/week
    c. 21 and 14 units/week
    d. 25 and 18 units/week
31. Blackout is due to:
    a. Alcohol intoxication
    b. Cocaine toxicity
    c. LSD toxicity
    d. Cyanide poisoning
32. Disulfiram is useful in:
    a. Alcohol dependence
    b. Heroin dependence
    c. Cocaine dependence
    d. Cannabis dependence
33. Most common symptom of alcohol withdrawal is:
    a. Body ache
    b. Tremor
    c. Diarrhea
    d. Rhinorrhea
34. Wernicke-Korsakoff's syndrome is due to the deficiency of:
    a. Pyridoxine
    b. Thiamine
    c. Vitamin B_{12}
    d. Riboflavin
35. A 55-year-old man presents with a 10-day history of confusion. His friend mentions that he drinks 15 units of alcohol per day. Which of the following strongly suggests a diagnosis of Korsakoff's psychosis:
    a. Delusional beliefs
    b. Poor long-term memory
    c. Auditory hallucinations
    d. Confabulation
36. True about alcohol paranoia:
    a. Tremors
    b. Fixed hallucinations
    c. Fixed delusions
    d. Wrist and foot drop
37. Criminal responsibility of an intoxicated person is under:
    a. Section 82 IPC
    b. Section 84 IPC
    c. Section 85 IPC
    d. Section 90 IPC

38. Widmark's formula is used for measurement of blood levels of:
    a. Benzodiazepines
    b. Barbiturates
    c. Alcohol
    d. Cocaine
39. The most reliable method of estimating blood alcohol level is:
    a. Cavett's test
    b. Breath alcohol analyzer
    c. Thin layer chromatography
    d. Gas liquid chromatography
40. The chemical used for qualitative and quantitative assessment of alcohol in the expired air is:
    a. Aniline
    b. Diphenylamine
    c. Potassium ferrocyanide
    d. Potassium dichromate
41. In contaminated liquor poisoning, all of the following are true, *except*:
    a. Metabolic alkalosis
    b. Blindness
    c. Treatment is with ethanol
    d. Toxicity is due to methanol
42. Ethanol is used for ethylene glycol poisoning because it is a:
    a. Competitive inhibitor of aldehyde dehydrogenase
    b. Higher affinity for alcohol dehydrogenase
    c. Chemically combines and neutralizes ethylene glycol
    d. Competitive inhibitor of alcohol dehydrogenase
43. Antidote for ethylene glycol poisoning:
    a. Methyl violet
    b. Fomepizole
    c. Fluconazole
    d. Ethyl alcohol
44. The police brought a person from railway platform. He was talking irrelevant, had dry mouth with hot dry skin, dilated pupils, staggering gait and slurred speech. Most probable diagnosis is:
    a. Alcoholic intoxication
    b. Datura poisoning
    c. OPC poisoning
    d. Aconite poisoning
45. In datura poisoning, 9 'Ds' include all, *except*
    a. Diarrhea
    b. Dysphagia
    c. Drowsiness
    d. Dilated pupil
46. Treatment of datura poisoning is done with:
    a. Pilocarpine
    b. Naloxone
    c. Physostigmine
    d. Neostigmine
47. All are true about atropine poisoning, *except*:
    a. Dilated pupils
    b. Decreased temperature
    c. Dysarthria
    d. Dysphagia
48. A patient presented with bronchodilatation, increased temperature, constipation and tachycardia. Probable diagnosis is poisoning with:
    a. Mushroom
    b. Atropine
    c. Arsenic
    d. Organophosphorus
49. Most common substance abuse in India:
    a. Cannabis
    b. Tobacco
    c. Alcohol
    d. Opium
50. Not a form of cannabis:
    a. Bhang
    b. Charas
    c. Afeem
    d. Ganja
51. Most potent form of cannabis:
    a. Bhang
    b. Charas
    c. Ganja
    d. Hash oil
52. Run-amok is:
    a. Running-away from stressful situation
    b. Killing people randomly
    c. Feeling of insects running under skin
    d. Ingesting corrosive in rage
53. Following are complications of cocaine poisoning, *except*:
    a. Myocardial infarction
    b. Epileptic seizures
    c. Hypothermia
    d. Hypertension

54. An addicted patient presenting with visual and tactile hallucinations, has black staining of tongue and teeth. The agent is:
   a. Cocaine
   b. Cannabis
   c. Heroin
   d. Opium
55. A person feels that small insects are creeping on the skin giving rise to itching sensation; the condition is seen in:
   a. Cocaine poisoning
   b. OPC poisoning
   c. Morphine poisoning
   d. Alcohol withdrawal
56. Itai-itai disease is caused by:
   a. Arsenic
   b. Barium
   c. Cadmium
   d. Chromium

ANSWERS

1. c	2. c	3. a	4. a	5. c	6. c	7. b	8. a	9. c	10. d
11. b	12. d	13. a	14. c	15. a	16. a	17. c	18. c	19. d	20. a
21. c	22. c	23. a	24. a	25. b	26. b	27. b	28. a	29. c	30. c
31. a	32. a	33. b	34. b	35. d	36. c	37. c	38. c	39. d	40. d
41. a	42. d	43. b	44. b	45. c	46. c	47. b	48. b	49. a	50. c
51. d	52. b	53. c	54. a	55. a	56. c				

CHAPTER 31

Cardiac Poisons

KEY WORDS

Nicotine, *Nerium odorum*, cerbera thevetia, digoxin, aconite, hippus.

FM10.1 Describe general principles and basic methodologies in treatment of poisoning: Decontamination, supportive therapy, antidote therapy, procedures of enhanced elimination with regard to: Cardiovascular toxicology cardiotoxic plants—oleander, odollam, aconite, digitalis.

NAME SOME IMPORTANT CARDIAC POISONS? (FM10.1)

Poisons which are primarily cardiotoxic and acts directly on the heart are:
- *Nicotiana tabacum* (tobacco)
- *Digitalis purpurea*
- *Aconite* (Monk's hood)
- *Nerium odorum* (white oleander)
- *Cerbera thevetia* (yellow oleander)
- Cerbera odollam and quinine.

WRITE SHORT NOTES ON NICOTINE? (FM10.1)

Nicotiana tabacum (Tobacco)

- The plant is widely cultivated throughout the world for preparation of tobacco.
- It is a shrub with blue flowers; the leaves contain the active principal nicotine which is volatile and bitter in taste.
- Tobacco is smoked, sniffed and also chewed; nicotine is a CNS stimulant.

Absorption

- Each cigarette contains about 15 to 20 mg of nicotine, of which 1 to 2 mg is absorbed through the alveoli during smoking.
- Nicotine is rapidly absorbed through mucus membranes, lungs and skin.
- About 80 to 90% of the absorbed nicotine is metabolized in liver and excreted through kidneys.

Chronic Poisoning

Chronic tobacco users usually get addicted to nicotine; symptoms include dyspnea, wheezing, tremors, insomnia, anxiety, palpitation, headache, irregular heartbeat and angina pain; these individuals have increase chances of bronchitis, oral cancer, lung cancer and chronic heart diseases.

Withdrawal Symptoms

- Intense urge to smoke, headache, anxiety, impaired concentration and memory, muscle cramps and sleep disturbances are usually present.
- Nicotine replacement therapy (NRT) by chewing gum, electric cigars, nasal spray and inhalers are used during the withdrawal phase; it may take a few weeks to completely get adopted.
- **Fatal dose:** 50 to 100 mg of nicotine; 15 to 30 g of tobacco.

Postmortem Findings

Signs of asphyxia, brown froth in moth and nostrils, patchy hemorrhages on stomach mucosa and pulmonary edema may be noticed; fragments of tobacco may be present in the stomach, if ingested.

Forensic Significance

- Tobacco is the commonest abused drug worldwide.
- Most cases of death are due to accidental over dosage, either consumption of large doses or heavy smoking.
- Rarely tobacco is used for **malingering**; tobacco is soaked in water and held beneath the axilla the whole night by a bandage; symptoms of poisoning occur in the morning. The axillary areas are stained with tobacco and the odor of tobacco can be perceived on the skin.

WHAT IS DIGITALIS? (FM10.1)

Digitalis purpurea is a cardiotoxic poisonous plant; active principals are digitalin, digoxin, digitoxin and many more glycosides, they are more concentrated in the leaves and seeds.

Signs and Symptoms

- **GIT:** Nausea, vomiting, anorexia and diarrhea.
- **Visual:** Photophobia, diplopia and blurring of vision. Skin: Urticaria.
- **CNS:** Headache, fatigue, anxiety, depression, confusion, disorientation, drowsiness and sometimes delirium and hallucinations.
- **Cardiac:** Arrhythmias, tachycardia, ventricular fibrillation, atrial flutter, SV and AV block. Death occurs due to cardiovascular collapse.
- **Fatal dose:** 5 mg of digitoxin; 10 mg digoxin; 15 to 30 mg of digitalin and leaves 2 g.
- **Fatal period:** Few hours to one day, depending on the dose.

Treatment

- Stomach wash with tannic acid. Bowel evacuation followed by activated charcoal.
- Digoxin specific fragment (**FAB**) therapy.
- In the absence of FAB, injection **lignocaine and propranolol** are given.
- Other supportive treatment include—potassium salts to reduce extrasystole and arrhythmias; bradycardia with atropine and trisodium EDTA to lower serum calcium.

WRITE ABOUT ACONITE? (FM10.1)

What is Hippus?

- *Aconitum ferox* is an herb with purple flowers widely grown in the foothills of Himalayas (**Fig. 31.1**). The root contains the active principal aconitine (**Monk's hood**, devil's helmet).
- The dry root is conical and tapering, and shows scars of broken rootlets.

Signs and Symptoms

- Tingling and numbness on contact with the skin, mouth and throat when swallowed.
- Nausea, salivation and vomiting.

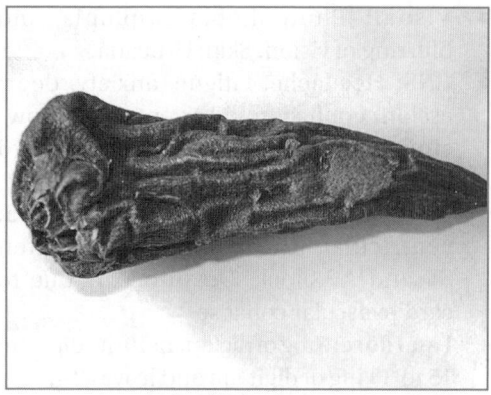

Fig. 31.1: Aconite root (Monk's Hood)
(For color version see Plate 21).

- Muscular weakness, headache, giddiness, profuse sweating and convulsions are present.
- **CVS:** Hypotension, arrhythmias and AV block; first there is tachycardia, later on due to AV block there is bradycardia. Death is due to cardiac arrest.

Hippus

- Alternative constriction and dilatation of the pupil (spasmodic pupil) is called as "hippus"; but the pupils remain dilated at later stage. There is dim of vision and diplopia.
- **Fatal dose:** 1 g of the root; 2 to 5 mg of aconitine.
- **Fatal period:** 2 to 6 hours.

Treatment

Gastric lavage with warm water and weak solution of potassium iodide or tannic acid; atropine 1 mg may be useful; rest are all symptomatic management.

Postmortem Appearance

- Not characteristic, except for signs of asphyxia.
- The stomach and duodenum show congestion and ecchymosis.
- **Heart:** Subepicardial petechio-ecchymotic hemorrhage on the left ventricle and other regions of the heart is a frequent finding.

Circumstances of Poisoning

- Accidental poisoning by eating the roots mistaking for horseradish root.
- **Homicide:** Aconite is said to be ideal homicidal poisons, as it difficult to detect by chemical analysis and symptoms resemble a natural disease (cardiac arrest).
- Occasionally aconite is mixed with liquor to enhance the kick.
- Used as an abortifacient; and is a constituent of many folk remedies, mainly ayurveda.
- Aconite is a cattle poison and is also used as a arrow poison.

WHAT ARE OLEANDERS? WHAT ARE THE TYPES? (FM10.1)

- *Nerium odorum* is white oleander.
- *Cerebera thevetia* is yellow oleander.
  Nerium odorum is white oleander, shown in **Figure 31.2**.
- *Nerium odorum* is an ornamental shrub widely grown all over India; it bears flowers in terminal clusters; flowers are

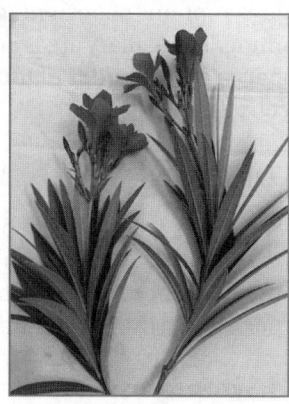

Fig. 31.2: Nerium odorum
(For color version see Plate 22).

white or pink in color. Leaves are narrow, lanceolate and dark green in color. Seeds are long, narrow and cylindrical of 5 to 10 cm long.
- All parts of the plant are poisonous, particularly leaves, root and stem; active principal is **Nerin** and **Oleandrin**.

Cerebera thevetia is yellow oleander (pila kaner)
- It is a large, bushy ornamental shrub, grows to 6 to feet in height; leaves are oblong; flowers are tubular and yellow in color. Fruits are green and globular in shape; 3 to 5 seeds are present inside the fruit and they are vaguely heart shaped.
- All parts of the plant are poisonous and exude milky white juice; the seeds and leaves are more toxic contains **glycosides thevetin, thevetoxin** and **neriifolin** as active ingredients.

WHAT ARE THE SIGNS AND SYMPTOMS AND TREATMENT OF OLEANDER POISONING? (FM10.1)

Signs and Symptoms

- Numbness in the mouth, burning sensation and dryness in the mouth and throat.
- Nausea, vomiting and diarrhea.
- Difficulty in swallowing, abdominal pain and diarrhea.
- Headache, giddiness, loss of muscular power and fainting.
- Pulse is rapid, weak and irregular; fall in BP, hypotension, heart block and collapse.
- Ventricular fibrillation, hypotension, AV block and death due to cardiac failure.
- Pupils are dilated, drowsiness, muscular twitching and spasms.
- Death is due to peripheral circulatory failure.
- **Fatal dose:** 15 to 20 g; 5 to 15 leaves; seeds: 5 to 8; fatal period: 24 hours.

Treatment

- Stomach wash; ECG monitoring.
- IV sodium molar solution and 5% dextrose to combat shock.
- Atropine 1 mg, adrenaline 0.2 mL and noradrenaline 2 mg IV or infusion.

Circumstances of Poisoning

- Commonly used as a suicidal poison. Homicide is rare.
- Used as an abortifacient and as a cattle poison.

MULTIPLE CHOICE QUESTIONS

1. **On autopsy shows signs of asphyxia in which of the following poisons:**
    a. Strychnine
    b. Aconite
    c. Nicotine
    d. All of the above
2. **One of the following is not a cardiac poison:**
    a. Aconite
    b. Curare
    c. Oleander
    d. Nicotine
3. **Hippus occurs in _____ poisoning.**
    a. Opium
    b. Curare
    c. Aconite
    d. Datura

ANSWERS

1. d   2. b   3. c

32
CHAPTER

Asphyxiants

KEY WORDS

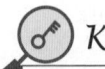

Asphyxiants, carbon monoxide, carboxy hemoglobin, cherry red discoloration, cyanide, cyan methemoglobin, cytochrome oxidase, nitrites, war gases, simple asphyxiants, tear gases.

FM9.6 Describe general principles and basic methodologies in treatment of poisoning: Decontamination, supportive therapy, antidote therapy, procedures of enhanced elimination with regard to ammonia, carbon monoxide, hydrogen cyanide and methyl-isocyanate, tear (riot control) gases.

WHAT IS THE MECHANISM OF ACTION, SIGNS AND SYMPTOMS AND TREATMENT OF CARBON MONOXIDE POISONING? (FM 9.6)

- Carbon monoxide is chemical asphyxiants; CO combines with hemoglobin and forms carboxyhemoglobin (CO-Hb).
- Hemoglobin has 2100 times more affinity to CO than oxygen and hence, hemoglobin readily combines with CO, even if oxygen is present.
- Combustion of any carbon particle results in the formation of carbon dioxide; but when there is incomplete combustion it results in the production of carbon monoxide.
- In any combustion process there cannot be complete combustion and hence in all such situations there is liberation carbon monoxide also, to some extent; there are more chances of formation of CO when, there is wetness on the carbon particle (trees, plants and wood).

Sources

Coal gas, smoke from fire, fumes from defective heating appliances, fumes of internal combustion engines, cigarette smoking, motor car exhaust, etc.

Properties of CO

CO is a colorless, odorless and tasteless non-irritant gas; it is lighter than air, insoluble in water and burns with a blue flame.

Mechanism of Action

- CO is absorbed across the alveoli, readily combines with hemoglobin displacing oxygen and forms CO-Hb; reduces oxygen content of the blood and results in anemic anoxia and produces rapid death.

- CO is a cellular toxin; it inhibits electron transport by inhibiting cytochrome A and cytochrome p450 enzyme systems and thus interferes with cellular respiration.
- **Elimination:** CO is eliminated through lungs; about one percent is converted to carbon dioxide.

Signs and Symptoms

- CO directly damages the CNS causing headache and monoplegia or hemiplegia.
- Impairment of higher intellectual functions.
- Cerebellar changes and personality changes.
- Parkinsonism.
- Subcutaneous bullae common in the regions of calves, buttocks, wrists and knees.

Table 32.1 is depicted the signs and symptoms of CO poisoning.

Treatment

- Remove from the source of exposure and expose to fresh air.
- 100% oxygen therapy through tight fitting mask or by using endotracheal tube.

TABLE 32.1: Signs and symptoms of CO poisoning.

CO %	Symptoms produced
0 to 10%	No symptoms
10 to 20%	Headache and shortness of breath
20 to 30%	Headache, shortness of breath, nausea and dizziness
30 to 40%	Severe headache, fatigue and vomiting
40 to 50%	Mental confusion, increased heart rate and respiratory rate
50 to 60%	Passing out, seizures and coma
60 to 70%	Rapidly fatal

- Hyperbaric oxygen (HBO) is the antidote but should be used with caution as there are serious risks like gas embolism, visual defects, pulmonary edema and convulsions.
- Complete rest and prophylactic antibiotics.
- Treat cerebral edema by giving steroids, mannitol and fluid restriction.

WHAT IS THE POSTMORTEM FINDINGS AND CIRCUMSTANCES OF CO POISONING? (FM9.6)

Postmortem Appearance

- Cherry red discoloration of the skin, mucous membrane, conjunctiva, nail bed, blood and internal organs.
- Cutaneous blisters on the skin of calf, buttock, wrist and knees.
- Lungs are congested with pink colored blood in the alveoli; pulmonary edema.
- Heart may show areas of focal necrosis on the myocardium.
- Brain is edematous; bilateral symmetrical necrosis and cavitation of basal ganglia may be seen; hemorrhages in the meninges and cortex may also be present.

Circumstances of Acute CO Poisoning

- Accidental is the commonest mode of death due to CO poisoning; an individual trapped inside the burning house or due to automobile exhaust, etc.
- Homicide and suicide are rare in occurrence.
- Since, CO is nonirritant and pleasant gas, the individual is totally unaware that he is inhaling CO and hence he may not get away from that place and soon becomes unconscious and death is ensured.

WHAT ARE THE CIRCUMSTANCES OF CHRONIC CO POISONING? (FM9.6)

- Chronic poisoning results from inhalation of relatively higher concentration of CO (below 20%) in respired air, commonly encountered as an occupational hazard, especially in individuals working in automobile and smelting industries.
- Symptoms of chronic poisoning are headache, confusion, weakness, paresthesias, hypertension, hyperthermia and palpitations.

WHAT IS THE SPECIMEN TO BE PRESERVED AND TESTS FOR DETECTION OF CO? (FM9.6)

Specimens

Note:
- Liquid paraffin should be added to the top of the sample of blood, to prevent evaporation of carbon monoxide. 100 mL of blood with sodium fluoride as preservative.
- If blood is not available, then spleen or muscles can be used as sample.
- In badly burnt bodies, the body fluids or bone marrow can be used as specimen.
- Other methods of detection in the laboratory are nondispersive infrared spectrophotometry and gas chromatography.

Test for Detection of CO

- Add 2 drops of sample blood to 15 mL of water in a test tube and seen through light, it will appear pink if carbon monoxide is present.
- **Kunkel's test:** If tannic acid is mixed with the sample, it gives a cherry red color.
- Spectroscopic examination of blood reveals bands of carboxyhemoglobin.

- **Note:** In smokers the concentration of CO at all times is 6 to 8% (<4% in nonsmokers).

WHAT ARE SYMPTOMS OF CO_2 POISONING? (TABLE 32.2)

TABLE 32.2: Concentration of carbon dioxide (CO_2) in air and symptoms.

Concentration of CO_2 in air	Symptoms
1%	Drowsiness
3%	Mild narcosis, reduced hearing, increased BP and heart rate
5%	Headache, confusion, dizziness and shortness of breath
8%	Profuse sweating, muscular tremors, dimmed vision and unconsciousness

WHAT ARE THE PROPERTIES, USES AND SOURCES OF HYDROCYANIC ACID? (FM9.6)

Properties

- Cyanide exists in the form of gas (hydrogen cyanide), liquid (hydrocyanic acid or prussic acid) and solid (salts of cyanide as potassium cyanide, sodium cyanide, etc).
- Hydrogen cyanide has a bitter almonds odor, which is not perceived by 40% (mostly males) of the world population, inherited as sex linked recessive trait.

Uses

- **Industrial:** Electroplating, photography, rubber and plastic industries.
- **Agricultural:** Rodenticide and insecticide.
- **Therapeutic:** Cancer (amygdalin), antihypertensive (sodium nitroprusside).

Sources

- **Plants:** A wide variety of plants (almonds, apricot, apple, peach, cherry, plum, etc.) possess cyanogenic glycosides; on hydrolysis of these glycosides in the GI tract, hydrocyanic acid is released.
- Burning plastics, silk, wool, cigarettes, etc., results in liberation of cyanide.

WHAT IS THE MECHANISM OF ACTION, SIGNS AND SYMPTOMS AND TREATMENT OF HCN? (FM9.6)

Action

- Cyanide inhibits cytochrome oxidase and carbonic anhydrase enzyme systems, thus interferes with the cellular respiration; it blocks the final step of oxidative phosphorylation and prevents formation of ATP.
- There is formation of **cyanme-themoglobin** and the blood is bright red in color. Oxygen will be available in the blood, but the tissues are unable to utilize oxygen, since cytochrome oxidase is necessary for uptake of oxygen by the tissues.
- Color of reduced blood is blue, normal blood is red in color. Color of oxygenated blood is scarlet red; in cyanide it is bright red (more pronounced) and in CO it is cherry red (most pronounced).

Signs and Symptoms

- The most rapidly acting poison and hence used by terrorists to commit suicide.
- When inhaled in gaseous form, action is instantaneous. When consumed as a salt, the symptoms are proportional to the dose; when a massive dose is ingested, there is sudden loss of consciousness and immediate death due to respiratory arrest; sometimes the symptoms are delayed for a few minutes.
- **CNS:** Headache, vertigo, perspiration, anxiety, confusion, drowsiness, convulsions, coma and death.
- **GIT:** Bitter burning taste, numbness, nausea and rarely vomiting.
- **RS:** Smell of bitter almonds in breath, tachyapnea, later slowing of respiration.
- **CVS:** Tachycardia, hypotension and collapse.
- **Skin:** Perspiration and subcutaneous bullae; pupils are dilated and there is acidosis.
- **Fatal dose:** 50 to 60 mg of acid; 200 to 300 mg of salt; concentration of 1:500 in air.
- **Fatal period:** Immediate by inhalation; half an hour with salts.

Treatment of Cyanide Poisoning

- The principal of treatment is to reverse cyanide-cytochrome combination.
- Treatment should be started immediately and stomach wash at later stage even if ingested.
  - **Amyl nitrite inhalation** for 15 to 30 minutes and repeated if necessary.
  - **Sodium nitrite** 0.3 mg in 10 mL distilled water by slow IV injection. There is formation of methemoglobin which competes with cytochrome oxidase for cyanide ions, thus protecting cytochrome oxidase.
  - **Sodium thiosulphate** 25 g as 15% solution by slow IV over a period of 3 minutes; it converts cyanide into nontoxic thiocyanate. All these are repeated when necessary.

Other Treatment Measures

- Hydroxocobalamine 4 to 5 g by slow IV as infusion. It detoxifies cyanide by giving a hydroxyl group, binds a cyanyl group from the cyanide; forming nontoxic cyanocobalamin, which is excreted in urine.

- Dicobalt EDTA acts by chelating cyanide to form harmless compound and is excreted in urine.
- Gastric lavage using 1:5000 potassium permanganate.
- Ventilation with 100% oxygen.
- Methemoglobin more than 50% is an indication for exchange transfusion.

WHAT ARE THE POSTMORTEM FINDINGS AND FORENSIC SIGNIFICANCE OF CYANIDE?

Postmortem Appearance

- Postmortem staining and blood will be bright red in color.
- All the signs of asphyxia are present.
- Jaws may be tightly closed and blood-stained froth may be present in mouth and nostrils, and will be also present inside the bronchial tree.
- The cranial cavity is opened first, as the smell of bitter almonds may be perceived better in the brain.

Forensic Significance

- Usually suicidal by those who have the access to the salts like people engaged in gold industry or laboratories. Sometimes, accidental or the fumes could be inhaled.
- **Homicide:** Cases are reported from time to time, where deaths have been successfully accomplished by administration of cyanide salts.
- Viscera should be preserved in tight containers, as it is lost during storage.

WRITE SHORT NOTES ON WAR GASES? (FM9.6)

- These are a group of chemical substances which are harmful to human beings and are mostly used in war times.
- Irritant gases, simple asphyxiants and tear gases are used to control riots in emergency situations by the authorities to disperse the crowd of people.

Vesicants

- Volatile liquids mainly mustard gas and lewisite are used as vesicants (blistering gases).
- Mustard gas causes irritation of the eyes, nose and respiratory passages; they also produce nausea, vomiting and abdominal pain. It can penetrate the clothing and thus produce intense itching, redness, vesication and ulceration.
- **Treatment:** Wash the affected area with plenty of water; eyes are irrigated with sodium bicarbonate solution, if necessary BAL is given.

Tear Gases or Lachrymators

- These substances produce severe irritation of the eyes and produce copious amount of tears.
- Chloroacetophenone (CAS), ethyl Iodoacetate (KSK) and bromobenzyl cyanide (BBC) are used as tear gases.
- They are fired in artillery shells or pen guns, the vapors produced causes severe irritation of the eyes and results in production of excessive tears, followed by spasm of the eyelids and temporary blindness. These gases also irritate the air passages; continued exposure is associated with nausea and vomiting and may also cause skin blisters.

Treatment

- All the effects are transitory and are reversible on removal from the source of exposure.
- The patient is removed to fresh air; eyes are washed with normal saline or boric

acid; sodium bicarbonate is applied to the affected areas of skin and blisters.

RESPIRATORY IRRITANTS OR SIMPLE ASPHYXIANTS

- Chlorine and phosgene (gases) and chloropicrin and diphosgene (liquids) are released in gas shells. Chlorine has mild toxicity; phosgene and chloropicrin have more potent toxic effects.
- **Action:** These gases when inhaled produces cough, dyspnea, a feeling of tightness of chest, and shortness of breath. They also produce irritation of the eyes, headache, nausea, vomiting, restlessness and the patient may sometimes collapse.
- Death may result in 48 hours due to acute pulmonary edema.
- **Treatment:** Eyes are washed with boric acid solution; adrenaline and oxygen inhalation are given. Antitussives and antibiotics may also be necessary and beneficial.

Nasal Irritants or Sternutators

- Organic compounds arsenic used as nasal irritants and are fired using artillery shells.
- They are composed of diphenyl chlorarsine (DA), diphenylamine chlorarsine (DM) and diphenyl cyanarsine (CD).
- The vapors cause irritation of the nasal mucosa and sinuses, resulting in sneezing, severe headache and nose pain; they also produce nausea, excessive salivation, vomiting and prostration.
- Diphenylamine chlorarsine (DM) is called as "sickness gas" and acts specifically on the vomiting center in the brain.
- **Treatment:** Remove from the source of exposure and symptomatic treatment.

Nerve Gases

- They are colorless and odorless volatile liquids, resembling phosphate esters in action.
- They are well absorbed through skin, conjunctiva, lungs and GIT.
- They inactivate cholinesterase and acetylcholine, resulting in nerve block.

MEDICO-LEGAL SIGNIFICANCE OF WAR GASES

Apart from usage of various types of these gases in wars depending on the necessity, vesicants and tear gases are used to control riots in the public. Rarely some cases may end up in fatality.

MULTIPLE CHOICE QUESTIONS

1. **Cherry red postmortem staining is seen in poisoning with:**
   a. Cyanide
   b. Carbon dioxide
   c. Carbon monoxide
   d. Phosphine gas
2. **Bluish green postmortem staining is seen in:**
   a. Hydrogen sulfide
   b. Carbon monoxide
   c. Hydrogen cyanide gas
   d. Phosphorus
3. **Treatment of carbon monoxide poisoning is:**
   a. Ascorbic acid
   b. Intravenous methylene blue
   c. 100% oxygen
   d. None of the above
4. **Cyanide inhibits:**
   a. Sulfhydryl group of enzymes
   b. Cytochrome oxidase
   c. Pyruvate kinase
   d. Acetyl choline

ANSWERS

1. c   2. a   3. c   4. b

CHAPTER 33

Miscellaneous Poisons

 KEY WORDS

Food poisoning, toxins, mushroom, botulism, marine food, food allergy, ptomaines.

FM8.6 Describe the general symptoms, principles of diagnosis and management of common poisons encountered in India.

DEFINE FOOD POISONING: WHAT ARE THE COMMON CAUSES OF FOOD POISONING? (FM8.6)

Definition

- WHO defines food poisoning as "diseases usually either infectious or toxic in nature caused by agents that enter the body through ingestion of food".
- It includes all illnesses which results from ingestion of food containing bacterial or nonbacterial products.

Causes of Food Poisoning

- Bacteria and their toxins
- Poisons of vegetable origin
- Poisons of animal origin
- Chemicals.

WRITE SHORT NOTES ON BACTERIAL FOOD POISONING: WHAT IS BOTULISM?

Infectious Type

- Symptoms of poisoning are produced by multiplication of the pathogenic organisms inside the human body transferred from food. Example: *Salmonella, Vibrio*, etc.
- Commonly results in symptoms of gastroenteritis (vomiting and diarrhea).

Toxin Type

- Ingestion of food in which poisonous substances have been formed due to bacterial proliferation.
- **Example:** Exotoxins of staphylococci and botulinum; meat, fish, egg, milk, canned,

preserved meats and imperfectly or uncooked food.
- These exotoxins resist boiling and disintegration by intestinal enzymes.
- Produces diarrhea, nausea, abdominal cramps and vomiting.
- **Diagnosis:** Diagnosis of bacterial food poisoning is by the history, clinical symptoms and isolation of the organisms from the remnants of food materials consumed by the patient.
- **Treatment:** Stomach wash and purgatives, IV fluids, antibiotics and other supportive measures.

Botulism
- It is food poisoning with *Clostridium botulinum*.
- There are no symptoms of gastroenteritis.
- *Clostridium botulinum* does not grow in the body, but produce a potent neurotoxin which is absorbed through the alimentary canal; these toxin are destroyed by heating at 100°C for 10 minutes.
- The toxin inhibits acetylcholine, there by blocking nerve impulses at the myoneural junction, resulting in paralysis of nerve endings.

Signs and Symptoms
- The incubation period is 12 to 36 hours, sometimes prolonged up to 72 hours.
- Initially nausea, vomiting and abdominal pain may be present but are not severe.
- Later on, there are symptoms of sore throat, difficulty in accommodation, diplopia; respiratory insufficiency and urinary retention; progressing onto descending bilateral symmetrical motor paralysis.
- Patient is conscious till death; death is preceded by delirium and coma.

Differential Diagnosis
- Botulism has to be differentiated from encephalitis, Gullian Barre syndrome, tetanus and elapid snake bite.

- Botulism toxin is one of the most potent toxins affecting the human body and the mortality rate is as high as 25%. After death, if liver and kidneys are subjected histopathological examination, they may reveal thrombosis formation.
- **Diagnosis:** It is made out from the history, clinical symptoms, demonstration of toxin in the blood, vomitus and feces of the patient and by demonstration of *Bacillus* and toxins in the remnant food materials.

Treatment
- Gastric lavage, purgatives and whole bowel irrigation.
- Activated charcoal.
- Botulinum antitoxin slow infusion in normal saline.
- Botulism immune globulin (BIG) daily till the patient recovers completely.
- Adequate respiration measures.

WHAT IS FOOD ALLERGY? (FM8.6)
- It is due to some intrinsic abnormalities in the immune system of the body; they are not due to poisonous food materials.
- Some individuals may have hypersensitivity to certain proteins; example: fish, meat, milk, egg or to some vegetables like brinjal.
- The symptoms developed are relatively harmless like urticaria, rashes, asthmatic attacks, or symptoms of gastroenteritis like nausea, vomiting and diarrhea.

WHAT ARE PTOMAINES?
- Ptomaines are alkaloid bodies formed as a result of bacterial decomposition of proteins. When these ptomaines are formed in dead bodies they are called as "cadaveric alkaloids".
- Those alkaloids which are secreted by living cells during metabolism are called "leucomaines".

- Ptomaines are not bacterial poisons and are not derived from the bacteria; they are only formed from the decomposition of proteins.
- These are detectable only when the food is decomposed and disagreeable to be eaten.
- Most of these ptomaines formed are nontoxic, except a few namely, neurine and mydalein. They have mild toxic effect resembling atropine only when injected into the animal body and not when ingested. These ptomains do not cause any food poisoning.

WRITE SHORT NOTES ON MUSHROOM POISONING? (FM8.6)

- Mushrooms are grown widely in moist woody areas. Some species are nonpoisonous and are used as food, while *Amanita phalloides* and *Amanita muscaria* are well known poisonous mushrooms. Poisonous mushrooms have bitter acid taste and contain some alkaloids as the poisonous ingredient.
- *Amanita phalloides* contains phalloidin which is a powerful inhibitor of cellular protein synthesis; *Amanita muscaria* contains muscarine which stimulates the parasympathetic postganglionic nerve fibers.

Signs and Symptoms

- The toxic alkaloids act both as irritant and neurotic poisons. Some cases may present predominantly with symptoms of irritation, some may present with neurotic symptoms and rarely mixed symptoms in some patients.
- First there are symptoms of irritation up to 12 hours; there is constriction of throat, burning pain in the stomach, nausea, vomiting and diarrhea; followed by sweating, slow pulse, bradycardia, labored respiration and collapse.
- Neurotic symptoms are headache, giddiness, delirium, muscle twitching and cramps, convulsions and coma.
- **Fatal dose:** 2 to 3 mushrooms; fatal period: one day.

Treatment

Stomach wash with potassium permanganate, atropine, fluid replacement and hemodialysis; rest is symptomatic treatment.

Postmortem Findings

- Inflammation of GIT and remnants of mushroom particles may be present inside the stomach. Sometimes fatty degeneration of liver, kidneys and heart may be present. Signs of asphyxia may be evident.
- Poisoning is usually accidental and rarely homicidal or suicidal.

WRITE SHORT NOTES ON FISH AND MARINE ANIMALS POISONING? SHORT NOTES ON: CIGUATERE; TETRODON; JELLYFISH POISONING?

- Marine fish are inherently poisonous, mainly ciguatera poisoning and tetradon poisoning.
- Poisoning could result from bacterial growth in partially decomposed fish.
- By eating some types of sea fish which are by themselves poisonous to humans, like catfish, lion fish, dragon fish (potent neurotoxin).

Ciguatera Poisoning

It affects the GIT and nervous system; produces symptoms are abdominal pain, nausea, vomiting, diarrhea, numbness of tongue and lips; death due to respiratory paralysis.

CHAPTER 33: Miscellaneous Poisons

Tetrodon Poisoning

- Globe fish, balloon fish and blowfish.
- It affects GIT and nervous system; causes neurotoxicity and muscle paralysis.

Shellfish Poisoning

Affects the nervous system, causes muscle paralysis, blurred vision, low BP, unable to breath and results in death.

Venomous Fish

Some sea fish have extremely sharp spines equipped with large poisonous sacs; cooking doesn't destroy the poison; it may cause punctures with swelling which bleed readily.

Box Jellyfish

This is the world's most venomous animal; it has dermal, neurotic and cardiotoxic poison.

MULTIPLE CHOICE QUESTIONS

1. **Drug of choice for muscarine poisoning:**
   a. Atropine
   b. Physostigmine
   c. Adrenaline
   d. Carbachol
2. **Botulinum affects all, *except*:**
   a. NM junction
   b. Preganglionic junction
   c. Postganglionic *jelly fish* junction
   d. CNS
3. **Which poisoning can be prevented by an antitoxin:**
   a. *Staphylococcus aureus*
   b. *Clostridium botulinum*
   c. *Salmonella typhimurium*
   d. *Bacillus cereus*
4. **A young male developed fever of 101.3°F fahrenheit, diarrhea and vomiting after eating chicken salad 24 hours ago after an outing. Two other friends also developed same symptoms. What is the diagnosis?**
   a. *Bacillus cereus* poisoning
   b. *Salmonella enteritis* poisoning
   c. *Staphylococcus aureus* poisoning
   d. *Vibrio cholera* poisoning
5. **Dysarthria, diplopia, dysarthria are characteristics features of food poisoning from:**
   a. *Bacillus cereus*
   b. *Salmonella typhimurium*
   c. *Clostridium botulinum*
   d. *Vibrio cholera*
6. **Epidemic dropsy is caused by:**
   a. Kesari dhal
   b. Argemone oil
   c. Poisonous mushroom
   d. Shellfish
7. **Epidemic dropsy is caused by which toxin?**
   a. Beta oxyl amino alanine
   b. Sanguinarine
   c. Aflatoxin
   d. Pyrrolidine
8. **The following have exotoxins, *except*:**
   a. Cholera
   b. Pertussis
   c. Diphtheria
   d. Hemophilus influenza
9. **BOAA is the active principle of:**
   a. Toor dal
   b. Masoor dal
   c. Kesari dal
   d. Moong dal
10. **The most common type of fish poisoning happens from which type?**
    a. Ciguatera
    b. Tetraodon
    c. Gymnothorax
    d. Scombroid

ANSWERS

1. a   2. d   3. b   4. b   5. c   6. b   7. b   8. d   9. c   10. a

SECTION 8

Practical Examination

SECTION OUTLINE

Exercise 1: Age Estimation by Dentition
Exercise 2: Age Estimation by Radiology
Exercise 3: Examination of Skeletal Remains
Exercise 4: Wound Certificate
Exercise 5: Drunkenness
Exercise 6: Sexual Offence Certificates
Exercise 7: Examination of the Accused of Rape
Exercise 8: Fetal Examination
Exercise 9: Leave Certificate and Certificate of Fitness
Exercise 10: Death Certificate
Exercise 11: Postmortem Certificate
Exercise 12: Spotters

Introduction

The pattern of practical examination differs for various universities, but the total number of marks and set of practical exercises to be covered is made uniform throughout the country as per the CBME curriculum. It may be in the form of major exercise with viva, short cases, objective structured practical examination (OSPE) and spotters. All the practical exercises are covered with sample exercises to enable the students to prepare easily for the practical examinations.

AGE ESTIMATION

Whenever a conflict of age arises in the procedure of investigation, the help of the medical expert is sought for to determine the age of the individual. Each age has got a medico-legal importance and therefore determination of age plays a crucial role in both civil and criminal cases. As far as possible the age estimated should fall within a range of 2 years (Example: 16 to 18 years). After the age of 21 years, it is very difficult to estimate the age of an individual within a range of 5 years (Example: 21 to 25 years).

Example

A victim of sexual offence is referred for age estimation, her alleged age is 18 years; after the radiological examination if the estimated age falls between 17 to 19 years, it is of no use to the court, it rather adds more contradiction that the victim could be <18 years. Here the court wants to know whether she <18 years or more than 18 years of age. Hence, caution should be taken by the expert before arriving at the final opinion regarding the age.

To estimate the age of an individual the following data are taken into consideration:

- **General physical development:** Height, weight chest and abdominal measurements.
- Teeth eruption and completion of root calcification.
- Radiological examination of all the joints (more reliable).
- Secondary sexual characteristics (helps to narrow down the estimated age).
- Closure of skull sutures and degenerative changes (after 25 years).

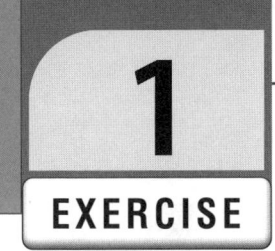

EXERCISE 1

Age Estimation by Dentition

FM14.4 Conduct and prepare report of estimation of age of a person for medico-legal and other purposes and prepare medico-legal report in a simulated/supervised environment.

The eruption of teeth both temporary and permanent has a chronological order and is used for age estimation.
- At birth there are 44 germ tooth presents inside the jaw of a full term baby (20 + 24).
- By 3 years there are totally 20 teeth all are temporary.
- By 6 to 7 years: There are 24 teeth (20 temporary + 4 permanent).
- From 6 to 12 years total number of teeth remains as 24 (mixed dentition).
- By the end of 12 years the total number teeth is 24 (all are permanent).
- By 14 years there are about 28 teeth.
- By 17 to 25 years, there are 32 teeth. Many people do not have 32 teeth, because many a times one of more of the 3rd molar gets impacted; since, there is less space for the 3rd molar to erupt.

From the germ tooth the crown is formed and then erupts outside in the oral cavity; after the eruption of the teeth, the root formation takes place. In the case of temporary teeth, the root resorption takes place and the unsupported crown falls off. In a short while, the respective permanent teeth erupt that pace. In the case of permanent teeth, after the teeth eruption, the root calcification gets completed after 2 years of eruption of the respective teeth and it is 3 years for the 3rd molar tooth. While examining X-rays or OPG, the root of the last erupted tooth and the crown of the next to erupt tooth are taken into consideration to determine the age of an individual. There is wide variation in the eruption of 3rd molar and hence not useful for age estimation.

Eruption of temporary teeth tabulate in **Table E1.1** and eruption of permanent teeth tabulated in **Table E1.2**.

The age of eruption of various teeth is as follows:

TABLE E1.1: Eruption of temporary teeth.

Teeth	Age of eruption	Average age (for remembering easily)
Central incisor—lower	6–8 months	7 months
Central incisor—upper	7–9 months	8 months

Contd...

Contd...

Lateral Incisor —upper	8–10 months	9 months
Lateral incisor—lower	9–11 months	10 months
1st molar	12–14 months (1 year)	12 months (1 year)
Canine	16–18 months (1½ years)	18 months (1½ years)
2nd molar	24–30 months (2 to 2 ½)	2 to 2½ years

TABLE E1.2: Eruption of permanent teeth.

Teeth	Age of eruption	Average age
1st molar	6–7 years	6 years
Central incisor	6–8 years	7 years
Lateral incisor	7–9 years	8 years
1st premolar	8–10 years	9 years
2nd premolar	9–11 years	10 years
Canine	10–12 years	11 years
2nd molar	12–14 years	12–14 years
3rd molar	17–25 years	17–25 years

Charting of Teeth (Figs. E1.1 to E1.4)

Federation Dentaire Internationale (FDI) System

Each tooth is identified by a two-digit number in which, the proximal digit indicates the quadrant and the distal digit indicates the actual tooth. While numbering the permanent teeth 1, 2, 3, 4 are used for designating right upper, left upper, left lower and right lower quadrants respectively. Whereas the quadrants are numbered as 5, 6, 7, 8 for the corresponding temporary teeth.

Permanent Teeth

18	17	16	15	14	13	12	11	21	22	23	24	25	26	27	28
48	47	46	45	44	43	42	41	31	32	33	34	35	36	37	38

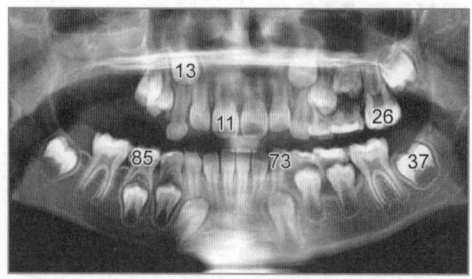

Fig. E1.1: OPG: 1st permanent molar, central and lateral incisors have erupted in all the quadrants. 1st premolar has erupted only in right upper quadrant. Age is 8 to 10 years.

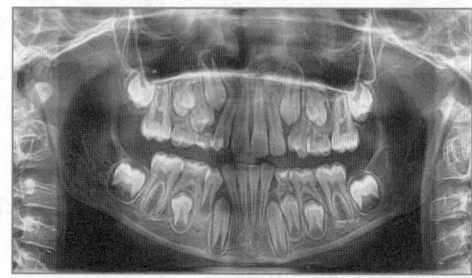

Fig. E1.2: OPG: 1st permanent molar, central and lateral incisors have erupted in all the quadrants. 1st premolar has erupted only in right lower quadrant. Age is 8 to 10 years.

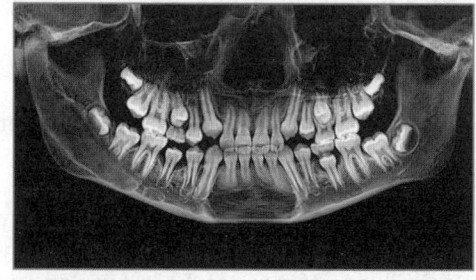

Fig. E1.3: OPG: 1st permanent molar, central incisors, lateral incisors, canines and 1st premolars erupted in all the quadrants. 2nd premolar erupted in lower quadrants and not erupted in upper quadrants. Age is more than 10 years and <12 years.

Temporary Teeth

		55	54	53	52	51	61	62	63	64	65		
		85	84	83	82	81	71	72	73	74	75		

EXERCISE 1: Age Estimation by Dentition

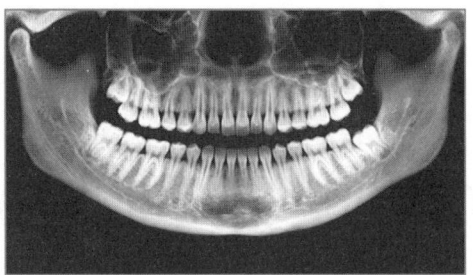

Fig. E1.4: All the permanent teeth up to 2nd molar erupted. 3rd molar erupted in right lower quadrant and root calcification also completed. 3rd molar erupting in all the other quadrants. Age is more than 20 years.

Note: The 3rd molar most of the times gets impacted since there is lack of space for eruption. Also wide range in eruption and hence not useful for age estimation.

Performa for Age Estimation

Department of Forensic Medicine

Name of the individual:
- Age:____ years (as alleged by him)
- Parent/Guardian's name:
- Residential address:
- Person accompanying:
- Time, date and place of examination:
- Informed consent:
- Identification marks:
- Physical examination:
- Height:
- Weight:
- Chest measurement (at the level of nipple)
- Abdominal girth (at the level of umbilicus)
- Examination of eruption of teeth:
- Examination of hair:
- Scalp hair, beard and moustache, axially hair, pubic and hair on other parts of the body.
- Examine the X-rays for appearance and fusion of ossification centers:
- Opinion of age:

Place: Signature of the medical officer.
Date:

Sample Exercise: 1

A dental charting or living individuals or OPG or mandibles wound be provided to the student and asked to estimate the age of the individual from the eruption status of the teeth.

	16	**55**	14	**53**	12	11	21	22	**63**	24	**65**	26	
	46	**85**	44	**83**	42	41	31	32	**73**	34	**75**	36	

Interference: The 1st permanent molar, central and lateral incisors and 1st premolar teeth have erupted. 2nd temporary molars and temporary canines are still present in the oral cavity. While calculating the age, the last erupted tooth and the next to erupt tooth are taken into consideration. 1st premolar erupted (8 to 10 years) and 2nd premolar has not erupted (9 to 11 years) and hence the age is above 8 years and below 11 years.

Sample Exercise: 2

	16	15	14	13	12	11	21	22	**63**	24	25	26	
	46	45	44	**83**	42	41	31	32	**73**	34	35	36	

Permanent canines have erupted in upper right quadrant and all other canines are temporary. All the other teeth are permanent in the oral cavity. The age is 10 to 12 years and any age estimated by dental examination has to be confirmed by radiological examination.

I have seen babies with 2 and 4 teeth present at birth and 8 to 12 teeth by 6 months. Tooth formation and bone development are directly dependent on genetic and the nutritional status of the individual. Age estimation by dentition is always used as corroborative finding. However, it's very useful to narrow down the estimated age in the period of mixed dentition (6 to 12 years).

EXERCISE 2

Age Estimation by Radiology

- Estimation of age is based on the appearance and fusion of various secondary ossification centers in the body.
- The process of bone formation and development is called ossification. The bones of human body develop from a number of ossification centers.
- At 11-12th week of intrauterine life, there are 806 centers of ossification.
- At birth there are about 450 centers; whereas the adult human skeleton carries only 206 bones.
- After birth, the growth of the bone takes place by formation of various secondary ossification centers tabulated in **Table E2.1**. The bone growth gets completed by fusion of the ossification center with the shaft of the respective bones.
- The appearance and fusion of various secondary ossification centers have a sequence and time period; this chronological sequence is used for determination of age **(Table E2.1)**.

On radiological examination of the various joints, the age of the individual is estimated by examining the status of various ossification centers **(Fig. E2.1)**. Shoulder joint depicted in **Figures E2.1 to E2.4**. Elbow joints described in **Table E2.2**, **Figures E2.5 to E2.11**, Wrist joint described in **Table E2.3**, **Figures E2.12 to E2.20**. Hip joint described in **Table E2.4**, **Figures E2.21 to E2.26**. Knee joint described in **Table E2.5**, **Figure E2.27** and ankle joint described in **Table E2.6** and **Figure E2.28**.

Whereas Other important centers tabulated in **Table E2.7** and centers of sternum tabulated in **Table E2.8**.

Students should by heart the table so that he can directly find out the age of any X-ray.

TABLE E2.1: Appearance and fusion of various ossification centers of the body.

Ossification center	Appearance	Fusion
Shoulder joint:		
Head	1 year	
Greater tubercle	3 years	18–19 years
Lesser tubercle	5 years	
Coracoid process	10–11 years	16–18 years
Acromion process	14–15 years	17–18 years
Medial end of clavicle	18–19 years	20–22 years
Articular facets of ribs		25 years

EXERCISE 2: Age Estimation by Radiology

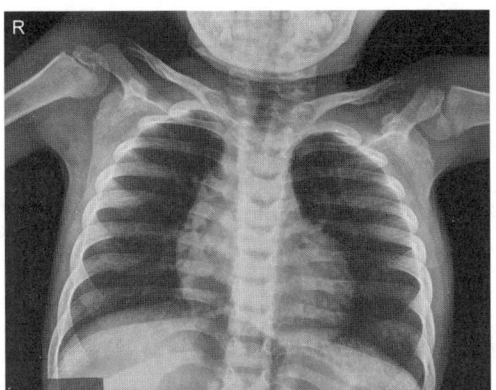

Fig. E2.1: *X-ray shoulder joint:* Center for head of the humerus appeared. Other centers not appeared. Age is more than 1 year and less than 3 years.

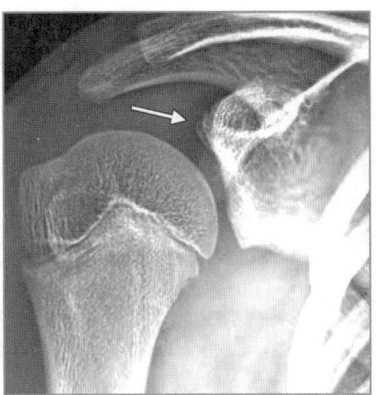

Fig. E2.3: *X-ray shoulder joint:* Ossification centers for head, greater tubercle and lesser tubercle have appeared and conjoint fusion has taken place; center for coracoid process appeared and tip of acromion has not appeared. Age of the individual is more than 10 years and less than 15 years.

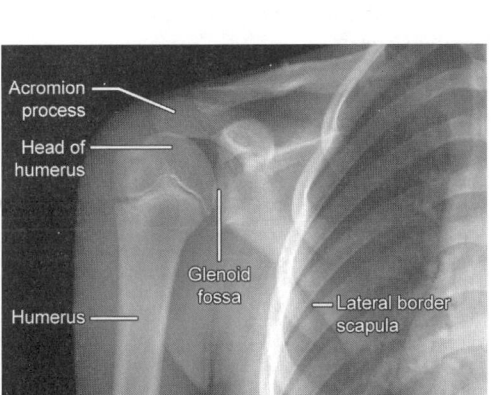

Fig. E2.2: *X-ray shoulder joint:* Ossification centers for head, greater tubercle and lesser tubercle have appeared and conjoint fusion has taken place; center for coracoid process and tip of acromion has not appeared. Age of the individual is more than 5 years and less than 10 years.

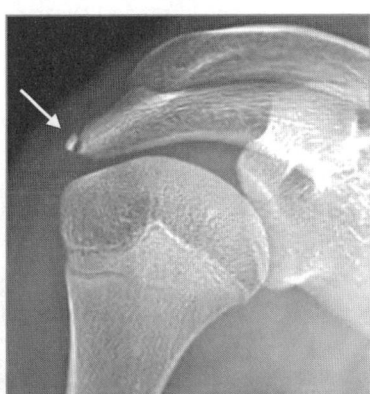

Fig. E2.4: *X-ray shoulder joint:* Ossification centers for head, greater tubercle and lesser tubercle have appeared and conjoint fusion has taken place; center for coracoid process tip of acromion appearing. But none of the centers have fused. Age of the individual is more than 15 years and less than 18 years.

TABLE E2.2: Elbow joint.		
Elbow joint	*Appearance*	*Fusion*
Capitulum	1 year	14–16 years
Medial epicondyle	6–7 years	14–16 years
Trochlea	9–11 years	14–16 years
Lateral epicondyle	11 years	14–16 years
Upper end of radius	5 years	16–17 years
Olecranon process of ulna	9 years	16–17 years

SECTION 8: Practical Examination

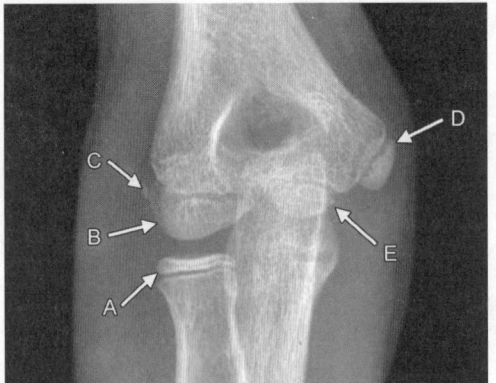

Fig. E2.5: *Elbow joint:* X-ray showing ossification centers of elbow joint. (A) Upper end of radius; (B) Capitulum; (C) Lateral epicondyle; (D) Medial epicondyle and (E) Trochlea and olecranon process of ulna. All the centers have appeared but lateral epicondyle is appearing and not appeared fully. Age is more than 9 years and less than 12 years.

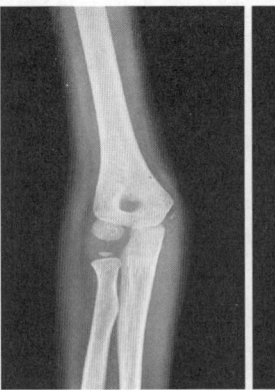 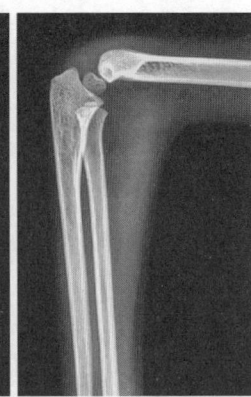

Fig. E2.7: *Elbow joint:* Ossification centers for capitulum and upper end of radius have appeared. The center for medial epicondyle appearing, trochlea, upper end of ulna and lateral epicondyle has not appeared and none of the centers have fused with the shaft. Age is more than 2 years and less than 6 years.

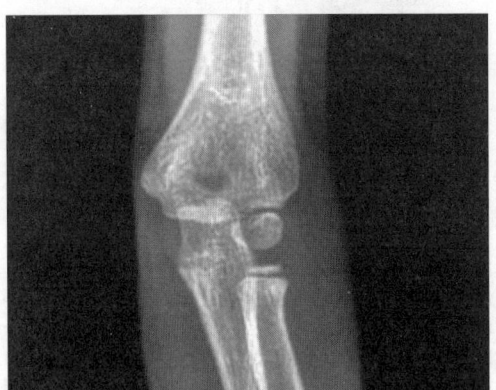

Fig. E2.6: *Elbow joint:* Ossification centers for capitulum and upper end of radius have appeared. The center for medial epicondyle, trochlea, upper end of ulna and lateral epicondyle has not appeared and none of the centers have fused with the shaft. Age is more than 2 years and less than 6 years.

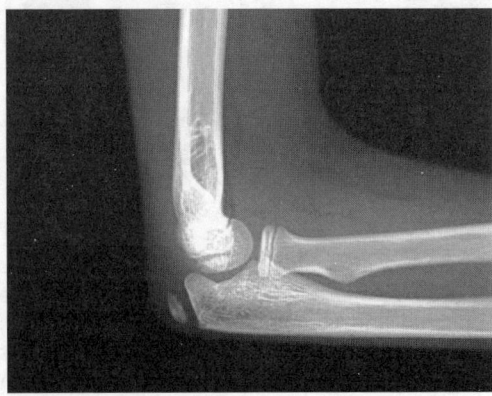

Fig. E2.8: *Elbow joint:* Ossification centers for capitulum, upper end of radius and upper end of ulna appeared, upper end of ulna visible only in flexed lateral view. Lateral epicondyle not appeared. Age is more than 9 years and less than 12 years.

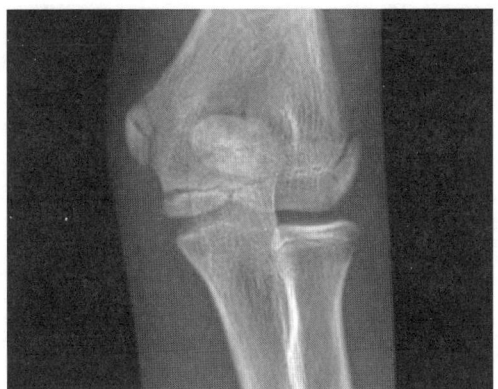

Fig. E2.9: *Elbow joint:* All the centers including lateral epicondyle has appeared and none of the centers have fused with the shaft. Age is more than 11 years and less than 16 years.

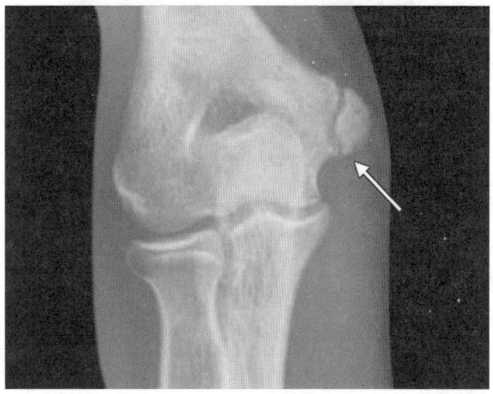

Fig. E2.10: *Elbow joint:* All the ossification centers have appeared; center for capitulum, lateral epicondyle and upper end of ulna have fused. The center for upper end of radius fusing and center for medial epicondyle not fused. Age is 14 to 16 years. (Note: As per the data we follow all the centers of elbow joint fuse by 14 to 16 years, but my experience I come across cases where the medial epicondyle fuses last).

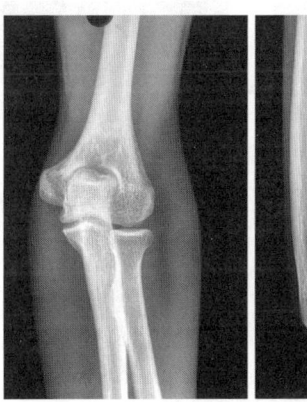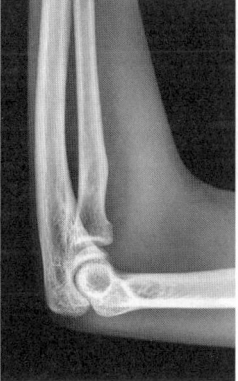

Fig. E2.11: *Elbow joint:* Ossification centers for all the centers appeared and completely fused with the shaft. Age is more than 16 years.

TABLE E2.3: Wrist joint.

Wrist joint	Appearance	Fusion
Lower end of radius	2 years	18–19 years
Lower end of ulna	5–6 years	17–18 years
Capitate	2 months	
Hamate	2 years	
Triquetral	3 years	
Lunate	4 years	
Trapezium	6 years	
Trapezoid	4–5 years	
Scaphoid	4–5 years	
Pisiform	10–12 years	
Base of 1st metacarpal	2–3 years	15–17 years

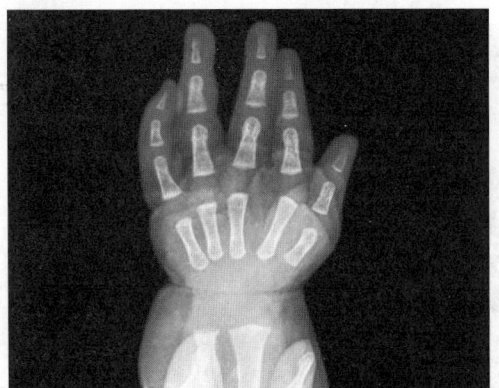

Fig. E2.12: *Wrist joint:* None of the carpal bones have appeared. Age is less than 2 months.

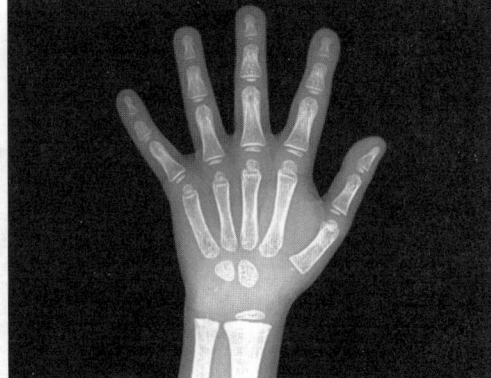

Fig. E2.13: *Wrist joint:* Two carpal bones have appeared, center for lower end of radius appeared and base of 1st metacarpal bone not appeared. Age is more than 2 years and less than 3 years.

EXERCISE 2: Age Estimation by Radiology

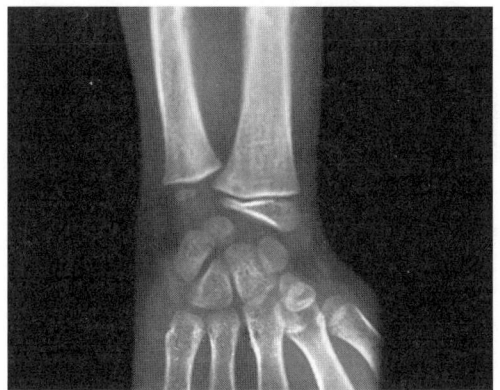

Fig. E2.14: *Wrist joint:* Six carpal bones have appeared, trapezium not appeared, center for lower end of radius appeared and ulna just appearing. Age is more than 5 years and less than 7 years.

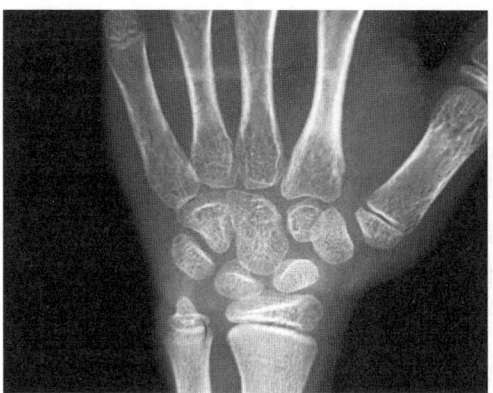

Fig. E2.16: *Wrist joint:* Seven carpal bones have appeared, pisiform not appeared, center base of 1st metacarpal, lower end of radius and ulna have appeared. Age is more than 6 years and less than 12 years.

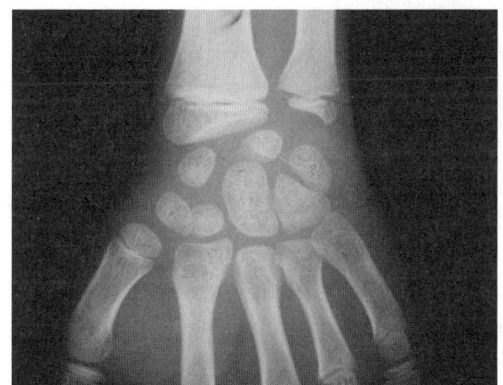

Fig. E2.15: *Wrist joint:* Seven carpal bones have appeared, pisiform not appeared, center for base of 1st metacarpal, lower end of radius and ulna have appeared. Age is more than 6 years and less than 12 years.

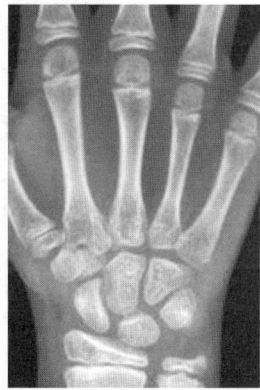

Fig. E2.17: *Wrist joint:* Seven carpal bones have appeared, pisiform not appeared, center base of 1st metacarpal, lower end of radius and ulna have appeared. Age is more than 6 years and less than 12 years.

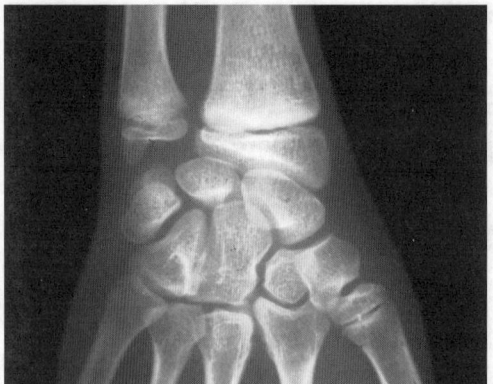

Fig. E2.18: *Wrist joint:* All the carpal bones including pisiform have appeared. Pisiform always is seen as overlapping shadow on trapezoid. The lower end of radius and ulna appeared but not fused. Base of first metacarpal not fused. Age is more than 10 years and less than 15 years.

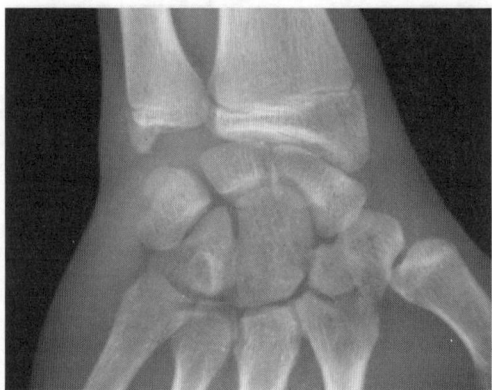

Fig. E2.19: *Wrist joint:* All the carpal bones including pisiform have appeared. The lower end of radius and ulna appeared but not fused. Base of first metacarpal fused. Age is more than 15 years and less than 18 years.

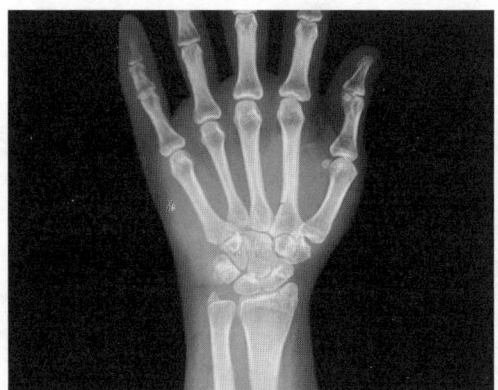

Fig. E2.20: *Wrist joint:* All the carpal bones have appeared. All the centers have fused with the shaft. Age is more than 18 years.

TABLE E2.4: Hip joint.		
Hip joint	**Appearance**	**Fusion**
Ischio-pubic ramus		6th year
Triradiate cartilage		13–15 years
Ischial tuberosity	16–18 years	20–22 years
Iliac crest	14–16 years	20–21 years
Head of femur	1 year	17–18 years
Greater trochanter	4 years	17–18 years
Lesser trochanter	12–14 years	17–18 years

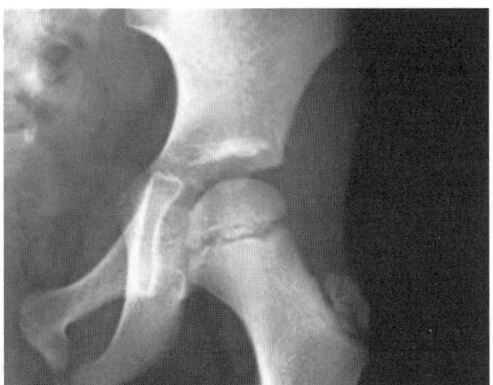

Fig. E2.21: *Hip joint:* Ossification center for head of femur appeared and greater trochanter appeared. Ischiopubic ramus not fused. Age is more than 4 years and less than 6 years.

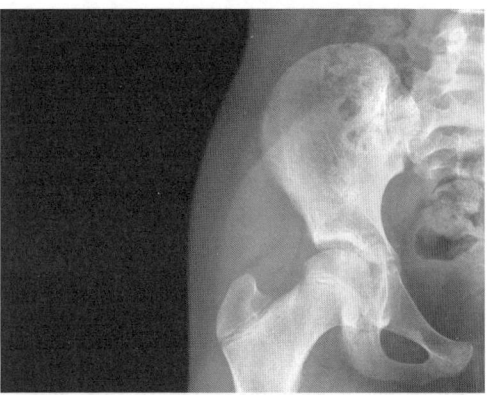

Fig. E2.23: *Hip joint:* Ossification center for head, greater trochanter and lesser trochanter of femur appeared, but not fused. Schiopubic ramus fused. Triradiate cartilage fusing. Age is more than 12 years and less than 15 years.

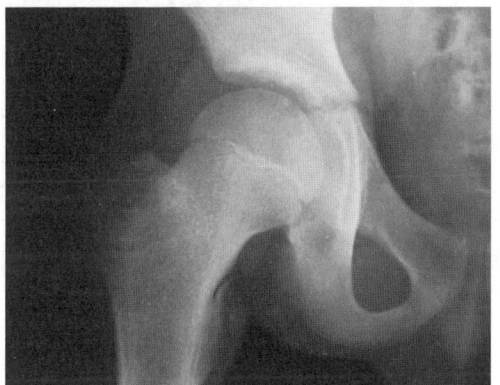

Fig. E2.22: *Hip joint:* Ossification center for head, greater trochanter and lesser trochanter of femur appeared, but not fused with the shaft. Ischiopubic ramus fused. Triradiate cartilage not fused. Age is more than 12 years and less than 15 years.

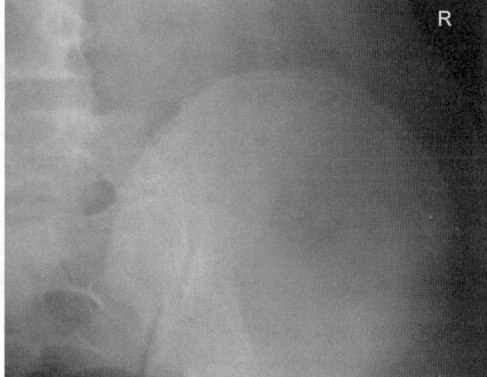

Fig. E2.24: *Hip joint:* Ossification center for iliac crest has appeared. Triradiate cartliage fused. Ischial tuberosity not appeared. Age is more than 14 years and less than 18 years.

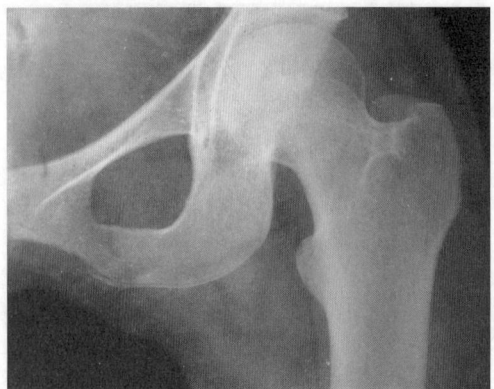

Fig. E2.25: *Hip joint:* Ossification center for ischial tuberosity appeared (16 years). Center for head, greater trochanter and lesser trochanter of femur has fused with the shaft. Age is more than 17 years and less than 20 years.

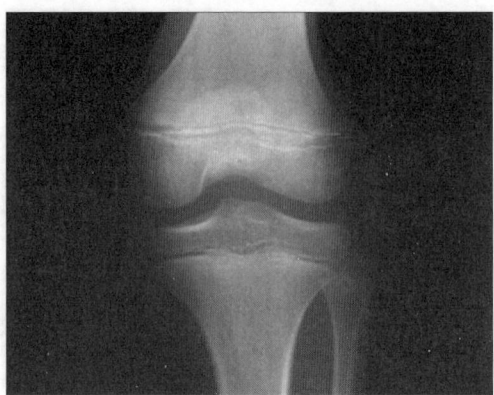

Fig. E2.27: *Knee joint:* Center for lower end of femur and upper end of tibia have appeared but not fused. Age is less than 18 years.

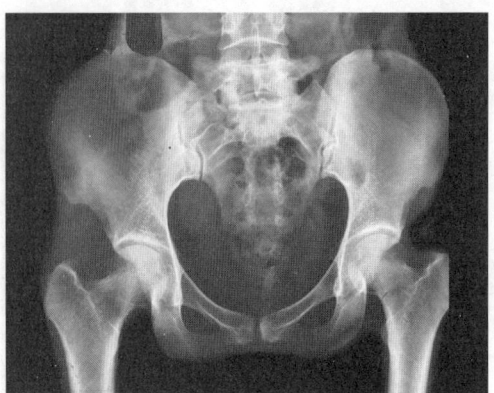

Fig. E2.26: *Hip joint:* All the ossification center have appeared and fused. Age is more than 20 years.

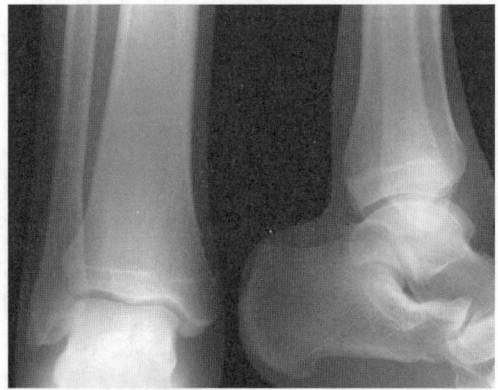

Fig. E2.28: *Ankle joint:* Center for lower end of tibia and fibula have fused. Note: The line of fusion (recently fused). Age is more than 16 years.

TABLE E2.5: Knee joint.		
Knee joint	**Appearance**	**Fusion**
Lower end of femur	9th IU month	18–19 years
Upper end of tibia	At birth	18–19 years
Upper end of fibula	4 years	18–19 years

TABLE E2.6: Ankle joint.		
Ankle joint	**Appearance**	**Fusion**
Lower end of tibia	1 year	16–17 years
Lower end of fibula	1 year	16–17 years

TABLE E2.7: Other important centers.

Other important center	Appearance	Fusion
Basi-sphenoid fuses with the basiocciput		18–20 years
Calcaneum	5th IU month	
Talus	7th IU month	

TABLE E2.8: Centers of sternum.

Sternum		
1st segment	5th IU month	Old age
2nd segment	5th IU month	14–25 years
3rd and 4th segments	7th IU month	14–25 years
5th segment	10 months (at birth)	14 years
Last segment	3 years	40 years

Sample Exercise

X-ray of all the joints is given as photographs and determination of age is discussed.

VIVA Questions (Both for Dental and Radiological Examination)

- Eruption of teeth (temporary and permanent teeth).
- How to differentiate temporary from permanent teeth.
- Mixed dentition.
- Gustafson's method.
- Consent:
  - When any excise is given X-rays, dental examination, wound certificate, drunkenness or sexual offence certificate, everyone should be thorough with consent. Every student is expected to know the definition, types, rules and application of consent for medical practice and medico-legal cases. Consent is discussed in detail in theory, refer Chapter 4.
- Medico-legal importance of various age groups; mainly age 7, 12, 14, 16 and 18 years. Discussed in Chapter 5.

EXERCISE 3

Examination of Skeletal Remains

> **FM14.9** Demonstrate examination of and present an opinion after examination of skeletal remains in a simulated/supervised environment.

A cluster of bones could be brought for examination; the doctor should examine each bone separately and gain as much knowledge as possible about the individual bone, document all the findings separately and then give a collective opinion. All the bones should be examined for features of sex and age. Sex differentiation in skull tabulated in **Table E3.1** and **Figures E3.1** and **E3.2**.

Some other information could be gained depending on the individual bones, e.g., skull for race and long bones for stature. Undergraduate students must be able to examine skull, mandible, pelvis and femur. Sex difference in pelvis bone tabulated in **Table E3.2.** and **Figure E3.3 to E3.6**.

Sacrum depicted in **Figures E3.7**. Sex difference in mandible tabulated in **Table E3.3** and **Figure E3.8**.

Age estimation from skull is started from the base and then the vault is examined for suture closure: The basisphenoid fuses with the basiocciput by 18 to 20 years. Then, the teeth are examined and lastly the fusion of skull sutures is examined to arrive at the age of the given skull. Closure of skull sutures tabulated in **Table E3.4.** The skull sutures starts fusion first on the inner surface, endocranially the fusion starts 5 to 10 years earlier than the ectocranium. Hence, during examination the inner table is first examined using a torch light through the foramen magnum. Some of the indices useful to determine the sex are described in **Table E3.5** and sex difference in femur described in **Table E3.6** and **Figures E3.9 to E3.10**.

In cases of examination of bones, the doctor should be able to answer the following:

WHETHER THE GIVEN BONES BELONG TO HUMAN OR ANIMAL?

By the morphological appearance and knowledge of anatomy it can be easily found out as the bones are of human origin or animal origin.

In case of long bones, when the entire bone is available there exists no difficulty in finding out the origin of the bone, but when the ends are not present and only the shaft

TABLE E3.1: Sex differentiation in skull.

Features	Male	Female
General appearance	Larger, rough with more prominent muscular markings in the temporal and occipital areas	Smaller and smooth
Capacity	1500 cc	1400 cc
Frontal eminence	Slopping	Vertical
Parietal eminence	Less pronounced	More pronounced
Occipital protuberance	Prominent	Less prominent or absent
Glabella	More prominent	Less prominent and smooth
Supra-orbital ridges	More prominent	Less prominent or absent
Fronto-nasal junction	Distinct angulation	Smooth curved
Orbits	Square shaped, placed relatively low on face, margins are rounded	Rounded, higher on face, margins are sharp
Cheek bones	Heavy, broad and laterally arched	Light, small and compressed
Zygomatic arch	More prominent	Less prominent
Mastoid process	Large and rounded	Small and pointed
Digastrics groove	Deep	Shallow
Condylar facets	Long and slender	Short and broad
Foramen magnum	Large	Small
Palate	Large, broad and 'U' shaped	Small and parabola in shape
Tooth sachets	Large	Small

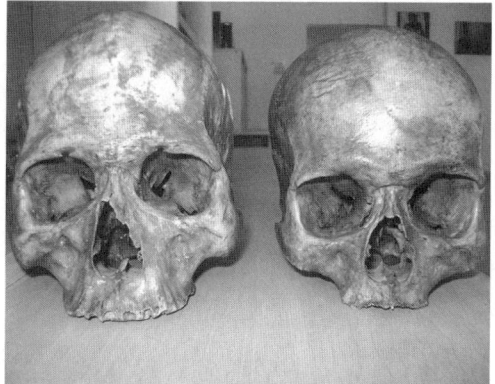

Fig. E3.1: *Skull:* Male and female skull: Sloping forehead, square and low placed orbits, large cheek bones and prominent supraorbital ridges—features of male skull; steep forehead, highly placed orbits, less prominent supraorbital ridges and less prominent muscular markings—features of female skull *(For color version see Plate 22).*

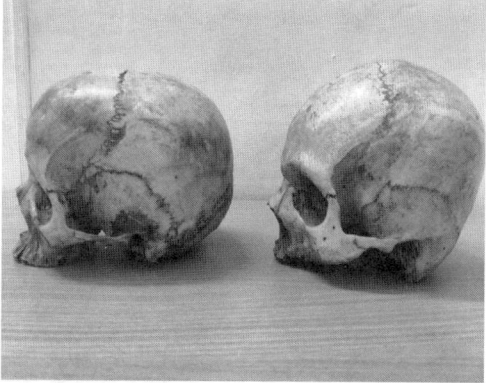

Fig. E3.2: *Skull lateral view:* Female and male skull: Vertical forehead, more prominent parietal eminence and less prominent zygomatic arch—features of female skull; sloping forehead, less prominent parietal eminence and more prominent zygomatic arch—features of male skull *(For color version see Plate 22).*

TABLE E3.2: Sex difference in pelvis bone.

Features	Male	Female
General body	Heavy, rough and deep funnel shaped	Light, smooth and flat bowl shaped
Ileum	Less vertical, curve of the crest reaches higher level and is more prominent	More vertical, height of the curve of the crest is less and not prominent
Preauricular sulcus (attachment of anterior sacroiliac ligament)	Not frequent, narrow and shallow	More frequent, broad and deep
Acetabulum	Large, 52 cm in diameter and directed laterally	Small, 46 cm in diameter and directed anterolaterally
Obturator foramen	Oval and large	Triangular and small
Greater sciatic notch (diagnostic)	Narrow, deep and 'V' shaped. The angle fits into index finger and middle finger	Wide, shallow and 'U' or 'L' shaped. Fits into the thumb and index finger
Ischial tuberosity	Inverted	Everted and widely separated
Subpubic angle	'V' shaped and angle is 70 to 75	'U' shaped and angle is 90 to 100
Pelvic cavity	Heart shaped and conical	Oval, spacious, broad and rounded
Sacroiliac articulation	Large and extends 2.5 to 3 segments	Small and extends 2 to 2.5 segments
Sacrum	Tall and narrow. Uniformly curved and body of 1st vertebra larger	Short and wide. Upper half almost straight and lower half curves forward. 1st sacral segment is small
Coccyx	Less movable	More movable

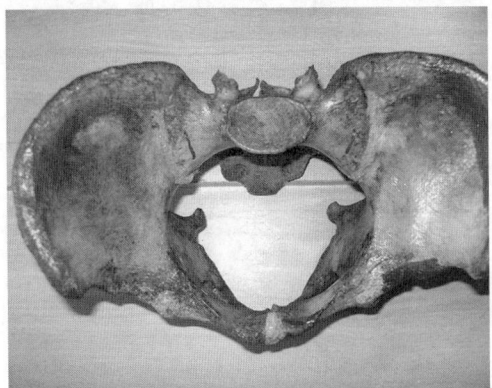

Fig. E3.3: *Male pelvis:* Deep funnel shaped and small pelvic inlet *(For color version see Plate 22).*

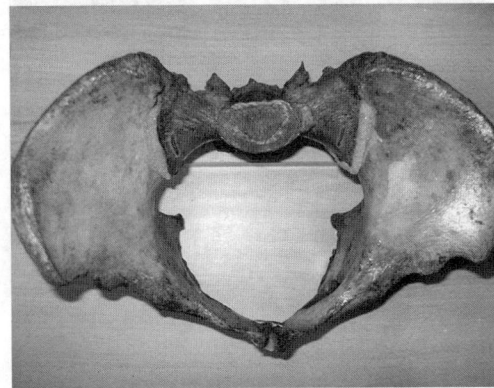

Fig. E3.4: *Female pelvis:* Flat bowl shaped and large pelvic inlet *(For color version see Plate 23).*

EXERCISE 3: Examination of Skeletal Remains

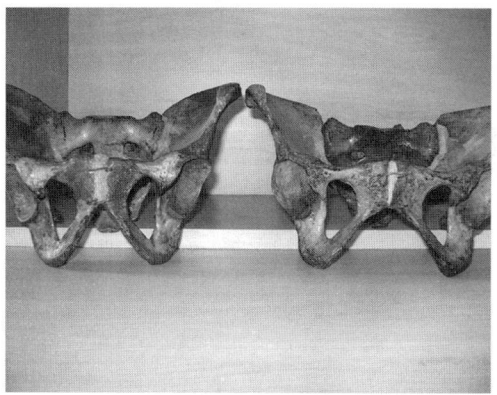

Fig. E3.5: *Male and female pelvis:* Less vertical ileum and "V" shaped subpubic angle in male. More vertical ileum and "U" shaped large subpubic angle in female *(For color version see Plate 23).*

TABLE E3.3: Sex difference in mandible.

Features	Male	Female
General	Large and thick	Small and thin
Chin	Square shaped	Rounded
Height	Taller	Smaller
Condyles	Large	Small
Ramus	Broad	Small
Angle of body and ramus	Less obtuse and everted	More obtuse and inverted

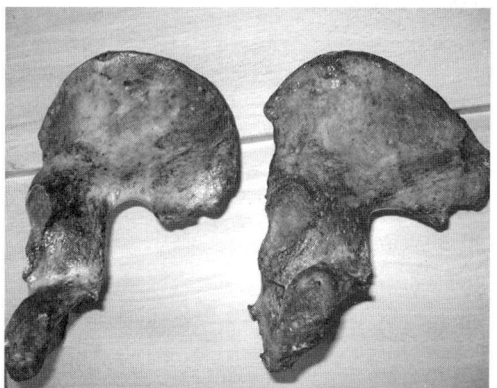

Fig. E3.6: *Male and female pelvic bone:* Note the sciatic notch; narrow, deep and "V" shaped in male; wide, shallow and "U" shaped in female. The only sex diagnostic feature in bones even before puberty, as the pelvic bone by nature is designed for delivery in females *(For color version see Plate 23).*

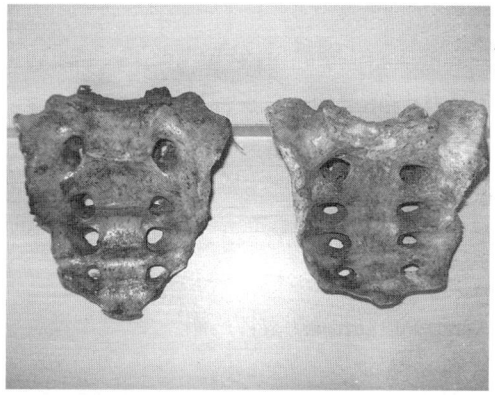

Fig. E3.7: *Sacrum:* Male and female; tall, narrow and uniformly curved in male and short, broad and curved only in the lower portion in female *(For color version see Plate 23).*

is available and also in cases of small bones like carpal and metacarpal bones, there exists difficulty in finding out whether the bones are of human origin.

In those circumstances, we can do a precipitin test to find out the origin of the bones.

WHETHER ALL THE GIVEN BONES BELONG TO THE SAME INDIVIDUAL?

- By finding out the sex and age of each individual bone, we would be able to say, whether all the bones belong to the same individual or different individuals.

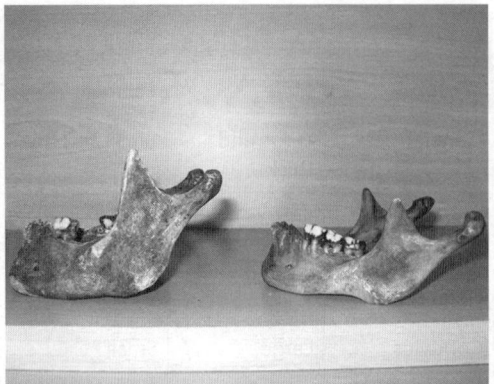

Fig. E3.8: *Mandible:* Male and female; large condyles and less obtuse angle of ramus in male and small condyles and more obtuse angled in female *(For color version see Plate 24).*

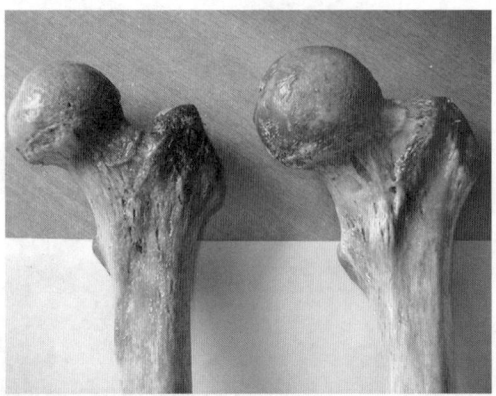

Fig. E3.9: *Femur:* Female and male; head is small, less obtuse angle with the shaft and the head forms less than two third of the sphere in female. Head is large, more obtuse angle with the shaft and the head forms more than two third of the sphere in male *(For color version see Plate 24).*

TABLE E3.4: Closure of skull sutures.	
Sagittal suture: Posterior 3rd	30–40 years
Anterior 3rd	40–50 years
Middle 3rd	50–60 years
Coronal suture: Lower half	40–50 years
Upper half	50–60 years
Lambdoid suture: Upper half	50–60 years
Lower half	60–70 years
Temporal suture	80 years

TABLE E3.5: Some of the indices useful to determine the sex.			
Index	Formula	Male	Female
Sciatic notch index	Width of the notch/Depth x 100	4–5	5–6
Ischiopubic index	Pubic length/Ischial length x 100	73–94	91–115
Sternal index	Length of manubrium/Length of the body x 100	46.2	54.3
Corporo-basal index of sacrum	Breath of 1st sacral vertebra/Breath of base of sacrum x 100	45	40.5
Medullary index	Diameter of the medulla/Diameter of the whole bone x 100		

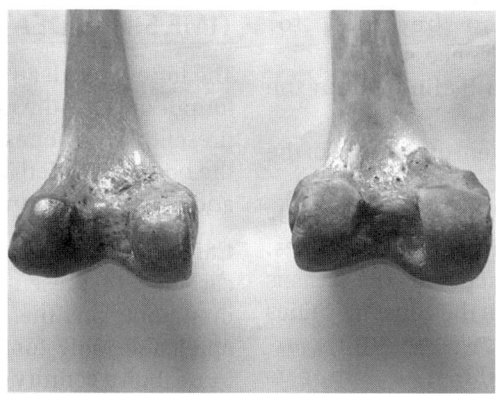

Fig. E3.10: *Condyles of femur:* Female and male; condyles are small and the bicondylar width is 67 to 76 mm in female. Condyles are large and the bicondylar width is 74 to 89 mm in male *(For color version see Plate 24).*

TABLE E3.6: Sex difference in femur.		
Features	*Male*	*Female*
General	Long, heavy, with more prominent muscular markings	Light and smooth
Head	Large, forms more than 2/3 of sphere and vertical diameter is more than 47 mm	Small, forms less than 2/3 of sphere and diameter is less than 45 mm
Neck shaft angle	Obtuse angle with the shaft, more than 125	Less obtuse, almost at right angle
Bicondylar width	More (74 to 89 mm)	Less (67 to 76 mm)
Angulation of the shaft with the condyles	Around 80	Around 75
Popliteal length	More (around 145 mm)	Less (around 106 mm)

- When the bones are of different sex and/or different age groups, then we can directly opine that the bones belong to more than one individual,
- If all the bones are of same sex and same age group, then we can say that all the bones may belong to the same individual. To confirm this, we can do ABO grouping (screening test) and DNA analysis (confirmatory).

CAUSE OF DEATH

If there are any injuries found on the bones, we would be able opine about the cause of death. The bones can be subjected to chemical analysis for detection of any poisons (heavy metals like arsenic and lead). The bones can also be subjected to diatoms test to find out whether death could be due to drowning.

ANY ADDITIONAL INFORMATION COULD BE PROVIDED?

- The **skull** can be used to find out the **race** and the approximate stature of the individual. The height of the skull with mandible × 8, will give the approximate stature of the individual.

- Skulls can also be used for superimposition if necessary.
- Race is identified by finding out the cephalic index.
- If any **long bone** is given, the **stature** of the individual can be calculated.

There are two types of formulae commonly used to find out the stature from long bones; only femur would be discussed. The basis is same for all the bones, but the constant values differ for different bones.

- **Percentage formula:** The femur is about 27% of the height of an individual. Multiplication of length of femur × 3.6–3.8 will give the height of the individual.
- **Pearson's regression formula:**
  - Males: 81.306 + 1.88 × F (Length of femur)
  - Female: 72.884 + 1.943 × F

TIME SINCE DEATH

The time since death could be approximately found out by the soft tissue attachments present on the bones. But in the examination, the bones provided are laboratory specimens and hence TSD cannot be ascertained.

Carbon dating: The amount of radio-active carbon $C14$ present in the bones is useful in finding out the age of the bones; it is applicable only for those bones which are more than a century old, as the half-life of $C14$ is 5,600 years.

EXERCISE 4

Wound Certificate

FM14.1 Examine and prepare medico-legal report of an injured person with different etiologies in a simulated/supervised environment.

Every doctor in his profession has to come across cases of injuries. There are various treatment modes for different types of injuries, but the legal implications of injuries are the same for any form of injury.

In the practical examination in UG course, you would be given a set of data and you will have to frame the certificate. But in real time practice, the scenario is different.

NAMING THE INJURY

By knowledge and experience, you have to find what injury it is? When you have named the injury, then you will automatically know what type of force is involved in causation of the injury and many a times you can find out the weapon also. Next you have to find out the time of infliction of the injury. Finding out up to this level is basic for any doctor. I have seen plenty of doctors documenting cut injuries as laceration and the case starts losing from that stage itself. Because all these benefits of doubts would be given to the accused only.

To learn those basic skills, first read the chapter on injuries and then the excise becomes so simple.

You will be given a set of data and would be asked to frame an AR copy and/or wound certificate.

ACCIDENT REGISTER (AR COPY)

This is a legal document made by the casualty medical officer, who receives any MLC (medico-legal case). In all these cases you are the first reliable and expert witness to the court. Sometimes, the patient may be seriously injured and lifesaving measures are given priority over legal duties.

Fill up the preliminary particulars in the AR copy.

History as narrated by the patient or the attender is documented briefly with relevant particulars. Document all the injuries from head to toe with reference to the type of injury, accurate dimension and the exact location on the body.

SAMPLE EXERCISE 1

AR No   345/2023 (Year) Dated: 01.10.2023.

Name: Age and sex: Address:
Accompanied by: History Narrated by: The patient himself

History

On 01.10.2023, at 5 AM, while he was walking on a road near his residence, he was assaulted by four people, out of whom two people were known to him. They have assaulted him using the fist and also weapons wooden club, iron rod and a pocketknife. He sustained injuries on face, left forearm, right hand, abdomen, right thigh and left knee. He has pushed those people away and has escaped from there in an auto.

General Examination

Height, weight, chest and abdominal girth; pulse, BP, heart rate.
CVS, RS, CNS and P/A examination.

Injuries

- Lacerated wound 3 × 2–1 cm × bone deep, on left side of the forehead.
- Reddish contusion 5 × 4–3 cm × muscle deep, on the right cheek.
- Reddish, irregular abrasion 8 × 4–3 cm, vertically oblique on back of left forearm.
- Stab wound 1.5 × 0.3 × 3 cm, on upper part of right side of the abdomen; peritoneum intact.
- Linear incised wound 7 × 0.5 × 1–0.5 cm, on inner aspect of right palm.
- Abraded contusion 6 × 4–3 cm × muscle deep, horizontally oblique, on front and outer aspect of upper third of right thigh.
- Multiple, reddish, irregular abrasion of size varying from 0.2 × 0.2 cm to 0.5 × 0.4 cm on the front of left knee, over an area of 6 × 4 cm.

Investigations Advised

X-ray skull, abdomen, right hand and right thigh.

Date: Signature of the doctor.
Place: (Name in block letters, with designation and registration number)

INJURY/WOUND CERTIFICATE

The doctor who was treating the patient should issue the wound certificate **Table E4.1**. The objective of the wound certificate is to certify:
- Which of the injuries and simple and which are grievous.
- If the weapon is known/made available for examination, then which all the injuries could have been caused by which weapon. If the weapon is not known to the investigation agency, then the doctor has to opine the probable weapon/force involved in causation of the injuries.
- The time of infliction of the injuries.

After Writing the Preliminary Particulars

Draw a table with seven columns. From the AR copy, document the injuries in the table. Arrive at the opinion. (The previous AR copy is used here to prepare the sample wound certificate).

Opinion: (In all medico-legal cases the opinion should be framed in this following way)

On examination of Mr ___, ___Years, Male/Female, residing at No: _____, bearing the following identification marks,

EXERCISE 4: Wound Certificate

TABLE E4.1: Wound certificate

Sl. No.	Type of injury	Size	Location	Simple/ grievous	Weapon involved	Time of injury	Remarks if any
1.	Laceration	3 × 2–1 cm × BD	Left side of the forehead	Grievous	Iron rod/ wooden club	Fresh	
2.	Contusion	5 × 4–3 cm × muscle deep	Right cheek	Simple	Fist/(Blunt force)	Fresh	
3.	Abrasion	8 × 5–4 cm	Vertically oblique on back of right forearm	Simple	Wooden club/Iron rod	Fresh	
4.	Stab wound	1.5 × 0.3 × 3 cm	Right side of the abdomen	Simple	Pocket-knife	Fresh	
5.	Incised wound	7 × 0.5 × 1–0.5 cm	Inner aspect of right palm	Simple	Knife	Fresh	
6.	Abraded contusion	6 × 4–3 cm × muscle deep	Horizontally oblique on middle third of right thigh	Simple	Iron rod/ wooden club	Fresh	
7.	Multiple abrasion of size 0.2 × 0.2 to 0.5 × 0.4 cm	Over an area of 6 × 4 cm	Front of left knee	Simple	Blunt force	Fresh	

- A black mole on upper part of right side of the chest, 1 cm above the nipple.
- A black mole on outer aspect of middle third of right forearm.
- A raised black mole 0.3 cm in diameter, with a few hair follicles present on the center of the mole, on outer aspect of right side of the jaw, 6 cm below the right mastoid process two ID enough.

I am of the opinion that:
- **Injury no:** 1 is grievous and injuries no: 2, 3, 4, 5, 6 and 7 are simple in nature.
- Injuries no: 1, 3 and 6 could be caused by iron rod/wooden club; injury no: 2 could be caused by blow with the fist; injury no: 4 and 5 could be caused by pocketknife and injury no: 7 could be caused by fall on the ground.
- All the injuries are fresh in nature and hence the time of infliction could be less than 6 hours.

Date: Signature of the doctor
Place: (Name in block letters, with designation and registration number)

VIVA QUESTIONS

1. Definition of injury.
2. Classification of mechanical injuries.
3. Grievous hurt; Section 320 IPC (must know).
4. Endangering injury.
5. Dangerous weapon.
6. Defense injury, self inflicted injury, hesitation cuts and fabricated injury.

All these are discussed in detail in theory, Chapter no: 12 and 14.

EXERCISE 5

Drunkenness

> **FM14.16** To examine and prepare medico-legal report of drunk person in a simulated/supervised environment.

DEFINITION

"Drunkenness is a condition produced in a person, who has consumed alcohol in sufficient quantities, so as to lose control over his faculties to such an extent, that he is unable execute the occupation safely, in which he is engaged at the material time".

Drunkenness is a clinical condition; blood alcohol concentration (BAC) is only corroborative and should not be fully relied upon. An acute alcoholic person who is consuming alcohol for the first time in life with BAC 80 mg/mL could be under the influence of alcohol and a person who consumes alcohol for 10 years with BAC 240 gm/mL could be normal and will be able to perform all the tests properly.

Hence certification of drunkenness can be done only by physical examination by a medical expert.

BAC estimated from dead bodies is useful to find out whether he has consumed alcohol or not and the approximate quantity of alcohol consumed, but cannot conclusively say whether he was under the influence of alcohol or not.

The preamble of the report consisting of general particulars like name, age, sex, accompanying police constable are filled up in the routine way.

General Examination

Height, weight, chest measurement at the level of nipple, abdominal girth at the level of umbilicus, pulse rate, respiratory rate and blood pressure are recorded.

Systemic examination of CVS, RS, CNS and per-abdominal examination are done.

Specific examination is focused on:
- **State of clothing:** Whether well-dressed or not, neatness, stains of vomitus on the clothing, etc., are noted.
- **Smell of alcohol in breath:** If smell of alcohol is present in breath, it indicates he has consumed alcohol.
- **Speech:** The individual may be too much talkative; or he may be over précised, will answer you in one or two words.

EXERCISE 5: Drunkenness

- **Behavior:** Note his behavior whether neatly behaving or he may behave too much rude
- **Eyes:** Checked for congestion and nystagmus and state of the pupil.
- **Tests for muscular coordination:** The opinion of drunkenness is mainly based on **smell of alcohol in breath** and the **tests for muscular coordination**. These tests are easy to perform and elicit the findings thus enabling the medical expert to give a direct positive opinion is cases of drunkenness.
- **Finger nose test:** Ask the person to stand straight and stretch his right hand on the side; now ask him to touch the tip of his nose with the tip of his index finger multiple times; if he is under the influence of alcohol, then he may not be able to do it properly rather he may pock into the nose or wrongly pock his own eyes.
- **Finger-finger test:** The individual is asked to touch the tips of all the fingers one by one.
- **Picking up small objects from the floor:** *Very useful test:* Throw some tiny objects like broken pieces of broom stick or thin match sticks on the floor and ask the individual to pick up those small objects one by one. If by chance, he may take a right object but not every time. When he is under the influence of alcohol there will be diplopia and he end up picking wrong images and not the real object.
- **Buttoning and unbuttoning of shirt:** Better not to do it you are a lady doctor.
  If you ask the individual to unbutton and button the shirt fast and repeatedly, he may not be able to do it and may he also button the shirt on wrong holes also.
- **Romberg's sign:** The individual is asked to stand straight with both feet together, stretch his hands apart and then close the eyes. He cannot perform the test properly rather he will sway if he is under the influence of alcohol.
- Walk in a straight line (**Gait**—Staggering gait)
- **Reaction time:** The individual is asked to perform an act and then interpreted with a new command; the time taken to change over from one muscular activity to the other is called the reaction time.
  Example: When the individual is walking in a straight line, give a new command like stop, turn right, etc., the time taken to change over to the new command will be delayed, if he under the influence of alcohol.
  The delay in reaction time is one of the main reasons for road traffic accidents. The time taken to change over from accelerator to brake and clutch etc., would be delayed.
- Deep tendon reflexes like knee jerk are tested; they would be initially exaggerated but later on diminished as the BAC increases.

Opinion

The opinion is based on whether smell of alcohol is present in breath or not and whether he is able to perform the tests for muscular coordination.

After examination there are three types of opinions which could be arrived at:
1. The individual has not consumed alcohol (when smell of alcohol in breath is absent and he is able to do all the tests for muscular coordination properly).
2. He has consumed alcohol, but not under the influence of alcohol (when smell of alcohol is present in breath, but he is able to do all the tests for muscular coordination properly).

3. He has consumed alcohol and is under the influence of alcohol (when smell is present and he is unable to perform the tests for muscular coordination).

VIVA QUESTIONS

1. Define drunkenness
2. Delirium tremens
3. Korsakov's psychosis and Wernik's encephalopathy.
4. Mc Evans sign.
5. Widmark's formula.

All are discussed in theory; Chapter no. 30.

6 EXERCISE

Sexual Offence Certificates

FM14.14 To examine and prepare report of an alleged accused in rape/unnatural sexual offence in a simulated/supervised environment.

Every medical expert must possess in them the basic knowledge of how to derive and frame opinions in any case of sexual assault. Both the accused and the victim are presented for examination.

In case of accused we should certify about his potency and find out whether there are any evidence which could suggest that he has taken part in recent sexual intercourse?

In case of victims, we should certify whether there are any evidences suggestive to say that the female has taken part in recent sexual intercourse; also make attempts to find out whether such sexual intercourse was forceful?

In many a circumstances, the authorities may also request for an age estimation of both the victim and/the accused where ever necessary.

EXAMINATION OF VICTIM OF SEXUAL OFFENCE

Fill up the preliminary particulars and note down the accompanying person (relative) name; informed written consent is mandatory and any victim cannot be examined against her consent. Consent of the legal guardian is also obtained when the victim is <18 years of age.

MEDICO-LEGAL EXAMINATION OF RAPE VICTIM

Prerequisites

Requisition for examination from the concerned authority (investigating officer, court).

An authorized person (accompanying police constable) to identify the victim.

A proper written informed consent has to be obtained.

Presence of a female attendant is mandatory, if examined by a male doctor.

Proforma of Examination of an Alleged Victim of Rape

Preliminary data: It should contain the following details.

- Name
- Age
- Sex
- Address:
- Occupation:
- Brought by (police constable name and number):
- Accompanied by (the female attender):
- Date, time and place of examination:
- Written informed consent, signed by the guardian if the female is <18 years.
- Two identification marks:

Examination

A comprehensive history is essential and integral part of sexual offence examination. It includes general medical history, marital and obstetric history, and a thorough complete history of the alleged crime.

General Medical History

- Past history, e.g., bleeding disorders.
- Medication and allergies.
- Details of any medication or alcoholic intake during last 24 hours.

Marital and Obstetric History

- Age of menarche, frequency and regularity of menstruation.
- Date of last menstruation.
- History of previous sexual exposure.
- Married/unmarried and details of siblings if married.
- History of sterilization and use of contraceptives.
- **History of any STD:** Whether treated or not.

HISTORY OF THE ALLEGED CRIME

- Date, time and place of the alleged sexual assault.
- Specific nature of the assault; whether penetration has taken place or not? If yes, whether penetration was vaginal, oral or anal.
- Any instruments/objects were inserted?
- Any body fluids were left on the victim: Ejaculation, saliva, urination or defecation.

Post Incident

- Whether the victim has washed her genitals/taken bath/change of clothing?
- Number of assailants involved.

General Examination

- Height, weight, and general built.
- Abdominal girth at the level of umbilicus and chest circumference at the level of nipples.
- **Examination of BP:** Pulse, heart rate and respiratory rate.
- **Examination of teeth:** Eruption and injuries.
- Presence or absence of secondary sexual characteristics.

Examination of Clothing

The victim is made to stand on clean white sheet of paper, and to undress herself, and collect any material that falls onto the paper, if the victim has not washed her genitals, taken bath or changed her clothing.

Examine the clothing for tears, any stains (blood, semen, etc.) or any foreign bodies adherent to the clothing (sand, mud, etc.). If satins are present on the clothes, it has to be dried, preserved, packed, labeled and sent to the forensic science laboratory.

Examination of the Body Surface

The whole-body surface must be examined for injuries, old and new. Document everything with care, as to the nature of injury, size, shape and location with reference to prominent anatomical landmarks wherever necessary.

Specific attention for recent injuries (scratches and bite marks).

Examination of Skin

- Any soiled area on the body must be swabbed, preserved and sent for analysis to FSL.
- Use of ultra-violet lamp will reveal areas of fluorescence (seminal soiling).
- Search for loose foreign hair or any other foreign material on the skin.

Examination of Fingernails

- Ragged or broken nails.
- Blood, skin tags or any foreign bodies under the nails are checked for. Fingernail scrapings from all the fingers are taken in separate plastic bags and sent to the forensic science laboratory.

LOCAL EXAMINATION

External Genital Examination

- **Pubic hair:** Matted or not; if matted, the bunch of matted hair are cut and preserved separately. Combing of pubic hair to be done for any loose pubic hair, if present they are preserved separately. A bunch of pubic hair from the victim to be collected separately, for comparison purpose.
- Look for injuries like bruises, bite marks, nail scratches, etc., over the inner aspect of thigh and labia and should be properly documented.

Internal Examination

- Using a vaginal speculum:
  - Vaginal swabs are taken.
  - Examine the lining vagina.
  - Note for any abrasion, erosion, bruise or tears.

Digital Examination

- Two fingers test which will reveal:
  - Areas of pain and tenderness in vagina.
  - Laxity of vaginal orifice (indicates previous penetration).
  - Elongation of posterior fornix (indicating habitual sexual intercourse).
  - The size of the vagina should be noted as admitting 1, 2 or 3 fingers as the case may be.

However, the significance and relevance of digital examination is highly controversial. Recent school of thought and some of the court judgments advice to dispense with this practice.

Vaginal washings and washings from the posterior fornix are to be collected separately and labeled to look for spermatozoa and prostatic secretions (acid phosphatase test).

Hymen

- Rupture of the hymen occurs with the first sexual intercourse.
- Tearing usually occurs in the 4 or 8 o'clock position, or in the middle.
- Soon after the act, the margins of the torn hymen are sharp and red, which bleed on touch.
- By 3 to 4 days, the edges are congested and swollen, which heal completely in 1 week.
- Rupture of the hymen due to sudden stretching can be caused by agents other than the penis, such as fingers. And therefore, evidence of local injury is not a proof of penetration.
- Frequently, in the absence of frank hymeneal tearing, there is abrasion and bruising of hymen, vaginal orifice and the vaginal canal.

Certification of Rape

Rape is a legal term and not a medical diagnosis and hence while issuing a certificate in cases of sexual assault, we should restrict ourselves within the boundaries of science.

Never use the word rape in the certificate.

The objective of our examination is to say, whether there are any evidence suggestive of recent sexual intercourse, if present then, whether such intercourse could be with mutual consent or whether there are evidence of struggle to say, such sexual intercourse was forceful.

Opinion

There are evidences suggestive of recent sexual intercourse/no signs of recent sexual intercourse.

There are evidences suggestive of recent sexual intercourse and it could be forceful (if evidence of struggle are present, with severe injuries in and around the genitals).

Proper documentation of all the injuries present on the body would automatically indicate that victim offered resistance.

It's for the court to decide whether such sexual intercourse was rape or not. Since, in a female who has delivered children, even forceful vaginal penetration may not leave any signs and we would be forced to opine as there are no evidence suggestive of recent sexual intercourse (especially, when laboratory reports are negative). Absence of injuries/no resistance doesn't mean that the victim had consented for such sexual act.

EXERCISE 7

Examination of the Accused of Rape

FM14.14 To examine and prepare report of an alleged accused in rape/unnatural sexual offence in a simulated/supervised environment.

It is almost similar to victim, only the examination of the genitalia vary.
- Preliminary particulars are filled up and the development of genitals is examined.
- History, mental state and general behavior.
- Influence of alcohol and/or drugs
- **Clothes:** Tears, stains, loss of buttons, etc.
- Hair/foreign material, cosmetic contact traces, etc.
- **Stains on the body:** Blood, semen or others.
- **Marks of struggle:** Scratches, bite marks, bruises etc. and age of injuries to be determined.

EXAMINATION OF GENITALS

Development with special reference to potency:
- **Injuries:** Scratches, bruise, tear of the frenulum and abrasion on the skin covering the glans penis and reddening of the glans.
- Dried blood stains may be found on the shaft of the penis, scrotum and adjoining skin.
- **Examination of glans for vaginal cells:** Lugol's iodine test (positive up to 4 days).
- Presence or absence of **smegma** (smegma is thick, white, cheesy material present beneath the skin of the glans penis of every male and would be absent if he is circumcised).
- Smegma is produced by Smegmatis bacilli which are normal inhabitant of the male genitalia. It is customary for every male to wash up the smegma during bathing.

INFERENCE

Absence of smegma suggests that he could have taken part in sexual intercourse or he has washed his glans penis recently. But presence of smegma strongly goes in favor of the accused as it suggests that he has not taken part in sexual intercourse recently.

Specimens to be Collected

- Swab from coronal sulcus and prepuce.
- Blood for grouping.
- Pubic hair combing, matted pubic hair and comparative sample of pubic hair.
- Nail scraping. Any loose hair found anywhere on the body.

OPINION

In examination of the accused, we have to opine whether there any evidences to say that the individual has taken part in recent sexual intercourse and also about his potency.

Certificate of Potency is always Given in a Double Negative Form

There is *nothing* to suggest that the individual is *incapable* of performing normal sexual intercourse. (or) There is *nothing* to suggest that he is *impotent*.

The double negative format is used because psychological impotence cannot be ruled out by routine physical examination.

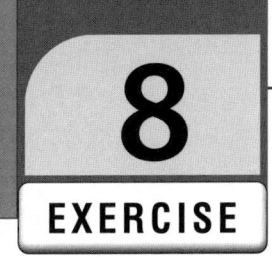

EXERCISE 8

Fetal Examination

FM14.13 To estimate the age of fetus by postmortem examination.

In real time cases, we would have to do a complete autopsy to find out dead born, still born or live born. But for undergraduate examinations, a fetus would be given you should examine and find out the age of the fetus and comment about viability.

To understand about infant deaths, refer Chapter 20.

GESTATIONAL AGE

The crown-heal length of the fetus is measured and the gestational age is calculated using Rule of Hasse. If the length is <25 cm, the square root value will give the approximate months of gestation; if the length of the fetus is more than 25 cm, the length divided by 5 will give the approximate age of gestation in months.

Example: If length is 9 cm, $\sqrt{9}$ + 3 months; if length is 40 cm, 40/5 = 8 months.

VIABILITY

Viability is the ability of a fetus to have a separate existence of its own, outside the mother's womb. It is due to certain physical development in the fetus, which makes it viable. Seven lunar months or 210 days is the minimum period of viability. When the crown-heal length is more than 35 cm, then it's a viable fetus. Rigor mortis does not appear in nonviable fetus (myofibrils are formed only by 7 months of IUL).

Sample Exercise

- **External appearance:** Color of skin, whether wrinkled.
- **Crown heal length:** 40 cm.
- **Weight of the fetus:** 1600 gm
- **Scalp hair:** Fully appeared, measures 1.2 cm
- **Body hair (Lanugo hair):** Well appeared (Not appeared/appeared/well appeared).
- **Eyebrow and eyelash:** Well appeared.
- **Fingernails and toe nails:** Appeared and covers up to the tip of the fingers.
- **Shape of chest:** Barrel shaped.
- **Meconium:** Found in the large intestine.
- **Position of the diaphragm:** At the level of 4th rib.

- **Sex:** Male/Female (differentiation easy after 14 weeks).
- **Umbilical cord:** Attached.
- **Ossification centers:** (check talus, calcaneus, sternum, lower end of femur).
- **Age of the fetus:** 8 months.
- **Viability:** Viable.
- **Cause of death:**

Date: Signature of the MO with seal
Place:

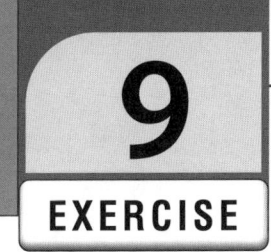

Leave Certificate and Certificate of Fitness

1. Certificate for medical leave/extension of leave (Sample certificate)

Medical Certificate for Leave/Extension of Leave

Signature of the candidate: _____

I (Dr_____) after careful personal examination of the case hereby certify that _____, Male/Female, whose signature is given above, working as _____, in the office of _____ _____, is/was suffering from _____, based on clinical condition and investigation done as it given below, and I consider that the period of absence from duty for _____ days, from _____, is/was absolutely necessary for the restoration of his/her health.

Station:

Date: (Authorized medical attendant)
                                                                     Signature and seal with Reg No

Clinical history

Investigations done:

Station:

Date: (Authorized medical attendant)
                                                                     Signature and seal with Reg No

2. Certificate of fitness to join duty (Sample certificate)

Medical Certificate of Fitness to Return to Duty

Signature of the candidate: _____

I (Dr _____) after careful personal examination of _____ _____, Male/Female, aged about _____ years, _____ working as _____, in the office of _____ _____, certify that, he/she has recovered from his/her illness and is fit to resume to duties from _____.

I have also verified the original leave certificate before arriving at the opinion.

Station:

Date:

                                                (Authorized medical attendant)

                                                Signature and seal with Reg No

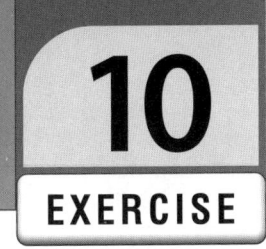

Death Certificate

While issuing death certificate the WHO format has to be used:

FORM NO 4A
(See Rule 7)
MEDICAL CERTIFICATE OF CAUSE OF DEATH
(For noninstitutional deaths. Not to be used for still births)
To be sent to Registrar along with form no 2 (death report)

I hereby certifiy that the deceased Shri/Smt/Km... son of/wife of/daughter of .... resident of ....was under my treatment from ....to ....and he/she died on .... at ....am/pm

NAME OF DECEASED					For use of statistical office
Sex	Age at death				
	Age in completed years	If less than 1 year age in months	If less than one month age in days	If less than one day, age in hours	
1. Male 2. Female					
CAUSE OF DEATH			Interval between on set and death approx.		
I. Immediate cause state the disease, injury or complication which caused death, not the mode of dying such as heart failure, asthenia, etc.		(a) ....Due to (or as a consequences of)			
Antecedent cause morbid conditions, if any, giving rise to the above cause, stating underlying condition last		(b) .... Due to (or as a consequences of)			
II Other significant conditions contributing to the death but not related to the disease or conditions causing II		(c)			
If deceased was female, was pregnancy the death associated with? 1. Yes 2. No If yes, was there a delivery? 1. Yes 2. No					

....
Name and signature of the medical attendant certifying the cause of death
_____
(To be detached and handed over to the related of the deceased)
Certified that Shri/Smt/Km.........................S/W/D of Shri..R/O ....was under treatment from...to.......................and he/she

Doctor...................................
Signature and address of Medical Practitioner/
Medical attendant with Registration No

The Medical data to be filled is designed as per the WHO norms and has two parts.
- **Part I:** Mentions the events which lead to death.
- **Part II:** Mentions the conditions which contributed to the death.

CAUSE OF DEATH

One cause is to be entered on each line. Underlying cause is to be filled on the lowest line. It is the condition that started the sequence of events which lead to immediate cause of death from normal health to immediate cause of death.

a. **Immediate cause of death:** Disease or injury or complication that precedes death.

   It's not the mode of dying e.g., heart failure, respiratory failure should not be entered.

c. **Due to (or as a consequence of):** If immediate cause occurred as a consequence of another condition it should be entered here. Antecedent condition might have just prepared the ground for immediate cause of death, even after a long interval.

c. **Morbid condition leading to the underlying condition.**

EXAMPLE 1

A patient died from bronchopneumonia following an intracerebral hemorrhage caused by cerebral metastases from a primary malignant neoplasm of the left main bronchus.

a. **Immediate cause:** Bronchopneumonia
b. **Antecedent cause:** Intracerebral hemorrhage.
c. **Underlying cause:** Cerebral metastases from squamous carcinoma of left main bronchus.

Note: While writing neoplasm, the exact pathological variant must be specified.

EXAMPLE 2

A 45-year-old chronic alcoholic patient, who was on regular treatment for diabetes, died from acute exacerbation of chronic pancreatitis.

Part I

a. **Immediate cause:** Acute exacerbation of chronic pancreatitis.
b. **Antecedent cause:** Chronic pancreatitis.
c. **Underlying cause:** Chronic alcoholism.

Part II

Contributory cause: Diabetes mellitus.

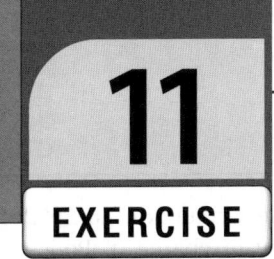

EXERCISE 11

Postmortem Certificate

FM14.14 Conduct and prepare postmortem examination report of varied etiologies (at least 15) in a simulated/supervised environment.

A set of findings could be given and the student is asked to frame the postmortem certificate; or a certificate would be given and the student is asked to write the opinion and answer some question about the basis of his opinion.

Logical and straight forward approach with the knowledge gained by reading this textbook would help any doctor to approach, dissect and opine with confidence in any case of postmortem.

A few models postmortem certificates are given for understanding.

Sample PM Certificate 1

PM No: 864/2022

POSTMORTEM CERTIFICATE

Date: 17.04.2022.

Regarding the body of a *male* aged about *34* years, named *Gopi*. Requisition received at *01.00 PM* on *17.04.2022.* from *Sub-Inspector of Police* of *T-14, Mangadu. Police Station* with the Crime No: *201/2022* dated *17.04.2022.* Body in charge of Police Constable No *WPC 3693* name *Mrs Hema*.

Identification and caste marks:
1. A black mole on the middle part of right side of the chest.
2. A black mole on the lower part of the left side of the chest.

The body was first seen by the undersigned at *01.20 PM* on ____ *17.04.2022.* ____ Its condition then was ____ *Rigor mortis present all over the body.* _____ Postmortem commenced at 01.20 PM on _____ 17.04.2022. _____ Appearances found at Postmortem: *Moderately nourished male body with bluish fingernails.*

Injuries:
1. An incomplete, asymmetrically oblique, well defined, brownish ligature abrasion 23 × 2 cm, on the front and sides of upper part of neck; on the front of the neck, ligature abrasion was above the level of the thyroid cartilage and was 5 cm below the chin and 7 cm above the suprasternal notch; on the sides of the neck, the ligature abrasion was 6 cm and 4 cm below the right

and left mastoid processes respectively; on the back of the neck, the ligature abrasion merges with the hairline; on dissection. The base of the ligature abrasion was pale and dry; subcutaneous soft tissues of the neck were pale; the hyoid bone and other laryngeal cartilages were intact.

There were no other external or internal injuries anywhere on the body.

Heart: Normal in size; C/S: Empty; Valves: Normal; Coronaries: Patent; Great Vessels: Normal. Lungs: Normal in size; multiple subpleural petechial hemorrhages on the surface of both the lungs. C/S: Congested. Larynx and trachea: Empty. Hyoid bone: Intact.
- **Stomach:** Contained 160 mL of brown fluid; no definite smell; Mucosa: Congested.
- **Intestines:** Contained brown chyme.
- **Liver, spleen and kidneys:** Normal in size; C/S: Congested. Bladder: Empty.
- **Pelvis and spinal column:** Intact.
- **Skull:** Intact. Brain: Normal in size; surface vessels congested.

Opinion as to cause of death:
The deceased would appear to have died of asphyxia due to hanging.

Station: Chennai -10   Name:
Date: 17.04.2022.   Rank:

Sample PM Certificate 2

PM No: 144/2022.

POSTMORTEM CERTIFICATE

Date: 18.01.2022.
Regarding the body of a *female* aged about 75 years, named *M Lakshmi*. Requisition received at *11.30 AM* on *18.01.2022.* from *Sub-Inspector of Police* of *T-10, Thirumullaivoyal* Police Station with the Crime No: *26/2022* dated *16.01.2022*. Body in charge of Police Constable *No HC 1538* name *Mr Haridoss*.

Identification and caste marks:
1. A raised black mole 0.5 × 0.5 cm, on right side tip of the nose.
2. A tattoo mark on right forearm.

The body was first seen by the undersigned at *11.40AM* on *18.01.2022*. Its condition then was *Rigor mortis present only in lower limbs*. Post-Mortem commenced at *11.40AM* on *18.01.2022*. Appearances found at Postmortem: *Moderately nourished female body*.

Greenish black discolouration with post-mortem peeling of cuticle in patchy areas on front of chest and abdomen, neck, face and both upper limbs.

There were no external or internal injuries anywhere on the body.

Heart: Normal in size; Flabby; C/S: Empty; Valves: Normal; Coronaries: Patent;

Larynx and trachea: Fine gritty mud particles mixed with brown froth adherent loosely onto the mucosal surface of larynx, trachea, primary and secondary bronchioles.

Lungs: Normal in size; C/S: Early decomposition changes. Hyoid Bone: Intact.
- **Stomach:** Contained 40 mL of brown fluid; no definite smell; Mucosa: Early decomposition changes. Intestines: Contained brownish black chyme.
- **Liver, spleen and kidneys:** Normal in size; C/S: Early decomposition changes.
- **Bladder:** Empty. Uterus: Normal in size; C/S: Empty.
- **Pelvis and spinal column:** Intact.
- **Skull:** Intact. Brain: Normal in size, softened and discolored gray.

Opinion as to cause of death:
The deceased would appear to have died of asphyxia due to drowning.

Station: Chennai -10, Name:
Date: 18.01.2022. Rank:

Sample PM Certificate 3

PM No: 02/2023.

POSTMORTEM CERTIFICATE

Date: 12.05.2023.
Regarding the body of a *male* aged about *56* years, named *Abath Sagayam*. Requisition received at *05.20 PM* on *12.05.2023.* from *Sub-Inspector of Police* of *C-5, Oragadam Police Station* with the Crime No: *147/2023* dated *12.05.2023*. Body in charge of Police Constable No: *HC 245* name *Mr. Pachaiyammal*.

Identification marks:
1. A black mole above the left eyebrow.
2. A black mole on the right side of abdomen.
The body was first seen by the undersigned at *05.30 PM* on *12.05.2023*. Its condition then was *Rigor mortis yet to set in. Postmortem* commenced at *05.30 PM* on *12.05.2023*. Appearances found at Postmortem *Well-nourished body of a male.*

Injuries:
1. Brown irregular abrasion 4 × 3-2 cm on inner aspect and front of left wrist, with deformity of the wrist joint; on dissection: Complete irregular fracture of lower end of both bones, with surrounding soft tissue bruising and extravasation of blood.
2. Dark blue contusion 8 × 6-5 cm on upper part of left knee; on dissection: Dark red muscle deep bruising of the underlying tissues.
3. **On reflection of the scalp:** Dark red, scalp deep, diffuse bruising on left fronto, parieto-temporal region of the scalp. Left temporalis muscle bruised. Two linear fissured fractures 6 cm and 5 cm on left fronto-temporal bones of the skull. On opening the calvarium: Thick film of subdural hemorrhage and diffuse subarachnoid hemorrhage on left fronto, temporoparietal region of the brain.
4. Midline, incised, surgical, sutured wound 53 cm, extending from the suprasternal notch to the symphysis pubis. On removal of the sutures: The wound margins were regular and gapping; Sternum has been opened by a cut incision on the midline. Both kidneys and the liver have been surgically removed and not in-situ.

There were no other external or internal injuries anywhere on the body.

Heart: Normal in size; C/S: Chambers were empty. Great vessels: Normal; Coronaries were patent.

Lungs: Normal in size; C/S: Congested. Larynx and trachea: Empty. Hyoid Bone: Intact.

- **Stomach:** Empty; Mucosa: Pale. Intestines: Contained brown chyme.
- **Spleen:** Normal in size; C/S: Congested.
- **Bladder:** Empty. Pelvis and spinal column: Intact.

Opinion as to cause of death:
The deceased would appear to have died of head injuries.

Station: Chennai -100, Name:
Date: 12.05.2023. Rank:

12 EXERCISE

Spotters

> **FM14.10** Demonstrate ability to identify and prepare medico-legal inference from specimens obtained from various types of injuries, e.g., contusion, abrasion, laceration, firearm wounds, burns, head injury and fracture of bone.
>
> **FM14.11** To identify and describe weapons of medicolegal importance which are commonly used, e.g., lathi, knife, kirpan, axe, gandasa, gupti, farsa, dagger, bhalla, razor and stick. Able to prepare report of the weapons brought by police and to give opinion regarding injuries present on the person as described in injury report/PM report so as to connect weapon with the injuries. (Prepare injury report/PM report must be provided to connect the weapon with the injuries).
>
> **FM14.12** Describe the contents and structure of bullet and cartridges used and to provide medico-legal interpretation from these.
>
> **FM14.17** To identify and draw medico-legal inference from common poisons, e.g., datura, castor, cannabis, opium, aconite copper sulphate, pesticides compounds, marking nut, oleander, Nux vomica, abrus seeds, snakes, capsicum, calotropis, lead compound and tobacco.

SEEDS

Undergraduate student should be able to identify and know the medico-legal importance of the following seeds (**Figs. E12.1 to E12.13**).

Irritants (FM14.17)

- Abrus precatorius
- Semecarpus anacardium (marking nut)
- Ricinus communis (castor)
- Croton tiglium
- Chilli seeds

Cardiac Poisons (FM14.17)

- Cerbera thevetia
- Digitalis

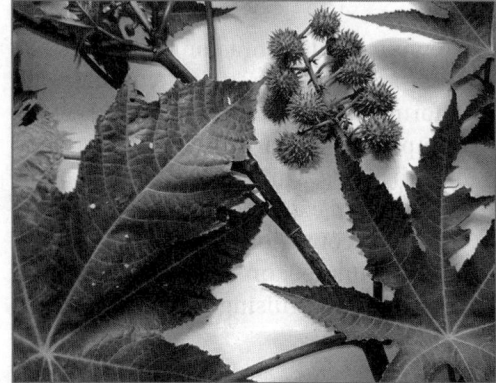

Fig. E12.1: Castor plant (ricinus communis): Fruits are born in clusters which contain the seeds. Oil extracted from the seeds are used as purgatives. The pressed cake retains the active ingredient resin—toxalbumin.

EXERCISE 12: Spotters

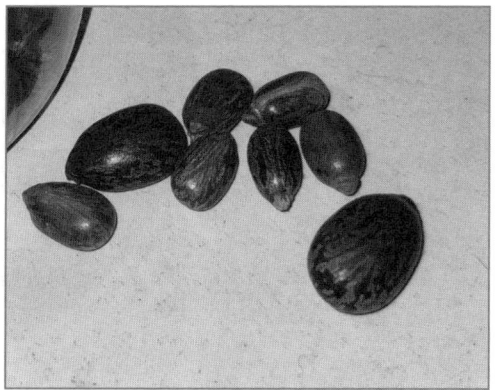

Fig. E12.2: Ricinus communis seeds.

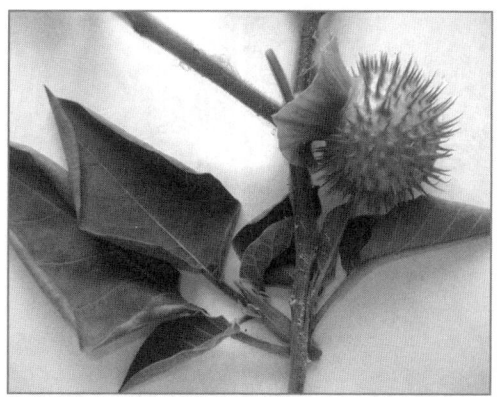

Fig. E12.5: Datura plant with fruit (thorn apple).

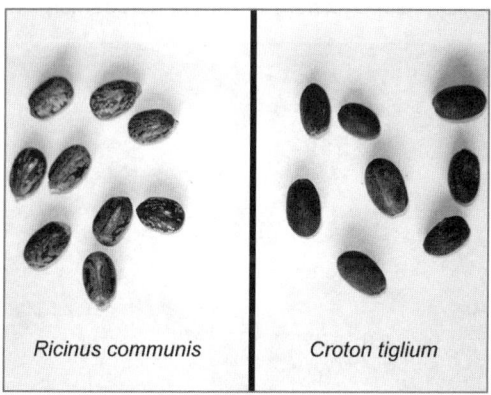

Fig. E12.3: Castor and croton seeds.

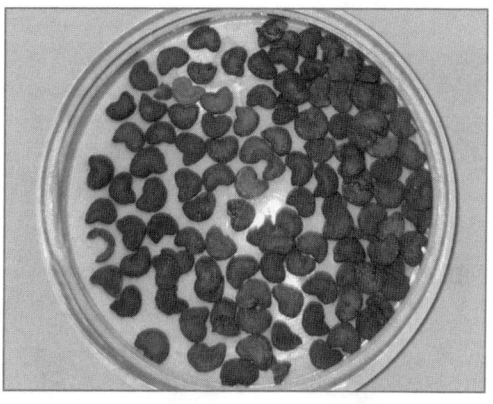

Fig. E12.6: Datura seeds.

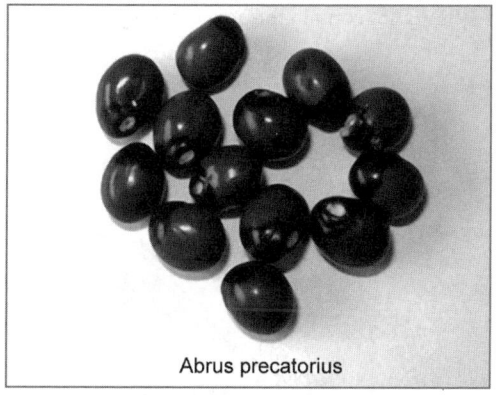

Fig. E12.4: Abrus precatorius.

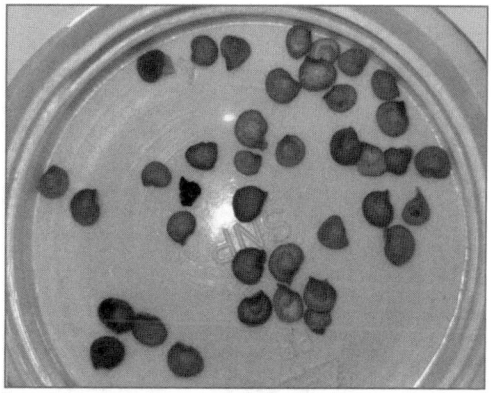

Fig. E12.7: Capsicum seeds.

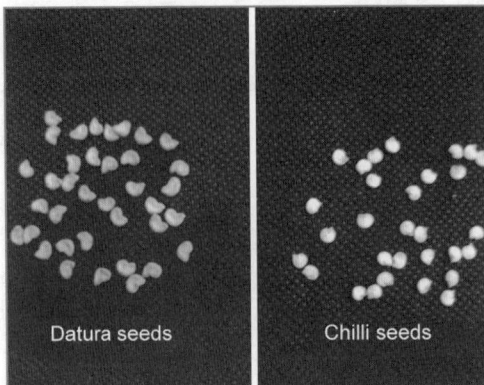

Fig. E12.8: Datura seeds and chilli seeds.

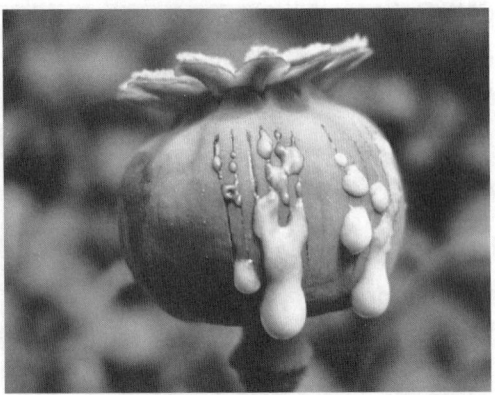

Fig. E12.11: Poppy capsule: Multiple superficial incisions made on the unripe poppy capsule, which yields a milky white juice. On drying it turns brown, which scrapped of from the capsule is crude morphine.

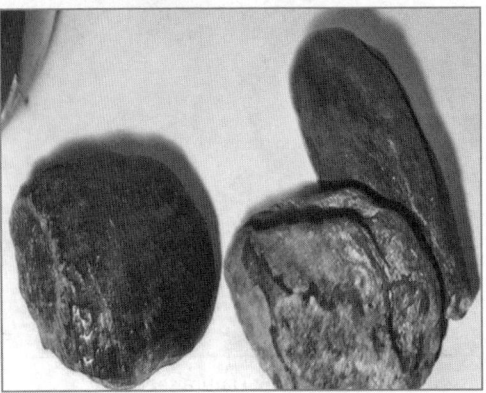

Fig. E12.9: Semecarpus anacardium (making nut).

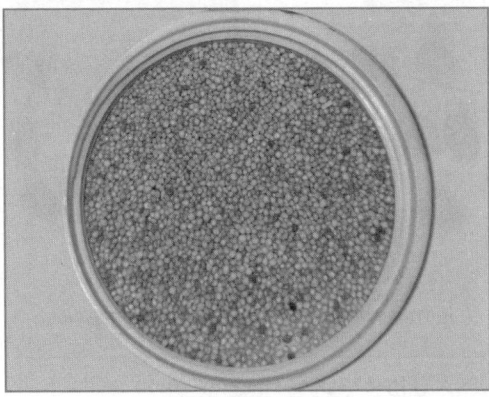

Fig. E12.12: Poppy seeds: The dried fruit is broken and the seeds are used for cooking curries. These seeds do not contain the active ingredient.

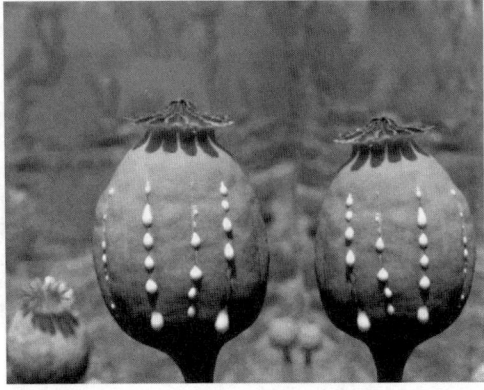

Fig. E12.10: Papaver somniferum: Somniferous poison.

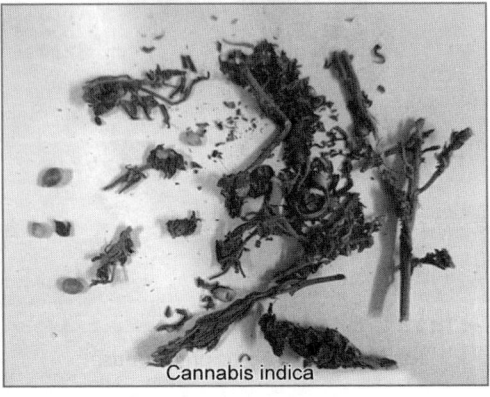

Fig. E12.13: Cannabis indica.

CNS Poisons (FM14.17)

- Poppy seeds (morphine)
- Nux vomica (strychnine—spinal poison) **(Fig. E12.14)**.

PLANTS

Irritants

- Calotropis **(Fig. 12.15)**
- Ricinus communis

Cardiac Poisons

- Nerium odorum **(Fig. E12.16)**
- Nicotine leaves
- Aconite root **(Fig. E12.17)**

Deliriant

- Datura (thorn apple)
- Cannabis

Chemicals

- Arsenic
- Lead salts

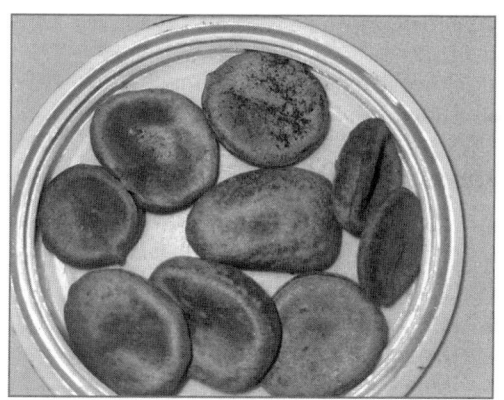

Fig. E12.14: Nux vomica seeds: Spinal poison, active ingredient is strychnine.

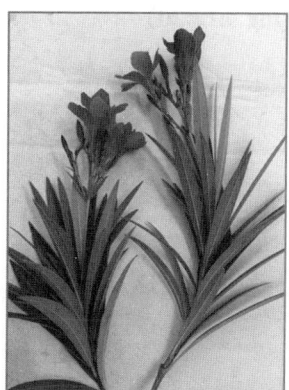

Fig. E12.16: Nerium odorum: Cardiac poison.

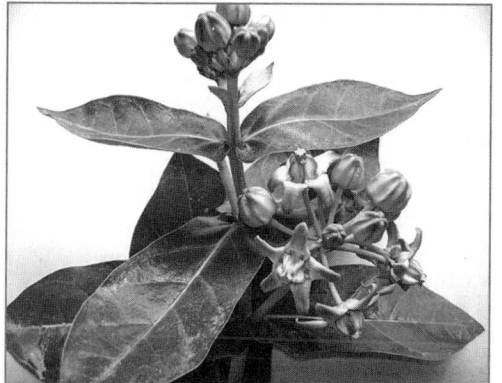

Fig. E12.15: Calotropis: Active ingredient, criminal use and medico-legal importance.

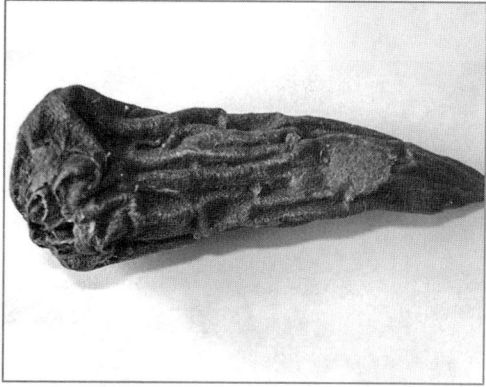

Fig. E12.17: Aconite root (Monk's hood): Cardiac poison.

- Copper sulphate **(Fig. E12.18)**
- Carbolic acid (phenol)
- Cleaning acid (sulfuric acid)
- Alcoholic beverage
- OPC compound

Soft Tissues (FM14.10)

- Intracranial hemorrhages
- Skull fractures
- Stab injury heart, lung and liver
- Cardiomegaly
- Scorpion
- Cobra **(Fig. E12.19)**
- Viper **(Fig. E12.20)**
- Krait

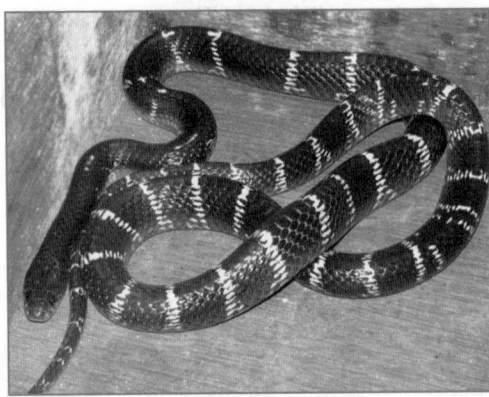

Fig. E12.20: Viper (viperidae): Hemotoxic snake.

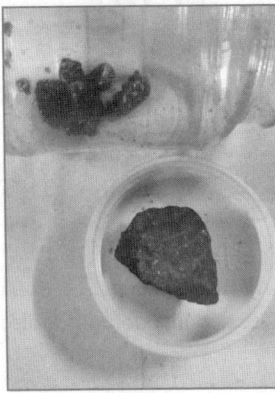

Fig. E12.18: Copper sulphate (blue vitriol): Metallic irritant poison.

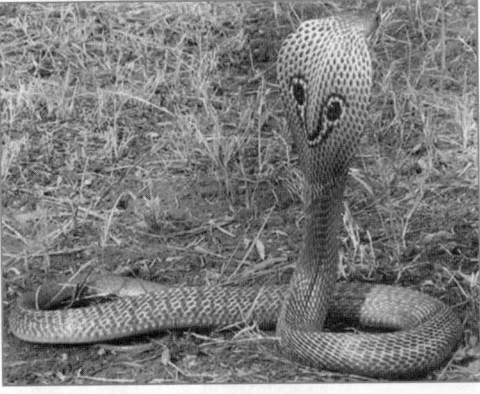

Fig. E12.19: Cobra (elapidae): Neurotoxic snake.

- Corrosive poisoning stomach
- Soot particles in trachea

Photographs

- **Hanging:** Complete and partial hanging
- Ligature abrasion
- Cyanosis
- Petechial hemorrhages: Lungs and heart
- Drowning
- Joule burns
- Postmortem staining
- Tattoo mark
- Scars and keloid

All the spotters' seeds, plants and photographs are discussed in detail in theory with necessary relevant photographs in the related chapters.

Weapons (FM14.11)

The weapons are examined with reference to:
- Name the weapon
- Blunt or sharp weapon
- Injuries produced

Blunt weapons like wooden club, iron rod, police lathi, etc., produces abrasion, contusion, laceration and fracture dislocation.

Sharp weapon could be light cutting weapon like hand knife or heavy cutting weapon like chopper or axe.

Light cutting weapons like hand knife or kitchen knife produces incised wounds (force is tangential) or stab wounds (force is perpendicular). Heavy cutting weapons like a long chopper produce cut wounds (force is perpendicular) or chop wounds (tangential force).

The following weapons are commonly used as weapon of assault and displayed for examination. (FM14.11)

- **Single edged knife:** Single edged light cutting weapon; produces incised wounds and stab wounds.
- Chopper
- Long chopper
- Axe

  All are heavy cutting weapons; produces cut wounds and fractures.

- **Sickle:** Curved single edges light cutting weapon; produces an incised wound and after a distance of intact skin, there could be a stab wound. Both the wounds are present along the same plane, indicating they were caused by a single strike; frequently the intact skin has a linear imprint abrasion.
- Wooden club
- Iron rod
- Police lathi

  All are heavy blunt weapons that produce abrasion, contusion, laceration and fracture dislocation.

- **Cycle chain:** Flexible heavy blunt weapon; produces imprint abrasion, patterned contusion (bruise), laceration and rarely fracture dislocation.
- Coir rope
- Nylon rope

  These are flexible blunt weapons; produces imprint abrasion (ligature mark or hanging and strangulation). These ropes are frequently used to tie the victim, to incapacitate him during assault or robbery.

- Hammer with nail plucker
- Wooden hammer

These are heavy blunt weapons with a small striking surface and hence produce depressed fracture of skull; on other parts of the body they could produce pressure/imprint abrasion, contusion, laceration and fracture dislocation. The nail plucker produces stab wounds.

- **Screw driver:** Pointed weapon and produces stab wounds. Sometimes when the hilt is used, it produces blunt force injuries.
- Short gun cartridge **(FM14.12)** (**Fig. E12.21**).

  Draw the diagram and label the parts.
  What is choking and why it is done?
  Choking (**Fig. E12.22**) is constriction of the terminal (muzzle end) portion of the barrel done in case of shot guns. Choking prevents early dispersion of pellets (shots).

- Bullet **(FM14.12)** (**Fig. E12.23**).

  Draw a labeled diagram.
  What is rifling and why it is done?
  The barrel of rifled firearm is scrolled inside by concentric spiral groves and it is called rifling. Rifling gives the bullet

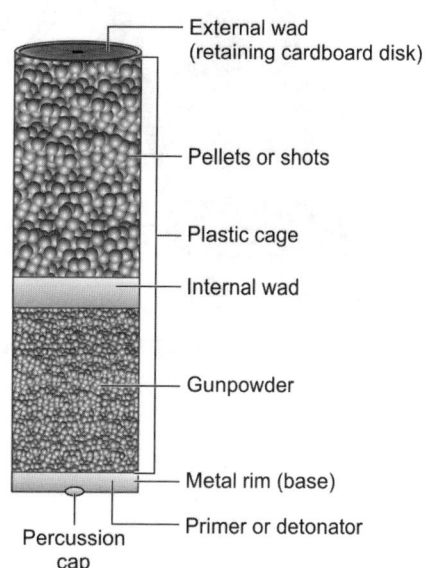

Fig. E12.21: Shotgun cartridge.

a spinning motion, thus increasing the penetration power of the bullet.
- Pistol **(FM14.12) (Fig. E12.24)**
- Revolver **(FM14.12)**
These are rifled firearms. They are handguns (low velocity firearms).

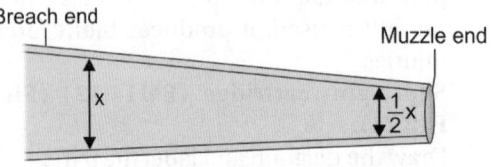

Fig. E12.22: Choking of a shotgun.

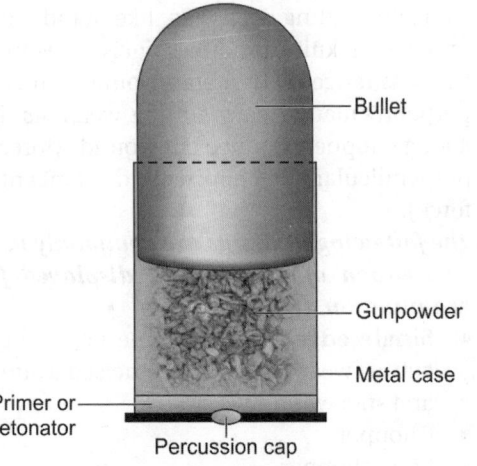

Fig. E12.23: Rifled cartridge.

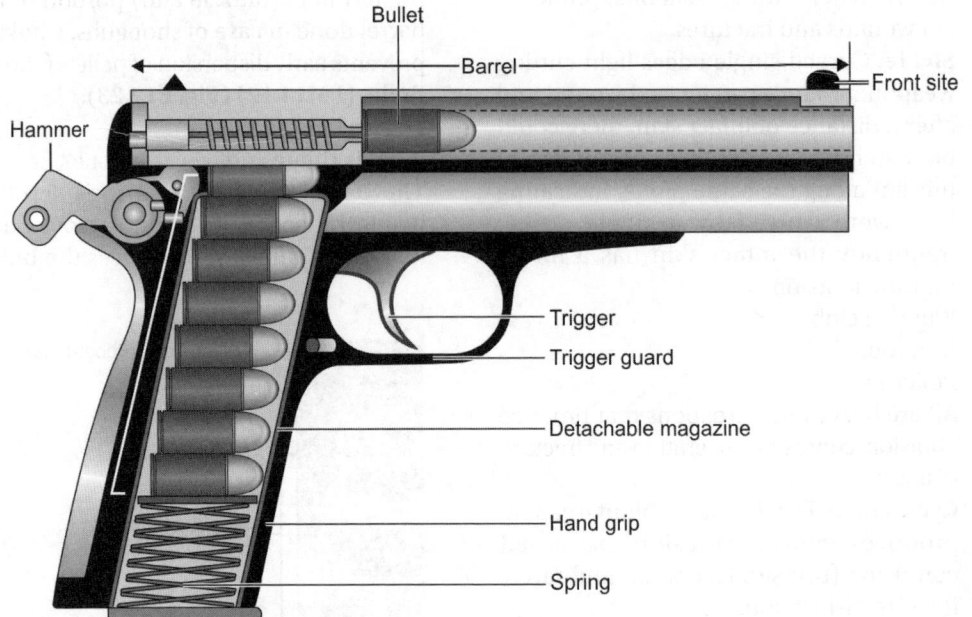

Fig. E12.24: Pistol (handgun—low velocity firearm).

Index

Page numbers followed by *f* refer to figure, *fc* refer to flowchart, and *t* refer to table

A

Abdomen scaphoid 161
Abduction fracture 147
Abortifacient 350, 389
　drugs 262
Abortion 29, 261, 265, 266, 373
　artificial 261
　complication of 261
　criminal 89, 261, 262, 264
　evidences of 261
　legal definition of 261
　natural 261
　recent 264
　stick 262, 263
Abortionists
　semiskilled 262
　types of 262
Abrasion 165-168, 177
　age of 167
　antemortem 169, 169*t*
　atypical 167
　collar 227
　healing of 167, 168*t*
　medico-legal importance of 167, 168
　postmortem 169, 169*f*, 169*t*
　types of 166
Abrus precatorius 343, 360, 361*f*, 461*f*
Abscess 76
Absent testis syndrome 65
Absolute infertility 249
　causes of 249
Absorption 339, 378, 382, 400
Accident register 439
Accidental ligature strangulation 144
Acconcher's hand 340
Acetic acid 320
Acetone 320
Acid 335
　phosphatase test 84
Aconite 314, 321, 400, 401
　root 402*f*, 463*f*

Aconitum ferox 401
Acrid 320
Acrodynia 350
Acrophobia 296
Acute arsenic poisoning 344, 345, 348*t*
　treatment of 345
Acute phosphorus poisoning
　mode of action of 354
　symptoms of 354
Acute poisoning 314, 344, 345, 348, 352, 355, 381, 386
　signs of 345
　symptoms of 345
Acute starvation 160
　death 161
　signs of 160
　symptoms of 160
Addiction 29, 387
Addison's disease 346
Adduction fracture 146, 147
Adenine 87
Adipocere 128
　formation 106, 129
Adrenal insufficiency 369
Adrenaline 372
Adultery 254, 283
Affective disorder 297
Age estimation 68, 419, 422
Agonal artefacts 101
Agoraphobia 296
Agrochemicals, classification of 328*fc*
AIDS 76
Air
　embolism 106
　insufflations 263
　mass movement of 203
Airway 379
Alcohol 110, 212, 321, 382, 386
　concentration of 382*t*
　influence of 442
　intoxication 49
　smell of 442, 443

Alcoholic beverages 382
Alcoholism 29, 298, 384
  complications of 384
Aldicarb 331
Aldrich Mee's lines 346
Algor mortis 120
Alkalies 341
  clinical features of 341
  postmortem findings of 341
  treatment of 341
  use of 341
Alkaline phosphatase, reaction of 217
Alkaloids 377, 411
  cadaveric 411
  natural 378, 378*t*
Alkyl phosphates 327
Alleged crime, history of 446
Aluminium phosphide 320, 333
  poisoning 333
Amanita
  muscaria 412
  phalloides 412
Amentia 298
American law institute test 304
Aminocarb 331
Ammonia, inhalation of 341
Ammonium hydroxide 341
Ammunition 223
Amniotic fluid
  embolism 265
  sac 255*f*
Amphetamine 394
Amygdalin 406
Amyl nitrite inhalation 407
Analgesic 378
Analytical toxicology 85, 312, 321
Anaphylactic reactions, early 371
Anaphylaxis 100
Anemia 113, 349
Anesthesia 207
  administration of 207
Angina pain 400
Angioma 193
Aniline 122, 319
Animal hair 83, 83*t*
Animal origin 83, 432
Ankle joint 430, 430*f*
Anonymity 43
Anorexia 401
Anoxia 113
  anemic 113
  types of 113

Anoxic anoxia 113
Antemortem 84, 103, 217
  abrasions 169, 169*t*
  burns 216*f*
    indicative of 217
    signs of 217
  injuries 201
  ligature abrasion 139*f*
  wounds 202, 202*t*
Anthropometry 67
Anticoagulant therapy 193
Antidote 316, 317, 385
  administration 314, 316, 329
  mechanism of action of 318*t*
Antiseptics 106
Antisnake venom 371
Antitussive 378
Antivenom
  composition of 370
  indications for 371
  injection, dosage schedule of 371
  reaction 371
    management of 372
  treatment, indications for 370
Anxiety 400, 407
  neurosis 297
Aorta
  coarctation of 65
  rupture of 194
Aphrodisiac 389
Apnea test 110
Apomorphine 378
Aprocarb 331
Aqua fortis 337
Arcus senilis 77
Arrhythmias 402
Arsenic 320, 343, 344, 347, 348
  effects of 346
  environmental sulfide of 343, 344
  ingestion, chronic 347
  poisoning 346, 348
    chronic 346
    diagnosis of 347
    medico-legal issues of 347
    postmortem findings of 347
  types of 344
Arsenicals, medicinal uses of 344
Arsine gas 344
  inhalation of 344, 345
  manifests 346
Artefacts 101
  kind of 102

types of 101
Arterial spurting test 116
Arteries, rupture of 338f
Artificial abortion 261
Artificial insemination 247, 249
    ethical and legal issues of 249
    indications of 249
    legal issues of 250
Artificial phalluses 285
Aryl phosphates 327
Asphyxia 113, 135, 138, 149
    causes of 135
    classical signs of 136
    combined 138
    form of 149
    signs of 144, 146, 149, 401
    traumatic 149
Asphyxial triad 136
Asphyxiants 314, 404
Aspiration 98, 101
    pneumonitis 339f
Assault 44, 198
Asthmatic attacks 411
Atavism 250
Ataxia 353
Atheroma 115
    localization of 115
Atomic absorption spectrometry 232
Atropine 318, 329
Attention 300
Attrition 70
Auditory hallucination 295
Auscultation 116
Auto-erotic asphyxia 150, 287
Autonomy 36
Autopsy 92, 93, 96, 102, 104-106
    clinical 94, 94t
    pathological 93, 94t
    psychological 94
    second 104
    surgeon 155
    types of 93
    verbal 94
Avulsion 175
Axillary hair 68

B

Bacillus 411
Bacterial food poisoning 410
    diagnosis of 411
Baldness 68

Ballistics 223
    intermediate 223
    terminal 223
Bansdola 149
Barberio's test 84
Barbiturates 110, 381, 386, 389, 394
    addiction 387
    automatism 386
    blisters 386
    classes of 386
    groups of 386
    poisoning 387
        signs of 386
        symptoms of 386
        treatment of 386
Barium poisoning 356
Barotrauma
    acoustic 204
    pulmonary 106
Barr body 64
Barrel, cross-section of 224f
Basic skin incisions 97
Battered baby syndrome 273
Beating heart donor 112
Bed side test 340
Behavior 300, 443
Benzidine test 147
Benzodiazepines 381
Benzylisoquinoline group 377
Bestiality 284, 285
Biological trace evidences 85
Biomedical research 38
Birth
    concealment of 259, 266
    natural 250
Bite mark 71, 367f
Black foot disease 346
Black gun powder 226
Blackmailing 254
Bladder emptying time 132
Blade, dimension of 182
Blast
    lung 204, 205
    wave 203
    wind 203
Bleeding disorders 368
Blindness, temporary 408
Blister formation 217
Blood 83, 132, 353, 379
    alcohol concentration 442
    clot 202

consistency of 202
microscopy of 202
collection of 194
discrasias 172
donor 42
extravasation of 147, 202
film 370
flow 99
groups 82
mercury level 351
stasis of 137
test 347
Blunt force injury 178
Body
condition of 128
cooling of 120
fat 161
floatation of 154
fluids 81
hair 451
internal examination of 131
mutilation of 155f
packer syndrome 380
part of 214
stuffing 380
surface, examination of 446
temperature 121
transaction of 175f
Bomb blast injuries 204
effects of 203
Bone
bundle of 102
cluster of 432
examination of 432
fracture of 103
marrow 132
Botulism 314, 410, 411
Box jellyfish 413
Boxers attitude 216
Brain 213, 321
abscess 138
compression of 113
concussion of 189
death certification, procedure of 111fc
fingerprinting 86
infarction of 138
mapping 86
stem 110
death 110, 112
functions 110, 116

tissues 97
tumor 193
waves 86
Brampton's cocktail 380
Breach loader 224
Breast 245, 256, 258
Breath 179, 442, 443
analysis 384
Breathing 379
Breathlessness 149
British anti lewisite 345
Broad ligature abrasion 139f
Broken tooth 70
Bromobenzyl cyanide 408
Bronchial tree, dissection of 154
Bronchioles
primary 98
secondary 98
Bronze diabetes 351
Brown atrophy 161
Brown sugar addiction 378
Bruise 146, 170, 172, 172f, 173, 173f
antemortem 174
artificial 171, 364
determine appearance of 172
false 172, 173
medico-legal importance of 171
postmortem 174
Brush burn 166, 167
Buccal coitus 284, 285
Buccal mucosa 64
Buggery 284
Bulbar paralysis 370
Bullet injury 187
Buprenorphine 378
Burking 148
Burning 227
pain 345
Burns 98, 213-215, 217, 219, 219t
antemortem 216f
classification of 214
epidermal 214
filigree 238
injury, age of 215
respiratory 219
surface 238
types of 214
Burnt rope 320
odor 391
Burtonian line 349

C

Cadaver, entomology of 130
Cadaveric
    donation 110, 112
    rigidity 123
    spasm 124, 124t, 154
Caecum 204
Caffey's syndrome 273
Calcium
    gluconate 332
    oxalate 340
Calotropis 343, 360, 361, 361f, 463f
    gigantea 361
    procera 361
    criminal use of 361
Camphor 320
Cancer 406
    oral 400
Cannabis 320
    abuse, chronic 391
    indica 390, 390f, 462
    preparations of 391
    signs of 391
    symptoms of 391
    type 394
Cantharides 373
Capsicum 360
    annum 343, 364
    seed 364f, 390, 390t, 461f
Carbamates 331
Carbofuran 331
Carbolic acid 320
    Poisoning
        clinical features of 338
        diagnosis of 338
        properties of 338
        treatment of 338
        use of 338
Carbolism 339
Carboluria 339
Carbon dioxide 113
    concentration of 406t
Carbon disulphide 320
Carbon monoxide 122, 314, 319, 404
    Poisoning
        mechanism of action of 404
        signs of 404
        symptoms of 404
        treatment of 404
    production of 404

Carbonic anhydrase enzyme systems 407
Carboxyhemoglobin 404
    elevated levels of 217
Cardiac arrest 402
Cardiac tamponade 194
Cardiomyopathies 115
Cardiovascular system 115
Cartridge 224
    brain of 226
Carunclunae
    hymenalis 246
    myrtiformis 246
Casper's dictum 127, 128
Castor 362
    plant 362f, 460f
    seeds 362f
Catamites 284
Cattle poison 350
Caustic soda 341
Cavity, abdominal 258f
Cells
    flattening of 139
    nucleus of 86
Cellular death 112
Cellular toxin 405
Central Forensic Science Laboratory 81
Cephalic index 62, 63, 63t
Cerbera
    odollam 400
    thevetia 400
Cerebera thevetia 403
Cerebral
    anemia 138
    concussion 100, 189
    edema 405
    liquefaction 138
    poisons 376
    softening 138
Cerebrospinal fluid 132
Cervical vertebra 103
    fracture dislocation of 138
Cervix 66, 256
    dilatation of 263
Charas 391
Charcoal 226
    activated 314, 315
Cheiloscopy 74
Chelation
    challenging test 351
    therapy 351

Chemical 463
  analysis 100, 101, 320
  antidotes 318
  asphyxiants 136
  examination 84
  injury 198
Chest, shape of 270, 451
Chilli seeds 390*f*, 462*f*
Chloral hydrate 381, 387
Chlorine 409
Chloroacetophenone 408
Chloropicrin 409
Chlorthion 327
Choking 225
  effects of 225*f*
Cholera 348, 348*t*
Cholinergic excess 328
Cholinesterase activity, depression of 329
Chop wound 176, 177, 177*f*
Chromatography, column 323
Chromosomal sex, disorders of 65
Chromosomes 87
Chronic arsenic
  ingestion 347
  poisoning 346
Chronic cannabis abuse, complications of 391
Chronic poisoning 314, 330, 340, 344, 352, 353, 355, 387, 400, 406
  symptoms of 406
Chvostek's sign 340
Ciguatera poisoning 412
Cincam 314
Cinderella syndrome 275
Circulation 379
  stoppage of 116
Civil case 7, 254
Civil negligence 51
Claustrophobia 296
Clinical death 112
Clinical Establishments (Registration and Regulation) Act 18
Clostridium botulinum 411
Clothes, examination of 215, 446
Clotting disorders 368
CNS 115
  effects 329
  poisons 463
CO
  detection of 406
  poisoning
    circumstances of 405

  signs of 405*t*
  symptoms of 405, 405*t*
  properties of 404
Cobra 366*f*, 464*f*
  snake, bite mark of 367*f*
Cocaine 380, 394
  bugs 295, 380
  desensitizes 380
Codeine 378
Cold 161
  effects of 211
  stiffening 124
Colic 349
Collapse 407
Colliquative putrefaction 124, 126
Colon 204
Coma 113, 191, 407
  cocktail 314, 315
  stage of 383
Common witness 13, 14
Commotio cerebri 189
Communication skills 37
Community health 26
Compartment syndrome 204
  clinical features of 372
Complexion 204
Compos mentis 17
Compression fracture 146
Computed automated system 85
Computed axial tomography 106
Concealed sex 64
Conception, products of 99
Concussion 190
  mercurialis 350
Conflict resolution techniques 37
Confusion 406, 407
Congeners 382
Congestion 137, 137*f*, 171, 172, 172*t*
Conjunctiva 409
Consciousness, period of 191
Consent 47, 302
  types of 48
Constipation 349
Consumer Protection Act 54
Consumption 384
  coagulopathy 366
Contact shot 229
Contracted pupil 77
Contre-coup injury 189
  mechanism of 189
Contre-coup lesion 189

Contusion 165, 170, 170*f*, 171, 172
   collar 227
   color changes of 170
   healing of 171*t*
   internal 171*f*
   true 172
   types of 170
Convulsions 362, 407
Copper 352
   acetoarsenite 344
   arsenite 344
   sulphate 352*f*, 464*f*
      poisoning 352
Cornea 120
Coronary artery
   bypass 207
   dissection of 99
Coronary occlusion 115
Coroner's court 8, 8*t*
Coroner's inquest 7, 8
Corporate negligence 53
Corpus delicti 62
Corrosive 314
   poisons 335
Coup injury 189, 190
Court 10
Cranial fossa, anterior 188*f*
Cranial nerve palsies 353
Creosote 320
Cribriform 244
Crime
   bullet 231
   scene of 74
Criminal abortion 89, 261, 262, 264
   complications of 264
   methods of 262
Criminal case 7, 49, 253
Criminal courts 10*fc*, 10*t*
Criminal Law Amendment Act 279
Criminal negligence 51
Criminal procedure code 7
Croton 360
   tiglium 343, 363
Crowned tooth 70
Crush
   injuries 194
   syndrome 204
Culpable homicide 200
Curren's rule 304
Current, amount of 235
Custody, chain of 15

Cut
   fracture 188
   throat injury 179
   wound 176, 177, 177*f*
Cutis anserina 153
CVS 353
Cyanide 122, 314, 318-320, 406, 407
   cytochrome combination 407
   forensic significance of 408
   inhibits cytochrome oxidase 407
   poisoning, treatment of 407
Cyanmethemoglobin 407
Cyanosis 136, 136*f*, 137
Cylindrical gun 225*f*
Cytochrome oxidase 407
Cytolytic toxins 366
Cytosine 87

D

Dactylography 73
Danbury's tremors 350
Dangerous weapon 199
Datura
   plant 388, 388*f*, 461*f*
   poisoning
      circumstances of 389
      signs of 389
      symptoms of 389
      treatment of 389
   seed 364, 388*f*, 389, 390, 390*f*, 390*t*, 461*f*, 462*f*
Davidson's bodies 64
Dead body
   preservation of 105
   process decomposition of 124
   reconstruction of 99
Dead born 268-270, 270*t*
Death 109, 160, 207, 235, 407
   accidental forms of 149
   anaphylactic 98
   asphyxial 99
   causes of 20, 101, 103, 128, 138, 143, 155, 161, 201, 214, 264, 345, 349, 437, 456
   certificate 30, 455
   delayed 138, 264
   investigation of scene of 88
   manner of 217
   mechanism of 151, 152, 213, 236
   mode of 113
   moment of 119
   natural 95, 100, 113, 114
   nonspecific external sign of 153*f*

presumption of 115
remote causes of 264
stage of 112
sudden 114, 115, 273
types of 112
unnatural 95, 113
Decomposed body 66
Decomposition, color changes of 124
Decontamination 314, 315, 329
Deep burns 214
Deep contusion 170*f*, 174
Defense
  injuries 177, 199
  wound 182, 205, 205*f*
Defloration 245
Degenerative diseases 98
Delayed bruising 173
Deliriants 377, 388, 463
  poisons 314
Delirium 294
  tremens 298
Delivery 253
  medico-legal aspects of 256
  recent 256, 257
Delusions 294
  types of 294
Dementia pugilistica 193
Demulcents 362
Dental examination 68
Dentin, second 70
Dentition 68
Deoxyribonucleic acid
  fingerprinting, applications of 86
  types of 87
  typing 87
    applications of 87
Depressant 377, 393
Depression, stage of 380
Depressive neurosis 298
Dermal
  collagen 182
  nitrate test 231
Dermatoglyphics 74
Dermo-epidermal burns 214, 216*f*
Detoxification, accelerated 318
Devil's helmet 401
Dextrose 315
Diacetyl morphine 378
Diaphragm
  level of 272
  position of 270, 451
Diarrhea 332, 345, 401, 410, 412

Diatoms 155
  isolation of 155
  medico-legal importance of 156
  test 155
Diazepam 362
Diazinon 327
Dichotomy 30
Digital examination 447
Digitalis 314, 321, 401
  purpurea 400, 401
Digitoxin 401
Digoxin 401
Dilated pupil 77, 331
Dildoes 285
Diphenyl chlorarsine 409
Diphenyl cyanarsine 409
Diphenylamine chlorarsine 409
Dipsomania 295
Direct violence 186
Discrimination 42
Disinfectant 320
Dissection methods 96
Distant shot 230
Distraction 299
District sessions court 9
Documentary evidence 16
Domestic violence 44
Dowry 45
  assaults 45
  death 8, 201
Drowning 98, 110, 151, 153, 154*f*, 155*f*, 156
  place of 156
  second 152
  sign of 153, 154*f*
  types of 151
Drowsiness 407
Drugs 393
  addiction 392, 393, 393*t*
  and Cosmetics Act 1945 313
  dependence 298, 392, 393
  dependence, types of 393
  habituation 392, 393
Drunkenness 384, 442
  certification of 442
Dry drowning 151, 152
Dry mouth 345
Dum dum bullet 230
Dura matter 190
Durham's rule 304
Dying declaration 17, 18, 18*t*
Dying deposition 18, 18*t*
Dynamic overpressure 203

Dysarthria 193
Dyspareunia 249
Dysphagia 332, 345
Dyspnea 400

E

Ear print 75
Ecchymosis 170
Ectopic
　bruise 170, 172
　contusion 172, 173*f*
Edema, acute pulmonary 409
Ejaculation, premature 247
Elapidae 365
Elastic fibers 182
Elbow joint 423, 423*t*, 424*f*, 425, 425*f*
Electric
　current, kind of 235
　injury 198, 235, 236*f*
Electricity 263
Electrocution 109, 235, 237
　mode of 235
Electrolysis 77
Embalming 105
　body after autopsy 105
　fluid 105
　method of 105
Embolism 115, 203
Embryo 66
Emesis 315
　indications for 315
Emphysema aquosum 154
Employees State Insurance Act 56
Encephalopathy 349
　hypoxic ischemic 138
Endocrine 112, 369
Endometrium 99
Endotoxin reactions 371
Entomo-toxicology 321
Entry wound 229, 229*t*
　features of 227
　general features of 227
Enzyme histochemistry 202
Epidural hemorrhage 190
　clinical features of 191
　features of 190
　medico-legal importance of 191
　salient features of 191
Epilepsy, effects of 299
Epileptic equilent 299
Epinephrine 372
Erotomaniacal delusion 294

Eruption, age of 419, 420
Erysipelas 76
Erythema 215
Erythroblastosis fetalis 269
Erythroderma 350
Esophagus 98
Ethanol 381, 382
　effects of 383
　poisoning 384
　　clinical features of 383
　use of 382
　usual fatal dose of 382
Ethical committee 40
Ethics
　code of 24
　historical emergence of 24
Ethyl iodoacetate 408
Eucalyptus 360
Eugenic 263
Euphoria 391
Euthanasia 26, 34
　classification of 34
　legal status of 34
　various forms of 34
Evidence 15
　speaks 52
　types of 15
Exaltation, delusion of 294
Excitement, stage of 378, 383
Exhibitionism 278, 286
Exhumation 103, 104*f*
　procedure of 103
Exhumed bodies 348
Exit wound 229, 229*t*
Exotoxins 410
Expert witness 13, 14
Extensive superficial burns 215*f*
Extraction 70, 377
Eye 120, 341, 443
　after death 120
　contact 337, 364
　medico-legal importance of 77
Eyebrow 451
Eyelash 451
Eyelids, dissection of 173*f*

F

Facial
　muscles, paralysis of 368
　pallor 349
Fallen masonry 150
Fallopian tubes 66

Family courts 11
Fang marks 367
Fasciotomy, criteria for 372
Fatal injury 199
Feather test 116
Federal rule 305
Federation Dentaire Internationale System 420
Feeler strokes 206
Feet, gangrene of 346, 368f
Fellate 285
Fellator 285
Femur 432, 436f
    condyles of 437f
Fertilization 253
Fetal heart sounds 254
Feticide 268
Fetishism 278, 286
Fetor hepaticus 355
Fetus compressus 255
Fever, infectious 113
Fibrillar necrosis 334
Fibroids 99
Filicide 268
Finger finger test 443
Finger nail 451
    cyanosis of 136f
    examination of 447
    test 116
Finger-nose test 443
Fingerprints
    removal of 74
    types of 73, 74
Firearm 223, 224
    choking of 225
    general makeup of 224
    injury 198, 350
        range of 227, 229
    mechanism of firing of 226
    types of 223
    wounds 166
Fireworks 354
First aid
    aims of 369
    methods 369
First information report 96
First-hand knowledge rule 13, 15
Fish and marine animals poisoning 412
Fitness, certificate of 453
Flash burn 237
Flexible rubber tube 317
Florence test 84

Fluid restriction 405
Foamy liver 127
Fodere's test 270
Folic acid 386
Folinic acid 386
Food allergy 411
Food poisoning 314, 410
    causes of 410
Foot, sole of 236f
Foramen fracture 187
Forensic
    ballistics 223
    deoxyribonucleic acid typing 86
    medicine 3
        clinical 3
        history of 4
        scope of 3, 4
    odontology 70
    pathology 3
    psychiatry 293
    science laboratories 281
        function of 81
    toxicology 312
Formaldehyde 100, 381
Formic acid 340
Formication 295
Fossa navicularis 244, 245
Foul smelling gases, evolution of 125
Fowler solution 344
Fracture 165, 188, 194
    ala signature 187
    antemortem nature of 147
    comminuted 187, 187f
    depressed 186, 187f
    diastatic 188, 188f
    fissured 186, 186f
    perforating 188
    sutural 188, 188f
Fragmented red cells 370
Freezing 105
Fresh water drowning 151
    pathophysiology of 152fc
Friction abrasions 167
Frigidity 248
    causes of 248
Frostbite 213
Frotteurism 286
Fugue state 296
Full surrogacy 251
Fulminant poisoning 314, 345
Fumigating pesticide 333

G

Gagging 151
Gait 300
Gallbladder 161
Galton system 73
Gangrene 76, 346, 368*f*
Garroting 149
Gas
    chromatography 324
    stiffening 124
Gastric lavage 315, 316, 316*t*, 331, 355, 362, 402
Gastritis, hemorrhagic 361
Gastroenteritis 345
Gastrointestinal corrosion 332
Gel electrophoresis 87
Gelsemium 314, 377
Gene 87
General violence 262
Genetic polymorphism 87
Geneva declaration 25
Genital examination 449
    external 447
Genital organs, female 243
Genital tract, female 99
Genitalia, external 66, 258
Genitourinary system 383
Gestation, period of 264
Gestational age 451
Gettler's test 155, 156
Giddiness 402
Gilroy test 231
Glans penis 280*f*
Glass jaw 355
Glassblowers tremors 350
Glory lily 360, 365
Glycosides thevetin 403
Gomorrah sin 285
Gonadal agenesis 65
Gonadal biopsy 64
Gonadal sex 65
    disorders of 65
Goose skin 153
Gradual hydrolysis 128
Grandeur, delusion of 294
Gravel rash 166, 169*f*
Gravity 335
    shifting contusion 172
Grazed abrasion 167, 169*f*
Grease collar 227
Grievous hurt 199
Guanine 87

Guard against therapeutic hazards 54
Guilty, verdict of 19
Gun powder 226
    composition of 226
Gunshot residues, tests for 231
Gustafson's method 70
Gustatory hallucination 295
Gutter fracture 187

H

Habitual passive agent 284
Haemin crystal test 83
Hair 68, 82
    analysis 351
    examination of 82
    follicles 75
    graying of 68, 83
    growth of 68*t*, 132
    medico-legal importance of 82
    medullary index of 83
    microscopy of 353
Hallucination 295
    types of 295
    visual 295
Hallucinogens 393
Hallucinosis, alcoholic 298
Handling pressure, principles of 38
Hanging 137, 138, 145, 147, 464
    atypical 138
    ligature
        abrasion of 139*f*, 140*f*, 145
        mark of 145, 145*f*
    partial 138
    types of 137, 138
Hangover 383
Harrison test 231
Hasee's rule 68
Hashish 391
    psychosis 391
Hasse rule 269
Hatter's shake 350
HCN
    mechanism of action of 407
    signs of 407
    symptoms of 407
    treatment of 407
Head injury 185, 191, 297, 297*t*
    signs of 204
Headache 400, 402, 407
    severe 409
Health, state of 161

Hearsay evidence 16
Heart 99, 237, 334, 347, 402
 burn 345
 contusion of 171*f*
 disease, chronic 114, 400
 dissection of 99
 rupture of 194
 wounds of 194
Heartbeat, irregular 400
Heat
 collapse 212
 cramps 211
 effects of 211
 exhaustion 211
 hematomas 216
 ruptures 216
 stiffening 124
 stroke 212
 syncope 212
 systemic effects of 211
 test 116
Heavy metals 106, 343
 chelating agents for 318
 poisoning 321
Helmet cell 370
Helsinki declaration 37, 39
Hematemesis 332
Hematocrit 370
Hematoma 170
Hemiparesis 248
Hemochromogen crystal test 83
Hemoglobin 371, 404
 concentration 370
Hemorrhage 97, 190, 191, 201, 202
 abdominal 204
 acute submucosal 213
 chronic subdural 192
 extradural 97, 190, 190*f*
 intracerebral 190, 193, 193*f*
 intracranial 115
 intrapulmonary 205
 intraventricular 237*f*
 multiple sub-endocardial petechial 237
 multiple sub-epicardial petechial 237
 multiple sub-pleural petechial 237
 petechial 136, 137, 137*f*
 petechio-ecchymotic 339*f*
 subarachnoid 190, 192, 192*f*
 subdural 190, 191
 sub-epicardial petechio-ecchymotic 99
 sub-pleural 98
 visible 101

Hemostatic abnormalities 371
Hemotoxic snake 464*f*
Hermaphroditism 65
Heroine, substitution therapy for 378
Hesitation cuts 206
Heterologous donation 112
Heterosexual intercourse 277
Hide and die syndrome 220
High court 9
High velocity guns 225
High-performance liquid chromatography 323
Hip joint 428, 428*t*, 429*f*, 430*f*
Hippocratic oath 24
 modified version of 25
Histotoxic anoxia 114
Homicidal 217
 cut throat injury 179, 180, 180*t*
 impulse 295
 injuries 199
 poisoning 356
 starvation 161
Homicide 44, 200, 402, 408
 attempted 44
 excusable 200
 justifiable 200
Homologous donation 112
Honeycomb liver 124, 127
Hospital smell 320
Hostile witness 16
Hot climate 131
Human bite mark 71*f*
Human hair 83, 83*t*
Human organs, storage of 110
Humanitarian 263
Hydrargyrism 350
Hydrocarbons 381
Hydrochloric acid 338
Hydrocortisone 372
Hydrocution 151, 152
Hydrocyanic acid, sources of 406
Hydrogen
 cyanide 406
 sulfide 122, 319, 320
Hydrophobia 296
Hydrostatic test 269, 271
Hydroxocobalamine 407
Hymen 244, 259, 447
 medico-legal importance of 246
 rupture of 245
 types of 244
Hyoid bone 103, 141, 146, 147

fracture 146, 147
    types of 147
Hyperbaric oxygen 405
Hypertension 406
Hyperthermia 406
Hypnosis 86
Hypnotism, effects of 303
Hypocalcemia 340
Hypochondriacal delusion 294
Hypoglycemia leads 220
Hypogonadism, female 65
Hypostasis, postmortem 121
Hypotension 402, 407
Hypothermia 110, 112, 212, 213
  pathophysiology of 212
  phases of 212
Hypovolemia 207
Hypoxia 113
Hysterical neurosis 297

I

I incision 97
Icard's test 116
Ideal homicidal poison, characteristics of 313
Ideal suicidal poison, characteristics of 313
Idiocy 298
Illusion 295
Immersion syndrome 151, 152
Imperforate hymen 244
Impotence 247
  causes of 248
Imprint abrasion 166, 167
Impulse 295
  types of 295
In vitro fertilization 251
Incest 284
Incised wound 176, 178, 178*f*
  features of 175, 176
  healing of 177
Indian Contracts Act 47
Indian Evidence Act 7
Indian Legal System 6
Indian Medical Council Act 27
Indian Penal Code 6
Indian Status on Drugs and Poisons 313
Indirect violence 186
Inebriant 376, 381
Inert complex formation 318
Infanticide 260
Infection 138, 203
Infectious diseases 31

Infertility 249
  absolute 249
Infidelity, delusion of 294
Inflammation 368
Influence, delusion of 294
Informed consent 48
  ingredients of 48
Infusion, intravenous 371
Ingestion 335, 364
Injury 165, 175, 179, 198, 439, 440
  accidental 199
  antemortem 201
  dangerous 199
  evidence of 217
  explosive 198
  fabricated 199
  legal
    classification of 199
    definition of 165, 198
  mechanical 165, 198
  medical
    classification of 198
    definition of 165
  medico-legal
    aspects of 198
    classification of 199
  nature of 76
  postmortem 201
  presence of 279
  primary 194, 203
  regional 185
  second 194, 204
  self-inflicted 199
  simple 199
  suicidal 199
  tertiary 204
  time of 441
  types of 441
Ink remover 340
Inorganic arsenic compounds 343
Inorganic irritants 343
  poisons 343
Inquest 7
  medical examiner system of 7-9
  superior type of 9
  types of 7
Insane
  criminal responsibility of 304
  general paralysis of 298
  restraint of 301
Insanity 297, 299

causes of 297
certification of 300
classification of 297
lucid interval of 297
observation of 300
true 301, 301t
Insecticide 333
Insomnia 400
Instantaneous rigor 124
Institutional Ethical Committees, functions of 40
Intense laryngeal spasm 336
Internal organs, dissection of 96, 96f
Intersex 64
classification of 65
Intestine 161, 379
Intoxication 383
stage of 383
Intracerebral hemorrhage 190, 193, 193f
causes of 193
Intracranial hemorrhage 115
types of 190, 191
Intranuclear inclusion bodies 64
Intraocular pressure 120
Intrauterine life 67
Intravenous push injection 371
Iris 75
Iron 351
poisoning 351
rod 440
Irresistible impulse test 304
Irritants 314, 343, 460, 463

J

Jatropha curcas 365
Jellyfish poisoning 412
Joule burn 236, 237
Judicial hanging 142
Judicial inquisition 302
Judicial magistrate courts 10
Juvenile justice courts 11

K

Kastle-Meyer test 83
Keloid formation 75f
Kennedy phenomenon 101, 231
Kerosene 320
poisoning 338f, 339f
Kevorkian sign 120
Kidney 98, 112, 347, 379
Klebsiella 203
Kleptomania 295

Klinefelter syndrome 65
Knee joint 430, 430t
Knockout drops 387
Korsakov's psychosis 298
Krogman's accuracy 66
Kunkel's test 406

L

Labia
majora 245, 256
minora 245, 256
Labor courts 11
Laceration 165, 174, 178, 178t
general features of 174
internal 194
medico-legal significance of 175
types of 175
Lachrymators 408
Lactational psychosis 299
Langer lines 182
Lanugo hair 451
Laparotomy, surgical incised wound scar of 75f
Laryngeal spasm, acute 152
Larynx
edema of 138
surface of 98
Laser beam 77
Latent tattoo marks 76
Law, medical aspects of 3
Lead 348
encephalopathy 349
lines 349
mechanism of action of 348
medico-legal significance of 349
osteopathy 349
palsy 349
ring 227
toxic compounds of 348
Leave
certificate 453
extension of 453
medical certificate for 453
Legal
classification 198, 199
duties 319
insanity 294
issues 259
responsibilities 283
Legitimacy 250
Lesbianism 284, 285
Leukocytic infiltration 217

Lie detector 85
Ligature 138
    mark 139, 141, 143
    material, fibers of 142
    strangulation 142, 143, 143f, 144f, 147
        symptoms of 143
    test 116
Lightening 238
    injuries 235
Lignocaine 401
Limbs 193
Lips, inner surface of 174f
Liquid paraffin 406
Litmus test 336
Live birth
    medico-legal aspects of 271
    signs of 269
Live born 271, 272, 272t
Live donation 112
Liver 98, 347, 379
Livor mortis 120, 121, 171
Locard's principle 81
Lochia 256, 257
    alba 257
    rubra 257
    serosa 257
Loco parentis 50
Long acting barbiturates 386
Long bone 438
Loperamide 378
Low velocity firearm 466f
Lower limb, paralysis of 193
Luminous gastric contents 355
Lungs 98, 155, 212, 237, 265, 270, 332, 347, 409
    cancer 400
    congestion of 137f
    cross section of 115f
    dissection of 154f
    edema of 138
    parenchyma 338f
Lust murder 286
Lynching 141

M

Maceration 269
    signs of 268
MacEwan's sign 383
Mad hatter 350
Magistrate
    court 8, 8t, 10t
    inquest 7, 8

Magnan's symptom 295, 380
Magnesium
    serum 155
    sulfate therapy 333
Magnus's test 116
Malingering 35, 364, 401
Malnutrition 160
Mandible 432, 435t, 436f
Maniac depressive psychosis 350
Mannitol 405
Marginal bruising 179
Marijuana 320
Marine fish 412
Marsh Berzelius test 346
Masked epilepsy 299
Masochism 278, 286
Mass
    disasters 67
    spectrometry 324
Masturbation 246
Maternity benefit 57
Mc Naughten's rule 304
McEwan's sign 383
Mechanical asphyxia 136
    causes of 135
Mechanical violence 262
Meconium 451
Medical
    degrees
        recognition of 28
        schedule of 28t
    ethics 4, 24, 25
    etiquette 24
    jurisprudence 3
    malpractice 50
    negligence 15, 47, 52, 54
    practice, corner stone of 48
    register, maintenance of 28, 29
Medical Termination of Pregnancy Act 18, 263
Medicine, legal aspects of practice of 3
Medico-legal autopsy 93, 94, 94t, 95
    aims of 95
    objectives of 95
Medullary index 67, 83
Memory 300
Meningeal artery, posterior 190
Meninges 97
Mental
    condition 299
    Health Act 18, 300
    illness 293

retardation 298
subnormality 298
Mentally ill person 293, 300, 302
Meperidine 378
Mercuria lentis 351
Mercurial erythrism 350
Mercurialentis 77
Mercury 98, 350
poisoning 351
Mesmerism 303, 344, 378, 382, 385
Metal fume fever 353
Metal tooth 70
Metallic irritant poison 343, 352*f*, 464*f*
Metastasis 193
Methadone 378
Methanol, ethanol inhibits metabolism of 318
Methyl alcohol poisoning
postmortem findings of 385
signs of 385
symptoms of 385
treatment of 385
Methyl parathion 327
Methyl salicylates 320
Micturition syncope 384
Mineral acids 335
Mini packer syndrome 380
Miosis 328
Mirror test 116
Missing tooth 70
Mitochondrial deoxyribonucleic acid 87
Mixed dentition 69
Mole bean 362
Molecular death 112
Monetary damages 19
Monk's hood 400, 401, 402*f*, 463*f*
Montgomery's tubercles 258
Mood 300
Morphine 110, 142, 321, 378, 393
clinical symptoms of 378
mechanism of action of 378
medico-legal importance of 380
pharmacokinetics of 378
poisoning 379
Mothballs 320
Motor car collisions 193
Mugging 148
Mummification 106, 128, 129
Munchausen's syndrome 272, 273
Munich beer heart 384
Murder 200
Muscarinic symptoms 329

Muscles 102
primary flaccidity of 119
Muscular coordination, tests for 443
Muscular weakness 402
Mushroom poisoning 412
Mustard gas 408
Mutilated bodies 102
examination of 102
identification of 203
Mutilation 128, 155*f*
Mutilomania 295
Mutism 299
Muzzle loader 224
Myocarditis 334
Myolytic phospholipases A2 366
Mysophobia 296

N

Nails 346
Naloxone 315
Naphthalene 320
Napoleon bonaparte 347
Narcoanalysis 85
Narcosis 378
stage of 379
Narcotic Drugs and Psychotropic Substances Act 313
Nasal irritants 409
National Commission 55
National Human Rights Commission 43
National Medical Commission
Act 18
constitution of 27
functions of 27
Natural abortion 261
causes of 261
Natural sexual offences 277
Nausea 401, 412
Near drowning 152
Neck
blood less dissection of 98
compression of 135
dissection 140, 144*f*
muscles trachea 144*f*
Necrophagia 278, 287
Necrophilia 278, 287
Necrotic toxins 366
Negligence 47
suit, components of 51
Neriifolin 403
Nerium odorum 400, 402, 402*f*, 463*f*

Nerve gases 409
Nervous poisons 314, 321
Nervous system 413
Neurosis 296, 297
Neurotic symptoms 412
Neurotoxic
  poisons 376
  signs 371
  snake 464f
Neurotoxins
  postsynaptic 367
  presynaptic 366
Neutron activation analysis 232
Nicotiana tabacum 400
Nicotinamide adenine dinucleotide phosphate 332
Nicotine 314, 400
  replacement therapy 401
Nicotinic
  effects 328
  symptoms 329
Nihilistic delusion 294
Nipples 256
Nitric acid poisoning 337
Nitrobenzene 122, 319, 320
Nitrocellulose 226
Nitroglycerine 226
Nonpoisonous snakes 365
Nontoxic cyanocobalamin 407
Nonvenomous snakes 365, 365t
Noscapine 378
Nostrils, bruising of 272f
Novus actus interveniens 51
Nulliparous uterus 258
Nux vomica seeds 394f, 463f
Nyctophobia 296
Nymphomania 278, 287

O

Obsession 295
Obsessive compulsive neurosis 298
Ochronosis 340
Odor 320
Oleander 402
  Poisoning
    signs of 403
    symptoms of 403
    treatment of 403
  types of 402
Olfactory hallucination 295
Open calvarium 97

Ophitoxaemia 367
Opiates 378, 378t, 393
Opioids 378, 378t
Opium 377
Oral consent 48
Oral feeds, use of 337
Organ, congestion of 136
Organic acids 335, 338
Organic arsenic compounds 343, 409
Organic irritants 343
  poisons 360
Organochlorines 331
Organophosphates 318, 327
Organophosphorus 320
  compounds poisoning 331
    clinical features of 327
    delayed symptoms of 330
    diagnosis of 327
    management of 327
    mechanism of action of 327
Oropharyngeal ulceration 332
Ossification center 422, 452
Ovaries 66, 265
Oxalic acid poisoning, systemic effects of 340
Oxaluria 340
Oxygen 343
  lack of 113

P

Pachymeningitis hemorrhagica interna 192
Pain, epigastric 387
Palatoprints 74
Palm rule 214
Palmer's notation 71
Palpitation 400
Panchanama 8
Pancreas 213
Papaver somniferum 377f, 462f
Papaverine 378
Paradentosis 70
Paradoxical respiration 370
Paraldehyde 381
Paralysis, respiratory 370, 379
Paraoxon 327
Paraphilias 277, 278
Paraplegia 248
Paraquat 332
  lung 332
  poisoning 332
Parathion 327
Paresthesias 406

Index

Paternalism 54
Paultaf's hemorrhages 98
Pearson's regression formula 438
Peculiar scars 75
Pederasty 284
Pedophilia 278, 287
Pellets, dispersion of 225f
Pelvis 432, 434f, 435f
    bone 434t
Penal erasure 32
Pentazocine 378
Pericardial fluid 99
Peripheral lymph edema 65
Peripheral poison 314, 376, 377
Peritoneum, bruising of 258f
Perjury 16
Permanent molar 420f
Permanent teeth 69, 69t, 71, 420
    eruption of 420t
Persecution, delusion of 294
Personality disorders 298
Pesticides 314
    classification of 328fc
Petechiae 170
Pethidine 378
Petrol 320
Pharmacokinetics 378
Phenanthrene group 377
Phenol 320
    marasmus 340
Phenotypic sex, disorders of 65
Philippine cobras 367
Phobia 296
    types of 296
Phobic neurosis 298
Phosgene 409
Phosphorus 122, 319, 320, 354, 355
    poisoning 354, 355
    use of 354
    varieties of 354
Phossy jaw 355
Physical evidence, preservation of 90
Physostigmine 389
Phytotoxin 362
Piggy back bullet 230
Pilocarpine 389
Pin point pupil 328
Pink disease 350
Pistol 226f, 466f
Placenta, medico-legal importance of 265
Plants 343, 407, 463

irritants 360
    penicillin 331
Plastic prints 74
Ploquet's test 270
Plumbism 349
Pneumococci 203
Pneumonia 113
POCSO Act 282
    complaint mechanism of 283
    salient features of 282
Poison 98, 122, 312, 314, 316, 321, 410
    absorbed 316
    action of 314
    agricultural 327
    anesthetic 321
    cardiac 314, 321, 400, 460, 463, 463f
    elimination 314
    information centers 312
Poisoning 89, 314, 318, 319, 349
    accidental 356, 402
    acute 314, 344, 345, 348, 352, 355, 381, 386
    chronic 314, 330, 340, 344, 352, 353, 355, 387, 400, 406
    circumstances of 350, 373, 402, 403
    clinical features of 360
    general considerations of 311
    mild 349
    moderate 349
    modes of actions of 314
    severe 349
    special circumstances of 321t
    stage of 314
    sub-acute 314
    suicidal 356
    symptoms of 410
    types of 314
Poisonous snakes 365
    families of 365
Police inquest 7, 8
    procedure of 7
Polygraph 85
Polymerase chain reaction technique 87
Polyneuropathy 330
Pond fracture 187
Poppy
    capsule 377f, 462f
    seeds 377f, 462f
Poroscopy 74
Postepileptic confusional state 299
Posterior commissure 245, 256
Posterior pharyngeal wall, extravasation on 146f

Postmortem 84, 95, 103, 217
 appearance 139, 143, 379, 386, 402, 405, 408
 artefacts 102
 blister formation 126*f*
 caloricity 121
 certificate 457-459
 changes 119, 131
 examination 19, 207, 269
  procedure of 319
 hanging 141
 incised wound 178
 lividity 121
 purge 126
 staining 121, 140, 171
 suspension 141
Post-traumatic stress disorder 204
Potassium 152
 chloride 122, 319
 cyanide 406
 hydroxide 341
 nitrate 226
Pralidoxime 330
Preanesthetic medication 378
Precipitin test 83, 84
Pregnancy 253, 254
 diagnosis of 255
 effects of 299
 medico-legal aspects of 253
 period of 264
 positive signs of 254
 presumptive signs of 254
 probable signs of 254
 toxemia of 269
Premature labor 261
Pressure
 abrasion 146*f*, 148*f*, 167
 immobilization method 369
 sores 169
Priapism 373
Procoagulant enzymes 366
Propranolol 401
Prostration 409
Proteus 203
Pseudocyesis 255
Pseudohermaphroditism 65, 66
 female 66, 66*f*
 male 66
Pseudomonas 203
Psychiatry and Mental Health Act, symptoms of 293
Psychomotor hallucination 295

Psychopath 296, 298
Psychopathic disorder 296
Psychosis 296-299
 organic 297
Ptomaines 411
Ptosis 368
Pubic hair 68
Pugilistic attitude 215, 216
Pulmonary air embolism 203
Pulse rate 356
Punch drunk syndrome 193
Pupillary reflex 110
Pupils 120
Puppy's rule 186
Pure gonadal dysgenesis 65
Putrefaction, modified forms of 128
Pyrethrins 332
Pyrethroids 332
Pyrogenic reactions 371
Pyromania 295

Q

Quantitative desferrioxamine color test 351
Quaternary injuries 204
Quinine 400

R

Race 62, 63
Radiation injuries 198
Radioactive carbon 132
Radiological examination 68
Radiology, applications of 69
Railway
 accidents 193
 spine 193
Rain drop pigmentation 346
Rape 44, 84, 168, 278
 certification of 447
 evidence of 283
 examination of alleged victim of 283
 proforma of examination of alleged victim of 445
 victim, medico-legal examination of 445
Rapid death 264
Rashes 411
Receptor site
 blockade 318
 competition 318
Rectum 347
Red cross emblem 33
Red velvety appearance 347

Reflux vagal inhibition 138
Registration certificate, display of 25
Rehabilitation 372
Renal failure, acute 204, 371
Replaced Indian Lunacy Act 300
Res ipsa loquitor 52
Respiration, stoppage of 116
Respiratory irritants 409
Respiratory system 115
Retina 75, 120
Retrograde amnesia 190
Ribs
    line of 204
    several 103
Ricinus communis 343, 360, 362, 362*f*, 460*f*
    seeds 461*f*
Ricochet bullet 230
Rifled cartridge 225*f*, 466*f*
Rifled firearm 224, 227
    injury 228
        exit wound of 229
Rigor mortis 120, 123, 124, 124*t*
Ring fracture 187
Road traffic accident 101, 150, 166*f*, 174*f*
Robbery 364
Robert's sign 269
Romberg's sign 443
Root
    resorption 70
    transparency of 70
Rotten egg 320
Rule of nine 214, 214*t*
Russell's viper 369

S

Sacrum 435*f*
Sadism 278, 286
Salicylates poisoning 321
Salivary stains 140
Sample PM certificate 457-459
Saponification 128
Saturnism 349
Satyriasis 278, 287
Scab 166
Scalds 218, 219, 219*t*
    injury
        circumstances of 219
        features of 218
        general features of 218
Scalp
    contusion 185*f*
    hair 451

Scar 75
    medico-legal importance of 75, 76
Scheele's green 344
Schizophrenia 297
Sciatic notch index 67
Scoptophilia 286
Scorching 227
Scorpions 372
Scratch abrasion 166, 167
Sea snakes 368
Sea water drowning 151, 154*f*
    pathophysiology of 152*fc*
Selenium 320
Semecarpus 360
    anacardium 343, 363, 363*f*, 462*f*
Seminal stains 84
Semi-somnolence 303
Septate 244
Septic inflammation 76
Septicemia 216*f*
Serum iron level 351
Sex
    behavior 300
    chromatin 64
    determination of 67
    differentiation 99
    highly probable evidence of 64*t*
    positive evidence of 64*t*
    presumptive evidence of 63*t*
Sexual abuse, forms of 282
Sexual asphyxia 149, 150, 287
Sexual assault 282
    forensic evidence kit 281
Sexual dysfunction 247
Sexual offences 83, 277, 279
    certificates 445
    examination of victim of 445
Sexual paraphilias 286
Sexual violence 279, 281
    examine victims of 279
    medical examination of 279
Shaken baby syndrome 274
Shallow water drowning 156
Sharp force injuries, types of 175
Shellfish poisoning 413
Shock 201
    delayed 203
    hypovolemic 201
    lung 340
    neurogenic 201
    primary 201
    second 203

septic 203
wave 205
Shotgun 224
    barrel of 225*f*
    caliber of 225, 226
    cartridge 225*f*, 465*f*
    choking of 225*f*, 466*f*
    entry wound, features of 229
Shoulder joint, X-ray 423*f*
Sickness gas 409
Silver nitrate test 333
Skeletal muscle breakdown 368
Skeletonization 127
Skills 24
    development of 37
Skin 102, 120, 341, 407
    blisters 408
    cherry red discoloration of 405
    destruction of 166
    examination of 447
    inflammation of 332
    irritation of 332
    lesions 169
    rash 353
    role of 212
    surface 167
Skull 432, 433*f*
    crack fractures of 274
    fractures 186
        base of 188, 188*f*
        mechanism of 185, 186
        types of 186
    superimposition of 77
    sutures 432
        closure of 436*t*
    types of 63
Sleep 300
Small intestine 204
Smegma 449
Smokeless gun powder 226
Smoky stool syndrome 355
Smooth muscle 378
Smothering 147
Smudging 227
    mode of 380
Snake
    bite, management of 369
    basic constituents of 366
Sodium
    bicarbonate solution 408
    carbonate 341
    cyanide 406
    hydroxide 341
    hypochlorite 341
    nitrite 407
    nitroprusside 406
    thiosulphate 407
Sodomy 168, 284
Soft tissues 102, 145, 146, 464
Solvent system 322, 382
Somatic death 112, 119
Somnambulism 303
Somniferous poison 462*f*
Somnolentia 303
Souvenir bullet 231
Spalding sign 269
Spark burn 237
Spasmodic pupil 402
Speech 300, 442
Speed ball 380
Spermatozoa 84
Spider's web 187
Spinal column 187, 193
Spinal cord, injury of 193
Spinal poisons 314, 376, 377, 394, 463*f*
Spleen 99, 347
Split laceration 175
Stab wound 179, 181*f*
    features of 179
    types of 179
Stabilization 314, 315
Stagnant anoxia 114
Stampede 150
Staphylococci 410
Starvation 160, 161
    acute 160
    chronic 160
    factors modifying effects of 161
    medico-legal aspects of 161
State Judicial Service 11
State Medical Council 28
    constitution of 28
    functions of 28, 29
Stature 67, 438
Stem cell
    research, ethical issues of 42
    research, legal issues of 42
Sterility 247
Sterilization 249
    medico-legal issues of 249
Sternum 431
    centers of 431*t*
Sternutators 409
Steroids 405

Stigma 42, 44
Still born 269, 270, 270t, 271, 272, 272t
Stockings fashion 140
Stomach 98, 161, 204, 333, 379, 412
    empty 344
    mucosa 336f
    wash 316, 351, 373
        procedure of 316
    wet blotting paper appearance of 337
Strangulation 142, 145
    horizontal ligature abrasion of 143f
    ligature mark of 145t
Streptococci 203
Stress 38
    management of 38
Stretch laceration 175
Strontium, serum 155
Strychnine 314, 321, 377, 394
Stupor, stage of 379
Subarachnoid hemorrhage 190, 192, 192f
    causes of 192
Subcutaneous tissues 274f, 368f
Substance abuse 392
Suffocation 149
Sugar, fermentation of 382
Suicidal cut throat 179, 180
    injury 180t
Suicidal impulse 295
Suicidal starvation 161
Suicide, attempted 44
Sulfur 226
Sulfuric acid 335
    poisoning 336f
        autopsy findings of 335
        clinical features of 335
        diagnosis of 335
        management of 335
        use of 336
Summons 11, 12
Sun stroke 212
Superfecundation 255
    medico-legal aspects of 255
Superfetation 255
    medico-legal aspects of 255
Superficial bruise 173
Superficial contusion 170, 170f
Supreme court 9
Surgical spirit 382
Surrogacy

    partial 251
    types of 251
Surrogate motherhood 251
    indications for 251
Sweat glands 75
Syncope 113, 114
Synthetic derivatives 378t
Syphilis 76
Syringing 263

T

Tache noire sclerotica 120, 120f
Tachycardia 407
Tactile hallucination 295
Takayama test 83
Tandem bullet 230
Tattoo mark 76, 76f
    complications of 76
    removal of 76
Tattooing 227
Tear
    gases 408
    laceration 175
Teeth 419, 420
    arrangement of 168
    artificial 70
    charting of 71, 420
    eruption of 68
    extractions of 70
Teichmann's test 83
Temporalis muscle 96
Temporary teeth 69, 69t, 71, 420
    eruption of 419t
Test tube baby 251
Testamentary capacity 303
Tetrodon poisoning 412, 413
Thallium 320, 352
    poisoning 352
    triad 352, 353
Thanatology 109
Thebaine 378
Thermal injuries 198, 210, 211
    classification of 211fc
Thermoregulation 212
    mechanism of 210
Thevetoxin 403
Thiamine 315
Thigh, crush laceration of 174f
Thin layer chromatography 321

applications of 322
disadvantages of 322
filter paper 322
mobile phase 322
plates 322
Thiosulfate 318
Thoracic cage, movement of 149
Thorn apple 388f, 461f
Thrombosis 115f
Thrombus 115
Throttling 142, 145, 146f
Thymine 87
Tiger skin 167
Time since death 95, 103, 130, 438
Tissues
    bridging of 174
    liquefaction of 126
Tobacco 400
Toe nails 451
Tongue 299
Total deprivation water and food 160
Total iron binding capacity 351
Toxalbumin 362
Toxemia 269
Toxic
    alkaloids act 412
    dust 204
    effect bypass 318
    parts 365
    principles 365
Toxicity 332, 344
    chronic 346
    mild 409
Toxicokinetics 327
Toxicological analysis 379
Toxicology 312
    clinical 312
    history of 312
    types of 312
Toxin 411
    type 410
Toxinology 312
Trace evidence 81, 82
Trachea, surface of 98
Tramadol 378
Transplantation of Human Organs Act 110
Transportation injuries 194
    types of 194
Transvestism 278, 286
Traumatic brain injury 204

Tremors 400
Trench foot 213
Troilism 286
Trousseau's sign 340
Truth serum 86, 387
Tuberculosis, chronic pulmonary 115f
Turner's syndrome 65
Tympanic membrane 204

U

Ulcer, decubitus 169
Ulceration 246
Ultrasonography 254
Umbilical cord 452
Unicellular algae 155
Universal antidote 317, 318
Universal flexion 216
Unnatural sexual offences 278, 284
Upper limb, paralysis of 193
Uremia 100
Urinary bladder 132
Urine 379
    analysis 384
Urticaria 411
Uterine cavity, dissection of 257
Uterus 99, 265
    inner surface of 257f, 258f
    multiparous 258
    rupture of 258f

V

Vagal inhibition 100, 113, 114, 143
    types of 114
Vagina 245, 256, 259, 265
Vaginal cells 449
Vaginal wall, bruising of 257f
Vaginismus 248
Veins, marbling of 125f
Venomous fish 413
Venomous snake 365, 365t, 366
    bite
        signs of 367
        symptoms of 367
Venous congestion 138
Venous pressure 194
Ventricular fibrillation 152
Vertigo 407
Vestibule 245
Vestibulo-ocular reflex 110
Violent asphyxial death 135, 145

Viper 365, 366*f*, 464*f*
   snake bite 361, 368*f*
Virgin, false 246
Virginity 243-245
   medico-legal importance of 246
   principal signs of 244
Virgo intacta 244
Viscera 321
Visceral organs, abdominal 185
Visual disturbances 385
Vitreous humor 132
Vitriolage 337
Volatile poisons 321
Vomiting 401, 409, 410, 412
Voyeurism 278, 286

W

War gases 408
   medico-legal significance of 409
Warfarin 193
Warm anoxic time 112
Washerwoman's hand 153, 153*f*
Washing soda 341
Weakness 406
Weapons 464
   wooden club 440
Wernicke's encephalopathy 298
Wet drowning 151, 152
Wheezing 400
Whiplash injury 193
White blood cell count 370
Widmark's formula 384
Willis circle 97
Winslow's test 116
Withdrawal symptoms 393, 394, 401
Witnesses 13
   types of 13
Workmen Compensation Act 56

Wound 165, 179, 198, 201
   antemortem 202, 202*t*
   ballistics 223
   biochemistry 202
   certificate 439, 440, 441*t*
   edges 202
   fabricated 182, 206
   fictitious 206
   invented 206
   multiple
      cut 205*f*
      incised 176*f*
      stab 181*f*
   penetrating 179
   postmortem 202, 202*t*
   self-inflicted 206
   tailing of 176, 176*f*
Wrist joint 426, 426*f*, 426*t*, 427*f*, 428*f*

X

Xanthoprotein reaction 337
Xerostomia 345

Y

Y incision 97
   modified 97
Yeast 382
Yellow oleander 400
Yoga 110

Z

Zahn lines 202
Zenanas 284
Zinc
   metalloproteinases 366
   phosphide 320, 334
Zygomatic arch 433*f*